2003

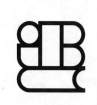

# HEALTH ISSUES IN THE
# LATINO COMMUNITY

# HEALTH ISSUES IN THE LATINO COMMUNITY

Marilyn Aguirre-Molina, Carlos W. Molina, and Ruth Enid Zambrana, Editors

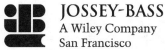
JOSSEY-BASS
A Wiley Company
San Francisco

Published by

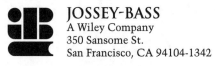

JOSSEY-BASS
A Wiley Company
350 Sansome St.
San Francisco, CA 94104-1342

www.josseybass.com

Jossey-Bass books and products are available through most bookstores. To contact Jossey-Bass
directly, call (888) 378-2537, fax to (800) 605-2665, or visit our website at www.josseybass.com.

Substantial discounts on bulk quantities of Jossey-Bass books are available to corporations,
professional associations, and other organizations. For details and discount information, contact
the special sales department at Jossey-Bass.

We at Jossey-Bass strive to use the most environmentally sensitive paper stocks available to us.
Our publications are printed on acid-free recycled stock whenever possible, and our paper always
meets or exceeds minimum GPO and EPA requirements.

**Library of Congress Cataloging-in-Publication Data**

Health issues in the Latino community/editors, Marilyn Aguirre-Molina, Carlos Molina,
Ruth Enid Zambrana.
    p. cm.
   Includes index.
   ISBN 0-7879-5315-6
     1. Hispanic Americans—Medical care—United States. 2. Hispanic Americans—Health and
   hygiene—United States. I. Aguirre-Molina, Marilyn. II. Molina, Carlos W. III. Zambrana, Ruth E.

RA448.5.H57 H395 2001
362.1'089'68073—dc21                                                    2001029048

*HB Printing*         10  9  8  7  6  5  4  3  2  1

# CONTENTS

## PART ONE: LATINO POPULATIONS IN THE UNITED STATES   1

# LIST OF TABLES AND FIGURES

## Tables

# Figures

# FOREWORD

This book, *Health Issues in the Latino Community,* comes at a critical juncture, both in terms of our nation's health objectives for the twenty-first century and the growing body of research on the health status of Latinos in the United States.

It has now become clear "that the health of the individual is almost inseparable from the health of the larger community and that the health of every community in every State and territory determines the overall health status of the Nation."[1] This is the underlying premise of the U.S. Department of Health and Human Services' nationwide health promotion and disease prevention agenda, accordingly entitled *Healthy People 2010: Healthy People in Healthy Communities.*

Consequently, the disparities in health among racial/ethnic population groups in the United States such as Latinos—soon to become the largest minority group in the United States—have a negative impact on the health of America as a whole. The United States, the richest country in the world, ranks only twentieth in quality and years of healthy life, lagging behind poorer countries such as Costa Rica, Greece, and Spain. Recent health gains for the U.S. population as a whole reflect achievements among the higher socioeconomic groups; lower socioeconomic groups continue to lag behind.

Thanks to the nationally recognized Latino researchers, scholars, educators, and activists—who through this publication have provided us with the most current health data, as well as in-depth and insightful analyses of the health issues

---

[1]U.S. Department of Health and Human Services. (2001). Hea*lthy people 2010: Understanding and improving health.* Washington, DC: U.S. Department of Health and Human Services, Government Printing Office.

and socioeconomic conditions affecting Latinos—we can see what is "critical" about this juncture.

Diabetes and other chronic conditions among Latinos, such as asthma, continue to present a serious obstacle in public health. Alcohol and other substance abuse, violence (homicide as well as suicide), and abusive behavior (such as domestic violence) continue to ravage Latino homes and communities across the country. Mental disorders among Latinos continue to go undiagnosed and untreated. Obesity among Latino children, adolescents, and adults has significantly increased over the past two decades. Smoking among Latino adolescents has increased in the past decade. And HIV/AIDS remains a serious health problem, now disproportionately affecting Latino women and youth. Furthermore, Latinos have the highest uninsured rates of all racial/ethnic groups in the United States, and have to navigate a health care system that is often unfamiliar with—and sometimes hostile to—their culture, language, and beliefs.

The contents of this publication also reintroduces us the "epidemiological paradox" (that is, high poverty but favorable infant mortality and low birth rates) among Mexican Americans as a way to remind us of two things: first, the importance of conducting intergenerational, longitudinal studies within groups; and second, how incomplete the picture of Latino health is, given the paucity of health data and research on the health status of the various Latino nationality groups— specifically, Central and South Americans, including Salvordoreans, Dominicans, Columbians, Guatemalans, and others.

Fortunately, unlike its earlier 1994 edition, *Latino Health in the U.S.: A Growing Challenge,* this publication is no longer the only book solely dedicated to the health of Latinos. It does, however, continue to be an important source of reference for students of public health and medicine, policymakers, academicians, health care professionals and advocates, as well as many other individuals and institutions concerned about the nation's health, not just Latino health.

One truism of public health is that knowledge gained from studying one group usually benefits many others. Therefore, the increased knowledge gained from research about the health status of Latinos will without a doubt result in findings that will contribute to the improvement of the delivery of health care services to— and the health of—all Americans.

*Raul Yzaguirre*
*President*
*National Council of La Raza*
*Washington, D.C.*

# PREFACE

This book represents a second effort to place between two covers a comprehensive and integrated review of the health and health status of Latinos living in the United States. Our earlier book, *Latino Health in the United States: A Growing Challenge* (1994), was and continues to be the first effort of its kind. Since that time, several developments have occurred. These developments provide the basis for a book that provides current analyses of events affecting the health of Latinos. Among recent developments are

- The increase in data sources that include ethnic identifiers and enable the inclusion of more and accurate data in this book.
- Changes in the health care market and the strong presence of managed care, which are affecting Latinos.
- Changes in federal immigration and welfare policies that have implication for the health and well-being of Latinos.
- Demographic changes that result in Latinos becoming the largest ethnic or racial group in the nation.

The purpose of the book is to

- Provide a profile—demographic and health status—of Latino populations in the United States by subgroup.
- Describe and analyze key issues affecting the health and health care of Latinos.
- Identify research needs, policy issues, and/or implications for programs and practice.
- Stimulate thinking on viable actions to address the needs of Latinos.

Very often books on Latino health focus on one aspect of their condition, such as mental health, women's health, drug abuse, and so on. While these efforts make important contributions to an understanding of the community's health needs, they often do not provide the reader with the "whole picture" or complete profile of Latinos. This book strives toward that end. It addresses key and critical health issues that affect Latinos' health so as to inform practice, program planning, research, and policy—good health policy and programs evolve from good information.

The book is divided into six parts. The first part, Latino Populations in the United States, defines Latinos and summarizes key health status indicators. Chapter One provides sociodemographic information and describes changes within the Latino community as it raises critical questions for the reader's consideration. It also provides an economic and demographic profile of Latinos by subgroups, with analyses of changing demographic patterns and their implications for the health and health care systems. The second chapter provides an overview of current available data sets as well as a discussion of the persistent lack of data on Latinos. The data on morbidity and mortality indicators (for children and adults) are summarized and the factors that influence their health status presented (including socioeconomic status, insurance coverage, and behavioral risk factors). Chapter Three looks at the changes in the health care market that are affecting consumers in numerous ways with regard to access to care and the quality of care rendered. This chapter describes and analyzes these changes as they affect Latinos. Special attention is given to issues such as the effects of managed care, devolution, insurance rates among Latinos, health care for immigrants, and so on.

Part Two, entitled Latino Life Stages and Health, reviews the special health needs of Latinos from birth through the golden years. In Chapter Four the authors review the available data on the health of Latino children and youth, ages zero to eighteen. They include an overview of access to care, preventive care (such as immunization), acute and chronic illnesses, intentional and unintentional injury, and infant health issues. Morbidity and mortality indicators for infants, children, and youth by subgroup and gender are also presented. The following chapters address the health status of Latinas with a focus on maternal and child health. Chapter Five examines behaviors during the prenatal period across groups and the influence of a number of socioeconomic variables, cultural factors, and the systems of care used by Latinas. The sixth chapter examines the health and social status of elderly Latinos with a particular emphasis on risk and protective factors, as well as the socioeconomic and sociocultural factors that affect their well-being. The last chapter in Part Two reviews and analyzes the empirical data on the mental health of Latinos. The authors review sociocultural factors, migration, and acculturation, among others, and their influence on diagnostic and treatment processes. They also present the limitations of existing research and identify areas in need of inquiry.

Part Three, Patterns of Chronic Diseases Among Latinos, reviews chronic conditions as they affect Latinos. The four chapters deal independently with cancer, cardiovascular disease, diabetes, and HIV/AIDS. Each chapter compares morbidity and mortality patterns across ethnic racial groups and describes their corresponding risk factors. The socioeconomic and sociocultural factors that play a role in each disease are also presented.

The two chapters in Part Four, Occupational Health and the Latino Workforce, examine data on the rates of occupational disease among urban and rural Latino workers who are employed in various industries and work settings. Chapter Thirteen on rural health goes beyond the health of workers in rural settings and examines the overall conditions of Latinos living in rural communities.

The fifth part, Alcohol, Tobacco, and Other Drug Use Among Latinos, contains three chapters that provide a comprehensive review of empirical studies describing patterns of alcohol, tobacco, and other drug use among Latinos. Each chapter examines the social, cultural, and other risk factors that influence specific drug use among Latinos. Chapter Fourteen presents public policy and other programmatic interventions for addressing alcohol problems. Chapter Fifteen analyzes the recent tobacco settlements and how it might affect Latinos. Drug use and its effect on Latino adults and youth is the focus of Chapter Sixteen.

Part Six brings the book to a close with a discussion of policy and programmatic interventions that are needed to address the needs of the Latino community.

Please note that the term "Latino" is used throughout this book instead of "Hispanic." Nevertheless, the reader should be aware of the fact that much epidemiological data have been collected using "Hispanic" as the operational label. For a discussion of these issues see Hayes-Bautista and Chapa (1987) and Treveno, 1987.

As we progress into the new millennium, our nation is on the cusp of a massive demographic transformation. Latinos are central to these changes. If our nation is to remain a productive leader of industrialized nations, then it cannot ignore the health and well-being of one of its largest and youngest population groups. If Latinos are not healthy, participating members of American society, then we all suffer as a nation. It is the humble desire of the editors of this publication that the materials contained herein serve to guide the formation of policies, programs, and research to ensure a healthy Latino citizenry.

*New York*                                                    *Marilyn Aguirre-Molina*
*New York*                                                         *Carlos W. Molina*
*Chevy Chase, Maryland*                                        *Ruth Enid Zambrana*
*March, 2001*

# ACKNOWLEDGMENTS

A project of this scale and scope can only be achieved by the goodwill and hard work of those who believe it is important. This proved to be the case in the preparation of this book. There are many that assisted in the production of this comprehensive volume on Latino health. The editors would like to acknowledge their contributions and express our appreciation.

I'd like to go back to the beginning of the project and thank those who not only supported the idea of a book on Latino health but also enabled it to become a reality. In some ways, they were the *padrinos* (godparents) of this project. In this instance, a special word of appreciation goes to Stephen Isaacs, a good friend and colleague from my days at The Robert Wood Johnson Foundation. Steve thought the book was important, and he facilitated discussions with Andy Pasternack, Senior Editor, Health Series, at Jossey-Bass Publishers. That first meeting resulted in our publisher's interest in this project.

One of our other *padrinos* was the U.S. Department of Health and Human Services, Office of Minority Health (OMH), under the direction of Nathan Stinson, Jr., Ph.D., M.D., MPH, Deputy Assistant Secretary for Minority Health. We'd like to thank the OMH for the support that enabled the preparation of the manuscript. They believed that this book was needed and that it would make an important contribution to the field. A very special word of thanks, *y un gran abrazo* (a big embrace), goes to Olivia Carter-Pokras, Ph.D., Director, Division of Policy and Data, OMH, who is the ultimate personification of the good *madrina* (godmother). She facilitated our process with the OMH and was a constant source of information, sharing existing and new data as they became available.

Thanks also to Jeannette Noltenius, Ph.D., Executive Director of the Latino Council on Alcohol and Tobacco, who was especially helpful in coordinating all of the administrative processes related to the OMH.

Of course this book would not exist if it were not for the contributions of the authors who wrote the chapters. We thank them for their hard work and for being such good colleagues. Their cooperation and response to our suggestions or requests for revisions made this process manageable and productive. Each and every one of them is respected for their contributions to the fields in which they work. We are especially proud that all are Latinos who are also contributing to a better understanding of Latinos in the United States. *Mil gracias* (many, many thanks) for your commitment to this project.

A special word of appreciation must be given to those who were of monumental help to the editors as we carried out the many activities—both editorial and administrative—that are required to produce a text of this magnitude. We'd like to thank Gina Arias, Maria Moreno, and Janna Stefanek, Graduate Research Assistants at the Mailman School of Public Health, Columbia University. Thanks also to Laura Logie, Research Project Coordinator in the Women's Studies Department at the University of Maryland.

I would be remiss if I did not acknowledge the support given to this project by my home institution, the Mailman School of Public Health at Columbia University. I greatly appreciate Jim McCarthy's encouragement (director, Division of Population and Family Health), and the gift of time that enabled me to work with my colleagues on the book.

In closing, *gracias* to Andy Pasternack at Jossey-Bass Publishers whose enthusiasm for the book from the beginning and his gentle and persistent prodding at the end got us through the home stretch.

M.A.M.

# THE EDITORS

**Marilyn Aguirre-Molina, Ed.D.**

Dr. Aguirre-Molina is currently a professor of public health at the Mailman School of Public Health, Columbia University in New York City. Prior to joining the Columbia faculty she served as the executive vice president of the California Endowment, and as a senior program officer at The Robert Wood Johnson Foundation. Preceding her work within philanthropy she was an associate professor in the UMDNJ-Robert Wood Johnson Medical School, Department of Environmental and Community Medicine. In this capacity she taught within the MD/MPH program and engaged in applied research.

The focus of Dr. Aguirre-Molina's work is on program development and applied research that address public health approaches to the prevention of alcohol, tobacco, and other drug problems among young people. She has published in this area of study. Dr. Aguirre-Molina is or has been a member of various national boards and committees, including the National Institutes of Health–National Advisory Council of the NIAAA, the NIAAA panel on College Drinking, and the National Council of the Center for Substance Abuse Prevention. She also serves on the National Board of the Alliance to End Childhood Lead Poisoning, and is on the editorial board of the *Journal for Public Health Policy*.

As a Kellogg Foundation Fellow, Dr. Aguirre-Molina traveled extensively in order to study the political economy of selected developing countries.

She currently serves as a consultant to The Robert Wood Johnson Foundation's substance abuse agenda. She also serves on the selection panel of the Johnson & Johnson Community Health Care Program (corporate giving).

In addition to her interest in substance abuse, Dr. Aguirre-Molina has worked extensively on and written about Latino health policy issues. This is her second edited book on the health of Latino populations in the United States. The first book, *Latino Health in the U.S.: A Growing Challenge,* was published in 1994.

Dr. Aguirre-Molina received a bachelor of science degree (*cum laude*) in health sciences from Hunter College–City University of New York. In addition, she attended Columbia University where she received a master of science degree in community health and a doctorate in health education and administration.

## Carlos W. Molina, Ed.D.

Dr. Molina is currently professor of community health education at York College of the City University of New York, where he has also served as the provost. The focus of his teaching and writings is on health administration, as well as behavioral health. From 1990 to 1992, he served as the CEO of Lincoln Hospital of the Health and Hospitals Corporation of New York City, the country's largest public hospital system. Dr. Molina is currently the president of the board of the Latino Council on Alcohol and Tobacco. He has served on the boards of directors of the national Planned Parenthood Federation of America, Alan Guttmacher Institute, SIECUS, as well as numerous other national and local boards and committees. In 1993, he was elected to a four-year term on the Executive Board of the American Public Health Association. Dr. Molina is on the editorial board of the *Journal of Public Health Policy.* He has written extensively on Latino health. His most prominent work on the subject is a book he co-edited in 1994, *Latino Health in the U.S.: A Growing Challenge.*

## Ruth Enid Zambrana, M.S.W., Ph.D.

Dr. Zambrana is currently a professor in the women's studies department at the University of Maryland. She was formerly the Elisabeth Shirley Enochs Professor of Child Welfare in the Social Work Program at George Mason University (1993–1999), a visiting senior research scientist at the Agency for Health Care Policy and Research (1992–1993), and a faculty member at the UCLA School of Social Welfare for ten years. Her work has focused on the multiple factors (poverty, psychosocial factors, and health behaviors) that contribute to the health status of low-income groups, with emphasis on maternal and child health, as well as on Latino children and families. Her book *Understanding Latino Families: Scholarship, Policy and Practice* (1996) is an edited volume that encourages a new discourse on the Latino population in the United States. She serves on several editorial boards and is a member of the board of directors of Family Support America. She completed a fellowship with the National Hispana Leadership Institute (1998–1999).

# THE CONTRIBUTORS

**Margarita Alegría, Ph.D.**

Dr. Alegría is professor of health services research and director of the Center for Sociomedical Research and Evaluation at the School of Public Health, University of Puerto Rico. Dr. Alegría is currently the principal investigator of the National Institute of Mental Health-funded Latino Research Program Project (LRPP), which focuses on research to improve the mental health care for Latino populations. She is part of a multisite collaborative on disparities in mental health care. Dr. Alegría has served as a consultant for the Secretary of Mental Health of the Commonwealth of Puerto Rico in the development of a strategic plan for AIDS prevention and in the design of mental health services. She serves on the board of directors for the Children's Foundation and the Felisa Rincón De Gautier Foundation. Her published works focus on the areas of mental health services research, conceptual and methodological issues with minority populations, and HIV risk behaviors.

**Hortensia Amaro, Ph.D.**

Dr. Amaro is professor of social and behavioral sciences at Boston University School of Public Health. For the last twenty years, Dr. Amaro has conducted research on social and behavioral factors related to HIV, mental health, and alcohol and drug abuse. She has developed and evaluated prevention programs targeted at adolescent and adult female populations. She has written on the central roles of gender, race, ethnicity, and culture in HIV risk among women and has articulated frameworks for understanding the context of women's risk. Her work includes "Love, Sex and Power: Considering Women's Realities in HIV Prevention," published in the *American Psychologist* in 1995 and "On the Margin: Power and Women's HIV Risk Reduction Strategies" (2000). Dr. Amaro has received awards from local, state, and national organizations for her work as a public health advocate and researcher.

## Kathryn Azevedo, Ph.D., ATRIC

Dr. Azevedo coordinates clinical trials as a postdoctoral fellow at Stanford University Medical Center and is a senior research associate at the Tomas Rivera Policy Institute in Claremont, California. Dr. Azevedo examined the issue of Latino underenrollment in California public insurance programs and ways to increase enrollment of eligible nonparticipating Latinos.

Her research focuses on community-based rehabilitation, disability issues, farm worker health, chronic pain, and access to medical services among California's rural poor. She has worked for the California Institute for Rural Studies, Centers for Disease Control, UCSF-Mt. Zion Hospital, Baylor College of Medicine, and other research centers.

## Joseph R. Betancourt, M.D., M.P.H.

Dr. Betancourt is an assistant professor of medicine and public health at New York Presbyterian Hospital-Weill Medical College of Cornell University. As associate director of Cornell's Center for Multicultural and Minority Health, Dr. Betancourt's research has focused on crosscultural medicine, minority recruitment into the health professions, and minority health and health policy. He currently is a principal investigator of several large-scale grants, including "Understanding Racial Differences in Lung Cancer Treatment." Dr. Betancourt serves on the New York Academy of Medicine's Racial/Ethnic Disparities Working Group, the Greater New York Hospital Association's Steering Committee on Racial/Ethnic Disparities, the New York Hospital Community Health Plan's Medical Management Committee, and the CDC's National Expert Council for the Diabetes Today Program. He is a reviewer for several medical journals and has published in the areas of crosscultural primary care and ethnic and racial disparities.

## Raul Caetano, M.D., M.P.H., Ph.D.

Dr. Caetano is a psychiatrist and epidemiologist who has been working in public health for twenty-two years. Presently, he is a professor of epidemiology and assistant dean, Dallas Master of Public Health Program, Houston School of Public Health, University of Texas.

From 1983 to 1998 he was at the Alcohol Research Group, Berkeley, California, where he was the director and principal investigator of a National Alcohol Research Center grant.

Dr. Caetano has written extensively about alcohol problems among U.S. ethnic minorities, especially among Latinos; his is the seminal research on Latinos and tobacco use. He currently is the principal investigator on a NIAAA/NIH MERIT Award to examine the relationship between alcohol and intimate partner violence across ethnic groups in the United States.

Dr. Caetano has served as a committee member for the Institute of Medicine of the U.S. National Academy of Sciences, and he has been a consultant for the National Institute on Alcohol Abuse and Alcoholism, the World Health Organization, and numerous other agencies. He is a member of various editorial boards, and he is also associate editor for *Addiction*.

## J. Emilio Carrillo, M.D., M.P.H.

Dr. Carrillo served in the faculties of Harvard Medical School and Harvard School of Public Health for ten years. He is now assistant professor of medicine at Weill Medical College of Cornell University.

In 1990, Dr. Carrillo was recruited through a national search to head the New York City Health and Hospitals Corporation. As the twelfth President of the nation's largest municipal hospital system, he implemented a multitude of health promotion efforts directed at minority communities.

In 1993, Dr. Carrillo joined the New York Hospital Network where he directs several research initiatives to promote primary care development and health promotion. He also helped develop a Medicaid Managed Care program for what is now the New York Presbyterian Hospital Network, where he serves as medical director.

## Olivia Carter-Pokras, Ph.D.

Dr. Carter-Pokras is the director of the Division of Policy and Data at the Office of Minority Health in the Department of Health and Human Services (DHHS). Dr. Carter-Pokras has more than nineteen years of experience in the collection, analysis, and presentation of health data; development of national health goals and objectives; and development of health policy. Dr. Carter-Pokras co-chairs the Working Group on Racial and Ethnic Data of the DHHS Data Council, and chaired the Hispanic work group of the federal Interagency Committee for the Review of the Racial and Ethnic Standards and the Healthy People 2000 Working Group for Hispanic Americans.

## Alberto Coustasse, M.D., M.B.A., M.P.H.

Dr. Coustasse is a research associate at the School of Public Health at the University of North Texas Health Science Center at Fort Worth. He also serves as Institutional Researcher at the Osteopathic Health System of Texas.

Dr. Coustasse served as the medical director of the Health and Rehabilitation Centers of the National Defense Pension Fund [CAPREDENA], the Chilean equivalent of the Veteran Affairs, from 1995 to 1999. From 1994 to 1995, he served as the national director of the same institution.

His research has focused on community interventions in cardiovascular disease and health administration issues.

## Angelo Falcón, M.A.

Falcón is the senior policy executive at the Puerto Rican Legal Defense and Education Fund (PRLDEF) in New York City, where he also directs the Institute for Puerto Rican Policy. As a political scientist, Falcón has written extensively on Puerto Rican and Latino policy issues and politics. He is the co-author of *Latino Voices: Mexican, Puerto Rican, and Cuban Perspectives on American Politics* (1992) and of *Latino Politics: A Select Research Bibliography* (1991). His research has been published in the *Journal of American Politics*, the *Hispanic Journal of Behavioral Science*, *New Community*, and other journals and books. He is a graduate of Columbia College and he completed his graduate work at the State University of New York at Albany, which awarded him the 1991 Distinguished Alumni Medal.

## Glenn Flores, M.D.

Dr. Flores is an assistant professor of pediatrics and public health at the Boston University Schools of Medicine and Public Health. He founded and is the director of the Pediatric Latino Clinic at Boston Medical Center. He is a Robert Wood Johnson Minority Medical Faculty Scholar, for which he received a four-year grant to examine avoidable hospitalizations in children. He has published more than thirty articles and book chapters on access barriers to health care for Latino children, the impact of ethnicity, family income, and parental education on children's health and use of health services, and cultural competency in health care.

Dr. Flores currently serves on the Health Care Research and Training study section of the Agency for Healthcare Research and Quality (AHRQ). He co-chairs the Latino Health Consortium of the American Academy of Pediatrics Center for Child Health Research. He was recently nominated to be a member of the Advisory Committee on Minority Health for the Secretary of Health and Human Services.

## George Friedman-Jiménez, M.D., Dr.P.H.

Dr. Friedman-Jiménez is currently an assistant professor with the New York University School of Medicine, Bellevue Hospital. Dr. Friedman-Jiménez currently directs the Bellevue Occupational Medical Clinic. He received his board certifications in internal medicine (1985) and preventive medicine (1990). Dr. Friedman-Jiménez's research interests lie in the field of occupational epidemiology.

## Frank Hector Galvan, M.S.W., Ph.D.

Dr. Galvan is currently a postdoctoral fellow (NIMH) with the Drew Center for AIDS Research, Education and Services at the Charles R. Drew University of Medicine and Science. He has written numerous publications on HIV/AIDS in Mexican and Mexican American men. He has worked extensively as a clinical social worker in the Los Angeles area.

## Aida L. Giachello, M.S.W., Ph.D.

Dr. Giachello is currently an associate professor at Jane Addams College of Social Work, University of Illinois at Chicago, and founder and director of the Midwest Latino Health Research Training and Policy Center.

She has worked with federal agencies such as the National Center for Health Statistics, Agency for Health Care Policy and Research, National Institutes of Health, Centers for Disease Control and Prevention, DHHS Office of Minority Health, and U.S. Office of the Surgeon General. Dr. Giachello has published extensively on maternal and child health and chronic conditions, such as asthma and diabetes, among Latinos.

## Andres G. Gil, M.S.W., Ph.D.

In 1994, Dr. Gil joined the faculty at the School of Family Studies at the University of Connecticut as an assistant professor. Currently he is an associate professor at the College of Health and Urban Affairs, and associate director for research in the School of Social Work, at Florida International University, Miami, Florida. His current research and publications continue to concentrate on adolescent substance use, including the study of risk, protective, and cultural factors associated with substance use and the treatment and prevention of substance use among Latino youth. He is also the co-author of *Drug Use and Ethnicity During Early Adolescence* (1999).

## Teresa Juarbe, R.N., Ph.D.

Dr. Juarbe is an assistant professor at the School of Nursing at the University of California, San Francisco. During the last twelve years, she has been involved in cardiovascular health research with Latinos. Her current research focuses on the promotion of heart health for aging Latina women, in particular the assessment of cardiovascular disease-related physical activity and dietary behaviors. She is also conducting research on breast cancer screening for underserved ethnic women. She is currently the principal investigator of the Latinas Heart Health Project.

## José Alejandro Luchsinger, M.D., M.P.H.

Dr. Luchsinger is currently an assistant professor of clinical medicine with Columbia University College of Physicians and Surgeons in New York City. He has received awards and honors including The Anne C. Gelman Award for Excellence in Epidemiology from Columbia University School of Public Health (1999); and The Best Scientific Abstract by a fellow with a paper on the use of antibiotics and risk of myocardial infarction at the Mid-Atlantic Regional meeting of the Society of General Internal Medicine, Washington, D.C. (1999). Dr. Luchsinger's current research interests are in the association between diabetes and insulin resistance and dementia and its mechanisms.

## Gerardo Marín, Ph.D.

Dr. Marín is currently a professor of psychology and senior associate dean for academic affairs in the College of Arts and Sciences at the University of San Francisco, where he has been since 1982.

He was the senior scientific editor of the 1998 Surgeon General's Report on Tobacco Use.

He has received numerous awards including Distinguished Research Award from the University of San Francisco (1995), Interamerican Psychology Award for Contributions to the Development of Psychology as a Science and a Profession in the Americas from the Interamerican Society of Psychology (1995), and Distinguished Lifetime Service Award from the University of San Francisco (1996).

Dr. Marín is involved in the Interamerican Society of Psychology, International Association for Cross-Cultural Psychology, National Hispanic Psychological Association, American Psychological Association, and International Association of Applied Psychology. His current research interests include identifying the predictors of tobacco use among Latino children and the study of acculturation.

## Gina Moreno-John, M.D.

Dr. Moreno-John is currently an assistant clinical professor of medicine at the University of California at San Francisco (UCSF), in the division of General Internal Medicine. She is also a co-investigator at the UCSF Resource Center for Aging Research in Diverse Populations, National Institute of Aging Grant. Other research includes improving strategies for the recruitment and retention of minorities into clinical research studies. In addition, she has been awarded a Junior Faculty Development Award with the UCSF National Center of Excellence in Women's Health, Community Outreach Project. Dr. Moreno-John's other academic interests include adolescent health care, smoking cessation and tabacco policy, and obesity and eating disorders.

## Rafael Moure-Eraso, Ph.D., C.I.H.

Dr. Moure-Eraso is a professor at the University of Massachusetts, Lowell, College of Engineering, Department of Work Environment. He has conducted research in work environment policy, cleaner production, and industrial hygiene since 1988. Dr. Moure-Eraso gained extensive experience in worker health issues during his fourteen years as an industrial hygienist of the Oil Chemical and Atomic Workers International Union and the United Automobile Workers.

Dr. Moure-Eraso has been a member of the National Advisory Committee for Occupational Safety and Health of the U.S. Department of Labor, OSHA. He serves on the Board of Scientific Counselors of the National Institute for Occupational Safety and Health and the Board of Advisors of the National Toxicology Program of the National Institute of Environmental Health Sciences.

## Hilda Ochoa Bogue, R.N., C.H.E.S., M.S.

Ochoa Bogue worked for ten years as a nurse in the Mexican Social Security System, and for two years at McDonough County Hospital in Illinois.

Her professional work has focused on increasing understanding of cultural differences in health care; improving the health status of the medically indigent; and assisting migrant farmworkers, refugees, and other Latino populations receive access to health services.

She received a one-year MATCH clinical fellowship from the National Association of Community Health Centers to learn clinical administration. She received didactic training at Johns Hopkins University and was placed at the Colorado Migrant Health Program. For the past seven years, she has served as coordinator of migrant health services for Community Health of South Dade, Inc., (CHI) operating two migrant health clinics near Homestead, Florida, and additional programs that provided primary health care and dental services to Haitian and Cuban refugees. She then worked as the coordinator of grants management and presently she is the director of planning and development for CHI.

## Eliseo Pérez-Stable, M.D.

Dr. Pérez-Stable is a professor of medicine at the University of California, San Francisco (UCSF) School of Medicine, and chief, Division of General Internal Medicine, Department of Medicine, UCSF. He completed a Henry J. Kaiser Family Foundation fellowship in general internal medicine. Dr. Pérez-Stable's research has focused on risk factor reduction interventions for Latino populations and health care issues of minorities.

Dr. Pérez-Stable has studied social and cultural factors in communication between Latino patients and their Anglo physicians by evaluating the effect of language ability on medical outcomes and culture-specific barriers to communication. Dr. Pérez-Stable is co-director of the University of California at San Francisco Medical Effectiveness Research Center for Diverse Populations (MERC) and director of the Center for Aging in Diverse Communities (CADC).

## Amelie G. Ramirez, Dr.P.H.

Dr. Ramirez is associate professor of medicine and deputy director, Chronic Disease Prevention and Control Research Center at Baylor College of Medicine, Houston, Texas. She also serves as associate director for Community Research and Program Leader for the Cancer Prevention and Health Promotion Program of the San Antonio Cancer Institute. Dr. Ramirez is a principal investigator for several grants of *Redes En Acción:* Cancer Awareness, Research and Training; program director of the replication of the *A Su Salud En Acción* Program; *Prevention;* and of a smoking prevention program funded by the Texas Department of Health and the Texas Higher Education Coordinating Board. From 1992 to 2000, she was principal investigator of the National Cancer Institute–funded National Hispanic Leadership Initiative on Cancer: *En Acción.*

Dr. Ramirez received a White House appointment to the National Cancer Advisory Board. She has served on the National Cancer Policy Board of the National Academy of Sciences, Institute of Medicine and Commission of Life Sciences.

Dr. Ramirez has received awards including the Dr. LaSalle D. Leffall, Jr., Cancer Prevention Award from the University of Texas M.D. Anderson Cancer Center.

## Lucina Suarez, M.S., Ph.D.

Dr. Suarez, a senior scientist at the Texas Department of Health, has worked in the field of epidemiology for twenty-five years. At the Texas Department of Health, she directs the Epidemiology, Biostatistics and Evaluation Research Section of the Office of the Associate Commissioner for Disease Control and Prevention. She has published extensively on cancer-related issues in Hispanic populations, including evaluations of community interventions, survey research, and cancer epidemiology. She has served on numerous special review committees for the National Cancer Institute (NCI), and is consultant to and co-chair of the Clinical and Research Committee for *Redes En Acción:* Cancer Awareness, Research and Training.

## Fernando M. Torres-Gil, Ph.D.

Dr. Torres-Gil is the associate dean for academic affairs and professor of social welfare and policy studies at the School of Public Policy and Social Research, University of California, Los Angeles, as well as director of the school's Center for Policy Research on Aging. Previously, he was a professor of gerontology and public administration at the University of Southern California.

Dr. Torres-Gil is an expert in the fields of health and long-term care, the politics of aging, social policy, ethnicity, and disability. He is the author of four books and more than seventy articles and book chapters, including *The New Aging: Politics and Change in America* (1992). He was elected a fellow of the Gerontological Society of America (1985) and the National Academy of Public Administration (1995). He served as president of the American Society on Aging (1989–1992) and is a member of the National Academy of Social Insurance. Dr. Torres-Gil is a winner of the National Council on Aging's Ollie A. Randall Award bestowed for leadership on behalf of older persons.

He served as the first-ever Assistant Secretary for Aging in the U.S. Department of Health and Human Services (HHS) and as a member of the president's Welfare Reform Working Group. He sits on the board of directors of the Families USA Foundation, the Older Women's League, and the AARP Andrus Foundation.

## Fernando M. Treviño, Ph.D., M.P.H.

Dr. Treviño is professor and founding dean of the School of Public Health at the University of North Texas Health Science Center at Fort Worth. He also serves as a past president of the World Federation of Public Health Associations, and was the executive director of the American Public Health Association in Washington, D.C., from 1993 to 1996, and executive editor of the *American Journal of Public Health*.

Dr. Treviño was one of the founders of the national Medicine and Public Health Initiative and served as co-chair from 1994 to 1996. He served as the co-chair of the National Congress on Medicine and Public Health held in March 1996; as a senior scientist at the American Medical Association from 1984 to 1986; and as a social science analyst at the National Center for Health Statistics from 1980 to 1984. At the National Center for Health Statistics, Dr. Treviño served as the principal consultant to the design, implementation, and analysis of the Hispanic Health and Nutrition Examination Survey.

Dr. Treviño has served on the National Committee on Vital and Health Statistics (was the founding chair of its Subcommittee on Minority Health Statistics); the Institute of Medicine's Access to Health Care Monitoring Panel; and the Institute of Medicine's Committee on Cancer Research Among Minorities and the Underserved, among others.

## Dellanira Valencia, M.A.

Valencia's research focuses on HIV/AIDS prevention, at Boston University and at the University of California San Francisco, Center for AIDS Prevention Studies (UCSF/CAPS). Currently, she is the project manager for a collaborative research study with UCSF/CAPS and the San Francisco Department of Public Health. This study examines the policy influence of California's HIV prevention planning groups on HIV/AIDS prevention policy. Her research includes examination of domestic and familial violence with a concentration on Latina

women, juvenile susceptibility to interrogation pressures and their understanding
of the Miranda warning, and others.

## Rodolfo R. Vega, Ph.D.

Dr. Vega is a senior consultant at JSI Research and Training, Inc. He also serves
as an adjunct professor in the School of Public Policy at the University of
Massachusetts, Boston, and at Simmons College. His research focuses in the areas
of migration, acculturation, mental health, HIV/AIDS, substance abuse prevention, and healthy communities.

## William A. Vega, Ph.D.

Dr. Vega is a professor of psychiatry at the University of Medicine and Den-
tistry of New Jersey—Robert Wood Johnson Medical School. His also holds the
position of associate director, Institute for Quality, Research, and Training, University of Behavioral Health Care. He was formerly a professor of public health
at the University of California, Berkeley.

Dr. Vega has conducted field research projects about health, mental
health, and substance abuse in various regions of the United States (East and West
coasts) and Mexico. His specialty is comparative health research, and immigrant
social adaptation and mental health adjustments that occur with adolescents
and adults. He has published more than 100 articles, chapters, and books on these
topics.

Most recently he was a member of the Institute of Medicine advisory group
on youth risk behaviors. Dr. Vega has served on numerous National Institutes of
Health technical committees and as a consultant to the World Health Organization for assessment of mental health problems.

## Valentine M. Villa, Ph.D.

Dr. Villa is an adjunct assistant professor with the University of California at
Los Angeles School of Public Health, Department of Community Health Sciences, and senior research associate with the University of California at Los
Angeles Center for Health Policy Research. Her primary areas of research are
aging, social policy and minority aging. The focus of her research is predictors
of health and economic differences between these population groups with an emphasis on the role that socioeconomic status, such as poverty, income, wealth, as
well as minority group membership, have on health and functioning.

Dr. Villa is a founding member and executive committee member of the Los
Angeles County Commission on Aging Organization (LAC/CAO), a research
advisor and consultant to the Los Angeles Area Agency on Aging, Los Angeles
Veterans Administration, and the Los Angeles Alzheimer's Association.

PART ONE

---

# LATINO POPULATIONS
# IN THE UNITED STATES

CHAPTER ONE

# LATINO HEALTH POLICY

## Beyond Demographic Determinism

Angelo Falcón, Marilyn Aguirre-Molina,
and Carlos W. Molina

As our knowledge of the Latino experience in the United States grows, so does our interpretation of it, and no less so when we are discussing the health status of the Latino community. Much of the research on Latino health has addressed socioeconomic linkages and the debate over class versus culture (Hunt, Tello, & Huerta, 1994; Molina & Aguirre-Molina, 1994; Link & Phelan, 1996; McCally, Haines, Fein, Addington, Lawrence, & Cassel, 1998; United States Commission on Civil Rights, 1999; United States Department of Health and Human Services, 1998; Williams & Collins, 1995). However, as demonstrated in this book, we currently possess sufficient information about these and other aspects of the Latino experience to engage in a more strategic analysis of this community's health and health care needs. The challenge before us is to consider the health of Latinos within the context of the demographic and social transformations that have begun and that will continue over the next several decades in the United States. Such a contextual analysis can serve to inform policy as well as empower Latinos as the strengths and potential of this community are identified.

This chapter is a departure from what is generally included in a book on Latino health and related issues. It raises a number of issues within a social and demographic context and examines the implications for the health and well-being of Latinos. The decision to take this approach was influenced by the frequently cited demographic imperative that warrants renewed scrutiny as it applies to the health of this population.

The chapter addresses several of the key social, demographic, and policy issues that are referred to throughout the book. The intent is to critically examine sociodemographic factors that have implications for the health of Latinos. First, a general yet selective overview of major demographic trends occurring in the Latino community in the United States over the last decade is provided with a summary of the issues they raise. Second, current perspectives on the Latino community and corresponding interpretations of the group's experience are presented. Third, some of these developments and issues are linked to their potential influence on Latino health and health care. The chapter concludes with a discussion of the broader policy implications and the need for a critical reexamination of the vision and strategies that are driving policy, research, and programs that respond to the needs of Latinos.

## Latino Communities at the Turn of the New Century

The Latino population is by all accounts growing dramatically and in the year 2000 became the country's largest "minority" group (United States Bureau of the Census, Census 2000 Redistricting Data). With the widespread recognition of the growing and enduring presence of Latinos in the United States has come an abundance of data and statistics used by government, the media, social scientists, politicians, and others to describe this population. (For examples of this statistical abundance, see Hornor, 1995; and Reddy, 1995.) Please refer to Table 1.1 for a statistical profile of Latinos. While important, these numbers have too often substituted for analysis, and in their repetition, especially by the media, they run the risk of numbing the intellect. Therefore, what is missing is a substantive analysis that would give the data some meaning.

### Emerging Latino Populations

In addition to growth due to natural increase, immigration from the Caribbean and South America is making significant contributions to the growth of the Latino population. As a result, relatively new Latino subgroups—such as Salvadorians, Dominicans, and the emerging presence of Mexicans in such untraditional places like New York—are increasing in the United States in large numbers. In 2000 (United States Bureau of the Census for Labor Statistics), the Latino population (excluding the close to four million Latinos who are U.S. citizens in Puerto Rico and the U.S. Virgin Islands) was 66.1 percent Mexican, 9 percent Puerto Rican, 4 percent Cuban, 14.5 percent Central and South American, and 6.4 percent "Other Latinos." Between 1980 and 2000 the size of the Central and South American population doubled from 7 percent to 14.5 percent, while the residual "Other Latino" category had the largest drop during the same period (from 14 percent to 6.4 percent (Figure 1.1).

During this time, the proportion of Mexicans, Puerto Ricans, and Cubans remained approximately the same. Notwithstanding the growth of these other groups from Central and South America, the U.S. Census has remained constant in the categories used in most of its data collection and reporting, focusing primarily on the three major Latino subgroups—Mexicans, Puerto Ricans,

## TABLE 1.1. STATISTICAL PROFILE OF LATINOS IN THE UNITED STATES: MARCH 1999.

| | Mexican Americans | Puerto Ricans | Cubans | Central and South Americans | Other Latinos | Total Latinos | African Americans | Asian Americans | Whites |
|---|---|---|---|---|---|---|---|---|---|
| Total persons (thousands) | 19,834 | 3,117 | 1,307 | 4,437 | 2,079 | 30,773 | 32,528 | 10,492 | 195,138 |
| Percent of total population | 6.9 | 1.1 | 0.5 | 1.5 | 0.7 | 10.6 | 11.3 | 3.6 | 67.5 |
| Percent of Latinos | 64.5 | 10.1 | 4.2 | 14.4 | 6.8 | 100.0 | NA | NA | NA |
| Percent of Latinos including Puerto Rico | 57.3 | 20.1 | 3.8 | 12.8 | 6.0 | 100.0 | NA | NA | NA |
| *Age Distribution of Group* | | | | | | | | | |
| Under 5 years old | 12.4 | 11.1 | 7.1 | 8.6 | 9.4 | 11.3 | 8.7 | 8.4 | 7.0 |
| 5–14 years old | 20.7 | 18.3 | 10.8 | 15.0 | 18.4 | 19.0 | 19.0 | 16.4 | 14.2 |
| 15–44 years old | 50.1 | 47.7 | 41.9 | 56.7 | 47.8 | 50.3 | 47.4 | 49.8 | 44.3 |
| 45–64 years old | 12.5 | 16.6 | 20.7 | 15.8 | 17.8 | 14.1 | 17.0 | 18.5 | 21.7 |
| 65 years old and over | 4.3 | 6.4 | 19.5 | 3.9 | 6.6 | 5.3 | 7.8 | 6.7 | 12.9 |
| *Educational Attainment* | | | | | | | | | |
| Persons 25 years old and over | 9,649 | 1,682 | 952 | 2,599 | 1,163 | 16,044 | 19,376 | 6,381 | 145,078 |
| Percent high school graduates or higher | 48.3 | 63.9 | 67.8 | 64.9 | 72.2 | 55.5 | 61.3 | 42.8 | 58.7 |
| Percent bachelor's or higher | 7.5 | 12.0 | 22.2 | 17.4 | 16.0 | 11.0 | 14.7 | 42.1 | 25.0 |
| *Labor Force Status* | | | | | | | | | |
| Civilians 16 years and over (000) | 13,216 | 2,080 | 1,062 | 3,215 | 1,497 | 21,070 | 24,373 | 7,689 | 171,478 |
| Percent in labor force | 68.8 | 60.0 | 61.3 | 72.9 | 65.3 | 67.9 | 65.6 | 68.5 | 67.3 |
| Unemployment rate | 7.3 | 8.3 | 6.0 | 6.1 | 7.8 | 7.2 | 8.9 | 4.6 | 3.9 |
| Male | 6.5 | 8.5 | 4.1 | 5.4 | 7.2 | 6.4 | NA | NA | NA |
| Female | 8.6 | 8.2 | 8.6 | 7.0 | 7.9 | 8.2 | NA | NA | NA |

*(Continued)*

# TABLE 1.1. STATISTICAL PROFILE OF LATINOS IN THE UNITED STATES: MARCH 1999. (*Continued*)

| | Mexican Americans | Puerto Ricans | Cubans | Central and South Americans | Other Latinos | Total Latinos | African Americans | Asian Americans | Whites |
|---|---|---|---|---|---|---|---|---|---|
| *Family Type* | | | | | | | | | |
| Total families (000) | 4,292 | 770 | 383 | 1,018 | 498 | 6,961 | 8,408 | 2,381 | 59,515 |
| Percent married | 72.1 | 53.9 | 80.7 | 67.6 | 59.8 | 69.0 | 46.6 | 81.7 | 80.8 |
| Percent single female household | 20.0 | 37.7 | 15.1 | 23.2 | 33.9 | 23.2 | 43.7 | 11.7 | 14.0 |
| Percent single male household | 7.9 | 8.4 | 4.2 | 9.1 | 6.2 | 7.8 | 6.7 | 6.6 | 5.3 |
| *Family Income in 1997* | | | | | | | | | |
| Total families | 4,292 | 770 | 383 | 1,018 | 498 | 6,961 | 8,408 | 2,391 | 59,515 |
| Less than $5,000 | 5.1 | 6.8 | 2.1 | 4.4 | 5.4 | 5.1 | 6.9 | 2.9 | 2.1 |
| $5,000–9,999 | 8.1 | 15.5 | 7.3 | 5.3 | 11.0 | 8.7 | 10.1 | 2.7 | 3.2 |
| $10,000–$14,999 | 11.6 | 10.5 | 11.5 | 8.7 | 8.8 | 10.9 | 9.8 | 5.3 | 5.1 |
| $15,000–$24,999 | 21.5 | 19.9 | 15.1 | 19.0 | 14.5 | 20.1 | 17.7 | 9.2 | 12.5 |
| $25,000–$34,999 | 16.0 | 11.9 | 11.5 | 16.1 | 15.5 | 15.3 | 14.2 | 9.8 | 12.7 |
| $35,000–$49,999 | 17.1 | 13.9 | 14.9 | 20.3 | 18.7 | 17.2 | 15.5 | 17.8 | 17.7 |
| $50,000 or more | 20.5 | 21.4 | 37.3 | 26.1 | 25.9 | 22.8 | 25.9 | 52.2 | 46.6 |
| median income | $27,088 | $23,729 | $37,537 | $32,030 | $30,130 | $28,141 | $28,602 | $51,850 | $46,754 |
| Percent of white median income | 57.9 | 50.8 | 80.3 | 68.5 | 64.4 | 60.2 | 61.2 | 110.9 | 100.0 |
| *Poverty* | | | | | | | | | |
| Families below poverty level (000) | 1,106 | 243 | 60 | 188 | 124 | 1,721 | 1,986 | 244 | 4,990 |
| Poverty rate for families | 25.8 | 31.6 | 15.7 | 18.5 | 24.9 | 24.7 | 23.6 | 10.2 | 8.4 |
| Persons below poverty level | 5,509 | 1,059 | 257 | 949 | 534 | 8,308 | 9,116 | 1,488 | 24,396 |
| Poverty Rate for Persons | 27.8 | 34.0 | 19.7 | 21.4 | 25.7 | 27.0 | 26.5 | 14.0 | 11.0 |

*Source: Current population survey: March 1999.* (United States Bureau of the Census). Please note that Puerto Rico and the U.S. Virgin Islands are not included in these data.

## FIGURE 1.1.  LATINOS IN THE UNITED STATES.

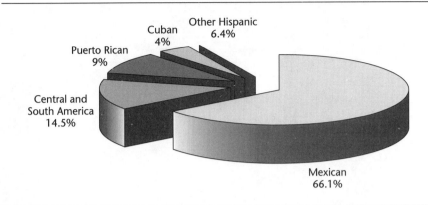

*Source:* Therrien, M., & Ramirez, R. R. (2000). *The Hispanic population in the United States: March 2000.*

and Cubans. The evident growth of other Latino groups, primarily from El Salvador, Nicaragua, and the Dominican Republic, raises question about the utility of this system of reporting and data collection. As they exist, there is only limited, and not of the best quality, information available on these growing populations.

At a time when the Latino population was growing, the proportion of Whites in the population has been decreasing. Whites made up 75.6 percent of the population in 1990, dropped to 73.6 percent by 1995, and to 67.5 percent by 1999 (Figure 1.2). During the period of projected growth of the Latino population, the percentage of growth of the White population is expected to stop by 2034 (Day, 1996). Much of the decrease will be due to deaths as more Whites enter older age groups in which the risk of mortality is greater.

The growth of the Latino population has implications for the composition of the workforce of the country. The Latino labor force is projected to grow 3.1 percent annually to a high of 17.4 million persons by 2006. This increase is more than that of any other group in the workforce. By 2006 it is expected that the Latino labor force will be greater than that of African Americans (Day, 1996; United States Bureau of Census, March 1999). This growth will be due to increased migration, and the increased participation of Latinas in the workforce.

The implications for the health and health status of Latinos are numerous due to the role Latinos will play in the economy of the nation. To ensure the highest-level functioning of this sector of the workforce, initiatives are currently needed to see that the health and health status of Latinos are attended to for future interests of this community as well as that of the economy as a whole. It will be important to monitor whether Latinos' access to insurance increases over this period and if this will correspond with employment in sectors where insurance is not only offered to its employees, but is affordable. At the present time the

## FIGURE 1.2.   PROJECTIONS OF THE RESIDENT POPULATION BY RACE AND  ETHNICITY (YEARS 2001 TO 2050).

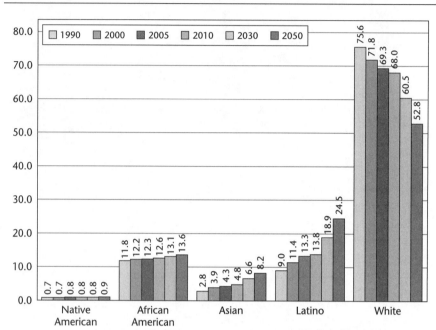

Source: Day, J. C. (1996). *Population projection for the United States by age, sex, race, and Hispanic origin; 1995–2050.*

Note: Source data for 2005; Population projections program, Population Divison, U.S. Census Bureau, January 2000.

very low rates of insurance coverage among Latinos poses a significant barrier to health care in this population.

Nationally, increases in the numbers of Central and South Americans may not appear to be a major shift, but it does manifest itself in significant ways locally, especially in many of the large urban centers where the composition of Latino subgroups is dramatically changing. For example, health care systems in Los Angeles can no longer assume that they are serving Mexicans, nor can those in New York City assume that their clients are primarily Puerto Rican. This means that when it comes to issues of health care, profiles and assumptions about health status attributed to known Latino groups may not apply and will require better documentation. This fact is raised throughout many of the chapters in this book.

### Diversity and Dispersion

Along the dimension of growth, the increasing diversity and dispersion of the Latino population will continue to have a significant effect on its development along several other dimensions. The diversity of Latinos has already been affected in major ways along at least two dimensions: (1) the number of different Latino national-origin groups with significant numbers in the population; and, (2) a growing social class diversity.

What makes the increasing diversity of the Latino experience especially complex is that it is occurring in different ways and at different rates in the various Latino national-origin groups. According to the census, in 1998 there was a wide range of socioeconomic diversity among Latinos. It ranged from the high poverty rates of more than 50 percent in Puerto Rico and 31 percent for Puerto Ricans in the United States, to the relatively low rate of 14 percent among Cuban Americans. Even though the aggregate poverty rate for Latinos has dropped (from 31 percent to 26 percent between 1993 and 1998), when compared to the total U.S. population it is still very high (26 percent compared to 13 percent in 1998) (Puerto Rican Legal Defense and Education Found (PRLDEF) Institute for Puerto Rican Policy, 2000; Rivera-Batiz & Santiago, 1996). (See Table 1.2.)

## Growth of the Latino Middle Class

The economic diversity of Latinos also appears to be growing. Despite a very high overall Latino poverty rate, the per capita income for Latinos has recently been growing faster than that for other groups. Between 1997 and 1998 Latino per capita income grew 4.5 percent compared to 3.3 percent for African Americans and 3.2 percent for Whites (Perez, 2000). This suggests the emergence of a small but growing Latino middle class that challenges the traditional view of Latinos as primarily poor and working class immigrants. Although Latinos continue to be significantly underrepresented in government employment, business ownership, and admissions into higher education, there nevertheless have been small gains in each of these areas. In turn, this is creating a critical mass that in the near future will provide the base for a socially significant professional and middle class (Trueba, 1999).

### TABLE 1.2.    POVERTY STATUS BY PROPORTION
### OF SUBGROUP POPULATION.

| Type of Origin | Proportion of Subgroup Population Below Poverty Level |
|---|---|
| Total Latinos | 22.8 percent |
| Mexican | 24.1 percent |
| Puerto Rican | 25.8 percent |
| Cuban | 17.3 percent |
| Central and South American | 16.7 percent |
| Other Latino | 23.6 percent |
| Non-Latino White | 7.7 percent |

*Source:* Therrien, M., & Ramirez, R. R. (2000). *The Hispanic population in the United States: March, 2000.*

United States Bureau of Census for Labor Statistics. (1999, March) *Current population survey (CPS).*

Large corporations, either Latino-owned or Latino-oriented, such as Goya Foods, Univision, Banco Popular, the U.S. Hispanic Chamber of Commerce, and others, have become important sectors of the economy. The formation of Latino-owned businesses is dramatic in places like Miami and Los Angeles (although surprisingly anemic in places like New York City). Latino leadership in areas such as education, social services, and the nonprofit sector has also grown, with such developments as Latinos leading major public school systems throughout the country, as well as large-scale nonprofit organizations such as the Independent Sector and others. During the Clinton Administration, we saw Latinos in the Cabinet serving in "non-Latino" posts such as Secretary of Housing and Urban Development, Secretary of Transportation, and head of the Small Business Administration.

This raises questions as to what the growth of this emerging middle class portends for the future of Latinos with regard to health status, access to decision-making positions, and influence on political processes. Some have begun to speculate (Zweigenhaft & Domhoff, 1998), but the prognosis is not at all clear. Will it result in an economic gap of significant proportion within the Latino community? Will these changes result in an increasing political leverage? Can these class differences be mediated across Latino subgroups? How will the changing class structure affect the health profile and health status of the community? Will this emerging class have better health outcomes as is anticipated with improvements in socioeconomic status?

In the African American community, this type of class differentiation is mediated by a tradition of civil rights struggle in the United States; but the Latino community does not have its equivalent in duration and depth. In terms of social conditions and public attitudes, Latinos are said to fall somewhere in between African Americans and Whites in the United States. While simplistic descriptions of this sort appear rather frequently in the news, media, books, and other sources, they belie the many complexities and project a certainty that does not exist. The African American experience, therefore, may not provide much of a guide in this respect, and we are left to speculate.

## Somos Latinos, Hispanic, or What?

The dramatic growing diversity of the Latino population over the past decade or so has raised difficult questions about the meaning of being Latino and what the term actually means. (For greater discussion on this issue, see, for example, Delgado & Stefancic, 1998; Darder & Torres, 1997; Flores, 2000; Romero, Hondagneu-Sotelo, & Ortiz, 1997.) No longer can we assume that Latino refers primarily to Mexicans, Puerto Ricans, or Cubans. These changes have raised debates over whether the term "Latino" or "Hispanic" is the most appropriate or accurate, and they have raised questions about whether these umbrella terms have any meaning at all (De la Garza, DeSipio, Garcia, Garcia, & Falcón, 1992).

Even at the level of national-origin labels—Mexican, Puerto Rican, Cuban, and so on—the dramatic changes in composition *within* these populations raise questions about the usefulness of these even more specific identifiers.

## A Panethnic Consciousness

The very meaning of "Latino" and "Hispanic," already ambiguous to many, will no doubt undergo significant changes in this century. While Latino outgroup intermarriage appears to be a steady trend (between 27–28 percent in the 1990s, as calculated from Table 65 of United States Bureau of the Census, 1999), there is evidence of increasing Latino subgroup intermarriage, especially among the younger generation. An indication is that in most metropolitan areas Latinos are more likely than any other group to identify, although in low single digits, as having two or more races (Minaya, 2000). This situation serves to strengthen panethnic consciousness among Latinos. The increasing intermarriage among members of Latino subgroups is not only the basis for a growing panethnic reality but has resulted in attempts to construct a new multiculturalism within the Latino experience, with terms such as "DomiRican," "MexiCuban," and others emerging. However, with more than a quarter of Latino marriages being to non-Latinos, how will this impact a panethnic identity as well as the ethnic identity of this community?

In addition to the factors within the Latino community to reinforce a panethnic identity, there are many other forces at work in the United States promoting such a consciousness among these groups (Fox, 1996; Oboler, 1995). These include corporations, both the English- and Spanish-language media, as well as government. Observing an expanding and lucrative ethnic market, corporations have developed strategies to aggregate this population, as well as differentiate it as needed to more easily market to it. Growing Spanish-language entertainment and news media, which are for the most part owned by U.S corporations, share a similar project. (For its racially discriminatory aspects, see Fletcher, 2000). The marketing of a Latino (or Hispanic) identity has become a powerful force in defining these diverse communities' realities in the United States but that still awaits serious critical analysis. (See Davila, 1997, for a useful starting point in the case of Puerto Rico.)

This, however, is a complex process worthy of preliminary analysis. The power of capitalism's commodification of experiences has its effects in homogenizing and disrupting sociocultural processes. As a result, while one can observe the effects of the commercialization of the Latino experience, one can also see processes variously described as the "Latinization" or "tropicalization" of U.S. society (Aparicio & Chávez-Silverman, 1997; Gonzalez, 2000). Whether this represents an authentic struggle for national affirmation by Latinos or a refining of U.S. cultural and social dominance may be too early to tell. But there is certainly much to explore and deliberate, especially the influence these processes will have on young Latinos whose identities are still in formation. In the same vein, the influences on Latino youth of such racialized cultural forms as hip-hop and rap and of such new technologies like the Internet may in the immediate future transform Latino cultural definitions in ways that are very different from today (Flores, 2000).

When it comes to corporate marketing interest, media influences, and the Internet, each poses challenges and opportunities for addressing the health and heath care needs of Latinos. For example, marketing activities that encourage disease-promoting behaviors such as tobacco or alcohol use—both issues that are addressed in detail in this book—pose significant challenges. On the other hand, the emergence and increase of Latino media outlets (radio, television, magazines, and so on) and the growing use of the Internet provide opportunities and can serve as vehicles for educating, informing, and empowering the community on a number of health issues. The real challenge faced by the health community is finding creative and viable ways of approaching and using these channels of communication to benefit Latinos.

## What's in a Name?

Without entering into the well-traveled territory of the by-now extraneous debate over the use of "Latino" versus "Hispanic" (Hayes-Bautista & Chapa, 1987; Trevino, 1987; Gimenez, 1989), a major issue is whether these overarching labels have any useful meaning. Survey after survey of Latinos have found that their preferred form of identification is through their specific national origin, that is, as Mexicans, Mexican Americans, Puerto Ricans, Cubans, Dominicans, and the like (De la Garza, DeSipio, Garcia, Garcia, & Falcón, 1992). The basis of their identification as "others" in U.S. society is through a nationalism and/or ethnicity grounded in their country of origin, whether born there or not. This creates the constant potential for transnational identities fed by very active international circular migrations, supporting such broad and to many obscure notions as "cultural citizenship" (Flores & Benmayor, 1997; see also Bonilla, Meléndez, Morales, & de los Angeles Torres, 1998) and other post-colonialist perspectives (Soja, 1996).

This is not to say that the debate over whether to use the term "Latino" or "Hispanic" instead of a group's national origin identification (hyphenated or not) is not important. The answers to this dilemma are not as straightforward as some would suggest. The meaning of words change and can be multiple, which suggests that their use needs to be carefully considered because a particular meaning or meanings can have important consequences. By understanding this we can better grasp the challenges before us as we try to capture the way we describe ourselves in a precise and necessarily dynamic way. The same is true for other umbrella terms such as "minority," a word that has often been used to refer to African Americans. Many in the Latino community see this as a deliberately imprecise term whose use frequently results in the interests of Latinos being compromised. This realization points to the fact that the Latino community needs to determine the process by which it self-defines, a process that cannot be ceded to others if it is to reflect its own reality.

The way in which Latinos are identified or classified has numerous implications on a variety of fronts. One is the health research arena. Categories and identifiers used to document and describe Latinos can greatly affect the kind and number of services and resources that are allocated by the public and other sectors for addressing Latinos' health needs.

## Immigrants or Ethnic and Racial Minorities?

Generational, racial, gender-based, and class-based issues and developments further complicate the Latino experience. Latinos are largely characterized by the media and in popular discourse as being newly-arrived immigrants (Suro, 1999). The facts that the majority of Latinos are U.S.-born (66 percent) or naturalized citizens (9 percent) (United States Bureau of the Census, 1993) and that a significant proportion of them are longtime residents of the United States are generally lost (Figure 1.3).

If the Latino experience is defined essentially as that of an immigrant group, analogous to that of earlier European immigrants, then responses to problems such as access to quality health care will be formulated accordingly. That is, Latino issues will be defined as problems common to new arrivals, and that once

**FIGURE 1.3.   NATIVITY AND CITIZENSHIP FOR SELECTED HISPANIC ORIGIN GROUPS: 1990.**

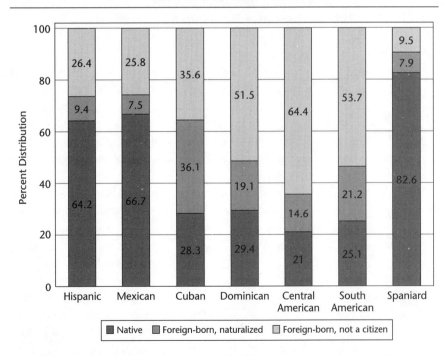

*Source:* United States Bureau of Census. (1993).

acculturated, Latinos will be able to navigate the system and become members of the American mainstream. Whatever its merits, the acculturation model does not easily adapt to the Latino population.

If the issues are defined from the perspective of Latinos as newcomers who need to quickly acculturate to American society, this approach may be shortsighted and possibly counterproductive. Studies have documented that rapid acculturation to American values and behaviors could result in negative health outcomes for Latinos (Abraído-Lanza, Dohrenwend, Ng-Mak, & Turner, 1999). It is increasingly realized that Latino newcomers to the United States bring with them certain culturally protective factors from their countries of origin. These protective factors serve to shield them from many high-risk health behaviors.

Despite the fact that Latinos report to "feel more ill" than Whites (Hajat, Lucas, & Kington, 2000), and are less satisfied than Whites and African Americans with the quality of care they receive (Collins, Hall, & Neuhaus, 1999), Latino newcomers tend to live longer, have less heart disease, and exhibit lower rates of breast cancer among women (Hayes-Bautista, 1992; Markides & Coreil, 1986; Sorlie, Backlund, Johnson, & Rogat, 1993). The "Hispanic paradox" demonstrates that the effects of social economic status (SES) on health indicators is modified by the acculturation status of the individual (Scribner, 1996). In other words, health behaviors for Latinos worsen with increased levels of acculturation, regardless of SES. While this "paradox" has not been fully analyzed, the "Healthy Migrant" effect appears to be the result of the socioeconomic and psychological selectivity of the immigration process. Nevertheless, it does provide an imperative for health professionals and researchers to reassess strategies and interventions that preserve culturally determined protective factors that maintain high levels of wellness.

There are as well many misconceptions about Latinos held by health care policy makers and professionals that create problems. Most appear to center on the definition of Latino health problems as solely those of the new immigrant. If the dominant response to the health problems faced by Latinos is shaped by an immigrant focus when the majority of Latinos are not immigrants, then one can readily see the many problems this might create in terms of policy and practice. Further, the characterization of Latinos as immigrants results in the continued perception that they are "outsiders" with none of the entitlements that come with citizenship or resident status.

In addition, if the question of health care access for Latinos is largely defined in terms of language and sociocultural barriers in health settings, then interventions that are developed on this basis will only affect a small part of this community. The 1990 Census found that about 78 percent of Latinos spoke Spanish at home, and half of those reported speaking English "very well." This means that overall, approximately 73 percent of Latinos reported speaking English "very well"; 22 percent reported speaking no Spanish (United States Bureau of the Census, 1993). Programs that address the language needs of non-English speakers are important and needed. However, their impact is on a limited percentage of the total Latino community (perhaps about one-third or so). Despite this, language proficiency should be taken into consideration when designing programs for Latinos, because there are great variations in the levels of English-language proficiency among different Latino subgroups. Many of the authors in this book recommend the delivery of health programs and services by linguistically proficient professionals. But while a significant problem, language does not appear to be *the* central barrier to Latino access to health care. (For an excellent overall discussion of the language policy debate in the United States, see Schmidt, 2000.) Several of the chapters in the book discuss the multiple of factors that create barriers, some of which are related to the lack of appropriate services and programs, the changes that have given rise due to managed care, and the lack of adequate resources to address the need.

Some conservatives and neo-liberal authors see the central issue for Latinos in the United States today as the need to resolve the ambivalence between viewing themselves as immigrants or as a racial minority group in this society (Skerry, 1993; Chavez, 1991; Falcón, 1995; Schmidt, 2000; and for a critique of Skerry, see Magaña, 1994). At the same time, the usefulness of race as compared to ethnicity for exploring group differences in areas such as health policy has also been opened to question. Some argue that ethnicity, as the broader concept of the two that encompasses both genetics and culture, is the most analytically powerful. The ethnic dimension of the Latino experience, therefore, can be seen as bridging many analytical divides that can take us beyond black and white formulations of social processes. (Angier, 2000)

It is becoming increasingly clear that the issues and difficulties that Latinos face in U.S. society are not amenable to simplified formulas or explanations. As immigration continues from South America and the Caribbean, the nature of Latino communities will be affected in unpredictable ways. The fact that this is all occurring in a society that perceives itself as "color blind" yet perceives at the same time that race is central to a number of processes adds another layer of complexity to these social processes for Latinos, who are a racially diverse population. The result is a multifaceted and dynamic Latino reality that is becoming increasingly difficult to characterize in simple overarching terms (Flores, 2000; on the dialectics of Latino realities and health, see Levins & Lewontin, 1985). The past and the experiences of previous immigrant groups or that of the African American community may not serve as a helpful guide, or for that matter may not be relevant in the case of Latinos.

## On Becoming the Largest "Minority"

The United States Bureau of the Census (Census 2000 Redistricting Data) reported that there were more than 31 million Latinos in the United States in the year 2000, a number that is predicted to *triple* in the next fifty years to more than 96 million. This would result in an increase of Latinos from 11 percent to 25 percent of the total population. In the year 2000, the number of Latinos surpassed the number of African Americans, making up 12.5 percent and 12.0 percent of the population, respectively (United States Bureau of the Census, Census Redistricting Data). Thus, Latinos became the nation's largest ethnic or racial minority group at the turn of the new millennium. Including the close to four million Puerto Ricans who are U.S. citizens living in the U.S. territories of Puerto Rico and the U.S. Virgin Islands brings the total U.S. Latino population to almost forty million during the twenty-first century. This is compared to an estimated thirty-four million African Americans. (Day, 1996; United States Bureau of the Census, January 2000).

But what exactly does being the largest "minority" mean? For Latinos, it means that the lack of visibility over which many have expressed concern over the decades becomes much harder to sustain by American society as a whole. There was a time when Latino leaders could legitimately claim that U.S. society was ignoring their community. Now this is no longer the case with the so-called Latin music explosion (see Watrous, 2000, on its waning after only a year or so) and new attention given to the Latino voter at the onset of this new century (Falcón, 2000). The Latino part of the electorate has grown to the point where it can be an important "swing vote" in national and state elections. This raises a different set of issues, primarily over defining the terms of agenda setting. It also means that the notion of Latinos as newcomers and temporary immigrants to the United States (a blip, if you like, on the American reality) will also be much harder to sustain.

For some African Americans, being "replaced" as the country's largest minority group is a cause for concern because the transfer of this status may mean that Latinos will benefit from the African American civil rights struggle and that African American issues will be bypassed by a socially mercurial American public. For many Whites, it may simply mean that the underlying Anglo-Saxon and European roots that are at the core of American society are eroding and that the threat of Spanish becoming the first language will become a reality. For others it may simply be perceived as a trivial matter, where food, music, culture, and community create a dynamic commodity to be enjoyed by all. (For current evidence of this process, see Johnson, 2000).

When referring to Latinos as becoming the largest "minority" in the United States, there appear to be a number of assumptions that either need to be made explicit or questioned. The first assumption is that "Latinos" (or "Hispanics"), a collection of communities from more than twenty Spanish-speaking countries and territories, will be acting and thinking cohesively on issues that are of importance to the community. A second is that the meaning of the term "Latino" (or "Hispanic") today will have the same meaning in fifty years, as will the racial component that affects them. A third is that ethnic and racial minority-majority group relations will be governed by the same values and rules in the future. These are better suited as questions than assumptions.

The notion of a panethnic consciousness among Latinos has undergone some systematic examination (Delgado & Stefancic, 1998; Padilla, 1985; de la Garza, DeSipio, Garcia, Garcia, & Falcón, 1992; Jones-Correa & Leal, 1996), and while it can be argued, as previously stated, that it is growing and real, to what extent this is the case and what it will actually mean in the future are generally unknown. While there are many policy issues that unite Latinos, such as bilingual education because of a common language, there are others in which there are differences. For example, continuing the embargo of Cuba and the support of NAFTA. But will policy and political differences emerge between those Latinos who are U.S. citizens and those who are not? This and a growing middle class within the Latino community may present challenges to a unified policy agenda.

With challenges to affirmative action, bilingual education, and other racially focused policies, the terms by which ethnic and racial relations are defined may be changing in important ways. The dramatic increases in the size of not only the Latino but also the Asian American population will challenge the continuing utility of viewing many American social issues from a binary Black White perspective. This would represent a major discontinuity in the country's dominant racial discourse. In addition, there are other indications that there may be potentially powerful changes in the ways race relations are viewed in the United States in the near future. They include the rise of conservatism in the African American community; the growth of large Latino-owned businesses; and the continued global dominance of the English language (through robust new media such as the Internet).

In the end, being the largest ethnic and racial "minority" at a time when there may be no more "majorities" may not mean much at all. But this raises important questions of relevance for the future well-being of Latinos. Will African Americans, Asian Americans, and Latinos form effective coalitions (Piatt, 1997)? Will Latinos divide more clearly between those who follow a "racial minority" agenda and those who follow a more accommodationist "immigrant" one? And are these viable alternatives?

The prognosis for these various scenarios is difficult to determine given current crosscutting developments. Will there be a major African American backlash to the growing presence of Latinos? Will political and economic special interests pursue divide-and-conquer tactics against communities of color? Will immigration from the Caribbean and South America subside and be replaced by immigration from other parts of the world, creating a stronger second-generation reality for Latino communities in the United States (Portes, 1996)?

While all of these social and demographic dynamics are evolving, what will it mean for the health of Latinos? Will there be added mental health problems as an increasingly diverse Latino population and its young people attempt to navigate its way through the changes? Can the culturally protective factors of family, social support networks, and health behaviors that produce the "Hispanic paradox" be preserved? Will this growing community be cohesive enough and politically influential enough to advocate for a health agenda that responds to their collective needs? These are all unknowns, requiring the serious attention of the health policy sector, researchers, health professionals, and service providers, as well as community advocates as they look to the future.

## Implications for Latinos and Health

As the chapters in this volume confirm, there are many basic and recurring issues surrounding the health disparities faced by Latinos in the United States. These include the issues of

- Financial barriers to care and health insurance.
- The availability of appropriate health, mental health, and preventive services across the life cycle.
- The disproportionate rates, for example, of diabetes, alcohol use, and mortality due to cancer and heart disease.
- Barriers to services due to language, gender, and other forms of discrimination (Centro Legal para Derechos Reproductivos y Políticas Públicas, 1997; Colectiva del Libro de Salud de la Mujeres en Boston, 2000; Delgado, 1997).
- Underrepresentation of Latinos and Latino-sensitive individuals in medical and health professions, or in the training pipeline (Kehrer & Burroughs, 1994).
- The lack of recognition of health practices based in Latino cultures (Molina, Zambrana, & Aguirre-Molina, 1994).
- The continuing lack of adequate health data on Latinos and Latino subgroups in particular (Collins, Hall, & Neuhaus, 1999).

A recent report by the National Center for Health Statistics (2000) found that 18 percent of African Americans and 15 percent of Latinos reported having poor-to-fair health, compared to the lower rate of 9 percent for Whites (Figure 1.4). The danger of the apparent persistence of this state of affairs is that it seems as though it has become an unalterable fact of life for the Latino community (and American society in general). On the surface, the health problems faced by Latinos in the United States are so tied to their poor socioeconomic status and lack of political power that to some it may appear hopeless to achieve any major changes. While these issues are complex in and of themselves, an unfortunate synergy is precipitated when placed in the context of the demographic transformation previously described and the historical context of ethnic and racial, class, and gender hierarchies in the United States' health system.

The highly complex and contingent realities that Latinos face in the United States are neither understood nor taken into consideration by the health care system. This assessment tends to leave no alternative but to promote what ultimately may be described as incremental changes in the nation's health care system. But is this where the situation starts and ends? This need not be the case. The answer lies within the strengths and resources of the community. This includes Latinos' growing numbers, their political and voting potential, and the human and organizational infrastructure of national groups, health professionals, and advocates. Collectively they can change the tide of events to the benefit and well-being of Latinos. The final chapter of this book more clearly defines a new direction for the Latino community of the future.

**FIGURE 1.4.   SELF-ASSESSED HEALTH STATUS BY HISPANIC ORIGIN SUBGROUP AND RACE FOR PEOPLE OF ALL AGES: UNITED STATES, ANNUALIZED FIGURES, 1992–1995.**

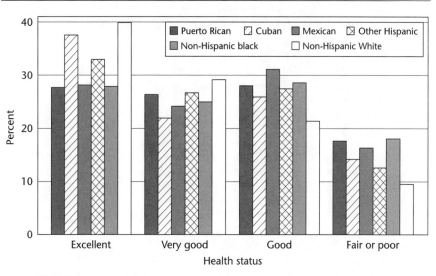

NOTE: Data are age related

*Source:* Advance Data No. 310, February 25, 2000, Vital and Health Statistics of the Centers for Disease Control and Prevention.

# References

Abraído-Lanza, A. F., Dohrenwend, B. P., Ng-Mak, D. S., & Turner, J. B. (1999, October). The Latino mortality paradox: A test of the 'Salmon Bias' and healthy migrant hypotheses. *American Journal of Public Health, 89,* 10, 1543–1548.

Angier, N. (2000, August 22). Do races differ? Not really, DNA shows. *The New York Times,* Science Desk. Section F, p. 1.

Aparicio, F. R., & Chávez-Silverman, S. (1997). *Tropicalizations: Transcultural representations of Latinidad.* Hanover, NH: University Press of New England.

Bean, F. D., & Tiendar, M. (1987). *The Hispanic population of the United States.* New York: Russell Sage Foundation.

Bonilla, F., Meléndez, E., Morales, R., & de los Angeles Torres, M. (1998). *Borderless borders: U.S. Latinos, Latin Americans, and the paradox of interdependence.* Philadelphia: Temple University Press.

Centro Legal para Derechos Reproductivos y Políticas Públicas. (1997). Mujeres del mundo: Leyes y políticas que afectan sus vidas reproductivas—América Latina y el Caribe. New York.

Chavez, L. (1991). *Out of the barrio: Toward a new politics of Hispanic assimilation.* New York: Basic Books.

Colectiva del Libro de Salud de la Mujeres en Boston. (2000). *Nuestros cuerpos, nuestras vidas: La guía definitiva para la salud de la mujer Latina.* New York: Seven Stories Press.

Collins, K. S., Hall, A., & Neuhaus, C. (1999). *U.S. minority health: A chartbook.* New York: The Commonwealth Fund.

Darder, A., & Torres, R. D. (1997). *The Latino studies reader: Culture, economy & society.* Malden, MA: Blackwell.

Davila, A. M. (1997). *Sponsored identities: Cultural politics in Puerto Rico.* Philadelphia: Temple University Press.

Day, J. C. (1996, February). Population projections of the United States by age, sex, race, and Hispanic origin: 1995–2050. Washington, D.C.: U.S. Bureau of the Census, Current Population Reports, U.S. Government Printing Office, 25–1130.

De la Garza, R. O., DeSipio, L., Garcia, F. C., Garcia, J., & Falcón, A. (1992). *Latino voices: Mexican, Puerto Rican & Cuban perspectives on American politics.* Boulder, CO: Westview Press.

Delgado, J. (1997). *¡Salud! A Latina's guide to total health—Body, mind, and spirit.* New York: Harper Collins Publishers.

Delgado, R., & Stefancic, J. (1998). *The Latino/a condition: A critical reader.* New York: New York University Press.

Falcón, A. (1995). Puerto Ricans and the politics of racial identity. In H. W. Harris, H. C. Blue, & E.E.H. Griffith (Eds.), *Racial and ethnic identity: Psychological development and creative expression.* (pp.193–208). New York: Routledge.

Falcón, A. (2000, February 14). Vote for me, amigos. *The Nation.* p. 20.

Fletcher, M. A. (2000, August 3). The blond, blue-eyed face of Spanish TV. *Washington Post.* p. A01.

Flores, J. (2000). *From bomba to hip-hop: Puerto Rican culture and Latino identity.* New York: Columbia University.

Flores, W., & Benmayor, R. (1997). *Latino cultural citizenship: Claiming identity, space, and rights.* Boston: Beacon Press.

Fox, G. (1996). *Hispanic nation: Culture, politics, and the constructing of identity.* Secaucus, NJ: Carol Publishing.

Gimenez, M. E. (1989). Latino/"Hispanic": Who needs a name? The case against a standardized terminology. *International Journal of Health Services, 19,* 3, 557–571.

Gonzalez, J. (2000). *Harvest of empire: A history of Latinos in America.* New York: Viking.

Hajat, A., Lucas, J. B., & Kington, R. (2000). *Health outcomes among Hispanic subgroups: United States, 1992–1995.* Advance data from vital and health statistics, n. 310.

Hayes-Bautista, D. E. (1992). Latino health indicators and the underclass model: From paradox to new policy models. In E. Furino (Ed.), *Health policy and the Hispanic.* Colorado: Westview Press.

Hayes-Bautista, D., & Chapa, J. (1987). Latino terminology: Conceptual bases for standardized terminology. *American Journal of Public Health, 77,* 61–68.

Hornor, L. L. (1995). *Hispanic Americans: A statistical sourcebook.* Palo Alto, CA: Information Publications.

Hunt, J. P., Tello, G. E., & Huerta, E. E. (1994). *Hispanic-American health, current bibliographies in medicine 94-6: January 1990 through July 1994.* Bethesda, MD: National Library of Medicine.

Johnson, G. (2000, August 13). Beyond burgers: New McDonald's menu makes run for the border. *Los Angeles Times.*

Jones-Correa, M., & Leal, D. L. (1996, May). Becoming "Hispanic": Secondary panethnic identification among Latin American-origin populations in the United States. *Hispanic Journal of Behavioral Sciences, 18,* 2, 214–254.

Kehrer, B. H., & Burroughs, H. C. (1994). *More minorities in health.* Menlo Park, CA: Henry J. Kaiser Family Foundation.

Levins, R., & Lewontin, R. (1985). *The dialectical biologist.* Cambridge: Harvard University Press.

Link, B. G., & Phelan, J. C. (1996, April). Editorial: Understanding sociodemographic differences in health—The role of fundamental social causes. *American Journal of Public Health, 86,* 4, 471–472.

Magaña, L. (Ed.). (1994). *Mexican Americans: Are they an ambivalent minority?* Claremont, CA: The Tomás Rivera Center. [The Tomás Rivera Policy Institute].

Markides, K. S., & Coreil, J. (1986). The health of Hispanics in the southwestern United States: An epidemiologic paradox. *Public Health Reports, 101,* 3, 253–265.

McCally, M., Haines, A., Fein, O., Addington, W., Lawrence, R. S., & Cassel, C. K. (1998, November 1). Poverty and ill health: Physicians can, and should, make a difference. *Annals of Internal Medicine, 129,* 9, 726–733.

Minaya, E. (2000, August 7). Latest census survey finds Hispanics more likely to claim two races. *Hispanic Link Weekly Report.* p. 2.

Molina, C., & Aguirre-Molina, M. (1994). *Latino health in the U.S.: A growing challenge.* Washington, D.C.: American Public Health Association.

Molina, C., Zambrana, R. E., & Aguirre-Molina, M. (1994). The influence of culture, class, and environment on health care. In C. Molina & M. Aguirre-Molina (Eds.), *Latino health in the U.S.: A growing challenge.* Washington, D.C.: American Public Health Association.

National Center for Health Statistics. (2000, February 25). Health outcomes among Hispanic subgroups: Data from the National Health Interview Survey, 1992–1995. *Advance Data,* 310.

Oboler, S. (1995). *Ethnic labels, Latino lives: Identity and the politics of (re)presentation in the United States.* Minneapolis: University of Minnesota Press.

Padilla, F. M. (1985). *Latino ethnic consciousness: The case of Mexican Americans and Puerto Ricans in Chicago.* South Bend, IN: University of Notre Dame Press.

Perez, S. M. (Ed.). (2000). *Moving up the economic ladder: Latino workers and the nation's future prosperity.* (State of Hispanic America). Washington, D.C.: National Council of La Raza.

Piatt, B. (1997). *Black and brown in America: The case for cooperation.* New York: New York University Press.

Portes, A. (Ed.). (1996). *The new second generation.* New York: Russell Sage Foundation.

Puerto Rican Legal Defense and Education Fund (PRLDEF) Institute for Puerto Rican Policy. (2000, April). Puerto Ricans and other Latinos in the United States: March 1999. *IPR Datanote on the Puerto Rican Community,* 24.

Reddy, M. A. (Ed.). (1995). *Statistical record of Hispanic Americans* (2nd ed.). New York: Gale Research.

Rivera-Batiz, F. L., & Santiago, C. E. (1996). *Island paradox: Puerto Rico in the 1990s.* New York: Russell Sage Foundation.

Romero, M., Hondagneu-Sotelo, P., & Ortiz, V. (1997). *Challenging fronteras: Structuring Latina and Latino lives in the U.S.* New York: Routledge.

Schmidt, Jr., R. (2000). *Language policy and identity politics.* Philadelphia: Temple University Press.

Scribner, R. (1996). Paradox as paradigm—The health outcomes of Mexican Americans. *American Journal of Public Health, 86,* 3, 303–305.

Skerry, P. (1993). *Mexican Americans: The ambivalent minority.* New York: The Free Press.

Soja, E. W. (1996). *Thirdspace: Journeys to Los Angeles and other real-and-imagined places.* Malden, MA: Blackwell Publishers.

Sorlie, P. D., Backlund, E., Johnson, N. J., & Rogat, E. (1993). Mortality by Hispanic status in the United States. *Journal of the Medical Association, 270,* 20, 246–2468.

Suro, R. (1999). *Strangers among us: Latino lives in a changing America.* New York: Vintage Books.

Therrien, M., & Ramirez, R. R. (2000). *The Hispanic population in the United States: March 2000.* Current Population Reports, P20–535. U.S. Census Bureau, Washington, D.C.

Trueba, E. (H.). (1999). *Latinos unidos: From cultural diversity to the politics of solidarity.* Lanham, MD: Rowman & Littlefield Publishers.

Trevino, F. M. (1987). Standardized terminology for standardized populations. *American Journal of Public Health, 77,* 69–72.

United States Bureau of the Census. (1993, September). *We the American . . . Hispanics.* Washington, D.C.

United States Bureau of the Census. (1999). *Statistical abstract of the United States: 1999* (199th ed.). Washington, D.C.

United States Bureau of the Census (2000). *Census 2000 Redistricting Data* (P.L. 94–171), Summary File for states.

United States Bureau of the Census. (2000, January 13). *Projections of the resident population by race, Hispanic origin and nativity, middle series, 2001–2005.* www.census.gov.

United States Bureau of the Census for Labor Statistics (1999, March). *Current population survey.* Washington, D.C.

United States Commission on Civil Rights. (1999). *The health care challenge: Acknowledging disparity, confronting discrimination, and ensuring equality* (Vol. I: The role of governmental and private health care programs and initiatives, and Vol. II: The role of federal civil rights enforcement efforts). Washington, D.C.

United States Department of Health and Human Services. (1998, October). *Racial and ethnic disparities in health: Response to the president's initiative on race.* Washington, D.C.

Watrous, P. (2000, August 6). Much of Latin pop, aging and sterile, isn't keeping pace. *New York Times,* Arts & Leisure Section. p. 27.

Williams, D. R., & Collins, C. (1995). U.S. socioeconomic and racial differences in health: Patterns and explanation. *American Review of Sociology, 21,* 349–386.

Zweigenhaft, R. L., & Domhoff, G. W. (1998). *Diversity in the power elite: Have women and minorities reached the top?* New Haven, CT: Yale University Press.

CHAPTER TWO

# LATINO HEALTH STATUS

## Olivia Carter-Pokras,* Ruth Enid Zambrana

Health status data for Latinos have become increasingly available, and significant progress has been made in data collection methods over the past decade. This chapter provides an overview of national data on morbidity and mortality among Latino populations in comparison with such data on African Americans and Whites.

The writing of this book takes place at the outset of a major shift in national health policy. Launched in January 2000 (see United States Department of Health and Human Services [DHHS], 2000), the national disease prevention and health promotion agenda for the year 2010 have an overarching goal of eliminating disparities. For the first time, the same targets have been set and baseline and monitoring data are presented for all racial and ethnic groups. To achieve this ambitious goal of eliminating disparities requires a considerable effort to better understand the reasons underlying the disparities. However, medical and non-medical factors that are associated with health disparities have not been adequately studied for Latinos. Primarily, this can be attributed to three major factors: comprehensive national Latino data have only recently become available; most published studies analyze only secondary databases; and the focus of research has been on "acculturation" as a proxy for English language proficiency and poverty, in contrast to measuring culture-specific protective factors and structural risk factors.

---

*The views expressed in this paper do not necessarily reflect the views of the Office of Minority Health or the United States Department of Health and Human Services.

## Current Data: Limitations and Promise

Latinos can be identified by Spanish surname, Spanish origin or heritage, Spanish language usage, birthplace in a Latin American country, or parentage. However, the size and composition of the group depends upon which one of these identification methods is used (Marín & Marín, 1991). For example, a person who speaks Spanish or has a Spanish surname is not necessarily of Latin American heritage, birth, or family origin (say, a Filipino). Furthermore, using a Spanish surname may exclude people of Latin American heritage who do not possess typical Spanish surnames or who have changed their names through marriage (Molina and Aguirre-Molina, 1994). Latinos may be of any race and may speak languages other than Spanish. In Mexico and Guatemala, about 1 percent of the population is Black, while in Nicaragua 10 percent are English-speaking Blacks (Pan American Health Organization, 1994). Spanish is neither the primary language nor the language spoken by a significant percentage of indigenous people in countries such as Bolivia, Ecuador, Guatemala, and Peru. Latinos have had a long-standing presence in North America and represent a dynamic and vastly heterogeneous group (Acosta-Belen & Santiago, 1998).

Despite the historic presence of Latinos in the United States, Latinos have remained largely invisible in the national scientific and public discourse on health (Flack et al., 1995; Surgeon General's Latino/Latina Health Initiative, 1993; Heckler, 1985). In 1976, the passage of Public Law 94-311 called upon the DHHS to collect and publish statistics on Americans of Spanish origin or descent (Committee on National Statistics, 1976). Federal standards for racial and ethnic data were first issued soon afterward (Office of Management and Budget, 1978). Although the first comprehensive Latino health survey in the United States, the Hispanic Health and Nutrition Examination Survey (HHANES), was conducted in 1982–1984, the leading causes of death for all Latinos were not published in the DHHS annual report to Congress until 1993. State-recommended standard registration certificates for births and deaths did not include a Latino identifier until 1989. In addition, Latinos could not be identified from Medicare beneficiary files until the middle of 1994 (National Committee on Vital and Health Statistics, 1999; for a review see Zambrana & Carter-Pokras, 2001).

During the past decade, there have continued to be significant improvements in federal and state data systems. A review of almost 200 data systems of the DHHS demonstrated that more than 90 percent of these systems collect information on Latino origin (United States Department of Health and Human Services [DHHS] Data Council, 2000). The Office of the Assistant Secretary for Planning and Evaluation [of the DHHS] (2000) recently completed an assessment of the strengths and limitations of fifteen major federal data sets for analyses of Latino and Asian or Pacific Islander subgroups and Native Americans. This assessment demonstrated that many federal data systems have sufficient numbers of Latinos to provide reliable estimates by Latino subgroup. Some federal household surveys now oversample Latinos in order to reduce sampling errors. Several years of data for a particular survey can be combined if the methods and questions asked are similar (see, for example, Hajat, Lucas, & Kington, 2000; Zambrana, Breen, Fox, & Gutierrez-Mohamed, 1999; Zambrana, Scrimshaw, Collins, & Dunkel-Schetter, 1999).

Focusing on one year of data, the aforementioned DHHS assessment found that all of the data systems studied could provide at least simple distributions for the largest Latino subgroup, Mexican Americans. The National Survey of Family Growth, National Health and Nutrition Examination Survey, Medicare Current Beneficiary Survey, and Early Childhood Longitudinal Study are examples of federal surveys that have insufficient numbers of Puerto Ricans, Cubans, or Central Americans to provide reliable estimates. The assessment also found that some of the federal surveys do not ask Latino respondents to identify themselves or report a specific subgroup. In general, the reviewed databases collect Latino subgroup information using the following categories: Mexican American, Puerto Rican, Cuban, or Other Latino. Central and South Americans can be identified from a few surveys. Questions on Latino origin vary between federal surveys, although they tend to be the same within the same survey over several years. Several federal surveys collect information on respondents' U.S. citizenship status, the year respondents entered the United States, and/or respondents' birthplace (for example, the National Health Interview Survey, National Survey of Family Growth, National Immunization Survey, Third National Health and Nutrition Examination Survey [NHANES III], Current Population Survey, American Community Survey, National Household Education Survey, and Early Childhood Longitudinal Study).

Several limitations still exist in the collection of national and state data. First, the most recent NHANES III only included Mexican Americans. For the second-largest group of Latinos, Puerto Ricans, who have consistently shown least-favorable health status, national morbidity data are generally not available (Hajat, Lucas, & Kington, 2000; Zambrana, 1996). Second, state data systems also show significant improvement, but data gaps still remain for Latinos. For example, infant mortality rates for the combined years of 1996–1998 are not reliable for Latinos in thirteen states and the District of Columbia because there were fewer than twenty infant deaths reported for Latinos in these areas (Mathews, Curtin, & MacDorman, 2000). Previous studies suggest that some underreporting exists for Latinos in mortality statistics (Lindan et al., 1990; Hahn, Mulinare, & Teutsch, 1992; Scott & Suagee, 1992; Sorlie et al., 1993). In addition, data for emerging Latino subgroups such as Dominicans and Salvadorans are not disaggregated. Although these growing groups of Latinos are likely to be at higher risk of adverse health outcomes due to lower education, income, and insurance coverage, they are essentially "below the national radar screen" because they cannot be identified easily in national data systems.

An equally important issue arises from the fact that the majority of surveys have been conducted in English with ad hoc and sporadic translation into

Spanish (for instance, use of a family member to translate). Thus the issue of representativeness of these survey data with respect to the inclusion of Latino respondents with limited English proficiency is a serious limitation (Hajat, Lucas, & Kington, 2000). For example, the core National Health Interview Survey (NHIS) instrument was not translated into Spanish until 1998 when the United States Bureau of the Census, which administers the survey, hired bilingual interviewers. The standard translation of all national survey instruments into Spanish is an important future step to ensure the inclusion of all segments of the increasing Latino population in the United States. In addition, the informed consent process for all studies involving human subjects should also be responsive to language and literacy needs to ensure a true informed consent. The use of English-only informed consent forms and data collection instruments in human subject studies excludes or raises serious data quality concerns for at least one-third of the total Latino population, an even higher rate of certain Latino subgroups, and a significant portion of the lower socioeconomic population (Hajat, Lucas, & Kington, 2000). For example, among adults eighteen to sixty-four years old who are monolingual Spanish speakers, more than half are living in or near poverty (Stevens, 2000).

## Mortality

The most important health problems in a community often are identified through an examination of mortality data. Mortality data by Latino origin have been available from almost all states since 1990.

Table 2.1 shows the ten leading causes of death in 1998 for Latinos of all ages, the total population, Whites, and African Americans (Murphy, 2000; National Center for Health Statistics [NCHS], 2000). Although the top two leading causes of death for all these population groups are the same—heart disease and cancer—age-adjusted mortality rates for these two diseases are lower than rates for the total population, Whites, and African Americans. Latinos have higher mortality rates from diabetes, homicide, chronic liver disease, and HIV infection than the total population and Whites when differences in age distribution are taken into account. During 1990–1998, Latinos experienced a decline in mortality when age was taken into account for all leading causes of death except diabetes. Homicide is the seventh-leading cause of death for Latinos, but it is *not* ranked in the top ten leading causes of death for the total population. Chronic liver disease is the eighth-leading cause of death for Latinos and the tenth for the total population, although the gap in chronic liver disease mortality between Latinos and the total population narrowed during 1990–1998.

Although leading causes of death are not available by Latino subgroup at the national level, all-cause mortality rates are available by Latino subgroup, gender, and age (Table 2.2) (Murphy, 2000). Puerto Ricans (406.1 per 100,000) have higher all-cause mortality rates than Cubans (299.5 per 100,000) or Mexican Americans

## TABLE 2.1. TEN LEADING CAUSES OF DEATH: UNITED STATES, 1998.

| | Number |
|---|---|
| *Total Population, Both Sexes, All Ages* | |
| All causes (age adjusted) | 2,337,256 |
| Heart disease | 724,859 |
| Cancer | 541,532 |
| Stroke | 158,448 |
| Chronic obstructive pulmonary disease | 112,584 |
| Accidents | 97,835 |
| Pneumonia and influenza | 91,871 |
| Diabetes | 64,751 |
| Suicide | 30,575 |
| Kidney disease | 26,182 |
| Chronic liver disease | 25,192 |
| *Latinos, Both Sexes, All Ages* | |
| All causes (age adjusted) | 98,406 |
| Heart disease | 24,596 |
| Cancer | 19,528 |
| Accidents | 8,248 |
| Stroke | 5,587 |
| Diabetes | 4,741 |
| Pneumonia and influenza | 3,277 |
| Homicide | 2,978 |
| Chronic liver disease | 2,845 |
| Chronic obstructive pulmonary disease | 2,528 |
| Perinatal conditions | 1,987 |
| *Whites, Both Sexes, All Ages* | |
| All causes (age adjusted) | 1,912,802 |
| Heart disease | 609,256 |
| Cancer | 449,785 |
| Stroke | 131,039 |
| Chronic obstructive pulmonary disease | 101,274 |
| Pneumonia and influenza | 78,174 |
| Accidents | 73,669 |
| Diabetes | 46,884 |
| Suicide | 25,846 |
| Alzheimer's disease | 20,834 |
| Kidney disease | 20,372 |
| *African Americans, Both Sexes, All Ages* | |
| All causes (age adjusted) | 275,264 |
| Diseases of heart | 77,434 |
| Cancer | 60,642 |
| Stroke | 18,067 |
| Accidents | 12,617 |
| Diabetes | 11,278 |
| Homicide | 8,282 |
| Pneumonia and influenza | 8,246 |
| Chronic obstructive pulmonary disease | 7,131 |
| HIV/AIDS | 7,055 |
| Perinatal conditions | 4,674 |

*Sources:* Adapted from Murphy, 2000; National Center for Health Statistics, 2000.

**TABLE 2.2.   DEATH RATES AND AGE-ADJUSTED DEATH RATES BY LATINO ORIGIN, RACE, AND SEX: UNITED STATES, 1998.**

| | Age-Adjusted Rate | <1 | 1–4 | 5–14 | 15–24 | 25–34 | 35–44 | 45–54 | 55–64 | 65–74 | 75–84 | ≥85 |
|---|---|---|---|---|---|---|---|---|---|---|---|---|
| *Total Population* | 471.7 | 751.3 | 34.6 | 19.9 | 82.3 | 109.6 | 199.6 | 423.5 | 1030.7 | 2495.1 | 5703.2 | 15111.7 |
| Male | 589.4 | 818.2 | 37.6 | 23.4 | 119.3 | 151.7 | 258.5 | 542.8 | 1296.9 | 3143.7 | 7019.2 | 16763.4 |
| Female | 372.5 | 681.3 | 31.4 | 16.2 | 43.5 | 68.1 | 141.5 | 309.6 | 788.4 | 1967.7 | 4831.9 | 14427.5 |
| *White, Non-Hispanic* | 452.7 | 599.4 | 29.4 | 18.0 | 72.3 | 93.4 | 176.7 | 382.8 | 979.8 | 2468.7 | 5736.5 | 15567.8 |
| Male | 563.6 | 651.5 | 31.8 | 21.0 | 101.2 | 128.1 | 229.7 | 487.2 | 1224.0 | 3112.5 | 7072.8 | 17363.4 |
| Female | 359.1 | 544.6 | 27.0 | 14.9 | 41.9 | 58.7 | 123.7 | 280.5 | 751.3 | 1935.8 | 4847.8 | 14839.1 |
| *African American* | 710.7 | 1618.5 | 64.7 | 30.9 | 131.0 | 211.2 | 392.2 | 835.4 | 1756.0 | 3421.4 | 6869.9 | 14359.7 |
| Male | 911.1 | 1789.4 | 72.4 | 37.5 | 201.4 | 295.6 | 503.4 | 1120.4 | 2339.7 | 4291.9 | 8468.6 | 15808.6 |
| Female | 555.8 | 1443.0 | 56.8 | 24.2 | 60.3 | 135.9 | 294.9 | 600.6 | 1311.3 | 2792.4 | 5919.9 | 13759.7 |
| *Latino* | 342.8 | 624.7 | 30.4 | 17.2 | 83.3 | 101.5 | 163.0 | 334.9 | 739.8 | 1782.0 | 3718.3 | 8877.1 |
| Male | 442.7 | 678.5 | 33.1 | 20.2 | 128.8 | 148.4 | 226.6 | 449.3 | 966.3 | 2284.9 | 4564.6 | 9946.7 |
| Female | 255.5 | 568.7 | 27.6 | 14.1 | 34 | 51 | 96.7 | 225.8 | 543.6 | 1384.3 | 3140.1 | 8336.3 |
| *Mexican American* | 348.4 | 622.9 | 32.3 | 17.6 | 88.2 | 99.1 | 150.4 | 314.1 | 748.3 | 1819.9 | 3852.4 | * |
| Male | 425.1 | 687.3 | 34.9 | 21.0 | 134.8 | 145.8 | 208.2 | 410.7 | 933.2 | 2217.5 | 4424.2 | * |
| Female | 273.9 | 559.4 | 29.5 | 14.1 | 35.9 | 46.2 | 88.9 | 214.3 | 576.6 | 1471.1 | 3396.8 | * |
| *Puerto Rican* | 406.1 | * | 27.6 | 18.1 | 74.3 | 143.4 | 286.5 | 539.1 | 945.3 | 1911.2 | * | * |
| Male | 540.8 | * | * | 19.1 | 123.7 | 214.8 | 414.2 | 746.3 | * | * | * | * |
| Female | 296.3 | * | * | 17.1 | 27.3 | 89.0 | 167.7 | 353.0 | 641.0 | * | * | * |
| *Cuban* | 299.5 | * | * | * | * | 77.1 | 154.2 | 378.1 | 689.7 | 1483.2 | * | * |
| Male | 421.9 | * | * | * | * | * | 226.1 | * | * | * | * | * |
| Female | 203.1 | * | * | * | * | * | * | * | * | * | * | * |
| *Other Latino* | 325.0 | 676.2 | 27.3 | 15.9 | 74.2 | 95.5 | 144.9 | 286.1 | 626.5 | 1805.6 | 3859.3 | * |
| Male | 469.2 | * | 31.5 | 18.4 | 113.1 | 137.7 | 199.4 | 410.4 | 838.4 | * | * | * |
| Female | 235.1 | * | 22.9 | 13.5 | 34.3 | 50.1 | 89.4 | 188.3 | 465.9 | 1313.6 | * | * |

*Source:* Murphy, 2000.

(348.4 per 100,000) once differences in age distributions are taken into account. Puerto Rican twenty-five- to fifty-four-year-olds are particularly at increased risk of death compared to Whites, Cubans, and Mexican Americans.

National data presented in this chapter are mainly focused on all Latinos, or the largest subgroup of Latinos—Mexican Americans.[*] National data systems are often limited in their ability to present statistically reliable estimates for Latino subgroups other than Mexican Americans due to small sample/cell sizes. If a specific reference is not given, these data have been used to set baselines for the national disease-prevention and health-promotion goals, *Healthy People 2010*, and are available on the Internet at *www.healthypeople.gov.*

## Chronic Disease Measures

Although data from the most comprehensive study of Latino health, HHANES 1982–1984, are now almost twenty years old, new data from other surveys provide useful insights regarding the burden of disability and disease among the Latino population. One measure, self-perceived health status, is a commonly used indicator of overall health status (Table 2.3). A recently published report from the National Health Interview Survey found that 16.2 percent of all Mexicans, 14.1 percent of all Cubans, and 17.5 percent of all Puerto Ricans reported that they were in fair or poor health once differences in age distributions were taken into account by investigators (Hajat, Lucas, & Kington, 2000). These rates were much higher than for the total population (10.8 percent) or Whites (9.3 percent) and mirror the percentage of persons who reported that they were limited in their major activity.

The most recent data from the National Health and Nutrition Examination Survey show that Mexican Americans are more likely than Whites or the total population to have high blood pressure (National Center for Health Statistics, 2000). Data from the Surveillance, Epidemiology and End Results study show that the risk of the most common cancer sites—prostate, breast, and lung cancers— are lower for Latinos than they are for Whites (Wingo, Ries, Rosenberg, Miller, & Edwards, 1998). However, the incidence rate of cervical cancer was almost one

[*]Data were obtained from several national data systems including the National Vital Statistics System, Centers for Disease Control and Prevention Abortion Surveillance, National Survey of Family Growth, National Linked Infant-Death Data Sets, HIV/AIDS Surveillance, STD (Sexually Transmitted Diseases) Surveillance System, National Health and Nutrition Examination Survey, National Health Interview Survey, National Notifiable Disease Surveillance System, Active Bacterial Core Surveillance, National TB Surveillance System, National Immunization Survey, Epidemiologic Catchment Area Study, Behavioral Risk Factor Surveillance System, U.S. Renal Data System, Continuing Food Survey of Food Intake by Individuals, Current Population Survey, Mothers' Survey of Abbott Laboratories, Inc., National Household Survey on Drug Abuse, Youth Risk Behavior Survey, National Infant Sleep Position Study, and the Surveillance Epidemiology and End Results Study.

## TABLE 2.3. CHRONIC DISEASE MEASURES.

| | Total Population | Whites | African Americans | All Latinos | Mexican Americans | Cubans | Puerto Ricans | Other Latinos |
|---|---|---|---|---|---|---|---|---|
| Fair/poor self-perceived health status (all ages)[a] | 10.8 percent | 9.3 percent | 18 percent | 15.3 percent | 16.2 percent | 14.1 percent | 17.5 percent | 12.4 percent |
| Limited in major activity (all ages)[a] | 10.8 percent | 10.3 percent | 14.9 percent | 11.3 percent | 11.3 percent | 10.8 percent | 16.2 percent | 10.8 percent |
| Osteoporosis (50 years old and over)[b],* | 10 percent | 10 percent | 7 percent | — | 10 percent | — | — | — |
| High blood pressure (20–74 years)[c],* | | | | | | | | |
| Men | 25.3 percent | 24.4 percent | 35 percent | — | 25.2 percent | — | — | — |
| Women | 20.8 percent | 19.3 percent | 34.2 percent | — | 22.0 percent | — | — | — |
| Prostate cancer incidence per 100,000 (all ages)[d],* | 149.7 | 145.8 | 225 | 101.6 | — | — | — | — |
| Breast cancer incidence per 100,000 (all ages)[d],* | 109.7 | 114.0 | 100.2 | 68.9 | — | — | — | — |
| Cervical cancer incidence (all ages)[d],* | 8.9 | 8.4 | 11.7 | 15.3 | — | — | — | — |
| Lung cancer incidence per 100,000[d],* | 55.2 | 55.4 | 73.3 | 27.1 | — | — | — | — |
| Men (all ages)* | 73.3 | 71.9 | 111.1 | 38 | — | — | — | — |
| Women (all ages)* | 41.6 | 43.3 | 45.8 | 19.4 | — | — | — | — |
| Diabetes incidence per 1000 (all ages)[e],* | 3.5 | 3.0 | 5.9 | 5.7 | — | — | — | — |
| Major depression episode[f],* | — | 2.2 percent | 2.5 percent | 2.6 percent | — | — | — | — |
| Adolescent suicide attempts[g] | 2.6 percent | 1.9 percent | 2.9 percent | 3.0 percent | — | — | — | — |
| Schizophrenia[f],* | — | 0.6 percent | 1.2 percent | 0.4 percent | — | — | — | — |

(Continued)

| | | | | | | |
|---|---|---|---|---|---|---|
| Untreated dental decay[c] | | | | | | |
| 2–5 years old | 18.7 percent | 14.4 percent | 25.1 percent | — | 34.9 percent | — |
| 6–17 years old | 23.1 percent | 18.9 percent | 33 percent | — | 37.2 percent | — |
| 18–64 years old | 28.2 percent | 23.6 percent | 47.9 percent | — | 39.9 percent | — |
| 65–74 years old | 25.4 percent | 22.7 percent | 46.7 percent | — | 43.8 percent | — |
| Complete tooth loss (65–74 years old)[h] | 26 percent | 26 percent | 30 percent | 24 percent | — | — |

[a]National Health Interview Survey, 1992–1995 (Hajat, Lucas, & Kington, 2000).

[b]National Health and Nutrition Examination Survey, 1988–1994 (United States Department of Health and Human Services, 2000).

[c]National Health and Nutrition Examination Survey, 1988–1994 (National Center for Health Statistics, 2000).

[d]Surveillance, Epidemiology and End Results Study, 1990–1997 (Wingo, Ries, Rosenberg, Miller, & Edwards, 1998).

[e]National Health Interview Survey, 1994–1996 (United States Department of Health and Human Services, 2000).

[f]Epidemiologic Catchment Area Study (Regier et al., 1993).

[g]Youth Risk Behavior Survey, 1999 (United States Department of Health and Human Services, 2000).

[h]National Health Interview Survey, 1997 (United States Department of Health and Human Services, 2000).

*Age adjusted.

and a half times higher for Latino women than for White women. Latinos are also more likely to develop diabetes than are Whites (5.7 per 1,000 compared to 3.0 per 1,000).

## Mental Health

Latino adults are slightly more likely than White adults to report a major depression episode (Regier et al., 1993), and Latino adolescents are more likely than White adolescents to report a suicide attempt. Schizophrenia rates are slightly lower among Latinos than among Whites (Regier et al., 1993). (For greater detail, see Chapter Seven of this volume.)

## Infectious Disease

Table 2.4 shows case rates and percentages of selected infectious disease measures for the total population, Whites, African Americans, and Latinos. The AIDS epidemic has seriously affected the Latino community. During a twelve-month period ending in June 1999, 55.2 per 100,000 new AIDS cases were diagnosed among Latino men compared to seventeen per 100,000 among White men (National Center for Health Statistics, 2000). Latinos have a rate of gonorrhea and syphilis that is between the rates for Whites and for the total population, and a rate of chlamydia and pelvic inflammatory disease that is similar to that of the total population but higher than that for Whites. Latinos also have a higher risk than Whites of hepatitis B, which can be transmitted through sexual contact, intravenous drug use, or transfusions (Margolis, 1998). A greater likelihood of reporting a diagnosis of sexually transmitted disease by a public health clinic than a private practitioner may influence these comparisons. Because it is based on a sample of the population, the National Health and Nutrition Examination Survey may provide a more accurate assessment of the risk of sexually transmitted disease—the genital herpes infection rate reported for twenty- to twenty-nine-year-old Mexican Americans was identical to that of Whites.

Rates of other infectious diseases are higher for Latinos than for Whites. Rates of the food-borne hepatitis A were much higher for Latinos (24.2 per 100,000) than they were for the total population (11.3 per 100,000) or Whites (7.3 per 100,000). Tuberculosis cases were also twice as high for Latinos (13.6 per 100,000) than for the total population or Whites. Immigration from countries with higher tuberculosis rates, HIV coinfection in the United States, development of drug-resistant strains of tuberculosis, and less than optimal screening, treatment, and management of tuberculosis cases and contacts all play a role in the higher rates of tuberculosis among Latinos (Hornick, 1998).

Although elderly Latinos are less likely to be diagnosed as having pneumonia (forty-three per 100,000) than are the total population or Whites, they are also at greater risk due to not receiving flu or pneumonia vaccines. Slightly more than

## TABLE 2.4. INFECTIOUS DISEASE MEASURES.

| | Total Population | Whites | African Americans | All Latinos | Mexican Americans |
|---|---|---|---|---|---|
| New AIDS cases per 100,000[a] | | | | | |
| Men (13 years old and over) | 32.8 | 17 | 125.7 | 55.2 | — |
| Women (13 years old and over) | 9.2 | 2.4 | 49.5 | 14.6 | — |
| New chlamydia cases (women 15–24 years old) | | | | | |
| Family planning clinics[b] | 5 percent | 3.1 percent | 11.1 percent | 5.2 percent | — |
| New gonorrhea cases per 100,000[b] | 123 | 26 | 808 | 69 | — |
| Women | 119 | 32 | 714 | 72 | — |
| Men | 125 | 20 | 912 | 67 | — |
| New syphilis cases per 100,000[b] | 3.2 | 0.5 | 22 | 1.6 | — |
| Women | 2.9 | 0.5 | 19.3 | 1 | — |
| Men | 3.6 | 0.6 | 25 | 2.1 | — |
| Genital herpes infection (20–29 years old)[c] | 17 percent | 15 percent | 33 percent | — | 15 percent |
| Pelvic inflammatory disease (women 15–44 years old) | 8 percent | 7 percent | 11 percent | 8 percent | — |
| New hepatitis A cases per 100,000[e] | 11.3 | 7.3 | 6.3 | 24.2 | — |

*(Continued)*

**TABLE 2.4. INFECTIOUS DISEASE MEASURES. (Continued)**

| | Total Population | Whites | African Americans | All Latinos | Mexican Americans |
|---|---|---|---|---|---|
| New hepatitis B cases per 100,000[e] | | | | | |
| 19–24 years | 24 | 10.3 | 50.6 | 16.9 | — |
| 25–39 years | 20.2 | 10.2 | 34.1 | 16 | — |
| 40 years old and over | 15 | 7.1 | 28.4 | 18.1 | — |
| New pneumonia infections per 100,000[f] | | | | | |
| 0–5 years old | 76 | 63 | 154 | 59 | — |
| 65 years old and over | 62 | 61 | 83 | 43 | — |
| New tuberculosis cases per 100,000[g] | 6.8 | 2.3 | 17.8 | 13.6 | — |

[a]HIV/AIDS Surveillance, July 1, 1998–June 30, 1999 (National Center for Health Statistics, 2000).

[b]STD Surveillance System, 1997 (United States Department of Health and Human Services, 2000).

[c]National Health and Nutrition Examination Survey, 1988–1994 (United States Department of Health and Human Services, 2000).

[d]National Survey of Family Growth, 1995 (United States Department of Health and Human Services, 2000).

[e]National Notifiable Disease Surveillance System, 1997 (United States Department of Health and Human Services, 2000).

[f]Active Bacterial Core Surveillance, 1997 (United States Department of Health and Human Services, 2000).

[g]National TB Surveillance System, 1998 (United States Department of Health and Human Services, 2000).

half (51 percent) of Latino elderly received the annual flu vaccine, while about one-quarter (23 percent) received the pneumonia vaccine (see Table 2.5). A possible explanation for the lower self-report of pneumonia diagnosis, despite the lower rate of annual pneumonia vaccinations, is that elderly Latinos are less likely to be aware of having pneumonia due to their inaccessability to health care.

## Unintentional and Intentional Injuries

Even when differences in age distributions are taken into account, Latinos are found to be at higher risk of death due to homicide. As shown in Table 2.6, Latinos experience a homicide rate that is more than two to three times the rate for Whites—ranging from 7.9 per 100,000 for Puerto Ricans to 9 per 100,000 for Mexican-Americans. Rates of physical assaults, though, are lower for Latinos when compared to those of Whites. Puerto Ricans also have higher rates of death due to poisoning and residential fires than Whites, and Mexican Americans have higher rates of motor vehicle crash deaths than Whites.

## Oral Health

Due to the likelihood of having no health insurance and lower health care utilization, the rates of untreated dental decay are consistently higher for Mexican Americans than for Whites. For example, among six- to seventeen-year-olds, 37.2 percent of Mexican Americans had untreated dental decay compared to 18.9 percent of Whites. The rate of complete tooth loss among sixty-five- to seventy-four-year-olds, though, was similar.

## Reproductive Outcome Measures

As a relatively younger population, Latinas have a higher birthrate: 24.3 births per 1,000 populations compared to 12.3 per 1,000 for Whites and 18.2 per 1,000 for African Americans (Ventura, Martin, Curtin, Mathews, & Park, 2000). Latinas also have a higher abortion rate (26.8 abortions per 100 live births) than Whites (19.3 per 100 live births) (National Center for Health Statistics, 2000). Thirteen percent of Latino or White married couples had an impired ability to conceive or maintain a pregnancy in 1995 (Table 2.7).

Of all Latino births, 6.9 percent are to teenagers under the age of eighteen (National Center for Health Statistics, 2000). This is more than twice the rate for Whites (3 percent). The rate of low birth weight infants is similar for all Latinos compared to that for Whites (6.4 percent and 6.6 percent, respectively), but the rates for Puerto Ricans are higher (9.7 percent) (Ventura, Martin, Curtin, Mathews, & Park, 2000). The preterm birthrate is higher for all Latinos (11.4 percent) compared to that for Whites (10.2 percent) (Ventura, Martin, Curtin,

## TABLE 2.5. HEALTH CARE UTILIZATION MEASURES.

| | Total Population | Whites | African Americans | All Latinos | Mexican Americans | Cubans | Puerto Ricans |
|---|---|---|---|---|---|---|---|
| Percentage without health insurance (<65)[a],* | 17 percent | 14 percent | 20 percent | 33 percent | 39 percent | 21 percent | 19 percent |
| Percentage without usual source of care[a],* | 13 percent | 11 percent | 14 percent | 21 percent | 25 percent | 14 percent | 14 percent |
| Fully immunized 19- to 35-month-old children[b] | 73 percent | 76 percent | 67 percent | 69 percent | — | — | — |
| Receipt of annual flu vaccine (≥65)[a] | 64 percent | 66 percent | 47 percent | 51 percent | — | — | — |
| Receipt of pneumonia vaccine (≥65)[a] | 46 percent | 50 percent | 26 percent | 23 percent | — | — | — |
| Late or no prenatal care[c] | 3.9 percent | 2.4 percent | 7.0 percent | 6.3 percent | 6.8 percent | 1.2 percent | 5.1 percent |
| Early and adequate prenatal care[c] | 74 percent | 79 percent | 67 percent | 66 percent | — | — | — |
| Received Pap test in past 3 years (18 years old and over)[d],* | 79 percent | 80 percent | 83 percent | 74 percent | — | — | — |
| Received mammogram in past 2 years (40 years old and over)[d] | 66.9 percent | 68 percent | 66 percent | 60.2 percent | — | — | — |

| | | | | | | |
|---|---|---|---|---|---|---|
| Oral health care visit during past year (2 years old and over)[d] | 66.2 percent | 69.5 percent | 58 percent | 54.1 percent | — | — | — |
| Dental sealants[e] (8 years old) | 23 percent | 29 percent | 11 percent | — | 10 percent | — | — |
| (14 years old) | 15 percent | 18 percent | 5 percent | — | 7 percent | — | — |
| Adults with depression who have received treatment (≥18)[f] | 23 percent | 24 percent | 16 percent | 20 percent | — | — | — |
| Adults with schizophrenia who have received treatment (≥18)[f] | 60 percent | 63 percent | 41 percent | 42 percent | — | — | — |
| Proportion of diabetics who were previously diagnosed (20 years old and over)[e,*] | 68 percent | 73 percent | 67 percent | — | 55 percent | — | — |
| Annual glycosylated hemoglobin measurement among diabetics (≥18)[g,*] | 24 percent | 24 percent | 21 percent | 22 percent | — | — | — |
| Dialysis patients on transplantation waiting list[h] | 20 percent | 65 percent | 29 percent | 12 percent | — | — | — |

(Continued)

**TABLE 2.5. HEALTH CARE UTILIZATION MEASURES. (Continued)**

| | Total Population | Whites | African Americans | All Latinos | Mexican Americans | Cubans | Puerto Ricans |
|---|---|---|---|---|---|---|---|
| Proportion of hypertensives who have blood pressure under control (≥18)[e],* | 18 percent | 18 percent | 19 percent | — | 13 percent | — | — |
| Blood cholesterol check in past 5 years (18 years old and over)[d],* | 67 percent | 70 percent | 67 percent | 59 percent | — | — | — |
| Completed curative therapy for tuberculosis[i] | 74 percent | 75 percent | 72 percent | 73 percent | — | — | — |

[a]National Health Interview Survey, 1997 (United States Department of Health and Human Services, 2000).

[b]National Immunization Survey, 1998 (United States Department of Health and Human Services, 2000).

[c]National Vital Statistics System, 1998 (Ventura, Martin, Curtin, Mathews, & Park, 2000).

[d]National Health Interview Survey, 1998 (National Center for Health Statistics, 2000).

[e]National Health and Nutrition Examination Survey, 1998–1994 (United States Department of Health and Human Services, 2000).

[f]Epidemiologic Catchment Area Study, 1997 (United States Department of Health and Human Services, 2000).

[g]Behavioral Risk Factor Surveillance System, 1998 (United States Department of Health and Human Services, 2000).

[h]U.S. Renal Data System, 1995–1997 (United States Department of Health and Human Services, 2000).

[i]National TB Surveillance System, 1996 (United States Department of Health and Human Services, 2000).

*Age adjusted.

**TABLE 2.6. INJURIES.**

| | Total Population | Whites | African Americans | All Latinos | Mexican Americans | Cubans | Puerto Ricans |
|---|---|---|---|---|---|---|---|
| Unintentional injury deaths per 100,000[a] | 35.8 | 34.6 | 40.7 | 30.2 | 32.1 | 22.5 | 28.8 |
| Poisoning deaths per 100,000[a] | 6.8 | 6.9 | 8.2 | 5.9 | 5.1 | 4.3 | 12.0 |
| Suffocation deaths[a] | 4.1 | 4.1 | 4.4 | 3.1 | — | — | — |
| Motor vehicle crash deaths per 100,000[a] | 15.6 | 15.5 | 17.3 | 14.7 | 16.5 | 10.9 | 10.8 |
| Residential fire deaths per 100,000[a] | 1.2 | 1.0 | 3.0 | 0.9 | 0.9 | — | 1.2 |
| Deaths from falls per 100,000[a] | 4.7 | 4.9 | 3.2 | 3.7 | 3.6 | 3.3 | 3.4 |
| Drowning deaths per 100,000[a] | 1.6 | 1.5 | 2.4 | 1.5 | 1.5 | — | 1.0 |
| Homicides per 100,000[a] | 6.5 | 3.1 | 23.4 | 8.8 | 9.0 | 8.3 | 7.9 |
| Physical assault per 1,000 persons (12 years old)[b] | 31.1 | 31.0 | 33.8 | 25.9 | — | — | — |

[a]National Vital Statistics System, 1998 (United States Department of Health and Human Services, 2000).

[b]National Crime Victimization Survey, U.S. Department of Justice, 1998 (United States Department of Health and Human Services, 2000).

**TABLE 2.7. REPRODUCTIVE OUTCOME MEASURES.**

| | Total Populations | Whites | African Americans | All Latinos | Mexican Americans | Cubans | Puerto Ricans | Other Latinos | Central & South Americans |
|---|---|---|---|---|---|---|---|---|---|
| Crude birthrate[a] (live births per 1,000 pop) | 14.6 | 12.3 | 18.2 | 24.3 | 26.4 | 10.0 | 19.0 | — | 23.2 |
| Abortions per 100 live births[b] | 30.5 | 19.3 | 54.3 | 26.8 | — | — | — | — | — |
| Fertility problems[c] Among married couples | 13 percent | 13 percent | 14 percent | 13 percent | — | — | — | — | — |
| Teen births under 18 years old (percentage of live births)[d] | 4.6 percent | 3.0 percent | 9.0 percent | 6.9 percent | 7.2 percent | 2.9 percent | 9.2 percent | 8.8 percent | 3.6 percent |
| Infant mortality (per 1000 live births)[e] | 7.2 | 6.0 | 13.9 | 5.8 | 5.6 | 3.6 | 7.8 | 6.5 | 5.3 |
| Low birth weight (percentage of live births)[a] | 7.6 percent | 6.6 percent | 13.2 percent | 6.4 percent | 6.0 percent | 6.5 percent | 9.7 percent | 7.6 percent | 6.5 percent |
| Preterm birth[a] (percentage of live births) | 11.6 percent | 10.2 percent | 17.6 percent | 11.4 percent | 11.0 percent | 11.4 percent | 13.9 percent | 12.1 percent | 11.6 percent |
| Maternal mortality[f],* (per 100,000 live births) | 6.1 | 4.0 | 16.1 | 5.2 | — | — | — | — | — |

[a]National Vital Statistics System, 1998 (Ventura, Martin, Curtin, Mathews, & Park, 2000).

[b]Centers for Disease Control and Prevention Abortion Surveillance (National Center for Health Statistics, 2000).

[c]National Survey of Family Growth, 1997 (United States Department of Health and Human Services, 2000).

[d]National Linked Birth/Infant Death Data Set, 1998 (Mathews, Curtin, & MacDorman, 2000).

[e]National Vital Statistics System, 1998 (National Center for Health Statistics, 2000).

*Age adjusted.

Mathews, & Park, 2000). Infant mortality rates are slightly lower for all Latinos (5.8 infant deaths per 1,000 live births) than for Whites (6 per 1,000), but they are higher for Puerto Ricans (8.6 per 1,000) (Mathews, Curtin, MacDorman, 2000). Maternal mortality rates are higher for all Latinos (5.2 per 100,000 live births) than for Whites (4.0 per 100,000 live births).

## Health Care Utilization

Latinos are the most likely to be uninsured of all racial or ethnic groups: 33 percent of all Latinos compared to 14 percent of Whites and 20 percent of African Americans (see Table 2.5). These rates are higher for Mexican Americans (39 percent) than for Puerto Ricans and Cubans (19 percent and 21 percent, respectively). The percentage with a usual source of care, a good measure of access to health care, mirrors these health insurance coverage rates. Mexican Americans are the most likely to not have a usual source of care (25 percent).

Latinos are also less likely to use health care services for preventive care. For example, 69 percent of nineteen- to thirty-five-month-old Latinos are fully immunized and 51 percent of Latino elderly have received their annual flu vaccine. Mexican Americans and African Americans are more likely to receive late or no prenatal care than are Whites (Ventura, Martin, Curtin, Mathews, & Park, 2000). Rates of mammograms, Pap tests, and blood cholesterol checks are also lower for Latinos than for Whites (National Center for Health Statistics, 2000). Oral health care visits and use of dental sealants show even greater disparities in usage, and are diminished but still remain when poverty is taken into account (National Center for Health Statistic, 2000).

Moreover, Latinos with existing health and mental health conditions are less likely to use health services than are Whites. For example, Latinos with a mental illness (such as depression or schizophrenia) are less likely to receive treatment for their illness. Latinos with diabetes are less likely to know that they have the disease. The National Health and Nutrition Examination Survey (NHANES) found 45 percent of Mexican Americans with the condition were not previously aware that they had diabetes, compared to 27 percent of Whites. Among diagnosed hypertensives, 13 percent of Mexican Americans had their blood pressure under control compared to 18 percent of Whites.

## Health Behaviors

As shown in Table 2.8, rates of obesity and high blood pressure are higher among Mexican Americans than among Whites, and they are less likely to engage in leisure time physical activity. The higher rates of overweight are also seen among Mexican American children and adolescents. Latino adolescents are also less likely to engage in vigorous physical activity (United States Department of Health and Human Services, 2000). These rates of obesity and physical inactivity among children and adolescents raise concerns regarding the continuing higher risk of diabetes among Latinos.

**TABLE 2.8.  BEHAVIORAL RISK FACTORS.**

| | Total Population | Whites | African Americans | All Latinos | Mexican Americans |
|---|---|---|---|---|---|
| Cigarette smoking (18 years old and over)[a],* | | | | | |
| Men | 26.5 percent | 26.9 percent | 30.8 percent | 24.4 percent | 24.5 percent |
| Women | 22.1 percent | 24.1 percent | 21.9 percent | 13.7 | 11.9 percent |
| Environmental tobacco smoke exposure by nonsmokers 4 years and over[b],* | 65 percent | 63 percent | 81 percent | — | 53 percent |
| Pregnant women abstaining from cigarette smoking in past month (15–44 years old)[c] | 87 percent | 84 percent | 90 percent | 96 percent | — |
| Obese (20–74 years old)[d],* | | | | | |
| Men | 19.9 percent | 20.1 percent | 21.1 percent | — | 23.1 percent |
| Women | 25.1 percent | 22.5 percent | 37.7 percent | — | 34.6 percent |
| Overweight children (6–11 years old)[d] | | | | | |
| Boys | 14.7 percent | 13.1 percent | 14.7 percent | — | 18.8 percent |
| Girls | 12.6 percent | 11.9 percent | 17.7 percent | — | 15.8 percent |
| Overweight adolescents (12–17 years old)[d] | | | | | |
| Boys | 12.4 percent | 11.8 percent | 12.5 percent | — | 14.8 percent |
| Girls | 10.5 percent | 9.3 percent | 16 percent | — | 14.1 percent |
| Less than 30 percent calories from fat (2 years old and over)[e] | 33 percent | 33 percent | 26 percent | 36 percent | 33 percent |
| Two or more servings per day of fruit (2 years old and over)[e],* | 28 percent | 27 percent | 24 percent | 32 percent | 29 percent |
| Three or more servings per day of vegetables (2 years old and over)[e],* | 49 percent | 50 percent | 43 percent | 47 percent | 50 percent |
| Sodium intake less than 2,400 mg daily (2 years old and over)[d],* | 21 percent | 20 percent | 25 percent | — | 25 percent |

| | | | | |
|---|---|---|---|---|
| Food security among U.S. households[f] | 88 percent | 91 percent | 76 percent | 75 percent | 73 percent |
| High serum cholesterol (20–74 years old)[d],* | | | | | |
| Men | 17.5 percent | 17.3 percent | 15.7 percent | — | 17.8 percent |
| Women | 20.0 percent | 20.2 percent | 19.8 percent | — | 17.5 percent |
| Females who began pregnancy with at least 40 μg of folic acid each day (15–44 years old)[g] | 21 percent | 23 percent | 18 percent | — | 13 percent |
| Breastfeeding in early postpartum period[h] | 64 percent | 68 percent | 45 percent | 66 percent | — |
| Current alcohol drinkers[i] | | | | | |
| 18–44 years old | 68.7 percent | 74.5 percent | 53.7 percent | 58.3 percent | — |
| Men | 74.4 percent | 78.1 percent | 60.7 percent | 71.1 percent | — |
| Women | 63.1 percent | 70.9 percent | 47.9 percent | 44.1 percent | — |
| 45 years old and over | 54.5 percent | 57.2 percent | 41.3 percent | 46.2 percent | — |
| Men | 62.7 percent | 64.1 percent | 53.6 percent | 61.2 percent | — |
| Women | 47.5 percent | 56.3 percent | 32.2 percent | 33 percent | — |
| No alcohol or illicit drug use in past month (12–17 years old)[j] | 79 percent | 74.7 percent | 82.0 percent | 79 percent | — |
| Pregnant women abstaining from alcohol during past month (15–44 years old)[k] | 86 percent | 85 percent | 83 percent | 93 percent | — |
| Marijuana used during past month (18–25 years old)[j] | 14 percent | 15 percent | 15 percent | 9 percent | — |
| Cocaine used during past month (18–25 years old)[j] | 2.0 percent | 2.2 percent | 0.6 percent | 2.7 percent | — |
| Inhalant used (12–17 years old)[j] | 2.9 percent | 3.4 percent | 1.0 percent | 2.8 percent | — |
| No leisure time physical activity[j] (18 years old and over) | 40 percent | 36 percent | 52 percent | 54 percent | — |
| Vigorous physical activity (9–12 grades)[m] | 65 percent | 67 percent | 56 percent | 61 percent | — |
| Proportion of women at risk of unintended pregnancy using contraception[n] (15–44 years old) | 93 percent | 93 percent | 90 percent | 91 percent | — |

(Continued)

**TABLE 2.8. BEHAVIORAL RISK FACTORS. (Continued)**

| | Total Population | Whites | African Americans | All Latinos | Mexican Americans |
|---|---|---|---|---|---|
| Responsible sexual behavior (9–12 grades)[o] | 85 percent | 85 percent | 84 percent | 84 percent | — |
| Infants put to sleep on their backs[p] | 35 percent | 37 percent | 17 percent | 28 percent | — |
| Physical fighting among adolescents (9–12 grades)[o] | 36 percent | 33 percent | 41 percent | 40 percent | — |
| Carrying weapon (grades 9–12)[o] | 6.9 percent | 6.4 percent | 5.0 percent | 7.9 percent | — |

[a]National Health Interview Survey, 1995–1998 (National Center for Health Statistics, 2000).

[b]National Health and Nutrition Examination Survey, 1998–1994 (United States Department of Health and Human Services, 2000).

[c]National Vital Statistics System, 1998 (United States Department of Health and Human Services, 2000).

[d]National Health and Nutrition Examination survey, 1988–1994 (National Center for Health Statistics, 2000).

[e]Continuing Survey of Food Intakes by Individuals, 1994–1996 (United States Department of Health and Human Services, 2000).

[f]Current Population Survey, 1995 (United States Department of Health and Human Services, 2000).

[g]National Health and Nutrition Examination Survey, 1991–1994 (United States Department of Health and Human Services, 2000).

[h]Mothers' Survey of Abbott Laboratories, Inc., 1998 (United States Department of Health and Human Services, 2000).

[i]National Interview Survey, 1998 (National Center for Health Statistics, 2000).

[j]National Household Survey on Drug Abuse, 1998 (United States Department of Health and Human Services, 2000).

[k]National Household Survey on Drug Abuse, 1996–1997 (United States Department of Health and Human Services, 2000).

[l]National Health Interview Survey, 1997 (United States Department of Health and Human Services, 2000).

[m]Youth Risk Behavior Survey, 1999 (United States Department of Health and Human Services, 2000).

[n]National Survey of Family Growth, 1995 (United States Department of Health and Human Services, 2000).

[o]Youth Risk Behavior Surveillance System, 1999 (United States Department of Health and Human Services, 2000).

[p]National Infant Sleep Position Study, 1996 (United States Department of Health and Human Services, 2000).

Latinas are less likely to smoke cigarettes than are White women (National Center for Health Statistics, 2000). Data from the National Household Survey on Drug Abuse also do not support the premise that Latinos are more likely to use alcohol and illicit drugs. Latinas are less likely to use alcohol than White women (National Center for Health Statistics, 2000) and are also less likely to use alcohol or tobacco while pregnant. Among young adults, Latinos are less likely to have used marijuana during the past month (9 percent) than Whites (15 percent) but are slightly more likely to use cocaine (2.7 percent versus 2.2 percent) (National Center for Health Statistics, 2000). Latino twelve- to seventeen-year-olds are less likely to use inhalants than are White teens (2.8 percent versus 3.4 percent).

Given the higher rates of HIV infection and AIDS among Latinos, it is worrisome that only 84 percent of Latino adolescents practice responsible sexual behavior—either abstaining or practicing safe sexual practices. Food insecurity is also a concern—approximately one out of four Latinos reported that they sometimes did not have enough to eat.

## Protective and Risk Factors

The greater likelihood of living in poverty places Latinos at increased risk of disease and disability. Poverty is highly linked with residing in resource-poor neighborhoods, greater likelihood of being exposed to environmental and occupational hazards, and greater likelihood of intentional and unintentional injury (Ellen & Turner, 1997). As low-income Latino immigrants integrate into society, as measured by number of years in the United States, we observe an increase in risk factors, such as higher use of alcohol and cigarettes, and lower physical activity (LeClere, Jensen, & Biddlecom, 1994). Although these observations appear to be easily generalized for all immigrants, for Latino immigrants the decrease in protective factors increases their burden of disease and disability (Vega & Amaro, 1994).

Alternative explanations for the relatively good health outcomes of foreign-born Mexican Americans include the protective effects of strong family and cultural ties, favorable health behaviors, and underreporting of mortality and poor birth outcomes due to misclassification of Mexican Americans on death certificates (Hajat, Lucas, & Kington, 2000; LeClere, Jensen, & Biddlecom, 1994). Better health outcomes among more acculturated U.S.-born Mexican Americans may be a function of their higher socioeconomic status (SES) (Hajat, Lucas, & Kington, 2000). In contrast, the decrease in favorable outcomes over time among both less acculturated U.S.-born and foreign-born individuals of Mexican origin may be associated with both long-term poverty and the stress associated with the continual process of integration into U.S. society.

Repeatedly, studies of Mexican Americans tend to perpetuate the confusion between acculturation and SES. Acculturation as measured in many surveys is generally restricted to items on language use and place of birth. More complete measures of acculturation need to be designed to identify culture-specific factors that promote favorable health behaviors and reduce risk behaviors.

Ethnic-specific protective behaviors such as reliance on family members and friends for support, low-fat nutritious eating habits, attitudes and value on motherhood and children, and low use of alcohol, tobacco, and illicit substances have not been adequately measured, with few exceptions, in prior studies. These health behaviors and psychosocial resources represent important mediators in Latino health. Importantly, these factors may contribute to lower levels of perceived stress by the Latino community and may mitigate the detrimental effects of poverty on health status and outcome, particularly for Mexican immigrants. The term "epidemiological paradox" (exemplified by high poverty but favorable infant mortality and low birth weight rates) is most often applied to interpretation of results from studies of Mexican Americans that fail to consider important differences by birthplace and generation, SES, and/or more complete measures of acculturation (Markides & Coreil, 1986; Scribner, 1991, 1996; Magana & Clark, 1995; Fuentes-Afflick, Hessel, & Pérez-Stable, 1999; Abraido-Lanza, Dohrenwend, Ng-Mak, & Turner, 1999; Ventura, Martin, Curtin, Mathews, & Park, 2000).

The role of protective factors and the "healthy migrant effect" are well documented in studies of other immigrant groups. The knowledge the scientific and public health communities have gleaned from migrant studies of Japanese Americans has greatly improved our understanding of the role of certain risk factors for cardiovascular disease (Marmot et al., 1975). Several studies confirm that many of the protective factors noted previously in this section for Mexican-origin women mediate the effects of poverty on birth outcome (Amaro, Fried, Cabral, & Zuckerman, 1990; Sherraden & Barrera, 1996; Zambrana, Scrimshaw, Collins, & Dunkel-Schetter, 1999). Other studies have found that life events and perceived stress can influence birth outcome and use of alcohol, tobacco, and illicit substances (Amaro, Fried, Cabral, & Zuckerman, 1990; Rumbaut & Weeks, 1996; Zambrana, Scrimshaw, Collins, & Dunkel-Schetter, 1997; Zambrana & Scrimshaw, 1997). Chronic stress such as economic strain and worry, risk of violence and danger in the community, and institutional discriminatory practices are associated with community-level effects (Williams, 1996; Williams & Collins, 1995; Williams, Lavizzo-Mourey, & Warren, 1994; Williams, Yu, Jackson, & Anderson, 1997). Psychosocial antecedents, including stress and available social support as mediators in Latino health, merit inquiry.

Emerging national data demonstrate Latino heterogeneity and differences in health status and outcome. Progress in Latino data collection provides us with an important opportunity to offer a critique and a proposal for change to guide the new generation of research.

## New Generation of Research Designs for Latinos

Data from national data systems are limited regarding certain health outcomes such as kidney disease and heart disease incidence, partly because the overwhelming majority of studies on Latinos are cross sectional. Intergenerational longitudinal investigations are important to increase our knowledge of the multiple medical and nonmedical factors associated with health outcomes and the structural and individual processes involved in adverse health outcomes over time. Studies should be conducted that are developmentally age appropriate and community based, and include the life-history approach and within-group analyses.

Stern and Wei's (1999) recent analyses of the San Antonio Heart Study demonstrate that longitudinal designs can provide significant insights into biological, sociocultural, and structural processes that increase protection or risk of heart disease among Latinos. Although national mortality data suggest that Latinos have a lower risk of heart disease and stroke compared to that of Whites and the total population, this may not provide an accurate picture of heart disease and stroke risk among Latinos (see Table 2.8).

Information from the Framingham Heart Study has been used to predict cardiovascular disease risk among Mexican Americans in the San Antonio Heart Study (Stern & Wei, 1999). Although a greater risk of all-cause mortality and cardiovascular disease (CVD) mortality was predicted for Mexican Americans than Whites, national mortality studies show lower rates of CVD mortality among Mexican Americans than Whites (Goff, Ramsey, Labarthe, & Nichaman, 1993). Current research does not suggest that the risk factors for CVD are any different for Latinos than they are for Whites or the total population. There is also no evidence to suggest that the relative contribution of these risk factors to the development of CVD is any different. One possible explanation is that the lower rates of some risk factors, such as smoking, may be overriding such risk factors as obesity, diabetes, high blood pressure, and no leisure time physical activity. For example, Latinos are less likely to have high-risk cholesterol, and they are as likely or more likely to eat less than 30 percent of their calories from fat and to eat sufficient amounts of fruit and vegetables.

What is worrisome is that, with greater time in the United States and for subsequent generations, Mexicans and other Latinos become more likely to smoke, drink alcohol, be overweight, and have diabetes. Through follow-up of the San Antonio Heart Study, Stern and Wei (1999) confirmed a 38 percent higher all-cause mortality rate and a 30 percent higher CVD mortality rate for Mexican Americans as compared to that of Whites. This excess risk was confined to U.S.-born Mexican Americans. These authors concluded that immigrants from Mexico had very low mortality despite low SES due to a "healthy migrant effect," that is, the role of the protective factors that Mexicans bring with them. These findings point out the importance of conducting longitudinal studies for Latinos and analyzing results by birthplace and generation.

Intergenerational studies might also provide a more comprehensive picture of a child's health status through an examination of how family health behaviors and use of health care patterns contribute to a child's well-being. Examination of what we know about younger Latinos demonstrates the need to expand studies to include multiple generations. For example, Mexican American children and adolescents have higher rates of being overweight and are less likely to engage in vigorous physical activity than Whites. Thus, the study of these factors can contribute to a more complete understanding of how biological markers and family behaviors may influence, for example, the onset of adult diabetes. Larger studies of developmentally age-appropriate Latino subgroups must become a norm rather than an exception. All too frequently women fifteen- to forty-four years of age or all children, for example, are studied as an aggregate, and thus results become difficult to interpret at different stages in their life cycle. Heightened sensitivity to age-appropriate samples is important in generating more meaningful and applicable results to age-specific groups. This is central to improving our understanding of the health of poor Latina women and their offspring, in which the accumulated generational effect of economic and social disadvantages may reveal itself in different morbidity and mortality patterns in adolescence, during the childbearing years, and in older age. Further identifying culture-specific protective behaviors among Latina women during developmental periods, particularly maternal behaviors that effect their children's well-being, are important as we seek to broaden our understanding of the intersection of ethnicity, gender, SES, and maternal and child health outcomes (Zambrana, Scrimshaw, Collins, & Dunkel-Schetter, 1997; Zambrana, Scrimshaw, Collins, & Dunkel-Schetter, 1999; Scrimshaw, Zambrana, & Dunkel-Schetter, 1997).

In examining maternal and child well-being indicators, subgroup membership reveal different morbidity and mortality patterns and child health outcomes by SES (see Table 2.7). Comparative approaches that examine within and across Latino subgroups by SES can yield information on how protective and risk factors are linked with number of years in the United States, geographic location, gender, marital status, age, and other family and community variables. The process of retention or loss of culture-specific health behaviors over time requires investigation. Comparative approaches within the same ethnic community or same subgroup permit the identification of social, environmental, and psychosocial factors that contribute to differential health outcomes.

Community-based, ethnic-specific population level data are a prerequisite for planning and implementing subgroup and age-appropriate interventions by state and within communities. In reviewing low birth weight and infant mortality indicators by race and ethnicity, it is clear that some groups are at higher risk than others for unfavorable birth outcomes (see Table 2.7). Population-level, community-based data, obtained by using geo-coding methodologies or community surveys, reveal unique epidemiological patterns for different communities. Recent data on state-specific racial and ethnic maternal and child health indicators reveal wide disparities by state (National Center for Health Statistics, 2000). Because Latino population groups are highly concentrated in a few states and are highly segregated in a select number of distressed communities, population level data can be used to plan interventions that effectively target community-specific needs of Latinos.

In the study of Latino health outcomes there is a compelling need to identify vulnerable subgroups such as Mexican-origin migrant farmworkers or poor head-of-household Puerto Rican women. National health data tend to be presented for all Latinos or for the largest Latino subgroup, Mexican Americans.

Less information is available on Puerto Ricans, who were repeatedly identified by various health measures during the HHANES as being at greater risk than Mexican Americans and Cubans. Developmental life-history approaches can be particularly insightful for these groups rather than aggregating or simply comparing them to other racial/ethnic groups.

# Measurement

Appropriate ethnic-specific measurement of important variables, such as sources of social support, is an integral component in the development of reliable and useful data. Traditional social support measures may not be tapping into the instrumental sources of support that are useful (supportive) for low-income Latino groups (see Marín & Marín, 1991; Zambrana, 1992). The measurement of the following sets of variables can facilitate our understanding of Latino health outcome differences by subgroup:

- Minimum data on gender, age, birthplace and generation, education, and length of time in the United States should be collected and used for studies of Latinos. Previous studies have found important differences in health status and use of health services by birthplace and/or generation.
- Measures of assets and wealth are necessary for the identification of the economic status of the household, because racial and ethnic differences in wealth are much larger than those for income. At every income level, the net worth of Latino households is dramatically less than that of White households.
- Measures of childhood social class are at least as important as current social class in understanding the etiology of disease and illness. For certain diseases, even diseases that occur in adulthood, the childhood environment may be even more important than the adult environment.
- Measures of the community resource environment are needed in addition to individual measures of SES. The effect of social class on health varies by the context within which the individual lives (Ellen & Turner, 1997).
- Measurement of racism and institutional discrimination is central to understanding racial and ethnic disparities in health after adjusting for SES (Williams & Collins, 1995; Williams, 1996; Montgomery & Carter-Pokras, 1993). Studies reveal that Latinos routinely encounter racial discrimination (Telles & Murguia, 1990; Fix & Struyk, 1993; Todd, Samaroo, & Hoffman, 1993). Contributing racial and ethnic differentials in health status entirely to socioeconomic differences ignores the possible contribution of the experiences of racism and discrimination in the production of ill health (Smith & Egger, 1992).
- Measures of acculturation are used to assess a limited set of social and demographic characteristics (such as education, birthplace and generation, English language proficiency, and ethnic or national origin), but they do not address the process of change in the acquisition of norms that contribute to adverse health outcomes. Future investigations need to include measures that assess values,

beliefs, and attitudes regarding health behaviors so as to advance our knowledge of the role of culture on behavioral risk factors.

## Implications for Advancing the Latino Health Discourse

Significant progress has been made in mapping and profiling the overall health status of Latinos in the United States in the last decade. *Healthy People 2010,* the national disease-prevention and health-promotion agenda for the year 2010, now has "eliminating disparities" as one of its two overarching goals. For the first time, single targets are set for all racial and ethnic groups and baseline and monitoring data will be routinely published for Latinos and other racial and ethnic groups. Major methodological approaches to enhance the understanding of Latino health outcomes and expand our research portfolio include the development of more appropriate research designs and new measures. Recent public acknowledgments, by federal officials and academic scholars, of distinct differences in health outcomes by Latino subgroup emphasize the urgent need to examine a framework for understanding Latino health that will redirect a new generation of researchers (Hajat, Lucas, & Kington, 2000).

The recommendations presented here build on existing evidence on Latino health and synthesize prior recommendations to improve Latino data collection, analysis and dissemination (Heckler, 1985; PHS Task Force on Minority Health Data, 1992; Surgeon General's Hispanic/Latino Health Initiative, 1993; United States Department of Health and Human Services [DHHS] Data Council, 2000). The issues addressed by these previous recommendations have not gone away during the past fifteen years and are still pressing and relevant. If we want to achieve the goal of eliminating disparities by the year 2010, targeted resources are needed to fully support these recommendations.

## Recommendations

- Collect information on Latino subgroups to allow analyses in surveys and medical record data systems (for example, birth and death certificates, patient discharge forms, and primary and ambulatory care clinics). Analysis and dissemination should be subgroup-specific for state and local communities with a significant (5 percent or greater) Latino population.
- Increase Latino representation in the design, implementation, analysis, and dissemination of health-assessment and health-monitoring data systems, and in funding decisions affecting these systems, including the identification of health indicators specific for Latinos.
- Establish federal, state, and local laws to ensure confidentiality of respondents and to provide absolute protection of respondents from use of the identifying information by law enforcement and immigration authorities.

- Allocate funds in federal, state, and local health programs to pay for collection, analysis, and dissemination of Latino health data so that progress in improving Latino health status, and ultimately the health status of the nation, can be tracked. Government agencies that use these data but do not produce data should share in the expenses of data collection, analysis, and dissemination.
- Include the improvement of Latino data collection, analysis, and dissemination in federal, state, and local strategic plans, such as *Healthy People 2010,* Minority Health Activities, and Primary Care Access Plans.
- Increase Latino membership in committees, councils, and commissions appointed by county, state, and federal health departments; agency administrators, state and federal legislators, and governors to monitor data collection, analysis, interpretation, and dissemination.

# Conclusion

During the past decade, there has been a substantial improvement in the availability of data on the health status of Latinos in the United States. These newly available data highlight several key health areas for which Latinos are at increased risk and demonstrate important risk variations within the Latino community. Future research and public policy initiatives on Latino populations require acknowledgment of the heterogeneity between subgroups and the scientific importance of designing and conducting longitudinal and intergenerational studies to ensure the reliability of baseline data and to enable trends analyses over time.

Although many of these health issues for Latinos are not new, they are receiving national attention at a critical time with the launch of the nation's disease-prevention and health promotion agenda, *Healthy People 2010.* The adoption of the goal to eliminate health disparities by *Healthy People 2010* reflects a major shift in national health policy. Embraced by a wide variety of organizations including the American Public Health Association, major philanthropic organizations, and state legislatures, this shift in national health policy provides a unique opportunity to influence policy decision making at the national, state, and local levels to improve the health of what will soon become the largest minority group in the United States. It is imperative that this momentum to make change be seized to improve the health of the Latino community. These efforts to make change must address institutional barriers in health care and other sectors. Economic equity must accompany efforts to improve access to health care and outcome. Until these institutional barriers are eliminated, Latinos cannot rise out of poverty and their health status will continue to be compromised.

# References

Abraido-Lanza, A. F., Dohrenwend, B., Ng-Mak, D., & Turner, J. (1999). The Latino mortality paradox: A test of the "salmon bias" and healthy migrant hypothesis. *American Journal of Public Health, 89,* 10, 1543–1548.

Acosta-Belen, E., & Santiago, C. E. (1998). Merging borders: The remapping of America. In A. Darder & R. D. Torres (Eds.), *The Latino studies reader: Culture, economy, and society.* Malden, MA: Blackwell.

Amaro, H., Fried, L. E., Cabral, H., & Zuckerman, B. (1990). Violence during pregnancy and substance use. *American Journal of Public Health, 80,* 1491–1499.

Committee on National Statistics. (1976). 94th Congress, H. J. Res. 92, *Joint resolution relating to the publication of economic and social statistics for Americans of Spanish-origin or descent.* (Public Law 94-311). Washington, D.C.: U.S. Government Printing Office.

Ellen, I. G., & Turner, M. A. (1997). Does neighborhood matter? Assessing recent evidence. *Housing Policy Debate, 8,* 4.

Fix, M., & Struyk, R. J. (1993). *Clear and convincing evidence: Measurement of discrimination in America.* Washington, D.C.: Urban Institute Press.

Flack, J. M. et al. (1995). Panel I: Epidemiology of minority health. *Health Psychology, 14,* 7, 592–600.

Fuentes-Afflick, E., Hessol, N. A., & Pérez-Stable, E. J. (1999). Testing the paradox of low birth weight in Latinos. *Archives of Pediatric Adolescent Medicine, 2,* 147–153.

Goff, D. C., Ramsey, D. J., Labarthe, D. R., & Nichaman, M. Z. (1993). Acute myocardial infarction and coronary heart disease mortality among Mexican Americans and Whites in Texas, 1980 through 1989. *Ethnicity and Disease, 3,* 1, 64–69.

Hahn, R. A., Mulinare, J., & Teutsch, S. M. (1992). Inconsistencies in coding of race and ethnicity between birth and death in U.S. infants: A new look at infant mortality, 1983 through 1985. *Journal of the American Medical Association, 267,* 259–263.

Hajat, A., Lucas, J., & Kington, R. (2000). *Health outcomes among Hispanic subgroups: United States, 1992–95.* Advance Data from Vital and Health Statistics, No. 310. Hyattsville, MD: National Center for Health Statistics.

Heckler, M. (1985). *Report of the Secretary's Task Force on African American and minority health: Vol. I: Executive summary.* Washington, D.C.: U.S. Department of Health and Human Services.

Hornick, D. B. (1988). Tuberculosis. In B. N. Doebbeling & R. B. Wallace (Eds.), *Maxcy-Rosenau-Last public health and preventive medicine* (14th ed.). Stamford, CT: Appleton & Lange, pp. 208–217.

LeClere, F. B., Jensen, L., & Biddlecom, A. (1994). Health care utilization, family context, and adaptation among immigrants to the United States. *Journal of Health and Social Behavior, 35,* 370–384.

Lindan, C. P. et al. (1990). Underreporting of minority AIDS deaths in San Francisco Bay area, 1985–86. *Public Health Reports, 105,* 400–404.

Magana, A., & Clark, N. M. (1995). Examining a paradox: Does religiosity contribute to positive birth outcomes in Mexican American populations? *Health Education Quarterly, 22,* 1, 96–109.

Margolis, H. (1998). Viral hepatitis. In B. N. Doebbeling & R. B. Wallace (Eds.), *Maxcy-Rosenau-Last public health and preventive medicine* (14th ed.). Stamford, CT: Appleton & Lange, pp. 174–188.

Marín, G., & Marín, B. (1991). *Research with Latino populations.* Newbury Park, CA: Sage.

Markides, K. S., & Coreil, J. (1986). The health of Latinos in the southwestern United States: An epidemiologic paradox. *Public Health Reports, 101,* 253–265.

Marmot, M. G. et al. (1975). Epidemiologic studies of coronary heart disease and stroke in Japanese men living in Japan, Hawaii and California: Prevalence of coronary and hypertensive heart disease and associated risk factors. *American Journal of Epidemiology, 102,* 415–525.

Mathews, T. J., Curtin, S. C., & MacDorman, M. F. (2000). Infant mortality statistics from the 1998 period linked birth/infant death data set. *National Vital Statistics Reports, 48,* 12. Hyattsville, MD: National Center for Health Statistics.

Molina, C., & Aguirre-Molina, M. (1994). Latino populations: Who are they? In Molina & Aguirre-Molina, *Latino Health in the U.S.: A Growing Challenge*. Washington, D.C.: American Public Health Association.

Montgomery, L. E., & Carter-Pokras, O. (1993). Health status by social class and/or minority status: Implications for environmental equity research. *Toxicology and Industrial Health, 5,* 729–773.

Murphy, S. L. (2000). Deaths: Final data for 1998. *National Vital Statistics Reports, 48,* 11. Hyattsville, MD: National Center for Health Statistics.

National Center for Health Statistics (NCHS). (2000). *Health, United States, 2000, with Adolescent Health Chartbook*. Hyattsville, MD: Author.

National Committee on Vital and Health Statistics. (1999). *Appendix VII: Report and conclusions regarding the availability of racial and ethnic identifiers in the SSA/HCFA administrative record systems*. 1994 Annual Report of the National Committee on Vital and Health Statistics. Washington, D.C.: U.S. Government Printing Office, pp. 13–118.

Office of the Assistant Secretary for Planning and Evaluation [of the DHHS]. (2000). *Assessment of major federal data sets for analyses of Latino and Asian or Pacific Islander subgroups and Native Americans*. Prepared by Westat, Rockville, MD.

Office of Management and Budget. (1978). Directive 15: Race and ethnicity standards for federal statistics and administrative reporting. In *Statistical policy handbook: Office of federal statistical policy and standards*. Washington, D.C.: U.S. Department of Commerce, pp. 37–38.

Pan American Health Organization. (1994). *Health conditions of the Americas*. (Scientific Publication No. 549). Washington, D.C.: Author.

PHS Task Force on Minority Health Data. (1992). *Improving minority health statistics*. Washington, D.C.: Author.

Regier, D. A. et al. (1993). One-month prevalence of mental disorders in the United States and sociodemographic characteristics: The Epidemiologic Catchment Area Study. *Acta Psychiatrica Scandanavica, 88,* 35–47.

Rumbaut, R., & Weeks, J. R. (1996). Unraveling a public health enigma: Why do immigrants experience superior perinatal health outcomes? *Research in the Sociology of Health Care, 13B,* 337–391.

Scott, S., & Suagee, M. (1992). *Enhancing health statistics for American Indian and Alaskan Native communities: An agenda for action*. Report to the National Center for Health Statistics. St. Paul, MN: American Health Care Association.

Scribner, R. (1991). Infant mortality among Latinos: The epidemiological paradox. *Journal of the American Medical Association, 16,* 2065–2066.

Scribner, R. (1996). Paradox as paradigm—The health outcomes of Mexican Americans. *American Journal of Public Health, 86,* 303–305.

Scrimshaw, S. C., Zambrana, R. E., & Dunkel-Schetter, C. (1997). Issues in Latino women's health: Myths and challenges. In A. E. Clark, S. B. Ruzek, & V. L. Olesen (Eds.), *Women's health: Complexities and differences*. Columbus: Ohio State University Press, pp. 329–347.

Sherraden, M. S., & Barrera, R. E. (1996). Poverty, family support, and well-being of infants: Mexican immigrant women and children. *Journal of Sociology and Social Welfare, 2,* 27–53.

Smith, D. S., & Egger, M. (1992). Socioeconomic differences in mortality in Britain and the United States. *American Journal of Public Health, 8,* 1079–1081.

Sorlie, P. D. et al. (1993). Mortality by Latino status in the United States. *Journal of the American Medical Association, 270,* 2464–2468.

Stern, M. P., & Wei, M. (1999). Do Mexican Americans really have low rates of cardiovascular disease? *Preventive Medicine, 29,* 90–95.

Stevens, G. (2000). Including language minority populations in national studies: Challenges, opportunities, and best practices—An overview of the linguistic demography of the

United States. Paper presented at the NIH Conference on Inclusion of Language Minority Populations in National Studies: Challenges, Opportunities and Best Practices.

Surgeon General's Hispanic/Latino Health Initiative. (1993). *One voice, one vision: Recommendations to the Surgeon General to improve Latino/Latina health.* Washington, D.C.: U.S. Department of Health and Human Services.

Telles, E. E., & Murguia, E. (1990). Phenotypic discrimination and income differences among Mexican Americans. *Social Science Quarterly, 71,* 682–67.

Todd, K. H., Samaroo, N., & Hoffman, J. R. (1993). Ethnicity as a risk factor for inadequate emergency department analgesia. *Journal of the American Medical Association, 269,* 12, 1537–1539.

United States Department of Health and Human Services (DHHS). (2000). *Healthy People 2010* (Conference ed., in 2 vols.). Washington, D.C.: Author.

United States Department of Health and Human Services (DHHS) Data Council. (2000). Improving the collection and use of racial and ethnic data in HHS. Retrieved from http://ospe.os.dhhs.gov/datacncl/racerpt

Vega, W. A., & Amaro, H. (1994). Latino outlook: Good health, uncertain prognosis. *Annual Review of Public Health, 15,* 39–67.

Ventura, S. J., Martin, J. A., Curtin, S. C., Mathews, T. J., & Park, M. M. (2000). Births. Final data for 1998. National vital statistics reports; vol. 48, no. 3. Hyattsville, MD: National Center for Health Statistics.

Williams, D. R. (1996). Racism and health: A research agenda. *Ethnicity and Disease, 6,* 1–6.

Williams, D. R., & Collins, C. (1995). U.S. socioeconomic and racial differences in health: Patterns and explanations. *Annual Review of Sociology, 21,* 349–386.

Williams, D. R., Lavizzo-Mourey, R., & Warren, R. C. (1994). The concept of race and health status in America. *Public Health Reports, 109,* 1, 26–41.

Williams, D. R., Yu, Y., Jackson, J. S., & Anderson, N. B. (1997). Racial differences in physical and mental health. *Journal of Health Psychology, 3,* 335–351.

Wingo, P. A., Ries, L.A.G., Rosenberg, H. M., Miller, D. S., & Edwards, B. K. (1998). Cancer incidence and mortality, 1973–1995. *Cancer, 82,* 1197–1207.

Zambrana, R. E. (1992). The relationship between use of health care services and health status: Dilemmas in measuring medical outcome in low-income and racial/ethnic populations. In M. L. Grady & H. A. Schwartz (Eds.), *Medical effectiveness research data methods.* Rockville, MD: U.S. Department of Health and Human Services, pp. 103–114.

Zambrana, R. E. (1996). The relationship of health perceptions, physical and mental health, and language use to usual source of care. In M. E. Blanton, W. Leigh, & A. Alfaro-Correro (Eds.), *Achieving equitable access.* Washington, D.C.: Joint Center for Political and Economic Studies, pp. 75–96.

Zambrana, R. E., Breen, N., Fox, S. A., & Gutierrez-Mohamed, M. L. (1999). Use of cancer screening practices by Latino women: Analyses by subgroup. *Preventive Medicine, 29,* 466–477.

Zambrana, R. E., & Carter-Pokras, O. D. (2001). Health data issues for Hispanics: Implications for public research. *Journal of Health Care for the Poor & Underserved, 12,* 1, 20–31.

Zambrana, R. E., & Scrimshaw, S. (1997). Maternal prenatal factors associated with substance use behaviors in Mexican-origin and African American low-income women. *Pediatric Nursing, 3,* 253–275.

Zambrana, R. E., Scrimshaw, S. C., Collins, N., & Dunkel-Schetter, C. (1997). Prenatal health behaviors and psychosocial risk factors in pregnant women of Mexican origin: The role of acculturation. *American Journal of Public Health, 87,* 6, 1022–1026.

Zambrana, R. E., Scrimshaw, S. C., Collins, N., & Dunkel-Schetter, C. (1999). Mediators of ethnic-associated differences in infant birth weight. *Journal of Urban Health: Bulletin of the New York Academy of Medicine, 76,* 1, 102–116.

CHAPTER THREE

# LATINO ACCESS TO HEALTH CARE

## The Role of Insurance, Managed Care, and Institutional Barriers

J. Emilio Carrillo, Fernando M. Treviño,
Joseph R. Betancourt, and Alberto Coustasse

The health care system in the United States is the most expensive and yet arguably among the least cost effective in the developed world (Anderson, 1998). Despite the highest per person health care spending among the Organization for Economic Cooperation and Development (OECD) nations, the United States still ranks below many along a variety of health indicators (Woolhandler & Himmelstein, 1991). In a complicated health care system where the rules are many and economic forces drive both structure and function, the needs of vulnerable populations inevitably suffer. This chapter explores the consequences of these market forces on a vulnerable population—Latinos in the United States. First, the health insurance status of Latinos is reviewed in the context of employment trends and participation in various government-sponsored programs. Next, the chapter explores the impact of managed care on Latinos, as well as that of other institutional, organizational, and structural barriers that stand between this population and full access to health care.

The U.S. health care financing system is based on the premise that most working-age Americans (and their dependents) receive health insurance through their employment (Collins, Hall, & Neuhaus, 1999). A large proportion of citizens who are not covered through their employment are only partially covered by charity care, municipal health care facilities, or government-sponsored programs such as Medicaid and Medicare. Both of these assumptions break down in the case of Latinos, a population that tends to be clustered in jobs that are low paying, less stable, more hazardous, and less likely to have fringe benefits such as health care coverage (Del Pinal & Singer, 1997). In addition, as a result of several acts of legislation within the last few years, Latinos who are unregistered residents also fall through the health care "safety net." Even broad initiatives toward "universal coverage," such as those proposed by the Clinton Administration's Health Security Plan of 1992, left the undocumented without health care coverage. Lack of access to health care due to the widespread lack of insurance is arguably the most pressing health problem facing Latinos today.

Moreover, "access" to care through health insurance does not necessarily guarantee quality care. Researchers have tried to better define "access" by delineating where along the continuum toward obtaining quality health care specific barriers may exist (Bierman, Magari, Jette, Splaine, & Wasson, 1998). According to this perspective, "primary access" is defined as having health insurance. Latinos' higher uninsured rates clearly provide a primary barrier to health care. Latino populations that are insured yet at a socioeconomic disadvantage, or whose primary language and culture are not those of the mainstream, are subject to other powerful access barriers that are not as tangible as insurance status alone. For example, "secondary access" barriers occur for those who are insured yet face institutional, organizational, or structural barriers such as difficulty getting appointments, lack of access to after-hours medical advice, or long waiting times for referrals to necessary medical specialists (National Hispanic/Latino Health Initiative, 1993). "Tertiary access" barriers occur for those who are insured and secure a medical appointment yet face significant linguistic and cultural barriers in the medical encounter as they attempt to develop a successful and effective relationship with their health care provider.

In the 1980s employers and governments chose health maintenance organizations (HMOs) as a preferred vehicle for cost containment in health care. An HMO differs from a standard health insurance provider in that patients are required to see doctors and use hospitals and other facilities within the plan's network of providers. HMOs often require members to select a primary care physician who then controls what specialists can be seen. Managed care practices may exacerbate rather than relieve secondary and tertiary access barriers. Not only do patients with low literacy and limited English proficiency have difficulty with bureaucratically complex managed care enrollment and precertification practices for emergency room visits and hospitalizations, but they also face the hurdle of communicating with a provider who may not speak their language or value their cultural health beliefs and behaviors. The rapid spread of Medicaid managed care during the past decade poses a particular challenge to those who are not able to maneuver through a new and complicated health care system. In any of these settings, as is usually the case, the most educationally, economically, and educationally vulnerable patients will have the greatest difficulties navigating these complex systems. The rise of managed care in the 1980s and 1990s not only failed to relieve Latinos' rising uninsurance rates but also posed new challenges to the "safety net" that protects the uninsured through charity and municipal health care (United States Department of Health and Human Services and the Commonwealth Fund, 1999).

## Primary Barriers to Health Care

By 2025, the Latino population of the United States is expected to increase from thirty-one million (11 percent of the population) to fifty-nine million (18 percent of the population). Nearly 40 percent of Latinos under the age of sixty-five do not have health insurance. Latino children are perhaps the most vulnerable, making up 29 percent of the uninsured under age eighteen (compared to 11 percent of Whites in this age group). A quarter of the nation's forty-four million uninsured are Latino. In fact, Latinos are more than twice as likely to lack health insurance as the population overall. This gap persists despite a booming economy (Quinn, 2000). Cities with large Latino populations exemplify this trend. The four states with the highest concentration of Latino residents—California, Florida, New York, and Texas—account for 73 percent of all uninsured Latinos. Approximately 40 percent of Latinos living in California and Texas and more than one-third of Latinos in Florida and New York are uninsured (Quinn, 2000).

A major reason why so many Latinos lack health insurance is that their employers do not offer them coverage. Nearly nine million of the eleven million uninsured Latinos are in families in which at least one person works. This proportion is similar to or exceeds that of other racial and ethnic groups (Quinn, 2000). According to a study by Hall, Collins, and Glied (1999), based on the 1997 Current Population Survey, 69 percent of White workers aged eighteen to sixty-four have health insurance through their employer as compared to 52 percent of African American workers and 44 percent of Latino workers. There are several factors that contribute to Latinos' low rate of employer-sponsored health insurance. Citizenship appears to play a role, as workers who are not U.S. citizens have lower odds of being insured by their employer than do U.S. citizens. Educational status is also a contributing factor, since individuals with more than a college education are about twice as likely to have coverage than those with less than a high school education. Workforce characteristics are also important, because individuals employed in agricultural, mining, service, domestic, and construction industries are not as likely to be covered as those in manufacturing and "white-collar" industries. Many more Latinos are employed in the first four industries than in the latter two. Latinos also tend to have greater employment in small firms (those with less than 100 workers), which are less likely to provide health insurance to their employees than are larger firms. Within small firms or low-wage jobs, Latino workers are half as likely to have employer coverage and twice as likely to be uninsured as are White workers. Low-wage workers, regardless of firm size, are more likely than higher wage employees to be without insurance. The impact of lack of insurance is quite palpable (Quinn, 2000). In 1999, almost half of uninsured Latinos had not seen a doctor when sick, had gone without a prescription for needed medications, or went without recommended medical tests or treatments. About two-thirds had trouble paying their bills or were contacted by collection agencies for medical expenses.

## The Development of Managed Care

In the 1970s containing the cost of health became a national objective. The Health Maintenance Organizations Act of 1973 promoted HMOs as less costly and more efficient forms of health care delivery. The National Health Planning and Resources Act of 1974 created a certification system for these new types of organizations. HMOs began taking off in about 1976, as Congress reduced the mandatory benefits and other stringent requirements that had curtailed the program up until then.

By 1996 the total number of HMO members grew by an estimated 8.4 million people, to 67.5 million—or about one in four Americans. Since 1990, HMO enrollment has increased by 85 percent.

Commercial managed care organizations (MCOs) are not required by legislation or court mandate to collect racial and ethnic identifiers for people enrolled in their plans. In fact, the U.S. Health Care Financing Administration (HCFA), perhaps the largest health care payer and the one with the greatest leverage on MCOs, does not ask that racial or ethnic identifiers be provided under the Medicare program. In 1999, the Commonwealth Fund conducted an informal survey which found that not one of twelve large, for-profit MCOs collected race and ethnicity data (United States Department of Health and Human Services and the Commonwealth Fund, 1999). Some MCOs collect such data only as part of targeted quality-of-care research. Consequently, there is only a smattering of information on racial and ethnic profiles of commercial MCO members. A survey conducted in the states of Florida, Tennessee, and Texas revealed that 72 percent of low-income African Americans were enrolled in managed care as compared to 55 percent of Latinos and 63 percent of Whites (Leigh, Lillie-Blanton, Martinez, & Collins, 1999).

## Quality-of-Care and Performance Indicators

MCOs are evaluated by a series of quality-of-care and performance indicators. The National Center for Quality Assurance (NCQA), a nongovernmental organization founded by large health care payers for the purpose of evaluating MCOs on the basis of a set of measures of quality of care, has been the pioneer in this field. Their primary tool of evaluation, the Health Employment Data Set (HEDIS), measures a variety of quality indicators that are used to compare managed care plans. One key limitation of the current quality-of-care and performance indicators is that they fall short on key issues and measurements that may be particularly important to Latino populations. For example, HEDIS has no measures that evaluate health care workforce diversity, the presence of interpreter services, or the ability (in detail) of patients to successfully communicate with their providers. The Consumer Assessment of Health Plans Survey (CAHPS), a tool used by the HCFA to obtain the consumer's perspective on the health care they receive, is also largely devoid of measures that could be important to Latino health. To its credit, in the "Adult Supplemental Questions" packet, the CAHPS does attempt to address doctor-patient communication (one question) and the need for the presence of interpreter services (two questions). Fortunately, there is currently research being done on the development and psychometric testing of a "Spanish CAHPS," which should better capture the issues pertinent to Latinos. This remains a crucial endeavor, as the Commonwealth Fund Managed Care Survey of 1994 found that minority Americans are less satisfied with the quality of managed care plans compared to that of fee-for-service (FFS) plans (see Figure 3.1).

Along these lines, the Kaiser Family Foundation and the Commonwealth Foundation jointly sponsored a study of low-income population's health coverage that demonstrated certain patterns. Surveys in the states of Florida, Tennessee, and Texas showed that with some notable exceptions, patients' views on their access to care and patient satisfaction with care are similar among Latinos and African American managed care and FFS enrollees. African American managed care enrollees are twice as likely as their FFS counterparts to report problems getting required medical care. Another exception is that Latinos in managed care rate their physician's concern about them as "fair" or "poor" at twice the rate of those in FFS plans (Leigh, Lillie-Blanton, Martinez, & Collins, 1999). Neither managed care nor FFS plans were found to be particularly effective in ensuring that Latinos and African Americans have access to the health care system. Roughly one in four Latinos and African Americans rate as "fair" or "poor" his or her satisfaction with care, measured by overall service, waiting time required to get a doctor's appointment, and physician concern for the patient. Ironically, despite managed care's aspirations to provide primary care and continuity, this survey

### FIGURE 3.1.  MINORITY AMERICANS ARE LESS SATISFIED WITH QUALITY OF MANAGED CARE.

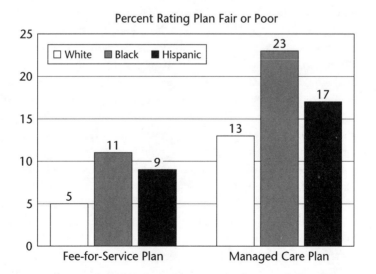

*Source:* The Commonwealth Fund Managed Care Survey, Louis Harris and Associates, Inc., 1994.

found that 42 percent of Latinos and 38 percent of African Americans in managed care plans did not have a regular provider, as compared with 52 percent of Latinos and 47 percent of African Americans in FFS plans. Spanish-speaking Latinos were nearly twice as likely as their English-speaking counterparts to lack a regular provider.

Continued efforts to better identify how Latinos define "quality" in the health care they receive will allow us to better develop systems to meet the needs of this young and growing population.

Several new initiatives directed toward developing quality measures that are responsive to the needs of minority populations have been launched in the last few years. The Henry Ford Health System and the Lovelace Clinic Foundation, in conjunction with the Center for Healthcare Improvement and the Commonwealth Fund, have begun working on and validating a "minority health report card" that would include various quality measures specific to Latino and other minority populations (Nerenz, 1999). As part of its Quality Improvement Standards in Managed Care, the Health Care Financing Administration (HCFA) has been working on "cultural competence quality measures," which include measurements of workforce diversity and patient satisfaction vis-à-vis doctor-patient communication, among others (Health Care Financing Administration, 1999). Finally, states have started to use their leverage in Medicaid managed care contracting to require MCO contractors to ensure that certain services and standards are put in place (interpreter services, diverse workforce) when they serve a part of the state that has a predominance of a particular population. For example, in California, as part the state's contracting with MediCal (a Medicaid MCO) contracting, specific requirements have been put into the contracts that address the needs of Latino patients. Health centers that receive a MediCal contract and that serve a predominately Latino population are mandated to maintain a diverse health care workforce and guarantee the presence of trained Spanish interpreters (Coye & Alvarez, 1999; Hinojosa, 1999). Similarly, some MCOs have begun to address the important issues of developing capacity to care for diverse patient populations. For example, Kaiser Permanente in California developed a National Diversity Council and targeted initiatives in interpretation and physician education to better serve that MCO's diverse patient population (Kaiser Permanente National Diversity Council, 1996). In addition, Harvard Pilgrim Health Care has begun "diversity training" and also piloted new interpretation services (Stern, 1999).

As was previously mentioned, a major barrier to developing quality measures that are responsive to specific issues relating to Latino health is the lack of race and ethnicity data being collected by the government and MCOs. To hold the health care system accountable for the delivery of care and subsequent outcomes, the collection of race- and ethnic-specific data is essential. There is currently great resistance to collecting such data because of the fear of infringement on patient confidentiality or the risk of exclusion of patients (redlining) from enrollment in managed care plans because of their race or ethnicity. It is only through the collection of race and ethnicity data that progress can be made toward the development of new measures in Latino health so that progress in improving care to this vulnerable population can be tracked.

## Medicaid and Medicaid Managed Care

Medicaid, enacted in 1965 as part of President Lyndon B. Johnson's "Great Society" program, is the largest health insurer in the United States in terms of eligible beneficiaries, covering medical services for some 41.3 million people. The Medicaid program is financed by the states and federal government and administered solely by the states. In 1997, Medicaid expended $159.9 billion, or 12.4 percent of the total national health care expenditures, to pay for covered services for low-income people who were elderly, blind, disabled, receiving public assistance, or among the working poor (Iglehart, 1999). The growth in Medicaid expenditures, which almost tripled from the 1980s to the mid-1990s, has recently slowed. The major factor accounting for the spike in Medicaid spending in the early 1990s was not enrollment growth but rather the states' use of disproportionate share hospital (DSH) payments and other contributions as a way to substantially increase the federal matching funds for the state.

Being poor does not automatically make a person eligible for Medicaid. In 1997, Medicaid covered only 44.4 percent of nonelderly persons with an income of less than $13,330 for a family of three. Each state sets its own criteria for eligibility, following broad federal guidelines (Iglehart, 1999). The Republican Congress of 1995 set a major policy goal of devolving federal authority and money to state governments, particularly in the realm of social welfare. The Personal Responsibility and Work Opportunity Reconciliation Act of 1996 granted states the authority to operate their own welfare and work (now called "workfare") programs, largely with federal resources. The new state laws that resulted from this legislation severed the link between Medicaid and public assistance. Many people who have moved from public assistance to workfare programs may not realize that they still qualify for Medicaid. This knowledge gap and the complex process of filling out a Medicaid application has resulted in dramatic declines in the Medicaid rolls—and of course there are many Latinos within this group (Iglehart, 1999). Those who go beyond workfare and enter into the workforce often find employment in low-paying positions that do not provide health coverage. These transitions may serve to increase the already alarming rates of uninsured in the Latino population. In New York City, where a large proportion of the Medicaid population is Latino, Medicaid rolls dropped by 12 percent (200,000) over the period 1995–1999. During this time, 105,000 children lost Medicaid coverage.

Since the 1980s, many states have implemented some form of Medicaid managed care, largely as a means of limiting Medicaid expenditures. Medicaid managed care plans are those whose enrollment is at least 75 percent Medicaid. Originally, enrollment into these managed care plans was patient-driven and voluntary. Understandably, enrollment grew slowly under voluntary conditions, as these plans could not articulate clear benefits for the targeted recruits. In fact, managed care would actually limit the individual's choice of physician and hospitals and also place limits on other benefits such as use of specialists. One of the fundamental principles of managed care is the relationship of one physician to one patient. This tenet is not necessarily held by the consumer, who values choice and alternatives.

Many states have implemented mandatory programs in which all Medicaid recipients, with some categorical exceptions, are phased into managed care. Such transitions from voluntary to mandatory status required a special clearance by HCFA until 1997, when congressional legislation gave the states the freedom to implement mandatory programs once certain federal guidelines are met.

More than eight million of the 13.3 million Medicaid beneficiaries enrolled in managed care programs have enrolled in HMOs as of mid-1996 (in forty-six states). Approximately 19.9 million Medicaid beneficiaries were enrolled in FFS plans. From 1991 through 1996, the number of Medicaid recipients enrolled in Medicaid managed care programs more than quadrupled, from 2.7 million to 13.3 million.

Similar to the situation previously presented for commercial MCOs, only some of the state Medicaid programs provide racial and ethnic data to Medicaid HMOs operating in their respective states. Massachusetts and California have provided such data to Medicaid plans, while Tennessee has provided only racial but not ethnic data.

Medicaid managed care poses particular challenges to the Latino patient, as the rules are so arcane and complicated that even health care industry administrators are often stymied by them. Enrollment brokers have been set up in many states to facilitate the enrollment process. Yet, despite these efforts, people with limited English-language proficiency and skills at negotiating bureaucratic processes cannot exert choice because they may not understand the complex presentation of the program. In fact, many patients are not even aware that they are in a managed care plan. People do in fact sense the impact of Medicaid managed care whenever they try to change doctors or plans and also whenever they request doctors and services not included in their particular plan. HCFA has attempted to address some of these concerns by closely monitoring states' compliance with guidelines and regulations that are part of the process of mandatory Medicaid managed care implementation. Provisions are made for grievance and fair hearing rights as well as external review processes. Some notable differences between Medicaid and commercial managed care plans have been reported. For instance, a survey of 154 health plans in eleven states and the District of Columbia showed that the Medicaid plans were more likely to target programs to the specific needs of the Medicaid population than were the commercial MCOs (Landon & Epstein, 1999).

## Access to the State Children's Health Insurance Program

Congress enacted the State Children's Health Insurance Program (S-CHIP) in 1997 as a method of increasing access to health care for uninsured children. This program allocated $20.3 billion in federal matching funds over five years to states to expand health insurance coverage to uninsured children under the age of nineteen in families with incomes below 200 percent of poverty. Children with private insurance or who are covered by or qualify for Medicaid are ineligible for S-CHIP. Undocumented and legally resident children arriving in the United States after August 22, 1996, are also ineligible for coverage but may qualify for emergency Medicaid assistance. States that choose to operate a separate state child health insurance program can establish eligibility based on geographic area, age, income and resources, residency, and disability status, as well as limit duration of coverage.

Poor and near-poor children are substantially more likely than middle- or high-income children to be uninsured. However, at each level of family income, Latino children are more likely to be uninsured than White or African American children. Poor and near-poor Latino children are least likely to have insurance (United States Department of Health and Human Services, Health Resources and Services Administration, 1998). The S-CHIP program was seen as a possible intervention to bridge this great disparity, yet states have struggled to promote it with various degrees of success. There may be large numbers of undocumented children who qualify for S-CHIP but who lack awareness of the program or access to the enrollment process. This could be particularly significant for Latino children because of social, cultural, and linguistic barriers.

## Balanced Budget Act of 1997: Consequences to the Safety Net

The Balanced Budget Act (BBA) was passed by Congress in 1997 in an effort to control overall spending and bring this nation's budget into balance. As part of this initiative, health care spending via HCFA and Medicare were targeted for reform. Through a series of new measures, cuts, and controls, the BBA is expected to result in significant savings to Medicare—some $393.8 billion over ten years. The Medicare reforms contributed significantly to the goal of a balanced budget; in fact, changes to the program account for 73 percent of total savings. Over a five-year period, BBA provisions reduce Medicare spending by $116.4 billion. Much of this reduction (67 percent) will be achieved by limiting growth rates in payments to hospitals and physicians under FFS arrangements. Academic health centers and hospitals serving a disproportionate share of low-income Medicare beneficiaries will also receive additional limits in payment growth.

To ensure access to care for the millions of uninsured people in this country, the U.S. health care system relies on a makeshift system of "safety net" providers— public hospitals, community health centers, local health departments, and rural health clinics, as well as special service providers such as AIDS-based and school-based clinics. They often provide specialized services such as trauma care and medical education. To remain financially viable, many of these facilities depend on a patchwork of grants and subsidies that have become increasingly uncertain and insufficient (Institute of Medicine, 1999). Such facilities serve predominantly low-income communities that include substantial caseloads of Medicaid and uninsured patients—and correspondingly small caseloads of privately insured patients. For example, community health centers (CHCs) serve as the entry point to the health care system for millions of Medicaid beneficiaries, the uninsured, and people residing in medically undeserved areas. Many of these users are members of minority groups and suffer disproportionately from health problems and disease. Of the ten million people served by CHCs in 1996, 41 percent were uninsured and another 33 percent were on Medicaid; also, 31 percent were Latinos and 27 percent were African American. Approximately 65 percent of CHC patients live below the federal poverty level, while another 20 percent live at 100–200 percent of the poverty level. According to the Bureau of Primary Health Care of the U.S. Department of Health and Human Services (DHHS), from 1990 to 1997 the number of uninsured patients at CHCs increased by 49 percent. Costs for uncompensated care at a sample of urban, safety net hospitals totaled $4 billion and represented 26 percent of total costs in 1996. These costs were financed through state and local government subsidies (59 percent), Medicaid disproportionate share hospitals (DSH) payments (29 percent), Medicare DSH payments (9 percent), and cost shifting from privately insured patients (3 percent). Aside from local tax appropriations for indigent care, the Medicare and DSH programs are an important source of financial subsidies for providers willing to care for the uninsured, the underinsured, and other low-income populations. The DSH program was originally intended to compensate hospitals for what were believed to be higher-than-average costs for treating low-income Medicare patients. The BBA cuts will have a significant financial impact on CHCs ability to serve these vulnerable populations.

In relation to public hospitals and academic health centers, the National Association of Public Hospitals and Health Systems (NAPH) reported that in 1995 Medicaid and uninsured patients made up 74 percent of discharges and 77 percent of outpatient visits in its member hospitals (Fagnani & Tolbert, 2000). Another study from 1996 found that Medicaid and uninsured patients accounted for 29 percent of discharges in academic medical centers in 1994. Public hospitals make up 7 percent of all hospitals in the nation's 100 largest cities but provide 18 percent of all outpatient visits and 19 percent of all emergency room visits, for an annual total in excess of 100 million visits (Coye & Alvarez, 2000). Furthermore, a 1998 NAPH survey of twenty-five urban safety net hospitals reported that 78 percent of its patients had incomes at or below 150 percent of the federal poverty level and that Latinos and African Americans had the highest number of visits, accounting for 31.7 percent and 40.9 percent, respectively. Coupled with declining local government appropriations and market forces that include managed care and an eroding Medicaid patient base, these BBA cuts will severely undermine the ability of safety net hospitals and academic health centers to remain financially viable. As a result of the BBA reforms, public hospitals and academic health centers are facing unprecedented fiscal challenges, which place their role as providers of care to vulnerable populations in great jeopardy.

Finally, the competition created by Medicaid managed care has also led to patients being siphoned away from their community providers, further endangering the safety net. A report on the health care safety net (Institute of Medicine, 1999) found that while patients did gain greater choice from Medicaid managed care, safety net providers lost 6 percent of their Medicaid primary care patients to competitors between 1995 and 1998. MCOs may also have financial incentives to exclude safety net providers from their networks because of the costly, high-risk, and very sick patients they serve. The fiscal pressures created by limits on public subsidies, expansions in Medicaid and Medicare managed care, and price competition in hospital markets may undermine the ability of safety net providers to fulfill their missions. If these challenges lead safety net providers to close, some communities could lose their only source of care. In summary, the BBAs impact on safety net hospitals, safety net providers, academic health centers, and graduate medical education has posed a clear and present challenge to the well-being of the health of Latinos and other underserved racial or ethnic groups.

## Secondary Barriers to Health Care

The fact that many Latinos are likely to lack health insurance clearly has a major impact on their overall health outcomes. It is difficult to imagine how a patient without insurance can get the necessary battery of preventive examinations such as mammography, Pap smears, and screening for diabetes and colon and prostate cancer, among others; or how a patient with hypertension can be examined and treated regularly to prevent the cardiovascular complications that result from this condition. As a result, despite the health-promotion and disease-prevention interventions that have improved the health of Americans in general, Latinos have benefited much less from these advances (National Hispanic/Latino Health Initiative, 1993). At the root of this problem is Latinos' lack of access to a source of primary care. Even Latinos who are fortunate enough to have "primary access" to care via some type of health insurance may face other barriers that preclude them from fully benefiting from what primary care has to offer. Ultimately, similar to their counterparts who are uninsured, many supposedly insured Latinos also have great difficulty accessing our health care system. There are several types of "secondary access" barriers to care—institutional, organizational, and structural—which greatly impact the Latino population's ability to get health care despite having insurance.

From the *organizational* standpoint, one factor that can impinge on both the availability and acceptability of health care is the degree to which the nation's health care professions reflect the racial and ethnic composition of the general population. The importance of racial and ethnic diversity in both the leadership and workforce of health care delivery systems has been well-correlated with the ability to provide quality care to socioculturally diverse patient populations. For example, for minority patients, it has been shown that in cases where there was racial concordance between the patient and the physician, patient satisfaction and self-rated quality of care was higher (Saha, Komaromy, Koepsell, & Bindman, 1999). Other work has established the preference of minority patients for minority

physicians (Moy & Bartman,1995; Komaromy et al., 1996). As it relates to identifying the root cause of these preferences, it has been shown that Spanish-speaking
Latino patients, for example, are more satisfied when their provider speaks Spanish (Cooper-Patrick et al., 1999), and in the case of African Americans, when their
physician employs a more participatory and inclusive style of decision making (Bureau of Health Professions, 1990).

A review of the data on racial and ethnic diversity of the U.S. health care
workforce reveals that Latinos made up only 2 percent of all physicians in 1990.
Approximately 24 percent of Latino physicians in office-based practices in
California care for patients with Medicaid as the primary insurer (versus 18 percent
of White physicians), and 9 percent care for patients who are uninsured (versus
6 percent of White physicians). In academic health centers, underrepresented
minorities (Hispanics, African Americans, and Native Americans) make up only
3 percent of the medical school faculty. Additionally, 53 percent of the Latino
faculty are those who teach in the medical schools in Puerto Rico, highlighting
the underrepresentation of Latino faculty on the mainland (Bureau of Health
Professions, 1990). Similarly, despite minorities comprising 30 percent of this
nation's population (United States Bureau of the Census, Census 2000
Redistricting Data), less than 16 percent of public health school faculty positions
are held by minority scholars, and only 17 percent of all city and county health
officers are from minority groups as well (Collins, Hall, & Neuhaus, 1999). The
prognosis for the future is not much brighter. Data from 1997 show that enrollment
of Mexican Americans and mainland Puerto Ricans into medical schools dropped
by 8.7 percent and 31 percent, respectively, and that in the same year only
11 percent of all graduates were from underrepresented minorities (Association of
American Medical Colleges, 1998). From 1996 to 1997, the drop in underrepresented matriculates has been greatest in states with new anti-affirmative action policies: California, 16 percent decline; Texas, 29 percent decline; Louisiana,
13 percent decline; and Mississippi, 13 percent decline (Association of American
Medical Colleges, 1998). Several initiatives of the Association of American Medical Colleges to address these disparities have come up short in the last few years.
For example, the "3000 by 2000 Project," founded on the goal of having 3,000 underrepresented minorities in medical schools by the year 2000, was unable to reach
its target.

The importance of diversity not only applies to the medical encounter but in
fact may be even more salient as it relates to leadership and representation within
an organization's administration. In cases where there is lack of diversity in the
leadership and workforce of health care organizations, the result may be structural policies, procedures, and delivery systems inappropriately designed or poorly
suited to serve diverse patient populations. In summary, increasing underrepresented minorities in the health professions is an important way to improve both
access to care and the health status of the nation's vulnerable populations.

From the *structural* standpoint, systems that provide care to Spanish-speaking
patients but lack interpreter services or do not provide culturally or linguistically

appropriate health education materials can severely compromise patient care to these populations. Doctor-patient communication, in the setting of even a minimal language barrier, is also recognized as a major challenge to health care delivery (Kirkman-Liff & Mondragon, 1991; Stewart, Grumbach, Osmond, Vranizan, Komaromy, & Bindman, 1997; Seijo, 1991; Pérez-Stable, Napoles-Springer, & Miramontes, 1997; Erzinger, 1991). Research in this area has shown that Spanish-speaking patients discharged from the emergency room are less likely than their English-speaking counterparts to understand their diagnosis, prescribed medications, special instructions, and plans for follow-up care (Crane, 1997); less likely to be satisfied with their care or willing to return if they had a problem; more likely to report problems with their care (Carrasquillo, Orav, Brennan, & Burstin, 1999); and less satisfied with the patient-provider relationship (Baker, Hayes, & Fortier, 1998). Physicians who have access to trained interpreters report a significantly higher quality of patient-physician communication than do physicians who used other methods (Baker, Parker, Williams, Coates, & Pitkin, 1996). Latino patients with language-discordant physicians are more likely to omit medication, miss office appointments, and visit the emergency room for care (Hornberger, Itakura, & Wilson, 1997).

These organizational, intrinsic, and systemic barriers oftentimes prevent minority, socioeconomically disadvantaged, and limited-English-proficient patients with insurance from having true access to health care. Some examples of barriers include those within health care systems that (1) lack interpreter services and language-appropriate health education materials and signage; (2) have bureaucratic, complicated intake processes, long waiting times for appointments, and limited operating hours (including after-hours availability); and (3) are located outside the community, making them difficult to reach via public transportation (National Hispanic/Latino Health Initiative, 1993). These barriers all clearly complicate Latinos' ability to obtain quality health care. The result is patient dissatisfaction, poor comprehension of critical health messages, nonadherence to health-promotion and disease-prevention interventions, lower quality of care, and poorer health outcomes, even in those Latinos who supposedly have access. MCOs, given their complex organizations, policies, procedures, and systems of care, although founded on principles of health maintenance, may pose particular challenges to Latinos.

## Tertiary Barriers to Health Care

Within the medical encounter, a physician's ability to communicate across language barriers and understand sociocultural variations in health beliefs, values, and behaviors is critical to the delivery of quality care to racially and ethnically diverse patient populations. Given the small proportion of Latino physicians, Spanish-speaking patients are very often cared for by physicians who may not speak their language, understand their social situation, or value their cultural beliefs. As a result, cultural and linguistic barriers in the medical encounter may lead to poor communication, patient dissatisfaction, and poor compliance (to both medications and health-promotion and/or disease-prevention interventions) (Manson, 1988; Stiles et al., 1979; Haynes, 1976; Stanton, 1987; Like & Steiner, 1986; Langer, 1999). Given this link between doctor-patient communication, patient satisfaction, compliance with diagnostic and therapeutic recommendations, and clinical outcomes, it might be hypothesized that in relation to health services, poor communication may lead to under- or overutilization of certain diagnostic and therapeutic procedures, and ultimately poorer outcomes. Although managed care tools such as "utilization management" may pick up instances of service overutilization, they are much less likely to detect the underutilization of services that often affects Latino populations. Two studies of California patients suggest that disparities in the treatment of Latinos compared to that of Whites may be similar to those found between African Americans and Whites. Giacomini (1996) found among California adult inpatients that Latinos were less likely than Whites to undergo three of nine procedures: coronary artery bypass graft (CABG), angioplasty, and kidney transplant. Carlisle, Leake, and Shapiro (1995) found that for ischemic heart disease patients in Los Angeles County, Latinos were less likely than Whites to receive CABG and angiography, but were equally likely to receive angioplasty.

Two separate studies that surveyed Latino patients' satisfaction with their ability to communicate with their provider also provide interesting findings. David and Rhee (1998, p. 396) state "in cases where language barriers existed between physicians and patients, test ordering may replace dialogue in the medical encounter." Similarly, Morales, Cunningham, Brown, Liu, and Hays (1999, p. 414) contend that "poor communication between a physician and a patient, as indicated by dissatisfaction with provider listening and answering of questions, may result in excessive ordering of medical tests as a provider attempts to establish a diagnosis in the absence of an adequate patient history." This second study showed that both Latino patients who spoke Spanish as a first language as well as those who spoke English as a first language were more dissatisfied with their ability to communicate with health providers, as compared to White patients. In essence, physicians who are unable to communicate effectively with Latino patients, either because of language barriers or because of cultural barriers other than language barriers, face great challenges in their attempts to deliver quality care to Latinos and others with similar situations. Two interventions aimed at diminishing these critical "tertiary access" barriers to care are gaining broader national attention. First, the Office of Civil Rights of the U.S. Department of Justice is attempting to strengthen Title VI of the Civil Rights Act so that interpreter services become more widely mandated in health care. Currently, there are several loopholes within the law (Title VI) that allow hospitals and other health care facilities to use volunteer, untrained interpreters for their medical encounters. These interpreters are selected either from the hospital workforce or from a volunteer pool. Most of the time, however, the AT&T Language Line, which is accessed via telephone, has served as a major source of interpretation services. Second, cultural competence training, a movement toward teaching medical students, residents, and physicians how to best understand and manage language barriers and sociocultural variations in health beliefs and behaviors, is rapidly growing in health care and medical education (Carrillo, Green, & Betancourt, 1999; Culhane-Pera, Like, Lebensohn-Chialvo, & Loewe, 2000; Culhane-Pera, Reif, Egli, Baker, & Kassekert, 1997). The overarching goal of cultural competence training is to provide physicians with the tools and skills to be able to deliver quality care to socioculturally diverse patient populations. Until the goals of these two interventions—interpreter services and cultural competence training—are realized, "tertiary access" barriers will persist and continue to compromise the care received by the "insured" portion of the Latino population.

## A New Latino Health Policy Agenda

A new Latino health policy agenda must address the primary, secondary, and tertiary barriers that this population faces in their pursuit of quality care. Efforts to improve primary access remain the most daunting task. The S-CHIP program is an intervention that if accessed to its fullest could significantly decrease the rolls of uninsured children. To date, however, S-CHIP has not reached its potential and has had particular trouble enrolling Latino children who stand to benefit the most from this policy. Similar initiatives, such as the Family Health Act of New York, a program to expand coverage to the working uninsured in a model similar to that of state children's health insurance programs, have prospered because of much popular and labor union support. These types of expansion of the safety net are needed, as is the need to closely guard the integrity of the safety net itself. Perhaps the intervention that could bring about the greatest benefit to the Latino population, however, is universal health care. Many have argued the merits of some type of universal health care coverage as being the foundation of any effort to improve minority health and eliminate racial and ethnic disparities (Woolhandler & Himmelstein, 1991). Given the current health insurance crisis facing Latinos in this country, any Latino health policy agenda must include strong advocacy of this major health care reform.

Despite some of the promising initiatives previously mentioned, several challenges currently persist. The BBA legislation poses a great risk to the health of the uninsured and underinsured, and could prove very harmful to academic medical centers and municipal health care facilities, which provide much of the uninsured care to the Latino population. The Medicaid programs, now in transition to managed care at the state level, have an entire new set of bureaucratic policies and procedures that preclude many Latinos, previously unused to such a complex health care system, from successfully accessing this care. Additionally, the lack of racial and ethnic identifiers at the governmental and private-sector level make it difficult to define quality of care for diverse patient groups and chart our progress in improving the care of our most vulnerable populations.

Various efforts that address secondary and tertiary barriers to care have been set forth over the last few years with the aim of improving the U.S. health care system, in general, and minority health care, in particular. For example, in 1998 President Bill Clinton set forth a major initiative to eliminate racial and ethnic disparities in health (the President's Initiative on Race; see United States Department of Health and Human Services and Grantmakers in Health, 1998). Six major areas of interest were delineated as targets of improvement: cardio-vascular disease, diabetes, HIV/AIDS, cancer screening and management, infant mortality, and immunization rates (United States Department of Health and Human Services, 1998; United States Department of Health and Human Services and Grantmakers in Health, 1998). As a result of this effort, a variety of new interventions have been developed to *eliminate* disparities in minority populations; improvements in diabetes, HIV/AIDS, and immunization rates stand to benefit Latino health the most. These goals are now reflected in the *Healthy People 2010* project, a departure from the previous goal of the *Healthy People* series that was simply to *reduce* disparities between racial and ethnic groups.

The Culturally and Linguistically Appropriate Services (CLAS) Project, sponsored by the Office of Minority Health of the U.S. DHHS, is also now being seen as a framework for culturally competent health care organizations (Fortier, 1998). Developed over two years with the assistance of national experts in cultural competence, the CLAS standards aim to be the first iteration of how health care systems can be better prepared to deliver quality care to diverse patient populations.

To overcome all the barriers explained in this chapter, a new Latino health policy agenda must rely on a strategic approach that identifies the common political leverage points for action and activism. Latino health care can only be defended and improved by constant vigilance and coordinated advocacy. Quantitative research guided by a solid qualitative understanding of the various Latino communities will yield the basic foundation upon which coordinated advocacy may yield legislative and judicial benefits.

Lack of insurance in the Latino community is clearly a critical health care issue, which should be addressed with great urgency. The BBA has only begun to exert its pressure on a system that is bending but on the verge of breaking, with particular serious implications for all Latino communities. Managed care operations and protocols are not going away, so we must also address all the peculiarities that arise as a result of this system of care and its subsequent policies and procedures. Institutional, organizational, and systemic barriers will continue to contribute to racial and ethnic disparities unless addressed immediately. Addressing all of these factors in a structured, strategic, and political fashion can make for an effective new Latino health policy agenda.

# References

Anderson, G. F. (1998). *Multinational comparisons of health care: Expenditures, coverage and outcomes.* New York: Commonwealth Fund.

Association of American Medical Colleges. (1998). *Minority students in medical education (Facts and Figures XI).* Washington, D.C.: Author.

Baker, D. W., Parker, R. M., Williams, M. V., Coates, W. C., & Pitkin, K. (1996). Use and effectiveness of interpreters in an emergency department. *Journal of the American Medical Association, 275,* 10, 783–788.

Baker, D. W., Hayes, R., & Fortier, J. P. (1998). Interpreter use and satisfaction with interpersonal aspects of care for Spanish-speaking patients. *Medical Care, 36,* 10, 1461–1470.

Bierman, A. S., Magari, E. S., Jette, A. M., Splaine, M., & Wasson, J. H. (1998). Assessing access as a first step toward improving the quality of care for very old adults. *Journal of Ambulatory Care Management, 21,* 3, 17–26.

Bureau of Health Professions. (1990). *Detailed occupation and other characteristics from the EEO file for the United States, 1990.* (Census of Population Supplementary Reports). Rockville, MD: U.S. Government Printing Office.

Carlisle, D. M., Leake, B. D., & Shapiro, M. F. (1995). Racial and ethnic differences in the use of invasive cardiac procedures among cardiac patients in Los Angeles County, 1986 through 1988. *American Journal of Public Health, 85,* 352–356.

Carrasquillo, O., Orav, E. J., Brennan, T. A., & Burstin, H. R. (1999). Impact of language barriers on patient satisfaction in an emergency department. *Journal of General Internal Medicine, 14,* 2, 82–87.

Carrillo, J. E., Green, A. R., & Betancourt, J. R. (1999). Cross-cultural primary care: A patient-based approach. *Annals of Internal Medicine, 130,* 829–834.

Collins, K. S., Hall, A., & Neuhaus, C. (1999). *U.S. minority health: A chartbook.* New York: Commonwealth Fund.

Cooper-Patrick, L., et al. (1999). Race, gender, and partnership in the patient–physician relationship. *Journal of the American Medical Association, 282,* 6, 583–589.

Coye, M., & Alvarez, D. (1999). *Medicaid managed care and cultural diversity in California.* New York: Commonwealth Fund.

Coye, M., & Alvarez, D. (2000). *Community health centers in a changing U.S. health care system* [policy brief]. New York: Commonwealth Fund. Retrieved from: http://www.cmwf.org/programs/minority/coye%Fculturaldiversity%Fbn%F311.asp.

Crane, J. A. (1997). Patient comprehension of doctor-patient communication on discharge from the emergency department. *Journal of Emergency Medicine, 15,* 1, 1–7.

Culhane-Pera, D. A., Like, R. C., Lebensohn-Chialvo, P., & Loewe, R. (2000). Multicultural curricula in family practice residencies. *Family Medicine, 32,* 167–173.

Culhane-Pera, K. A., Reif, C., Egli, E., Baker, N. J., & Kassekert, R. (1997). A curriculum for multicultural education in family medicine. *Family Medicine, 29,* 10, 719–723.

Current Population Reports. (1996). *Population of the United States by age, sex, race, and Latino origin: 1995 to 2050* (Series P25-1130). Washington, D.C.: Author.

David, R. A., & Rhee, M. (1998). The impact of language as a barrier to effective health care in an underserved urban Latino community. *Mount Sinai Journal of Medicine, 65,* 5–6, 393–397.

Del Pinal, J., & Singer, A. (1997). Generations of diversity: Latinos in the United States. *Population Bulletin, 52,* 3.

Erzinger, S. (1991). Communication between Spanish-speaking patients and their doctors in medical encounters. *Culture Medicine and Psychiatry, 15,* 91.

Fagnani, L., & Tolbert, J. (2000). *The dependence of safety net hospitals and health systems on the Medicare and Medicaid disproportionate share hospital payment programs.* Washington, D.C.: National Association of Public Hospitals and Health Systems; New York: Commonwealth Fund. Retrieved from: http://www.cmwf.org/programs/medfutur/fagnani_dependsafetynethospitals_351.asp

Fortier, J. P. (1998, June). *The development of standards for cultural and linguistic competence. Providing care to diverse populations: State strategies for promoting cultural competency in health systems.* Paper presented at the Agency for Health Care Policy and Research User Liaison Program, Charleston, SC.

Giacomini, M. K. (1996). Gender and ethnic differences in hospital-based procedure utilization in California. *Archives of Internal Medicine, 156,* 1217–1224.

Hall, A. G., Collins, K. S., & Glied, S. (1999). *Employer-sponsored health insurance: Implications for minority workers.* New York: Commonwealth Fund.

Haynes, R. B. (1976). A critical review of the "determinants" of patient compliance with therapeutic regimens. In D. L. Sackett & R. B. Haynes (Eds.), *Compliance with therapeutic regimens.* Baltimore, MD: Johns Hopkins University Press, pp. 26–39.

Health Care Financing Administration. (1999, May). *Report to the Cultural Competence Measures Review Panel.* Washington, D.C.: Abt Associates.

Hinojosa, M. (1999, June 10). *Providing care to diverse populations: State strategies for promoting cultural competency in health systems.* Paper presented at a conference in Charleston, South Carolina.

Hornberger, J., Itakura, H., & Wilson, S. R. (1997). Bridging language and cultural barriers between physicians and patients. *Public Health Report, 112,* 5, 410–417.

Iglehart, J. K. (1999). The American health system: Medicaid. *The New England Journal of Medicine, 340,* 5, 403–408.

Institute of Medicine (1999, March). *America's health care safety net: Intact but endangered.* Washington, D.C.: National Academy of Sciences.

Kaiser Permanente National Diversity Council. (1996). *A provider's handbook on culturally competent care: Latino population.* Oakland, CA: Author.

Kirkman-Liff, B., & Mondragon, D. (1991). Language of interview: Relevance for research of Southwest Hispanics. *American Journal of Public Health, 81,* 11, 1399–1404.

Komaromy, M. et al. (1996). The role of African-American and Latino physicians in providing health care for undeserved populations. *New England Journal of Medicine, 334,* 1305–1310.

Landon, B. E., & Epstein, A. M. (1999). Quality management in Medicaid managed care: A national survey of Medicaid and commercial health plans participating in the Medicaid program. *Journal of the American Medical Association, 282,* 1769–1775.

Langer, N. (1999). Culturally competent professionals in therapeutic alliances enhance patient compliance. *Journal of Health Care for the Poor and Underserved, 10,* 1, 19–26.

Leigh, W. A., Lillie-Blanton, M., Martinez, R. M., & Collins, K. S. (1999). Managed care in three states: Experiences of low-income African-Americans and Hispanics. *Inquiry, 36,* 318–331.

Like, R. C., & Steiner, R. P. (1986). Medical anthropology and the family physician. *Family Medicine, 18,* 2, 87–92.

Manson, A. (1988). Language concordance as a determinant of patient compliance and emergency room use in-patients with asthma. *Medical Care, 26,* 12, 1119–1128.

Morales, L. S., Cunningham, W. E., Brown, J. A., Liu, H., & Hays, R. D. (1999). Are Latinos less satisfied with communication by health care providers? *Journal of General Internal Medicine, 14,* 409–417.

Moy, E., & Bartman, B. A. (1995). Physicians race and care of minority and medically indigent patients. *Journal of the American Medical Association, 273,* 19, 1515–1520.

National Hispanic/Latino Health Initiative. (1993). *Public Health Reports, 108,* 534–558.

Nerenz, D. (1999, May). *New quality measures: A minority health report card.* Paper presented at the Commonwealth Fund-Harvard University Fellowship in Minority Health Policy Annual Meeting, Boston, MA.

Pérez-Stable, E. J., Napoles-Springer, A., & Miramontes, J. M. (1997). The effects of ethnicity and language on medical outcomes of patients with hypertension or diabetes. *Medical Care, 35,* 12, 1212–1219.

Quinn, K. (2000). *Working without benefits: The health insurance crisis confronting Hispanic-Americans.* New York: Commonwealth Fund.

Saha, S., Komaromy, M., Koepsell, T. D., & Bindman, A. B. (1999). Patient–physician racial concordance and the perceived quality and use of health care. *Archives of Internal Medicine, 159,* 997–1004.

Seijo, R. (1991). Language as a communication barrier in medical care for Latino patients. *Latino Journal of Behavioral Science, 13,* 363.

Stanton, A. L. (1987). Determinants of adherence to medical regimens by hypertensive patients. *Journal of Behavioral Medicine, 10,* 4, 377–394.

Stern, B. (1999, June). *Serving diverse populations: Real world examples. Providing care to diverse populations—State strategies for promoting cultural competency in health systems.* Paper presented at the Agency for Health Care Policy and Research User Liaison Program, Charleston, SC.

Stewart, A. L., Grumbach, K., Osmond, D. H., Vranizan, K., Komaromy, M., & Bindman, A. B. (1997). Primary care and patient perceptions of access to care. *Journal of Family Practice, 44,* 2, 177–185.

Stiles, W. B. et al. (1979). [Patient–physician communication and patient satisfaction with medical interviews from working papers]. Unpublished raw data, University of North Carolina at Chapel Hill, Health Services Research Center.

United States Bureau of the Census, Census 2000 Redistricting Data (P.L. 94-171), Summary File for states.

United States Department of Health and Human Services and the Health Resources Services Administration. (1998, July). *Access for all: Barriers to health care for racial and ethnic minorities. Access, workforce diversity, and cultural competence.* (Town Hall Meeting, Boston, MA).

United States Department of Health and Human Services. (1998, September). *Eliminating racial and ethnic disparities in health.* Potomac, MD: Author.

United States Department of Health and Human Services and Grantmakers in Health. (1998, February). *Racial and ethnic disparities in health: Response to the President's Initiative on Race.* Washington, D.C.: Authors.

United States Department of Health and Human Services and the Commonwealth Fund (1999). *Performance measurements in managed care and its role in eliminating racial and ethnic disparities in health.* (Summary meeting). Washington, D.C., and New York: Authors.

Woolhandler, S., & Himmelstein, D. U. (1991). The deteriorating administrative efficiency of the U.S. health care system. *New England Journal of Medicine, 324,* 18, 1253–1258.

PART TWO

## LATINO LIFE STAGES AND HEALTH

CHAPTER FOUR

# THE EARLY YEARS

## The Health of Children and Youth

Glenn Flores, Ruth Enid Zambrana

Latino children are the largest minority group and have the fastest growing poverty rates of all children in the United States (United States Bureau of the Census, 1999a). In 1996, there were twelve million Latino children in the United States, compared with 50.8 million White and 11.4 million African American children. Latino children currently constitute more than 15 percent of the total U.S. population of children, and 21 percent are under fourteen years of age (United States Bureau of the Census, 1999b). Both Latino (36 percent) and African American (37 percent) children are three times more likely to be poor than White children (11 percent) (United States Bureau of the Census, 1999b). Latino children in single female-headed households (31 percent) are also more likely than their African American or White counterparts to be poor (United States Bureau of the Census, 1999b).

Overall, Puerto Rican children are the poorest children both within Latino groups and across racial and ethnic groups. Puerto Rican children, both in Puerto Rico and in the United States, are especially affected by poverty: two in three (67 percent) are poor in Puerto Rico, while more than half (53 percent) live below the poverty level in the United States. Two in five (40 percent) Latino children in the United States are poor (National Council of La Raza, 1998). Although 87 percent of Latino children are U.S. citizens, either born or naturalized, limited accessibility exists to primary and preventive health services (Zuvekas & Weinick, 1999; Commonwealth Fund, 2000; American College of Physicians, 2000).

Good health for all children and youth is one of society's priorities. Adverse health events in childhood can result in premature death, lifelong disabilities, chronic diseases, preventable pain and suffering, increased societal costs and use of resources, and even multigenerational transmission of morbidity. Latino children (zero to eighteen years of age) in the United States are at extremely high risk for adverse health events. Latino children experience a disproportionate share of morbidity and suboptimal health status, and they often underutilize health services. Even after adjusting for family income and parental education, Latino children are significantly more likely than White children to have suboptimal health status, spend more days in bed for illness, and make fewer physician visits (Flores, Bauchner, Feinstein, & Nguyen, 1999).

Data on the health needs of Latino children and families are sparse due to the limited collection of state and national data by ethnic-specific identifiers (Zambrana & Carter-Pokras, 2001). Although data are usually presented in the aggregate for Latino children, Latino children are highly concentrated primarily in ten states: California, Texas, Arizona, New Mexico, New York, New Jersey, Colorado, Illinois, Florida, and Massachusetts (United States Bureau of the Census, 1999b). National and state data systems are limited in their collection of Latino child health indicators, particularly with regard to trend analysis, gender differences, Latino subpopulation data, and emerging issues such as environmental and immigrant health. Geographic clustering of Latinos suggests regional differences. However, because state-specific data are not readily available, data are derived predominantly from national data sets, studies conducted in specific states, and a comprehensive literature review. When available, differences by subgroup are noted and comparisons by race and ethnicity are also described.

The purposes of this chapter are to (1) critically examine the major health and health care issues confronting Latino children by developmental age—preschool, elementary school age, and adolescents; (2) examine interventions that have been shown to improve Latino child health; and (3) identify policy action points for improving the health services of Latino children.

## Access to Use of Health Services

Access to health care services is crucial to maintaining good health. A consistent theme that emerges in the literature on Latino children is their lack of access to care due to lack of insurance and lower quality of care once they enter the system. Because Latino children are dependent on their parents for both financial access and the ability to negotiate the health care system to ensure a favorable health outcome, Latino child health status must be examined within a family context as well as within an institutional context.

Problems with obtaining access to health care and lack of insurance coverage or inadequate coverage continue to be more severe among Latino children and adolescents than among the young of any other racial or ethnic group nationwide (Valdez, Giachello, Rodriguez-Trías, Gómez, & De La Rocha, 1993).

Latino children are more than twice as likely to not have health insurance than White children and about one-and-a-half times more likely to not have health insurance than African American children. Because Latino children are disproportionately poor and their parents are most likely to work in secondary labor markets that do not provide employment-linked health benefits (Halfon, Wood, Valdez, Pereyra, & Duan, 1997; Commonwealth Fund, 2000), Latino children are the least likely to have health insurance coverage. Mexican ethnicity (whether self-identified as Mexican American or Mexican-born) are the most likely to be uninsured compared to the total population and other Latino subgroups (Holl, Szilagyi, Rodewald, Byrd, & Weitzman, 1995). Overall, Latino children have one of the lowest rates of total private (42 percent) and employer-based insurance coverage and are at greatest risk of losing employee coverage, with a 16 percent reduction documented between 1988 and 1992 (Newacheck, Hughes, & Cisternas, 1995). Latino children consistently have higher rates of public insurance (consisting primarily of Medicaid) than White children, but lower rates than African American children (Guendelman & Schwalbe, 1986; Cornelius, 1993; Newacheck, Hughes, & Cisternas, 1995).

Evidence-based literature shows the following as persistent barriers to access in the last two decades: lack of a regular source of care (Guendelman, 1985; Cornelius, 1993; Lieu, Newacheck, & McManus, 1993; Halfon, Wood, Valdez, Pereyra, & Duan, 1997; Kass, Weinick, & Monheit, 1999), least likely to have physician contact (Guendelman & Schwalbe, 1986), lack of English proficiency (Wood, Hidalgo, Prihoda, & Kromer, 1993; Lewis, Rachelefsky, Lewis, Leake, & Richards, 1994), provider attitudes (Mikhail, 1994), excessive waiting time in clinics (Cornelius, 1993; Flores & Vega, 1998), transportation problems (Wood, Hidalgo, Prihoda, & Kromer, 1993; Lewis, Rachelefsky, Lewis, Leake, & Richards, 1994; Moore & Hepworth, 1994), decreased preventive screening opportunities, and receipt of proportionally fewer prescriptions (Flores, 2000a). Individually or in combination, these factors can impede preventive efforts and delay or compromise the outcome of clinical interventions. Table 4.1 provides a summary of those factors that have been consistently reported in the literature to be such barriers.

Lack of health insurance coverage is also highly associated with lack of a regular source of care (American College of Physicians, 2000). However, Latino children, even those with insurance, were less likely to have a regular source of care, including children with chronic illnesses (Newacheck, Stoddard, & McManus, 1993), asthma (Wood, Hidalgo, Prihoda, & Kromer, 1993), and those visiting pediatric emergency departments (Zambrana, Ell, Dorrington, Wachsman, & Hodge, 1994). In 1996, Latino children (17.2 percent), were more likely than African American children (12.6 percent) and three times more likely than White children (6 percent) to lack a usual source of care (Kass, Weinick, & Monheit, 1999). Lack of a regular source of care was a significant predictor of delayed diphtheria, tetanus, and pertussis (DTP) immunizations in Mexican

## TABLE 4.1.   SUMMARY OF ACCESS BARRIERS TO HEALTH CARE FOR LATINO CHILDREN IDENTIFIED IN THE REVIEW OF THE LITERATURE.

| Barrier | Supportive Evidence[a] |
|---|---|
| Health insurance | |
| Absence | ++ |
| Episodic | + |
| Low proportion of private insurance coverage | ++ |
| Loss of employee-based coverage | + |
| Poverty | ++ |
| Geography | |
| Area of residence (inner city/suburban/rural) | E |
| Region of residence | + |
| Parent educational attainment | ++ |
| Parent beliefs | + |
| Use of home remedies | + |
| Source of parent advice on child's illness | + |
| Folk medicine practices | E |
| Immigration status | E |
| Duration of parent residency in United States | 0 |
| Child's age | 0 |
| Child's gender | 0 |
| Family size | E |
| Parents' marital status (less than two parents living in the household) | E |
| Major Latino subpopulations | + |
| Provider practices and behaviors | |
| Reduced screening | + |
| Missed vaccination opportunities | + |
| Decreased likelihood of receiving prescriptions | ++ |
| Suboptimal management plans | + |
| Inadequate communication/patient education | ++ |
| Negative attitudes of staff | + |
| No regular source of care | ++ |
| Type of practice setting | E |
| Excessive waiting times | + |
| Transportation | + |
| Acculturation | E |
| Cultural differences | + |
| Language problems | + |

[a]Key:   + = evidence is present but supported by multiple studies, with or without control groups;
++ = evidence is strong, supported by multiple studies, usually with relevant control groups;
E = evidence is equivocal;
0 = no evidence.

*Source:* Adapted from G. Flores and L. R. Vega (1998).

American children (Gergen, Ezzati, & Russell, 1988). Among children under the age of 18, Latinos (7.8 percent) were almost twice as likely as African American children (4.2 percent) and close to three times as likely as White children (2.9 percent) to be in fair-to-poor health (Kass, Weinick, & Monheit, 1999). Thus inability to have access to care and a regular source of care places Latino children at risk for less preventive screening and detection services, more lost school days, and potential health problems in adulthood. However, access to the health care system does not ensure that appropriate services will be provided, nor that the child's health will improve.

More recent work has closely examined factors in the context of the health care institution that adversely affect the well-being of Latino children's health. These parental and institutional barriers include inability of the parent to communicate with the provider due to limited English-language proficiency, ethnic-specific parental beliefs, and attitudes associated with low socioeconomic status and possibly difficulties with literacy, as well as unhelpful provider attitudes.

Limited English-language proficiency can have a substantial impact on multiple aspects of Latino children's health outcomes. For example, children whose parents primarily or exclusively speak Spanish were significantly more likely to be in fair or poor health (by parental rating), less likely to have a usual source of medical care, and less likely to have visited a health care provider in the past year (Kirkman-Liff & Mondragón, 1991). Latino mothers report that staff not speaking Spanish was a major barrier to obtaining health care for their children in the past year (Zambrana, Ell, Dorrington, Wachsman, & Hodge, 1994). In another study, mothers of Latino children with asthma reported that limited English-language skills (25 percent) combined with attitudes of physicians and nurses (31 percent) presented difficulties in talking to physicians about managing their child's illness (Lewis, Rachelefsky, Lewis, Leake, & Richards, 1994). Among Latino mothers at an urban primary care clinic, 11 percent said that they had deferred a medical visit for their child because the doctors and nurses did not understand Latino culture (Flores, Abreu, Olivar, & Kastner, 1998). Lack of confidence in the health care staff was cited by 31 percent of Latino mothers in a pediatric emergency department as a major barrier to obtaining care for their child in the past year (Zambrana, Ell, Dorrington, Wachsman, & Hodge, 1994).

Since the majority of providers are English-speaking only and few interpreters are easily available in health care settings, parents with limited English-language proficiency are not able to effectively communicate the actual symptoms or the clinical history of their child's problem, nor can they understand the provider's instructions for ameliorating the conditions and follow-up for referral recommendations. Patient-provider communication in Latino families is oftentimes exacerbated by the low-income status of parents, fear and mistrust of providers, technical language and subsequent lack of familiarity of parents with medical terminology, and ethnic-specific parental beliefs and attitudes regarding childhood illnesses (Flores, Abreu, Olivar, & Kastner, 1998). Although limited English-language ability represents a barrier to patient-provider communication, ethnic disparities persist after data are adjusted for the patient's language (Wasserman, Croft, & Brotherton, 1992; Wood, Hidalgo, Prihoda, & Kromer, 1993; Hahn, 1995).

Equally important and powerful predictors of Latino child health can be the provider's knowledge and experience with this group and his or her attitudes regarding Latinos. Several studies show that provider attitudes can compromise quality of care for Latino children. In other words, these attitudes may impede a provider from recommending the best treatment possible for the condition due to concerns regarding cost to the family or their ability to effectively use the recommended treatment. Ethnic disparities in vision screening and receipt of prescription medications are two examples. A nationwide study of vision screening at 102 pediatric practices found that Latino children (56 percent) were screened by pediatricians significantly less often than were White children (Wasserman, Croft, & Brotherton, 1992). Among children aged six to seventeen years who had made an outpatient physician visit, only 52 percent of African American and 53 percent of Latino children received prescriptions, significantly less than the 66 percent of White children who did. Significant differences were also found among these groups in the mean number of prescribed medicines, with Latino (mean prescriptions = 1.5) and African American (1.7) children receiving fewer prescriptions than did White children (2.4). In a study of preschool children hospitalized for asthma, Wood, Hidalgo, Prihoda, & Kromer (1993) found that Latino children were seventeen times less likely than White children to be prescribed a nebulizer for home use at discharge. The reasons why providers may deliver lower quality of care to Latino children remain unexplained.

## A Developmental View of Latino Child Health Status

Multiple factors are associated with the morbidity and mortality patterns of Latino children and youth at different developmental stages. These include disproportionate numbers of families and children in poverty, formidable barriers to access to health care, and frequent residence in urban environments associated with disproportionate morbidity, suboptimal health, and underutilization of services. In this section we present available health information on infants and preschool children, school-age children, and adolescents. What is known about morbidity and mortality patterns is presented with particular attention to immunizations, tuberculosis, developmental conditions, child welfare, chronic diseases, unintentional injuries, and adolescent health problems. Environmental health hazards are discussed in a later section. Many of the issues described here affect more than one development stage unless otherwise noted.

## Infants and Preschool Children: Zero to Five Years of Age

Preventive health behaviors are usually practiced by adults and learned by children at an early age. Children aged zero to five years are most in need of well-baby checkups, immunizations, early exposure to nutritional foods and good eating habits, stimulation for physical and cognitive development, and a safe environment to prevent intentional or unintentional injury. Thus, these early years are an important time in which adults should strive to ensure the development of healthy behavior and access to preventive health services that promote a "healthy start" for the new generation of Latinos.

*Immunizations.* Latino children are less likely to be fully immunized than White children. Only 71 percent of Latino children are fully vaccinated (four doses of DTP vaccine, three doses of polio vaccine, one dose of measles-containing vaccine, and three doses of Hib [*Haemophilus influenzae* type b] vaccine) by age two compared to 80 percent of White children and 78 percent of African American children (United States Department of Health and Human Services, 1991). Several factors are associated with inadequate immunization status among Latino children. These include being other than the firstborn child, maternal report of poor child health status, inadequate maternal prenatal care, the mother living in a household without a close family member present, multiple family moves within a child's lifetime (Prislin, Suarez, Simspon, & Dyer, 1998), insurance coverage (Guendelman & Schwalbe, 1986; Gergen, Ezzati, & Russell, 1988) and parental level of acculturation (Waterman et al., 1996; Anderson, Wood, & Sherbourne, 1997; Prislin, Suarez, Simspon, & Dyer, 1998).

Two recent studies show that less acculturated mothers are more likely to have better-immunized children. In a study of mostly Mexican American families, data showed that with each point increase on a five-point acculturation scale (based on language use, ethnic identity, and generation status), the odds for inadequate immunization increased by a factor of 1.3 (Prislin, Suarez, Simspon, & Dyer, 1998). Similarly, a study that representatively sampled all Latino households in Texas (92 percent of which were Mexican American) found that the odds of inadequate immunization increased by 1.3 for each point increase on the aforementioned acculturation scale (Waterman et al., 1996). The least-acculturated mothers were 2.6 times more likely to have their child adequately immunized than were the most acculturated. Increased maternal acculturation level was associated with less positive parental attitudes toward immunization, a diminished sense of parental responsibility for getting children immunized, and a stronger perception that cost and time were barriers to children's immunization.

*Tuberculosis.* Recent data revealed that Latinos have the highest number of newly diagnosed tuberculosis cases (650) of any U.S. ethnic group of children under the age of fifteen years old. In 1994, 39 percent of all reported childhood tuberculosis cases in the United States occurred among Latinos, and the tuberculosis case rate for Latino children was more than thirteen times higher than that of White children. National data (Ussery, Valway, & McKenna, 1996) and local data (Watchi, Kahlstrom, Vachon, & Barnes, 1998), confirm that the majority of Latino children diagnosed with tuberculosis were born in the United States, suggesting that ongoing transmission in U.S. communities is a major concern. Children born in a Latin American country account for the largest proportion of foreign-born childhood tuberculosis cases. In 1994, 56 percent of foreign-born children diagnosed with tuberculosis had a Latin American country of origin, with Mexico by far accounting for the highest proportion. About half of all foreign-born children with tuberculosis were born in Mexico, and between 1986 and 1994 the proportion of foreign-born cases from Mexico rose dramatically, from 30 percent to 48 percent, due to increases in immigration.

***Developmental Conditions.***  Early screening and detection of developmental lags and of hearing and speech loss are crucial to the healthy growth and development of a child. Yet developmental issues for Latino children are absent from the literature with few exceptions (Garcia-Coll, 1990). Analysis of data from the Hispanic Health and Nutrition Examination Survey (HHANES [1982–1984]) revealed that Puerto Rican children have higher prevalence than Mexican American children of chronic developmental conditions (11 percent versus 7 percent, respectively), functional limitations (13 percent versus 8 percent), medical diagnoses (7 percent versus 3 percent), and developmental problems by parental report (20 percent versus 13 percent) (Arcia, Keyes, & Gallagher, 1994). Although the prevalence of moderate-to-severe functional limitations among Mexican American children (2 percent) is about the same as national estimates for all children (2.3 percent), the prevalence among Puerto Rican children is substantially higher (7 percent). Data for other Latino subgroups of children were not examined.

A second analysis of these data showed subgroup differences in presence of developmental conditions and parental perceptions of poor child health status (Arcia, 1998). A child currently having one or more developmental conditions (including mental retardation, a coordination problem, muscle weakness or paralysis, convulsions, a speech problem, and a psychological or behavioral problem) was significantly more likely to be rated in poor health by Mexican American parents than by Puerto Rican parents. Although the author concluded that Puerto Rican parents might be less likely to seek needed health care for children with developmental conditions, additional studies are needed to assess the severity of developmental conditions and the reasons for such differences in reported parental perceptions.

***Oral Health Care.***  Access to oral health care is a significant problem for poor Latino children. Regular screening and preventive services reduce dental problems, but such services are not always available to those children who most need them (Center for Medicaid and State Operations, 1999). Recent data show that close to one-third of Latino children two to four years of age have dental corrosion to their permanent teeth and almost 50 percent of children five to seventeen years of age have dental cavities (United States Department of Health and Human Services, 1999). National Health Interview Survey data show that only 53 percent of Latino children aged two years and over have accessed preventive dental services within the past year, compared to African American children, 56 percent, and White children, 68 percent. In 1996, only one in five children received a preventive dental service among those eligible under the Medicaid Early and Preventive Screening, Diagnosis, and Treatment (EPSDT) program (National Center for Health Statistics, 2000). Untreated tooth decay and dental caries impair the overall quality of life for children and youth, can cause disorders of eating, learning, and speech, and are responsible for fifty-two million lost school hours per year (Center for Medicaid and State Operations, 1999; National Center for Health Statistics, 2000). Although the percentage of adolescents affected by dental caries has been decreasing, substantial racial, ethnic, and socioeconomic disparities persist.

***Speech and Hearing Loss Conditions.***  Recent work demonstrates that Latino children who attend bilingual preschool, compared with those who remain at home, show equivalent gains in Spanish language development but greater gains in English proficiency (Winsler, Díaz, Espinosa, & Rodríguez, 1999). In a study of low-income Mexican American children, researchers found that the preschool children's Spanish proficiency matched that of their stay-at-home counterparts, but the preschoolers' English expressive skills improved significantly over time. These findings conclusively refute a prior finding that "language minority" children attending bilingual or monolingual English preschools rapidly lose native language proficiency, resulting in disruption of parent-child communication and placing the child on a high-risk developmental course (Wong Fillmore, 1991). Observation and noted empirical work suggest that detection of speech disorders may be hindered due to Spanish being the first language of many young Latino children.

Factors associated with childhood hearing loss appear to differ by Latino subgroup (Lee, Gomez-Marin, & Lee, 1997). Using HHANES (1982–1984) data reveals that the prevalence of hearing loss among Cuban children in the United States was greatest among those with parents with less than seven years of education and was associated with falling below the expected grade level. Hearing loss prevalence for Mexican American children was associated with being uninsured and was greatest among those with parents with less than seven years of education. None of the factors analyzed were significantly associated with hearing loss among Puerto Rican children. Interestingly, in a study of stress and coping among the parents of deaf children, Latino parents scored significantly higher than African American parents on six of eight measures (Mapp & Hudson, 1997).

Latino parents were found to score higher on "confrontive" coping, seeking social support, "planful" problem solving, and positive appraisal.

**Child Welfare.**  Child welfare refers to the physical, mental, and social well-being of a child and it is highly associated with family and community resources. According to the National Committee for Prevention of Child Abuse, approximately 10 percent of all abused children are Latino (National Research Council, 1993). Nationally, close to half of all substantiated child welfare cases are for neglect and about 25 percent for physical abuse (National Research Council, 1993b). About 57 percent of protective services referrals among Latino children are for neglect, 19 percent are for physical abuse, and 10 percent each are for sexual and emotional abuse (Ortega, Guillean, & Gutierrez-Najera, 1996). Multiple factors are associated with child abuse and neglect, including poverty, poor parenting skills, substance use, and economic stress (Child Welfare League of America, 1999). Lack of adequate economic resources (such as health insurance) and social support systems often hinder the ability of Latino parents to seek mental health and family support services.

For many Latino parents there are multiple barriers to accessing social services, including fear of removal, unavailable, inaccessible, or unacceptable service; lack of Spanish-speaking personnel and/or written materials; lack of a philosophy of family support; and lack of cultural congruence and competence with this population (Ortega, Guillean, & Gutierrez-Najera, 1996). A sizable proportion of children in the child welfare system come from families with psychosocial disabilities, and many of these children are special needs children with psychosocial, developmental, behavioral, and health problems of their own (Simms, Freundlich, Battistelli, & Kaufman, 1999; Santiago, 1995). Although few studies on child welfare have focused on Latino children, research suggests that there are notable disparities in the representation of Latino children in the child welfare system in states with large Latino populations (Zambrana & Capello, in press).

Current work on Latino child welfare is limited, but some data suggest that sexual abuse is lower among Latino children. In a Los Angeles study, the prevalence of childhood sexual assault was lower among Latinos (3 percent) as compared with Whites (9 percent) (Siegel, Sorenson, Golding, Burnam, & Stein, 1987). Latino respondents completing interviews in Spanish had a lower prevalence of childhood sexual assault (1 percent) than Latinos completing interviews in English (5 percent), suggesting that less acculturation might be protective. In one Los Angeles school-based clinic, at a high school where 95 percent of the students are Latino, 7 percent of the 922 students seen reported being sexually assaulted, and 89 percent of these victims were females (McGurk, Cárdenas, & Aldelman, 1993). Frequent feelings of depression were mentioned by 84 percent of students victimized by sexual assaults, and 47 percent had considered suicide at least once.

Almost 80 percent of child abuse and neglect victims are under seven years of age. Child maltreatment crosses all racial, ethnic, and class lines, but families living in poverty (which disproportionately affects Latino families) are more likely to have their children removed and placed in child welfare settings and to have parental rights terminated (Kamerman & Kahn, 1993; Vincent, 1999; White, Courtney, & Fifield, 1998). Thus, interventions to reduce poverty in the postnatal and early preschool years have the potential to significantly decrease abuse and neglect among young Latino children.

## School-Age Children: Ages Six to Thirteen Years

The school-age years represent an important developmental period for Latino children. Acute and chronic health conditions can contribute to a low sense of control in their environment, affecting cognitive and intellectual development, and undetected health conditions can hamper activities of daily living as well as participation in school and extracurricular activities. Although limited research exists on this age group, the emerging areas of import include nutrition and physical activity, chronic diseases, oral health, and mental health.

***Obesity, Physical Activity, and Nutrition.*** Recent national estimates of overweight in children aged six to eleven years indicate that Mexican American boys have the highest prevalence of obesity (19 percent), exceeding the proportions for both African Americans (15 percent) and Whites (13 percent) (Centers for Disease Control and Prevention, 1997); for Latino girls of that age, obesity prevalence is 16 percent, greater than the prevalence among Whites (12 percent) and exceeded only by figures for African Americans (18 percent) (Centers for Disease Control and Prevention, 1997).

A study of low-income Mexican American children of elementary school age showed that 27 percent of girls and 23 percent of boys were obese (using age- and gender-specific body-mass indices [BMIs]) (Suminski, Poston, & Foreyt, 1999). For all gender and age groups, the mean BMIs of Mexican American children exceeded those of a national reference group of age-matched peers. Compared with this national reference group, the mean BMI was 14 percent greater for Mexican American boys and 20 percent greater for Mexican American girls. Children at risk for developing obesity can be identified at an early age. Children with a BMI greater than or equal to 23.7 in kindergarten had a 91 percent chance of being obese in the fifth grade. Overweight children are at risk of developing chronic health problems in adulthood such as diabetes and heart disease. Ethnic-specific preventive and intervention measures in early childhood require identification and investigation in future studies.

***Chronic Diseases.*** Data indicate that there are important subgroup differences in the prevalence of chronic medical conditions among Latino children. In an analysis of data from the HHANES (1982–1984), mainland Puerto Rican children had the highest prevalence of chronic medical conditions at 6 percent, compared with 4 percent for Mexican Americans and 2 percent for Cubans in the United States (Garwick, Kohrman, Wolman, & Blum, 1998; Mendoza et al., 1991).

In a small qualitative study of families with children who have chronic diseases (Treviño, Marshal, Hale, Rodriguez, Baker, & Gómez, 1999), Latino (and African American) parents suggested that the cultural relevance of services and programs needed to be improved. (See their further suggestions in the discussion of asthma, to follow.)

*Diabetes.* An extremely high prevalence of risk factors for future type 2 diabetes mellitus was noted in a study of low-income Mexican American nine-year-olds in Texas (Treviño, Marshal, Hale, Rodriguez, Baker, & Gómez, 1999). A family history of diabetes mellitus, an indicator of genetic predisposition, was high, with 60 percent of the children having a first- or second-degree relative diagnosed with diabetes. Prevalence of overweight, another predisposing factor, was 21 percent for boys and 18 percent for girls, about double the national average in each case. Unacceptable physical fitness scores were noted for 38 percent of the children, and the mean percentage of body fat was substantially greater than national reference means. Study children also reported eating higher than recommended percentages of energy from fat and from saturated fat, and about half the recommended daily fruit and vegetable intake (Treviño, Marshal, Hale, Rodriguez, Baker, & Gómez, 1999).

*Asthma.* Of an estimated half-million Latino children who have symptoms of asthma, two thirds are Puerto Rican (Carter-Pokras & Gergen, 1993). The percentage of families with at least one asthmatic child was 24.5 percent for Latinos (mainly Puerto Rican), 17.7 percent for African Americans, and 9.6 percent for Whites (Beckett, Belanger, Gent, Holford, & Leaderer, 1996). Puerto Rican children have the highest prevalence of active asthma (11 percent) of any U.S. ethnic or racial group of children, exceeding by far the prevalence for African Americans (6 percent) and Whites (3 percent)(Carter-Pokras & Gergen, 1993). These national data also illustrate the importance of analysis by Latino subgroup, as Mexican American children were found to have the lowest prevalence of active asthma (3 percent) and Cuban children had a prevalence (5 percent) comparable to that of African Americans (Carter-Pokras & Gergen, 1993). Other studies from New York City (Colp et al., 1990) and Connecticut (Crain, Weiss, Bijur, Hersh, Westbrook, & Stein, 1994) confirm that Puerto Rican children have the highest prevalence of asthma, whether active or lifetime prevalence (diagnosed asthma without symptoms or impairment in the past twelve months) is considered.

The reasons for such dramatic subgroup differences in asthma prevalence have not been determined. Limited evidence suggests that the increased asthma risk among Puerto Rican children may in part be related to genetically determined differences in the inflammatory response. Studies have shown an increased risk of asthma among Puerto Rican children with abnormal variants of $alpha_1$-antitrypsin, a protein involved in inflammatory reactions (Colp et al., 1990; Colp, Pappas, Moran, & Lieberman, 1993). Studies have also demonstrated that Mexican American children have better lung function than their White and

African American counterparts, and researchers have hypothesized that Mexican American children's low asthma prevalence might be associated with larger airways that are less likely to wheeze (Hsu et al., 1979; Dodge, 1983; Carter-Pokras & Gergen, 1993). Among parents of Latino children with asthma, the main reported barriers in the management of their child's condition was inability to afford medicines (61 percent) (Lewis, Rachelefsky, Lewis, Leake, & Richards, 1994), payment for medicines (73 percent), and payment for visits to the doctor (Wood, Hidalgo, Prihoda, & Kromer, 1993). Uninsured Latino children are 1.3 times less likely than insured children to receive medical treatment for asthma (American College of Physicians, 2000) and 6.3 times more likely not to have taken a beta-antagonist inhaler or any anti-inflammatory medication before hospitalization (Wood, Hidalgo, Prihoda, & Kromer, 1993).

For Latino families with children who have chronic diseases, multiple barriers exist in accessing culturally appropriate and high-quality care. In one study Latino (and African American) parents reported on what would help them to better manage their child's condition. Specifically, the parents stated the following: include children from diverse backgrounds in teaching materials, provide resources in various languages, improve Latino interpreter availability, and disseminate information in communities of color (Garwick, Kohrman, Wolman, & Blum, 1998). Very limited information overall is available on the prevalence of chronic diseases among Latino children, etiology of disease, and how children and parents manage the chronic condition. Research attention needs to be focused on the risk factors that contribute to childhood diseases as well as to institutional responsiveness in helping Latino parents to manage their child's condition.

*Unintentional Injury.* Latino children are five times more likely to be involved in unintentional injury (Agran, Winn, Anderson, & Del Valle, 1996). For Latino children, pedestrian injury, motor vehicle accidents, drowning, and poisoning are the leading causes of morbidity and mortality (Agran, Winn, Anderson, & Del Valle, 1996). In a case-control study of primarily Mexican American children, eight factors were significantly associated with pedestrian injury resulting in hospitalization: poverty, household crowding, parental unemployment, one or more moves in the past year, the child does not speak English, the father does not speak English, the mother does not read well, and the father does not read well (Agran, Winn, Anderson, & Del Valle, 1998). Brown, Bell, Conrad, Howland, and Lang (1997) report that deaths from motor vehicle accidents are highest in states with high concentrations of Latinos, suggesting that social and economic factors are important. Using mortality data from the National Center for Health Statistics and the Census, researchers found that Latino children five to twelve years of age had a death rate 72 percent higher than the rate for their White counterparts (five per billion vehicle miles) and exceeded only by the rate for African American children (fourteen per billion vehicle miles) (Baker, Braver, Chen, Pantula, & Massie, 1998).

Poisoning is another leading cause of injury and hospitalization in Latino children (Agran, Winn, Anderson, & Del Valle, 1996). Poisoning may be more frequent among Latino children because many warning labels are in English and may be poorly understood by Latino parents who speak limited English. Latino families with children are less likely than non-Latino families with children to be aware of poison control centers and to keep ipecac (an over-the-counter medication to induce vomiting) in the house in case of poisoning (Agran, Winn, Anderson, & Del Valle, 1996). An ethnographic study of Mexican American families in California revealed that children are exposed to potential poisoning agents in 80 percent of homes, including bleach, cleansing powder, rubbing alcohol, and oven cleaner (Mull, Agran, Winn, & Anderson, 1999). Unintentional injury remains a significant concern for Latino children due to environmental conditions in which they live, stressors their parents confront, and lack of access to quality health services.

***Mental Health.*** Very little research has been conducted on the mental health of Latino children. Evidence from discharge data in California on children of elementary school age reveal that Latinos are significantly less likely than Whites and African Americans to be hospitalized for mental illness (Chabra, Chávez, & Harris, 1999). White and African American children were both about five times more likely than Latino children to be hospitalized for any mental health diagnosis. These findings persisted even after data were adjusted for Medicaid status. For all seven specific mental illness diagnostic categories, Latino children were also significantly less likely to be hospitalized. For example, compared with White children, Latino children were eight times less likely to be hospitalized for anxiety disorders, nine times less likely to be hospitalized for impulse control disorders, and eleven times less likely to be hospitalized for bipolar disorders. These patterns of underutilization of inpatient and outpatient mental health care among Latino children are consistent with reports of underutilization among Latinos adults (see Chapter Seven). Data suggest that culturally and economically accessible mental health services for Latino children are severely limited (United States Department of Health and Human Services, 1999).

Other research indicates that Latino children, indeed, have a higher prevalence and severity of certain psychopathologies. Among children five to twelve years old referred to a New York City outpatient child psychiatry clinic, investigators found that significantly higher proportions of Latinos than African Americans presented with morbid depression, phobias and fears, anxiety and panic, school refusal, and disturbances of relationships with other children (Canino, Gould, Prupis, & Shaffer, 1986). Although these disparities could be attributed to a lower prevalence of severe psychopathology among Latino children, the researchers argue that barriers related to ethnicity, culture, language, and socioeconomic status may play major roles. The outcome of untreated child and parental mental health problems all too often contributes to increased mental distress during adolescence.

## Adolescents: Ages Thirteen to Eighteen Years

Early adolescence is a critical transition period for Latino youth, characterized by risk taking and efforts to achieve increased independence. In these formative years, experiences of violence or abuse, risky sexual behaviors, access to health care, and supportive relationships can either enhance or undermine teen health, as well as shape the quality of life in years to come (Schoen, Davis, Collins, Greenberg, Des Roches, & Abrams, 1997). Recent data show a cluster of risky behaviors for Latino children and adolescents that may have important associations with patterns of morbidity and mortality. Threats to the health of Latino adolescents include pregnancy, sexually transmitted diseases (STDs), depression, substance use, and violence.

*Alcohol, Tobacco, and Other Drugs.* Multiple studies document high rates of illicit drug use, alcohol consumption, and tobacco use among Latino adolescents. Almost one-fourth of Latinos in tenth grade report heavy drinking and illicit drug use in the past thirty days, a proportion comparable to that of Whites and significantly higher than that of African Americans (Johnston, O'Malley, & Bachman, 1998). A 1997 national survey of adolescent girls found that Latinos and Whites were more likely than African Americans and Asian Americans to engage in risky behaviors (smoking cigarettes, consuming alcohol, using illicit drugs, bingeing and purging, or not exercising) (Schoen, Davis, Collins, Greenberg, Des Roches, & Abrams, 1997). Analysis by Latino subgroup of HHANES data on adolescents reveals that Mexican Americans (30 percent) and Puerto Ricans (28 percent) more often reported illicit drug use than did Cubans (16 percent), whereas the prevalence of alcohol consumption was roughly equivalent (15 percent, 12 percent, and 16 percent, respectively) (Sokol-Katz & Ulbrich, 1992).

Factors associated with present and future alcohol consumption were revealed in a survey of 1,410 Latino seventh graders in New York City (Epstein, Botvin, & Diaz, 1999). Increased alcohol consumption per drinking occasion was significantly associated with most friends drinking, siblings drinking, smoking cigarettes, marijuana use, finding it easy to obtain alcohol, and getting in trouble in the past month. Factors significantly associated with intent to drink in the future included most friends drinking, the mother drinking, getting into trouble in the past month, smoking cigarettes, and finding it easy to obtain alcohol.

The prevalence of smoking cigarettes among Latino adolescents is second only to that of White teens. Data from the National Longitudinal Survey of Youth reveal a 20-percent lifetime prevalence of cigarette smoking among adolescents, compared with 16 percent among African Americans and 27 percent among Whites (Griesler & Kandel, 1998). National findings from the Teenage Attitudes and Practices Surveys indicate that the factors associated with smoking initiation among Latinos—having friends who smoke, and positive attitudes and beliefs toward smoking—are similar to those for Whites and African Americans (Cowdery, Fitzhugh, & Wang, 1997).

*Sex and Sexuality.* The age of onset for sexual intercourse for Latino adolescents falls between that of African Americans and Whites: by the age of seventeen, 50 percent of Latino adolescents report having intercourse compared to age sixteen for African Americans and age eighteen for Whites. Latino males tend to initiate sex at 13.9 years of age, some two years earlier than Latino girls (Sonenstein, Stewart, Lindberg, Pernas, & Williams, 1997). Mexican American males are not significantly different from White males as regards the age of first sexual intercourse. Latina adolescents report an average age of fifteen for initiating sexual intercourse, with Mexican American Latinas starting slightly older, at age sixteen (Day, 1992). Latinas were the least sexually experienced of all gender and race groups. Among Mexican American and White female adolescents, White girls had had two or three partners, compared to one among the Mexican American teens (de Anda, Becerra, & Fielder, 1990). However, Latina adolescents are twice as likely as Whites to give birth, are less likely to be informed about human sexuality and birth control, and are less likely to use condoms during intercourse (Mayden, Castro, & Annitto, 1999). This highlights the importance of considering race and ethnicity in assessing sexual behavior trends.

Every year approximately three million adolescents acquire an STD. The most serious of these infections is HIV, with subsequent development of AIDS. Although Latinos comprise only 12 percent of the thirteen- to nineteen-year-old age group, they account for 18 percent of the cases of AIDS reported for this age group (Mayden, Castro, & Annitto, 1999). Youth Risk Behavior Surveillance data from California reveal higher incidence of HIV infection and AIDS among Latino boys and girls between thirteen and nineteen years of age than among their African American or White peers. Further, the higher prevalence of STDs among Latino adolescents suggest that they experience multiple barriers to quality STD prevention services, including lack of insurance, lack of transportation, discomfort with health education services designed for English-speaking teens, concerns about confidentiality, and cultural values (Mayden, Castro, & Annitto, 1999).

Contraceptive use at first intercourse has been on the rise. In 1982, 48 percent of adolescents reported some form of contraceptive use compared to 76 percent of adolescents in 1995 (Abma, Chandra, Mosher, Peterson, & Piccinino, 1997). Latino adolescents have less information available on sexuality and STD prevention and less access to contraceptives (Marcell, 1994), possibly accounting for the low level of contraceptive use among Latino adolescents. Latino adolescents (40 percent) are significantly less likely to report using a condom during sexual intercourse than their White (49.2 percent) or African American (58.9 percent) peers (Alan Guttmacher Institute, 1994). Sexually active adolescent Latino males reported using condoms inconsistently or not at all (71 percent) more often than their White (54 percent) and African American (53 percent) peers (Sonenstein, Stewart, Lindberg, Pernas, & Williams, 1997).

*Vehicular Injury.* In the last decade, major shifts have occurred in Latino adolescent morbidity and mortality patterns. Among teens thirteen to nineteen years old, Latinos had the highest motor vehicle occupant death rate compared to both African Americans and Whites (Baker, Braver, Chen, Pantula, & Massie, 1998). The higher death rates for Latino youth may be associated with the documented lower rates of safety belt and child restraint use among Latinos. This disparity in death rates would have been overlooked using traditional death rates per 100,000 people. Racial and ethnic differences in car ownership and amount of car travel can obscure significant differences in death rates per unit of travel.

*Violence.* Past and recent data suggest that Latino adolescents are at risk of experiencing and witnessing violence and are at higher risk of attempting or committing suicide at a younger age than either African American or White youth (Hovey & King, 1996; Blackford & Meade, 1999). Data since the 1990s suggest that Latino adolescent boys are 3.5 times more likely to die from violence (140.3 per 100,000) than Latino females (39.2 per 100,000). Latino males are also more likely to carry a weapon to school than are African American or White males. Because carrying a weapon increases the risks of intentional and unintentional injury, Latino males are at higher risk of being injured than African American or White males (Centers for Disease Control and Prevention, 1990). Violence in the community contributes to a persistent sense of worry about personal safety among both adolescents and their families. These persistent worries by the adolescent, coupled with high rates of poverty and resource-poor environments, contribute to feelings of limited hope and depression. Depression is highly linked with suicide and attempted suicide (Hovey & King, 1996).

*Depression and Suicide.* Studies suggest that Latino adolescents have the highest prevalence of depressive symptoms of any ethnic group. One study of high school students in a large Texas school district found that one-quarter of Latinos met criteria for clinical depression, compared with 18 percent for African Americans and 12 percent for Whites (Emslie, Weinberg, Rush, Adams, & Rintelman, 1990). For females, the differences were even more dramatic, with prevalences of 31 percent among Latinos, 22 percent in African Americans, and 16 percent in Whites.

Given that Latino youth suffer from a high prevalence of depression, it is not surprising that suicide is also a significant problem. For example, national data reveal that 15 percent of Latino adolescent girls attempted suicide in 1997, compared with 9 percent of African American and 10 percent of White adolescent girls (Schoen, Davis, Collins, Greenberg, Des Roches, & Abrams, 1997). A binational survey of depressive symptoms and suicidality revealed disturbing findings among more than 4,000 adolescents attending school in six Texan border cities and the neighboring Mexican state of Tamaulipas (Swanson, Linskey, Quintero-Salinas, Pumariega, & Holzer, 1992). A validated scale of depressive symptoms showed that 48 percent of the American students scored above the critical level for depression, compared with 39 percent of Mexican youths. About 23 percent of American adolescents reported current suicidal ideation, compared with 12 percent among Mexican students.

In a small study of high school students in a California bilingual program, 24 percent scored at a critical level on a suicide questionnaire, indicating potentially significant psychopathology and suicide risk (Hovey & King, 1996). A depressive symptomatology instrument revealed that 23 percent of the students scored at the critical level. In contrast, only 11 percent of the standardization sample for the suicide questionnaire scored at the critical level, and only 12 percent of the standardization sample scored at the critical level for depression. In multivariate analyses, acculturative stress and a low level of family functioning were significantly associated with depression, whereas acculturative stress, nonhopeful expectations of the future, and depression were significantly associated with suicidal ideation.

# Environmental Health

Increasing awareness of the vulnerability of children to environmental toxicants has contributed to pediatric environmental health emerging as a national priority in the *Healthy People 2010* initiative. Latino children disproportionately are exposed to a variety of environmental toxins, including air pollutants, hazardous chemical waste, pesticides, and lead (Metzger, Delgado, & Herrell, 1995; Mott, 1995). For example, to control air pollution, the U.S. Environmental Protection Agency (EPA) established National Ambient Air Quality Standards (NAAQS), which restrict ambient levels of particular pollutants that affect public health. Eighty percent of Latinos live in areas that fail to meet one of the NAAQS, compared with 65 percent of African Americans and 57 percent of Whites (Wernette & Nieves, 1992). Latinos consistently have the highest percentages of citizens living amid the worst levels of air quality (from failing to meet two to failing to meet four NAAQS) (Mott, 1995). This is particularly troubling because the American Lung Association (1993) found that 61 percent of pediatric asthma cases occur in children who live in areas failing to meet at least one of the NAAQS. Latinos also are substantially more likely than African Americans and Whites to live in EPA nonattainment zones for elevated particulate matter, ozone, and carbon monoxide (Wernette & Neives, 1992).

Three of the five largest hazardous landfills in the United States are located in Latino and African American neighborhoods, and the mean percentage of Latino and African American citizens residing in areas with toxic waste sites is twice that for areas without toxic waste sites (Commission for Racial Justice, United Christ Church, 1987). A pilot project by the California Department of Health Services examined the potential residential pesticide exposure of infants and children residing in homes within a quarter-mile of agricultural fields. Most farmworkers in the area are Latino, and half of the sampled homes had at least one farmworker residing there. Twelve different pesticides were detected in the house dust samples (Mott, 1995).

Lead poisoning is the most common pediatric environmental health problem in the United States (Agency for Toxic Substances and Disease Registry, 1988; National Research Council, 1993a). Lead toxicity is associated with learning disabilities, a poor attention span, and lower IQ scores (Needleman et al., 1990). The Third National Health and Nutrition Examination Survey (NHANES III) found elevated blood lead levels (greater than or equal to ten μg/dl) in 17 percent of Latino children but only in 6 percent of inner-city Whites and 3 percent of suburban Whites (Pirkle et al., 1994; Landrigan & Carlson, 1995). Data from NHANES III also indicate that Mexican American children (aged one to seven years) have a mean blood lead level (four μg/dl) that is significantly higher than that of Whites (three μg/dl) but lower than that of African Americans (six μg/dl) (Ballew, Khan, Kaufman, Mokdad, Miller, & Gunter, 1999). In the state of Florida, the prevalence of elevated blood lead levels (greater than or equal to ten μg/dl) in Latino children (7 percent) is about triple that of non-Latino children (2.5 percent) (Hopkins, Quimbo, & Watkins, 1995).

The San Diego Department of Health and Human Services found that 82 percent of children identified with elevated blood lead levels were of Latino ethnicity (Gersberg et al., 1997). Multiple cases of serious lead toxicity have been documented among Mexican American children treated with certain folk remedies (Bose, Vashistha, & O'Loughlin, 1983; Centers for Disease Control and Prevention, 1983, 1993; Trotter, 1985; Baer, Garcia de Alba, Cueto, Ackerman, & Davison, 1999). These folk remedies, called *greta, azarcón,* or *albayalde,* contain high concentrations of lead oxide and are used to treat the folk illness *empacho,* a condition in which certain substances are believed to cause gastrointestinal obstruction (Flores, 2000a). These lead oxide remedies were used by 11 percent of mothers in a study at a California clinic (Mikhail, 1994). Shops called *botanicas,* located in Latino and Caribbean communities throughout the United States, sell metallic mercury (*azogue*), as an ethnomedical remedy (Wendroff, 1990). Pediatric mercury poisoning can manifest itself as neurological disorders, personality changes, hypersensitivity of the palms of the hands and feet, fever, headache, and tremors (Grandjean, 1998).

## Interventions That Work

Evidence suggests that community-based organizations serving Latino families can play an effective role in providing health services to children and adolescents. A multilevel intervention to improve immunization rates among high-risk Latino preschoolers, designed as a combination of free walk-in immunization clinics, computerized reminders, provider education, community health promotion, and Women, Infants, and Children Program (WIC) referrals, resulted in significant improvements in overall vaccination rates (from 37 percent to 50 percent) for the targeted community (Waterman et al., 1996). A drop-in vaccination clinic was found to be effective at reaching extremely high-risk, underimmunized Latino children (Flores et al., 1999). Most Latino children who attended this urban clinic were very poor, uninsured, foreign-born, and severely underimmunized, and most of their parents were unemployed non-U.S. citizens with limited English proficiency.

Disease-specific community outreach programs have been shown to be effective in providing early diagnosis, treatment, education, and identification of children with previously undiagnosed disorders. For example, a New York City hospital-based outreach program was initiated to identify musculoskeletal disorders in mostly Latino underserved areas. Conducted at day-care centers, schools, and a health fair, the project screened more than 2,500 children, identifying 168 children with forty-five different musculoskeletal disorders. Children with these disorders were then referred to and treated by orthopedic specialists (Kasper, Robbins, Root, Peterson, & Allegrante, 1993).

Data indicate that a community-university partnership was successful in improving outcomes for poor Latino children with asthma in Los Angeles (Lewis, Lewis, Leake, Monahan, & Rachelefsky, 1996). The key intervention, a three-session family educational program to increase knowledge and skills regarding asthma, resulted in significant reductions in hospitalizations, emergency department visits, and asthma-related physician visits. An intervention to improve the quality of asthma care for Latino and African American children was effective in improving patient education, access, continuity, and quality of care. About 1,900 children at twenty-two New York City Bureau of Child Health clinics participated, and staff at the eleven intervention clinics received education and training on clinical practice guidelines, improved screening and continuity, and communication skills. Data revealed that intervention clinics, compared with control clinics, had significantly more new asthma patients, return visits for asthma, patients receiving effective drugs, and parents reporting asthma education from health care providers (Evans et al., 1997).

Several community-based interventions have been shown to be effective in promoting healthier lifestyles and reducing risk factors for obesity, diabetes, and cardiovascular disease among Latino children. Jump Into Action, a school-based, non-insulin-dependent diabetes mellitus (NIDDM) prevention program among Latino fifth-grade students was effective in increasing knowledge and self-efficacy regarding NIDDM prevention and in improving diet and exercise levels (Holcomb, Lira, Kingery, Smith, Lane, & Goodway, 1998). At follow-up one month after completion of this school-based educational intervention, these gains persisted. A school intervention for seventh-grade Latino and African American students, Dance for Health, was found to be an effective way to promote weight loss and physical fitness among girls (Flores, 1995). Female students randomized to the intervention group, consisting of dance-oriented physical education classes and a health education curriculum, experienced significant reductions in their BMI and resting heart rate, compared with the control group of females.

School-based clinics provide an opportunity to identify, refer, and treat Latino victims of sexual abuse. One Los Angeles public school, where 95 percent of the students are Latino, found that 7 percent of the 922 students visiting their clinic reported being sexually abused (McGurk, Cárdenas, & Adelman, 1993). In a fourteen-month period, only one of twenty-two students reporting sexual assault had received outside psychological treatment, despite being reported to the Department of Child Services. After visiting the school clinic, half of these students had joined group therapy at the school. In a study of inner-city Latino high school students, significantly more visits were made to a school-based clinic compared with a hospital-based pediatric clinic for counseling issues, including nutrition, stress reduction, substance abuse, smoking cessation, and contraception (McHarney-Brown & Kaufman, 1991).

Establishment of pediatric Latino clinics has been shown to be an effective approach to providing Latino children with culturally competent, linguistically appropriate health care. The Pediatric Latino Clinic at Boston Medical Center is a primary care "clinic-within-a-clinic," staffed by bilingual receptionists, medical assistants, nurses, and resident and attending physicians, many of whom also are bicultural. Data suggest that the Pediatric Latino Clinic has successfully eliminated many of the formidable barriers to health care access faced by Latino children (Flores, 2000b). A program evaluation indicated that the Pediatric Latino Clinic is providing needed services to the intended target population with good outcomes and high parental satisfaction. Preliminary data revealed high rates of recommended health maintenance visits, low rates of missed appointments, a significantly lower proportion of uninsured among repeat versus first-time patients, high rates of preventive screening, significantly higher immunization rates in repeat versus first-time patients, and universal parental satisfaction with care.

## Policy Issues

Table 4.2 summarizes what we consider to be the most significant policy action points needed to improve Latino children's health. To reduce the high proportion of Latino children with no health insurance, we recommend improved outreach and enrollment to the many uninsured children who are not being reached by the state Children's Health Insurance Programs (CHIPs). Expansion of Medicaid eligibility and employer-based coverage is needed to guarantee that all low-income working families can obtain health insurance for their children. Safety net plans, such as the Children's Medical Security Plan in Massachusetts, will guarantee universal coverage for children, especially undocumented citizens and those otherwise ineligible for other insurance plans.

We have identified seven policy action points for addressing priority Latino child health issues (Table 4.2). These issues include (1) reducing poverty; (2) reducing ethnic disparities in health care; (3) increasing the culturally competent

### TABLE 4.2.  POLICY ACTION POINTS FOR IMPROVING LATINO CHILDREN'S HEALTH.

| Health Needs of Latino Children | Suggested Policy Response |
|---|---|
| Reduce high proportion without health insurance | Improve outreach and enrollment to target populations in all state Children's Health Insurance Programs (CHIPs) |
| | Expand Medicaid eligibility |
| | Expand employer-based coverage to guarantee insurance for all low-income working families |
| | Provide safety net plans for children ineligible under other plans |
| Reduce poverty | Provide living wage for working poor |
| | Expand affordable day-care opportunities, particularly for welfare-to-work programs |
| | Evaluate and implement interventions to reduce excessive high school dropout rates |
| Reduce ethnic disparities in health care | Monitor for disparities in health care institutions and health plans |
| | Increase federal funding of interventions and programs to eliminate disparities |
| | Train culturally competent health care providers |
| Increase culturally competent delivery of health care | Require courses in health professions schools |
| | Use professional continuing education opportunities |
| Provide adequate medical interpreter services | Require third-party reimbursement for medical interpreters in areas with sizable limited-English-proficient populations |
| Increase research on improving health and health outcomes | Require recording Latino ethnicity on all birth and death certificates and in national surveys |
| | Enforce federal guidelines for inclusion of minorities and children in research |
| Reduce excess disease burden for key conditions, including asthma, tuberculosis, diabetes, adolescent risk behaviors, and child abuse | Encourage greater use of preventive screening and education among patients, clinicians, and community organizations |
| | Increase federal funding of interventions and programs to reduce target disorders |
| Reduce health inequities for immigrant children | Guarantee health insurance and adequate health care for immigrant children |

delivery of health care; (4) providing adequate medical interpreter services; (5) increasing research on improving the health and health outcomes; (6) reducing the excess disease burden for key conditions, including asthma, tuberculosis, diabetes, adolescent risk behaviors, and child abuse; and (7) reducing health inequities for immigrant children.

## Conclusions

Latino children in the United States are at extremely high risk for adverse health events. They experience a disproportionate share of morbidity, including high rates of asthma, tuberculosis, unintentional injuries, child abuse and neglect, developmental disorders, and mental health problems. Compared with other ethnic groups, Latino adolescents have among the highest rates of alcohol and illicit drug use, motor vehicle occupant death rates, carrying weapons, depression, and suicide. Latino children all too often face multiple barriers to access to health care, including poverty, absence of a regular health care provider, numerous cultural and linguistic barriers, and lack of health insurance. They frequently encounter ethnic disparities in health care, including a lower likelihood of getting necessary medical equipment for asthma management after hospital discharge, fewer laboratory and radiological tests when treated for gastroenteritis in the emergency department, less preventive screening, and receipt of fewer prescriptions.

Interventions, such as school-health and pediatric health clinics, tailored to Latino children can help to reduce or even eliminate health disparities. Federal and state policy initiatives, however, may be the only way to achieve equitable health for all Latino children. The most important health policy issues for Latino children include efforts to reduce poverty, insure more of the uninsured, and increase federal funding for research and ethnic-specific intervention programs. Latino children experience the serious health problems of all vulnerable, medically underserved children. Lessons learned from promoting the health of Latino children should prove useful in improving the health of any group of children suffering health inequities in the United States.

## References

Abma, J., Chandra, A., Mosher, W., Peterson, L., & Piccinino, L. (1997). Fertility, family planning and women's health: New data from the 1995 National Survey of Family Growth. *Vital and Health Statistics, 23,* 19.

Agency for Toxic Substances and Disease Registry. (1988). *The nature and extent of lead poisoning in children in the United States: A report to Congress.* Atlanta, GA: Author, p. 2.

Agran, P. F., Winn, D. G., Anderson, C. L., & Del Valle, C. P. (1996). Pediatric injury hospitalization in Latino children and White children in southern California. *Archives of Pediatric and Adolescent Medicine, 150,* 400–406.

Agran, P. F., Winn, D. G., Anderson, C. L., & Del Valle, C. P. (1998). Family, social, and cultural factors in pedestrian injuries among Latino children. *Injury Prevention, 4,* 188–193.

Alan Guttmacher Institute. (1994). *Sex and America's teenagers.* New York: Author.

American College of Physicians. (2000). *No health insurance? It's enough to make you sick* [White Paper]. American Society of Internal Medicine. Philadelphia: Author.

American Lung Association. (1993). *Breath in danger II. Estimation of populations at-risk of adverse health consequences in areas not in attainment with National Ambient Air Quality Standards of the Clean Air Act.* Washington, D.C.: Author.

Anderson, L. M., Wood, D. L., & Sherbourne, C. D. (1997). Maternal acculturation and childhood immunization levels among children in Latino families in Los Angeles. *American Journal of Public Health, 87,* 2018–2021.

Arcia, E. (1998). Latino parents' perception of their children's health status. *Social Science Medicine, 46,* 1271–1274.

Arcia, E., Keyes, L., & Gallagher, J. J. (1994). Indicators of developmental and functional status of Mexican-American and Puerto Rican children. *Journal of Developmental and Behavioral Pediatrics, 5,* 27–33.

Baer, R. D., Garcia de Alba, J., Cueto, L. M., Ackerman, A., & Davison, S. (1999). Lead-based remedies for *empacho:* Patterns and consequences. *Social Science and Medicine, 29,* 1373–1379.

Baker, S. P., Braver, E. R., Chen, L. H., Pantula, J., & Massie, D. (1998). Motor vehicle deaths among Latino and African American children and teenagers. *Archives of Pediatric and Adolescent Medicine, 152,* 1209–1212.

Ballew, C., Khan, L. K., Kaufman, R., Mokdad, A., Miller, D. T., & Gunter, E. W. (1999). Blood lead concentration and children's anthropometric dimensions in the Third National Health and Nutrition Examination Survey (NHANES III), 1988–1994. *Journal of Pediatrics, 134,* 623–630.

Beckett, W. S., Belanger, K., Gent, J. F., Holford, T. R., & Leaderer, B. P. (1996). Asthma among Puerto Rican Hispanics: A multi-ethnic comparison study of risk factors. *American Journal of Respiratory and Critical Care Medicine, 154,* 894–899.

Blackford, A. J., & Meade, P. D. (1999). *Boys to men: The impact of non-financial barriers on health care access for adolescent boys.* (Prepared for Boys to Men: A Roundtable on Improving Access to Health Care.) Washington, D.C.: Opening Doors—Resources for Reducing Sociocultural Barriers to Health Care.

Bose, V., Vashistha, K., & O'Loughlin, B. J. (1983). *Azarcón por empacho*—Another cause of lead toxicity. *Pediatrics, 72,* 106–108.

Brown, P. N., Bell, P., Conrad, J., Howland, J., & Lang, M. (1997). State level clustering of safety measures and its relationships to injury mortality. *International Journal of Health Services, 27,* 2, 347–357.

Canino, I. A., Gould, M. S., Prupis, S., & Shaffer, D. (1986). A comparison of symptoms and diagnoses in Hispanic and Black children in an outpatient mental health clinic. *Journal of the American Academy of Child Psychiatry, 25,* 254–259.

Carter-Pokras, O. D., & Gergen, P. J. (1993). Reported asthma among Puerto Rican, Mexican-American, and Cuban children, 1982 through 1984. *American Journal of Public Health, 83,* 580–582.

Center for Medicaid and State Operations. (1999). *Annual EPSDT participation report: FY 1996.* Baltimore: Health Care Financing Administration.

Centers for Disease Control and Prevention. (1983). Lead poisoning from Mexican folk remedies—California. *Morbidity and Mortality Weekly Report, 32,* 554–555.

Centers for Disease Control and Prevention. (1990). Weapon carrying among high school students—United States, 1990. *Morbidity and Mortality Weekly Report, 40,* 381–384.

Centers for Disease Control and Prevention. (1993). Lead poisoning associated with use of traditional ethnic remedies—California. *Morbidity and Mortality Weekly Report, 43,* 521–554.

Centers for Disease Control and Prevention. (1997). Update: Prevalence of overweight among children, adolescents, and adults—United States, 1988–1994. *Morbidity and Mortality Weekly Report, 46,* 198–202.

Chabra, A., Chávez, G. F., & Harris, E. S. (1999). Mental illness in elementary school-aged children. *Western Journal of Medicine, 170,* 28–34.

Child Welfare League of America. (1999). *Foster care in the next century.* Washington, D.C.: Author.

Colp, C., Pappas, J., Moran, D., & Lieberman, J. (1993). Variants of alpha$_1$-antitrypsin in Puerto Rican children with asthma. *Chest, 103,* 812–815.

Colp, C. et al. (1990). Profile of bronchospastic disease in Puerto Rican patients in New York City: A possible relationship to alpha$_1$-antitrypsin variants. *Archives of Internal Medicine, 150,* 2349–2354.

Commission for Racial Justice, United Church of Christ. (1987). *Toxic wastes and race in the United States: A national report of the racial and socioeconomic characteristics of communities with hazardous waste sites.* New York: Author.

Commonwealth Fund. (2000, March). *Working without benefits: The health insurance crisis confronting Hispanic Americans.* New York: Author.

Cornelius, L. J. (1993). Barriers to medical care for White, African American, and Latino American children. *Journal of the National Medical Association, 85,* 281–288.

Cowdery, J. E., Fitzhugh, E. C., & Wang, M. Q. (1997). Sociobehavioral influences on smoking initiation of Hispanic adolescents. *Journal of Adolescent Health, 20,* 46–50.

Crain, E. F., Weiss, K. B., Bijur, P. E., Hersh, M., Westbrook, L., & Stein, R. E. (1994). An estimate of the prevalence of asthma and wheezing among inner-city children. *Pediatrics, 94,* 356–362.

Day, R. (1992). The transition to first intercourse among racially and culturally diverse youth. *Journal of Marriage and the Family, 54,* 749–762.

de Anda, D., Becerra, R. M., & Fielder, E. (1990). In their own words: The life experiences of Mexican-American and White pregnant adolescents and adolescent mothers. *Child and Adolescent Social Work, 7,* 4, 301–318.

Dodge, R. (1983). A comparison of the respiratory health of Mexican-American and Non Mexican-American White children. *Chest, 84,* 587–592.

Emslie, G. J., Weinberg, W. A., Rush, A. J., Adams, R. M., & Rintelman, J. W. (1990). Depressive symptoms by self-report in adolescence: Phase I of the development of a questionnaire for depression self-report. *Journal of Child Neurology, 5,* 114–121.

Epstein, J. A., Botvin, G. J., & Diaz, T. (1999). Etiology of alcohol use among Hispanic adolescents. Sex-specific effects of social influences to drink and problem behaviors. *Archives of Pediatrics and Adolescent Medicine, 153,* 1077–1084.

Evans, D. et al. (1997). Improving care for minority children with asthma: Professional education in public health clinics. *Pediatrics, 99,* 157–164.

Flores, G. (2000a). Culture and the patient-physician relationship: Achieving cultural competency in health care. *Journal of Pediatrics, 136,* 14–23.

Flores, G. (2000b). The pediatric Latino clinic: An approach to providing culturally competent, linguistically appropriate health care to an under-served population. In *Child health in the multicultural environment* (Report of the Thirty-First Ross Roundtable on Critical Approaches to Common Pediatric Problems). Columbus, OH: Abbott Laboratories, Ross Products Division, 88–98.

Flores, G. Abreu, M., Olivar, M., & Kastner, B. (1998). Access barriers to health care for Latino children. *Archives of Pediatric Adolescent Medicine, 152,* 1119–1125.

Flores, G. et al. (1999). Addressing persistent pockets of need for childhood immunization: Use of an urban drop-in vaccination clinic by high-risk children. *Ambulatory Child Health, 5,* 3–13.

Flores, G., Bauchner, H., Feinstein, A. R., & Nguyen, U.D.T. (1999). The impact of ethnicity, income, and parental education on children's health and use of health services. *American Journal of Public Health, 89,* 1066–1071.

Flores, G., & Vega, L. R. (1998). Barriers to health care access for Latino children: A review. *Family Medicine, 30,* 196–205.

Flores, R. (1995). Dance for health: Improving fitness in African-American and Hispanic adolescents. *Public Health Reports, 110,* 189–193.

Garcia-Coll, C. T. (1990). Developmental outcome of minority infants: A process-oriented look into our beginnings. *Child Development, 60,* 270–289.

Garwick, A. W., Kohrman, C., Wolman, C., & Blum, R. W. (1998). Families' recommendations for improving services for children with chronic conditions. *Archives of Pediatric and Adolescent Medicine, 152,* 440–448.

Gergen, P. J., Ezzati, T., & Russell, H. (1988). DTP immunization status and tetanus antitoxin titers of Mexican American children ages six months through eleven years. *American Journal of Public Health, 78,* 1446–1450.

Gersberg, R. M. et al. (1997). Quantitative modeling of lead exposure from glazed ceramic pottery in childhood lead poisoning cases. *International Journal of Environmental Health Research, 7,* 193–202.

Grandjean, P. (1998). Health significance of metal exposures. In R. B. Wallace & B. N. Doebbeling (Eds.), *Public health and preventive medicine* (14th ed.). Stamford, CT: Appleton & Lange, pp. 502–503.

Griesler, P. C., & Kandel, D. B. (1998). Ethnic differences in correlates of adolescent cigarette smoking. *Journal of Adolescent Health, 23,* 167–180.

Guendelman, S. (1985). Children's health needs in seasonal immigration. *Journal of Public Health Policy, 6,* 493–509.

Guendelman, S., & Schwalbe, J. (1986). Medical care utilization by Latino children. How does it differ from African American and White peers? *Medical Care, 24,* 925–940.

Hahn, B. A. (1995). Children's health: Racial and ethnic differences in the use of prescription medications. *Pediatrics, 95,* 727–732.

Halfon, N., Wood, D. L., Valdez, R. B., Pereyra, M., & Duan, N. (1997). Medicaid enrollment and health services access by Latino children in inner-city Los Angeles. *Journal of the American Medical Association, 277,* 636–641.

Holcomb, J. D., Lira, J., Kingery, P. M., Smith, D. W., Lane, D., & Goodway, J. (1998). Evaluation of *Jump into action:* A program to reduce the risk of non-insulin-dependent diabetes mellitus in school children on the Texas-Mexico border. *Journal of School Health, 68,* 282–288.

Holl, J. L., Szilagyi, P. G., Rodewald, L. E., Byrd, R. S., & Weitzman, M. L. (1995). Profile of uninsured children in the United States. *Archives of Pediatric and Adolescent Medicine, 149,* 398–406.

Hopkins, R. S, Quimbo, R., & Watkins, S. M. (1995). Elevated blood lead prevalence in Florida two-year-olds. *Journal of Florida Medical Association, 82,* 193–197.

Hovey, J. D., & King, C. A. (1996). Acculturative stress, depression, and suicidal ideation among immigrant and second-generation Latino adolescents. *American Academy of Child and Adolescent Psychology, 35,* 1183–1192.

Hsu, K. H. K. et al. (1979). Ventilatory functions of normal children and young adults— Mexican-American, White and African American: I. Spirometry. *Journal of Pediatrics, 95,* 14–23.

Johnston, L. D., O'Malley, P. M., & Bachman, K. G. (1998). *National survey results on drug use from the Monitoring the Future study, 1975–1997.* (NIH Publication No. 98-4345). Rockville, MD: National Institute on Drug Abuse.

Kamerman, S. B., & Kahn, A. J. (1993). If CPS is driving child welfare, where do we go from here? *Public Welfare, 51,* 1, 41–43.

Kasper, M. J., Robbins, L., Root, L., Peterson, M.G.E., & Allegrante, J. P. (1993). A musculoskeletal outreach screening, treatment, and education program for urban minority children. *Arthritis Care and Research, 6,* 126–133.

Kass, B. L., Weinick, R. M., & Monheit, A. C. (1999). *Racial and ethnic differences in health, 1996.* Rockville, MD: U.S. Agency for Health Care Policy and Research.

Kirkman-Liff, B., & Mondragón, D. (1991). Language of interview: Relevance for research of Southwest Latinos. *American Journal of Public Health, 81,* 1399–1404.

Landrigan, P. J., & Carlson, J. E. (1995). Environmental policy and children's health. *The Future of Children, 5,* 2, Fall/Spring, 1–19.

Lee, D. J., Gómez-Marín, O., & Lee, H. M. (1997). Sociodemographic and educational correlates of hearing loss in Hispanic children. *Pediatric and Perinatal Epidemiology, 11,* 333–344.

Lewis, M. A., Lewis, C. E., Leake, B., Monahan, G., & Rachelefsky, G. (1996). Organizing the community to target poor Latino children with asthma. *Journal of Asthma, 33,* 289–297.

Lewis, M. A., Rachelefsky, G., Lewis, C. E., Leake, B., & Richards, W. (1994). The termination of a randomized clinical trial for poor Latino children. *Archives of Pediatric and Adolescent Medicine, 148,* 364–367.

Lieu, T. A., Newacheck, P. W., & McManus, M. A. (1993). Race, ethnicity, and access to ambulatory care among U.S. adolescents. *American Journal of Public Health, 3,* 960–965.

Mapp, I., & Hudson, R. (1997). Stress and coping among African American and Hispanic parents of deaf children. *American Annals of the Deaf, 142,* 48–56.

Marcell, A. (1994). Understanding ethnicity, identity formation, and risk behavior among adolescents of Mexican descent. *Journal of School Health, 64,* 8.

Mayden, B., Castro, W., & Annitto, M. (1999). *First talk: A teen pregnancy prevention dialogue among Latinos.* Washington, D.C.: CWLA Press [imprint of the Child Welfare League of America].

McGurk, S. R., Cárdenas, J., & Adelman, H. S. (1993). Utilization of a school-based clinic for identification and treatment of adolescent sexual abuse. *Journal of Adolescent Health, 14,* 196–201.

McHarney-Brown, C., & Kaufman, A. (1991). Comparison of adolescent health care provided at a school-based clinic and at a hospital-based pediatric clinic. *Southern Medical Journal, 84,* 1340–1342.

Mendoza, F. S. et al. (1991). Selected measures of health status for Mexican-American, mainland Puerto Rican, and Cuban-American children. *Journal of the American Medical Association, 265,* 227–232.

Metzger, R., Delgado, J. L., & Herrell R. (1995). Environmental health of Latino children. *Environmental Health Perspective, 103,* Suppl. 6, 25–32.

Mikhail, B. I. (1994). Latino mothers' beliefs and practices regarding selected children's health problems. *Western Journal of Nursing Research, 16,* 623–638.

Moore, P., & Hepworth, J. T. (1994). Use of perinatal and infant health services by Mexican-American Medicaid enrollees. *Journal of the American Medical Association, 272,* 297–304.

Mott, L. (1995). The disproportionate impact of environmental health threats on children of color. *Environmental Health Perspectives, 103,* Suppl. 6, 33–35.

Mull, D. S., Agran, P. F., Winn, D. G., & Anderson, C. L. (1999). Household poisoning exposure among children of Mexican-American born mothers: An ethnographic study. *Western Journal of Medicine, 171,* 16–19.

National Center for Health Statistics. (2000). *Health, United States 2000 with adolescent health chartbook.* Hyattsville, MD: Author.

National Council of La Raza. (1998). *U.S. demographic profile of Hispanics in the United States.* Washington, D.C.: Author.

National Research Council. (1993a). *Measuring lead exposures in infants, children, and other sensitive populations.* Washington, D.C.: National Academy Press.

National Research Council. (1993b). *Understanding child abuse and neglect.* Washington, D.C.: National Academy Press.

Needleman, H. et al. (1990). Low-level lead exposure and the IQ of children. *Journal of the American Medical Association, 263,* 673–678.

Newacheck, P. W., Hughes, D. C., & Cisternas, M. (1995). Children and health insurance: An overview of recent trends. *Health Affairs, 14,* 244–254.

Newacheck, P. W., Stoddard, J. J., & McManus, M. (1993). Ethnocultural variations in the prevalence and impact of childhood chronic conditions. *Pediatrics, 91,* 1031–1039.

Ortega, R. M., Guillean, C., & Gutierrez-Najera, L. (1996). *Latinos and child welfare/Latinos y el bienestar del niño: Voces de la comunidad.* Ann Arbor: University of Michigan, School of Social Work.

Pirkle, J. L. et al. (1994). The decline in blood lead levels in the United States: The National Health and Nutrition Survey Examination Surveys (NHANES II, 1976 to 1980, and NHANES III, 1988 to 1991). *Journal of the American Medical Association, 272,* 4, 284–291.

Prislin, R., Suarez, L., Simspon, D. M., & Dyer, J. A. (1998). When acculturation hurts: The case of immunization. *Social Science and Medicine, 47,* 1947–1956.

Santiago, A. M. (1995). Intergenerational and program-induced effects of welfare dependency: Evidence from the National Longitudinal Survey of Youth. *Journal of Family and Economic Issues, 16,* 2/3, 281–306.

Schoen, C. K., Davis, K. S., Collins, L., Greenberg, L., Des Roches, C., & Abrams, M. (1997). *The Commonwealth Fund Survey of the Health of Adolescent Girls.* New York: Commonwealth Fund.

Siegel, J. M., Sorenson, S. B., Golding, J. M., Burnam, M. A., & Stein, J. A. (1987). The prevalence of childhood sexual assault. The Los Angeles Epidemiologic Catchment Area Project. *American Journal of Epidemiology, 126,* 1141–1153.

Simms, M. D., Freundlich, M., Battistelli, E. S., & Kaufman, N. (1999). Delivering health and mental health care services to children in family foster care after welfare and health care reform. *Child Welfare, 78,* 166–183.

Sokol-Katz, J. S., & Ulbrich, P. M. (1992). Family structure and adolescent risk-taking behavior: A comparison of Mexican, Cuban, and Puerto Rican Americans. *International Journal of the Addictions, 27,* 1197–1209.

Sonenstein, F. L., Stewart, K., Lindberg, L. D., Pernas, M., & Williams, S. (1997). *Involving males in teen pregnancy: A guide for program planners.* Washington, D.C.: Urban Institute.

Suminski, R. R., Poston, W. S., & Foreyt, J. P. (1999). Early identification of Mexican American children who are at risk for becoming obese. *International Journal of Obesity, 23,* 823–829.

Swanson, J. W., Linskey, A. O., Quintero-Salinas, R., Pumariega, A. J., & Holzer, C. E. (1992). A binational school survey of depressive symptoms, drug use, and suicidal ideation. *Journal of the American Academy of Child and Adolescent Psychiatry, 31,* 669–678.

Treviño, R. P., Marshal, R. M., Hale, D. E., Rodríguez, R., Baker, G., & Gómez, J. (1999). Diabetes risk factors in low-income Mexican-American children. *Diabetes Care, 22,* 202–207.

Trotter, R. T., II. (1985). *Greta* and *Azarcón:* A survey of episodic lead poisoning from a folk remedy. *Human Organism, 44,* 64–72.

United States Bureau of the Census. (1999a). *Population projections of the United States by age, sex, race, and Latino origin: 1995 to 2050.* (Current Population Reports, Series P-25, No. 1130.) Washington, D.C.: U.S. Government Printing Office.

United States Bureau of the Census. (1999b). *March Current Population Survey.* (Current Population Reports, Consumer Income, Series P-60.) Washington, D.C.: U.S. Government Printing Office.

United States Department of Health and Human Services. (1991). *Healthy people 2000: National health promotion and disease prevention objectives.* (USDHHS Publication PHS 91-50212). Washington, D.C.: U.S. Public Health Service.

United States Department of Health and Human Services. (1999). *Mental health: A report of the Surgeon General.* Rockville, MD: U.S. Government Printing Office.

Ussery, X. T., Valway, S. E., & McKenna, M. (1996). Epidemiology of tuberculosis among children in the United States: 1985 to 1994. *Pediatric Infectious Disease Journal, 15,* 697–704.

Valdez, R. B., Giachello, A., Rodriguez-Trías, H., Gómez, P., & De La Rocha, C. (1993). Improving access to health care in Latino communities. *Public Health Reports, 108,* 534–539.

Vincent, A. M. (1999). The organizational culture of child protective services. *Family Resource Coalition Report, 16,* 2, 19–20.

Wasserman, R. C., Croft, C. A., & Brotherton, S. E. (1992). Preschool vision screening in pediatric practice: A study from the Pediatric Research in Office Settings (PROS) network. *Pediatrics, 89,* 834–838.

Watchi, R., Kahlstrom, E., Vachon, L. A., & Barnes, P. F. (1998). Pediatric tuberculosis: Clinical presentation and contact investigation at an urban medical center. *Respiration, 65,* 192–194.

Waterman, S. H. et al. (1996). A model immunization demonstration for preschoolers in an inner-city barrio, San Diego, California, 1992–1994. *American Journal of Preventive Medicine, 12,* Suppl. 1, 8–13.

Wendroff, A. P. (1990). Domestic mercury pollution. *Nature, 347,* 6294 (London), pp. 347–623.

Wernette, D. R., & Nieves, L. A. (1992). Breathing polluted air: Minorities are disproportionately exposed. *Environmental Protection Agency Journal, 18,* 16–17.

White, A., Courtney, J., & Fifield, A. (1998). Race, bias, and power in child welfare. *Child Welfare Watch, 3,* Spring/Summer, 1–16.

Winsler, A., Díaz, R. M., Espinosa, L., & Rodríguez, J. L. (1999). When learning a second language does not mean losing the first: Bilingual language development in low-income, Spanish-speaking children attending bilingual preschool. *Child Development, 70,* 349–362.

Wong Fillmore, L. (1991). When learning a second language means losing the first. *Early Childhood Research Quarterly, 6,* 323–346.

Wood, P. R., Hidalgo, H. A., Prihoda, T. J., & Kromer, M. E. (1993). Latino children with asthma: Morbidity. *Pediatrics, 91,* 62–69.

Zambrana, R. E., & Capello. (in press). Promoting Latino child and family welfare: Strategies for strengthening the child welfare system. *Children & Youth Services Review.*

Zambrana, R. E., & Carter-Pokras, O. D. (2001). Health data issues for Hispanics: Implications for public health research. *Journal of Health Care for the Poor and Underserved, 12,* 1, 20–31.

Zambrana, R. E., Ell, K., Dorrington, C., Wachsman, L., & Hodge, D. (1994). The relationship between psychosocial status of immigrant Latino mothers and use of pediatric emergency services. *Health Social Work, 19,* 93–102.

Zuvekas, S. H. & Weinick, R. M. (1999). *Changes in access to care; 1977–1996: The role of health insurance.* (USDHHS Publication 99-R054). Washington, D.C.: U.S. Department of Health and Human Services.

CHAPTER FIVE

# THE REPRODUCTIVE YEARS

## The Health of Latinas

Aida L. Giachello

Despite the rapid growth of the Latino population in the United States and the large percentage of Latinas in this population, data about the health and social well-being and the quality of health care being delivered to Latinas are still limited. Review of recent research and available data document their poor health as well as the barriers to their health care, which are due to financial, institutional, and cultural factors. It has been argued (Giachello, 1994a) that socioeconomic factors (for example, health insurance) appear to be the strongest determinants of Latino women's ability to enter the formal medical care system. Once they enter the medical care system, they experience linguistic, sociocultural, and systemic barriers. They encounter health care services that are often unresponsive to women's health needs. Many health care providers are biased against women in general and have stereotypical views of women of color in particular; moreover, they often have limited knowledge, understanding, or skills to meet the needs of populations who may have illnesses with which they are inexperienced and cultural practices or languages different from their own. These factors affect the quality of health services delivered to Latino women of all age groups, their adherence to medical treatment, and often their health outcomes and general well-being.

This chapter provides an overview of the health of Latino women, with emphasis on issues related to women in their reproductive years (ages fifteen to forty-four years). Specifically, the chapter (1) identifies the major factors affecting Latino women's health; (2) describes selected sociodemographic and economic factors affecting Latino women's health; (3) discusses some of the major health disparities, selected lifestyle practices, and medical risk factors of Latino women; (4) describes the use of selected health services related to pregnancy, delivery, and family planning, including abortion; (5) discusses some findings on selected pregnancy outcomes and infant health; and (6) concludes with program, policy, and future research recommendations.

## Sociodemographic Characteristics

Latinas comprise 51.5 percent of the total Latino population in the United States (Hajat, Lucas, & Kington, 2000). The sex distribution varies by Latinos of different national origins, with Puerto Rican women substantially outnumbering Puerto Rican men in the United States (54.3 percent versus 45.7 percent) (United States Bureau of the Census, 2000; Hajat, Lucas, Kington, 2000) (see Table 5.1). Latinos are one of the youngest population groups in the United States. Differences in median age by gender indicate that currently Latino women are slightly older as a group than Latino men but are mostly concentrated in much younger age groups than are White men and women. Latino women tend to be concentrated in two age groups—either they are extremely young (twenty-one years or younger) or they are in the prime age workers' group (twenty-two to fifty-five years). Very few of them are currently of retirement age. However, this situation is expected to change by 2025, when 18 percent of the Latino population will be sixty-five years of age and over (Kaiser Family Foundation, 1999).

Most Latino women are concentrated in low-paying occupations (for example, factories, restaurants, or clerical work). They experience twice the rate of unemployment, compared to that of Whites, and suffer from multiple social and economic disadvantages, such as low levels of education, low income, single parenting, and high levels of poverty, all of which impact their health and social well-being, and limit their access to and utilization of health services.

## Life Expectancy and Leading Causes of Death

Latino women's life expectancy in 1995 was higher (77.1 years) compared to that of Latino men (69.6 years), slightly lower than that of White women (79.6 years), but higher than that of African American women (74.4 years) (National Institutes of Health, 1998). These actuarial projections need to be interpreted with caution, however, considering (1) the trends and patterns of certain diseases affecting Latino women such as diabetes, HIV/AIDS, and cervical cancer; (2) the higher rates of women in the labor force and now entering nontraditional (more stressful) occupations, which might lead to an increase of heart disease and strokes; and (3) the poor health and quality of life of women who live longer, as they are most likely to experience acute symptoms of illnesses, chronic conditions, and short- and long-term disabilities (National Institutes of Health, 1992).

The leading causes of death of Latino women are heart disease, cancer, injuries, cerebrovascular diseases, diabetes mellitus, homicide, pneumonia and influenza, liver diseases, pulmonary respiratory problems, and HIV/AIDS (see Tables 5.2 and 5.3, and Figure 5.1) (Hoyert, Kochanek, & Murphy, 1999).

# TABLE 5.1. SELECTED CHARACTERISTICS OF LATINOS BY GENDER AND NATIONAL ORIGIN COMPARED TO THOSE OF WHITES: MARCH 1999.

| Characteristics | Total Latino | | | Mexican | | | Puerto Rican | | | Cuban | | | Central and South American[a] | | | White | | |
|---|---|---|---|---|---|---|---|---|---|---|---|---|---|---|---|---|---|---|
| | Male | Female | Total | Male | Female | Total | Male | Female | Total | Male | Female | Total | Male | Female | Total | Male | Female | Total |
| **Sex distribution** | 48.5 | 51.5 | — | 49.6 | 50.4 | — | 45.7 | 54.3 | — | 50.3 | 49.7 | — | — | — | — | 31.7 | 28.2 | 29.9 |
| **Not U.S. born** | b | — | 48.9 | — | — | 47.5 | — | — | 3.0 | — | — | 72.1 | — | — | 63.0 | — | — | 4.7 |
| **Age distribution** | | | | | | | | | | | | | | | | | | |
| <15 yrs | 31.1 | 30.1 | 30.6 | 32.6 | 33.1 | 32.8 | 31.7 | 26.3 | 28.9 | 15.8 | 16.6 | 16.2 | 27.7 | 24.7 | 26.2 | 20.5 | 18.7 | 19.6 |
| 15–19 yrs | 8.5 | 9.4 | 8.9 | 7.8 | 9.0 | 9.2 | 9.0 | 10.2 | 9.6 | 6.8 | 5.0 | 5.9 | 7.5 | 6.7 | 7.0 | 7.0 | 6.5 | 6.7 |
| 20–24 yrs | 8.9 | 8.3 | 8.6 | 9.6 | 8.8 | 9.2 | 8.3 | 7.1 | 7.7 | 3.4 | 5.1 | 4.3 | 8.6 | 8.8 | 8.7 | 6.3 | 6.0 | 6.1 |
| 25–29 yrs | 8.7 | 8.4 | 8.5 | 9.4 | 9.0 | 9.2 | 7.9 | 7.1 | 7.5 | 5.3 | 6.0 | 6.0 | 8.5 | 10.4 | 8.3 | 6.4 | 6.3 | 6.4 |
| 30–34 yrs | 9.2 | 8.7 | 8.9 | 8.9 | 8.5 | 8.7 | 7.3 | 9.1 | 8.3 | 9.2 | 7.7 | 8.4 | 12.0 | 11.3 | 11.3 | 7.0 | 6.9 | 6.9 |
| 35–44 yrs | 14.5 | 14.7 | 14.6 | 13.6 | 13.9 | 13.7 | 14.0 | 15.2 | 14.6 | 15.7 | 13.7 | 14.7 | 19.0 | 16.5 | 18.5 | 17.2 | 16.5 | 16.9 |
| 45–54 yrs | 8.7 | 9.3 | 9.0 | 7.9 | 8.0 | 8.0 | 10.5 | 10.9 | 10.7 | 13.0 | 12.2 | 12.6 | 11.3 | 7.2 | 10.5 | 14.1 | 13.9 | 14.0 |
| 55–64 yrs | 4.8 | 6.0 | 5.4 | 4.2 | 5.0 | 4.6 | 5.8 | 6.6 | 6.2 | 14.1 | 14.3 | 14.2 | 7.2 | 3.5 | 5.4 | 9.3 | 9.4 | 9.4 |
| 65–74 yrs | 3.1 | 3.8 | 3.4 | 2.6 | 3.1 | 2.9 | 3.6 | 5.0 | 4.3 | 11.5 | 8.2 | 10.2 | 2.6 | 3.5 | 3.0 | 7.0 | 8.1 | 7.6 |
| 75 yrs + | 1.6 | 2.3 | 1.9 | 1.4 | 1.6 | 1.5 | 1.8 | 2.5 | 2.2 | 5.1 | 9.8 | 7.6 | 1.1 | 1.3 | 1.2 | 5.2 | 7.8 | 6.4 |
| **Median age** | | | 26.6 | | | | | | | | | | | | | | | 38.4 |
| **Education (pop. 25+)** | | | | | | | | | | | | | | | | | | |
| <9 yrs | 28.1 | 27.4 | 27.1 | 33.2 | 32.2 | 32.7 | 17.4 | 17.3 | 17.4 | 19.2 | 21.6 | 20.4 | 24.3 | 22.8 | 23.5 | 4.5 | 4.4 | 4.5 |
| 9–12 (no diploma) | 15.9 | 16.3 | 16.1 | 16.9 | 18.2 | 17.6 | 19.6 | 18.1 | 18.8 | 10.5 | 8.2 | 9.3 | 12.7 | 12.3 | 12.5 | 7.8 | 7.8 | 7.8 |
| High school graduate | 27.2 | 26.6 | 26.9 | 26.6 | 25.9 | 26.2 | 31.4 | 29.1 | 30.1 | 28.2 | 28.1 | 28.2 | 24.2 | 26.7 | 25.5 | 32.1 | 36.3 | 34.3 |
| Some college or assoc. degree | 18.1 | 18.7 | 18.4 | 16.2 | 16.6 | 16.4 | 21.2 | 23.2 | 22.6 | 14.4 | 17.3 | 17.4 | 20.4 | 20.5 | 20.4 | 25.0 | 26.3 | 25.7 |
| Bachelor degree | 7.4 | 8.2 | 7.8 | 5.2 | 5.4 | 5.3 | 7.4 | 8.4 | 8.0 | 14.7 | 17.8 | 16.3 | 12.5 | 13.3 | 12.9 | 19.8 | 17.3 | 18.5 |
| 4 yrs of advanced degree | 3.3 | 2.8 | 3.1 | 1.9 | 1.7 | 1.8 | 3.1 | 3.3 | 3.2 | 10.1 | 7.0 | 8.5 | 5.9 | 4.3 | 5.1 | 10.8 | 7.6 | 9.1 |
| **Marital status (pop. 15+yrs)** | | | | | | | | | | | | | | | | | | |
| Married, spouse present | 54.7 | 51.0 | 52.8 | 46.3 | 51.0 | 49.6 | 45.5 | 35.9 | 40.3 | 61.3 | 54.0 | 57.5 | 45.7 | 47.6 | 46.7 | 54.7 | 51.0 | 52.8 |
| Married, spouse absent | 1.3 | 1.1 | 1.2 | 4.6 | 2.0 | 3.3 | 1.6 | 2.7 | 2.2 | 1.3 | 0.8 | 0.8 | 5.6 | 2.3 | 3.9 | 1.3 | 1.1 | 1.2 |
| Widowed | 2.5 | 10.0 | 6.4 | 1.4 | 5.6 | 3.5 | 0.8 | 6.0 | 3.6 | 1.5 | 10.8 | 6.3 | 1.1 | 5.3 | 3.3 | 2.5 | 10.0 | 6.4 |
| Divorced | 8.4 | 10.2 | 9.3 | 4.9 | 6.8 | 5.8 | 8.5 | 11.0 | 9.9 | 10.4 | 10.6 | 10.5 | 4.6 | 8.9 | 6.9 | 8.4 | 10.2 | 9.3 |
| Separated | 1.8 | 2.7 | 2.3 | 2.4 | 5.2 | 3.7 | 3.8 | 6.5 | 5.3 | 3.7 | 4.0 | 3.8 | 3.4 | 5.3 | 4.4 | 1.8 | 2.7 | 2.3 |
| Never married | 31.3 | 25.1 | 28.1 | 38.4 | 29.4 | 34.0 | 39.8 | 38.0 | 38.8 | 21.7 | 20.3 | 21.0 | 39.6 | 30.6 | 34.3 | 31.3 | 25.1 | 28.1 |

*(Continued)*

# TABLE 5.1. SELECTED CHARACTERISTICS OF LATINOS BY GENDER AND NATIONAL ORIGIN COMPARED TO THOSE OF WHITES: MARCH 1999. (Continued)

| Characteristics | Total Latino | | | Mexican | | | Puerto Rican | | | Cuban | | | Central and South American[a] | | | White | | |
|---|---|---|---|---|---|---|---|---|---|---|---|---|---|---|---|---|---|---|
| | Male | Female | Total | Male | Female | Total | Male | Female | Total | Male | Female | Total | Male | Female | Total | Male | Female | Total |
| **Type of family** | | | | | | | | | | | | | | | | | | |
| Married couple | — | — | 15.7 | — | — | 18.8 | — | — | 12.5 | — | — | 7.7 | — | — | 14.4 | — | — | 3.8 |
| Female householder | — | — | 43.7 | — | — | 46.9 | — | — | 48.0 | — | — | 25.3 | — | — | 31.6 | — | — | 20.7 |
| Male householder, nonspouse | — | — | 19.6 | — | — | 20.8 | — | — | 28.2 | — | — | 14.3 | — | — | 13.7 | — | — | 7.8 |
| **Labor force participation** | 78.4 | 55.8 | 67.0 | 80.4 | 55.2 | 68.1 | 66.3 | 52.6 | 58.8 | 73.4 | 49.2 | 60.8 | 80.8 | 61.8 | 70.7 | 74.3 | 60.3 | 67.1 |
| **Percent unemployment (pop. 16+)** | 6.0 | 7.6 | 6.7 | 5.9 | 8.6 | 7.0 | 7.4 | 7.3 | 7.3 | 4.7 | 5.3 | 4.9 | 6.4 | 5.3 | 5.9 | 3.8 | 3.3 | 3.6 |
| **Type of occupation** | | | | | | | | | | | | | | | | | | |
| Executive, administrative/managerial | 14.9 | 14.3 | 14.6 | 5.2 | 8.1 | 6.3 | 8.8 | 11.5 | 10.1 | 15.5 | 10.1 | 13.2 | 8.9 | 7.1 | 8.1 | 6.9 | 8.8 | 7.7 |
| Professional | 13.4 | 17.8 | 15.5 | 3.7 | 7.5 | 5.2 | 6.6 | 11.9 | 9.2 | 9.8 | 13.7 | 11.4 | 6.5 | 9.2 | 7.8 | 4.9 | 9.0 | 6.6 |
| Technical | 2.9 | 3.4 | 3.1 | 1.2 | 2.1 | 1.5 | 2.2 | 2.5 | 2.4 | 1.9 | 6.5 | 3.9 | 2.7 | 2.1 | 2.4 | 1.6 | 2.3 | 1.9 |
| Sales | 11.7 | 12.8 | 12.2 | 6.7 | 13.2 | 9.2 | 9.6 | 11.1 | 10.3 | 14.4 | 10.9 | 12.9 | 8.1 | 11.6 | 9.8 | 7.9 | 12.7 | 9.9 |
| Administrative support | 5.5 | 23.7 | 14.1 | 4.9 | 22.0 | 11.5 | 9.4 | 27.5 | 18.3 | 6.5 | 31.6 | 17.0 | 5.5 | 19.5 | 12.1 | 5.7 | 22.6 | 12.7 |
| Precision production, crafts, and repairs | 18.6 | 2.1 | 10.9 | 21.9 | 3.0 | 14.6 | 18.1 | 2.9 | 10.6 | 15.0 | 4.0 | 10.4 | 20.4 | 1.1 | 11.7 | 20.6 | 2.8 | 13.2 |
| Transportation | 6.8 | 4.4 | 5.7 | 7.3 | 1.1 | 4.9 | 9.4 | 9.4 | 9.4 | 8.2 | 5.4 | 7.0 | 9.6 | 9.3 | 9.5 | 10.3 | 9.1 | 9.8 |
| Handlers, equipment cleaners, laborers | 6.7 | 0.9 | 4.0 | 11.7 | 2.8 | 8.2 | 7.5 | 0.5 | 4.0 | 8.9 | 0.6 | 5.4 | 6.9 | 0.5 | 3.9 | 7.3 | 0.8 | 4.6 |
| Workers, private household | 6.0 | 1.6 | 4.0 | 0.1 | 3.3 | 1.3 | 8.2 | 2.7 | 5.5 | 9.8 | 1.6 | 6.4 | 10.5 | 3.5 | 9.2 | 10.8 | 2.8 | 9.5 |
| Workers, except private household | 0.1 | 1.3 | 0.6 | 15.6 | 24.8 | 19.1 | — | — | — | 0.4 | 0.9 | 0.4 | 0.2 | 10.5 | 5.0 | 0.1 | 4.0 | 1.7 |
| Farming, forestry, fishing | 10.0 | 16.7 | 13.1 | 10.9 | 2.3 | 7.6 | 17.6 | 19.7 | 18.6 | 11.3 | 14.6 | 11.3 | 17.0 | 24.5 | 20.6 | 15.7 | 23.6 | 19.0 |
| Machine operators, assemblers, inspectors | 3.5 | 1.0 | 2.3 | 11.1 | 9.8 | 10.6 | 2.5 | 0.4 | 1.5 | 0.7 | — | 0.7 | 3.5 | 0.6 | 2.1 | 8.1 | 1.5 | 5.4 |

| Persons with money earnings | | | | | | | | | | | | | | | | | |
|---|---|---|---|---|---|---|---|---|---|---|---|---|---|---|---|---|---|
| <$10,000 | 24.4 | 46.4 | 34.7 | 24.8 | 47.2 | 34.6 | 28.7 | 48.8 | 39.7 | 25.5 | 49.0 | 37.2 | 17.8 | 40.4 | 29.0 | 16.0 | 35.5 | 25.9 |
| $10,000–24,999 | 25.6 | 35.7 | 39.5 | 45.2 | 37.7 | 41.9 | 31.7 | 30.3 | 30.9 | 31.7 | 26.7 | 29.2 | 47.3 | 40.0 | 43.7 | 26.2 | 33.3 | 29.8 |
| $25,000 + | 29.8 | 16.9 | 23.8 | 27.8 | 14.3 | 22.3 | 46.3 | 19.5 | 27.0 | 35.6 | 23.7 | 29.6 | 31.3 | 18.6 | 25.2 | 47.2 | 28.7 | 37.8 |
| Median income | $17,252 | $10,862 | — | — | — | — | — | — | — | — | — | — | — | — | — | $29,862 | $15,217 | — |

**Poverty level:1998**

| | | | | | | | | | | | | | | | | | | |
|---|---|---|---|---|---|---|---|---|---|---|---|---|---|---|---|---|---|---|
| Families below poverty level | — | — | 10.0 | — | — | 24.4 | — | — | 26.7 | — | — | 11.0 | — | — | 18.5 | — | — | 6.1 |
| Married couple below poverty level | — | — | 5.3 | — | — | 18.0 | — | — | 12.5 | — | — | 7.7 | — | — | 14.4 | — | — | 3.8 |
| Family headed by female | — | — | 29.9 | — | — | 46.9 | — | — | 48.0 | — | — | 25.3 | — | — | 31.6 | — | — | 20.7 |

aIncludes Central and South Americans and other and unknown Latinos.

bData not available, February 2000.

*Sources:* United States Bureau of the Census. (1999, March). The Hispanic population in the United States. *Current Population Reports*, pp. 20–527. United States Bureau of the Census, Ramirez (1999, December); *Advance Data*, No. 3 (February 25, 2000), Table 2.; United States Bureau of the Census. *The Hispanic population in the United States. Current Population Reports* (March 2000). United States Bureau of the Census, Historical income tables: People (March); *Current Population Survey* (November 1999).

**TABLE 5.2.  AGE-SPECIFIC LEADING CAUSES OF DEATH BY TOTAL LATINO MEN AND WOMEN AND BY LATINO WOMEN'S AGE GROUPS COMPARED TO THOSE OF WHITES: 1997. (RATES PER 100,000)**

| Causes of Death | Total Latino | | | Latino Women's Age Groups | | | | | | White | | |
| --- | --- | --- | --- | --- | --- | --- | --- | --- | --- | --- | --- | --- |
| | Female | Male | Total | 1–4 | 5–14 | 15–24 | 25–44 | 45–64 | 65+ | Total Female | Total Male | Total |
| Diseases of the heart | 78.3 | 83.9 | 81.2 | NAa | NA | 1.2 | 5.2 | 68.6 | 975.2 | 292.5 | 295.3 | 293.8 |
| Cancer | 61.4 | 65.4 | 63.5 | 2.2 | 2.9 | 3.5 | 19.8 | 128.9 | 513.7 | 203.4 | 233.2 | 217.9 |
| Cerebrovascular diseases | 19.6 | 16.7 | 18.1 | NA | | NA | 3.0 | 20.1 | 228.4 | 76.9 | 51.6 | 64.6 |
| Diabetes mellitus | 17.2 | 13.8 | 15.5 | | | | 1.6 | 28.6 | 184.0 | 26.1 | 22.4 | 24.3 |
| Injury or accidents | 13.7 | 39.7 | 27.0 | 10.4 | 4.9 | 14.9 | 12.5 | 15.5 | 41.0 | 26.0 | 47.9 | 36.6 |
| Pneumonia and influenza | 10.6 | 10.7 | 10.6 | NA | NA | NA | 1.2 | 6.5 | 129.3 | 37.2 | 32.3 | 34.8 |
| Chronic obstructive pulmonary diseases | 7.8 | | 8.4 | | | NA | | 7.2 | 94.1 | 42.3 | 46.9 | 44.6 |
| Conditions related to the perinatal period | 5.8 | | | NA | NA | | | | | | | |
| Liver diseases and cirrhosis | 5.5 | 13.3 | 9.5 | | | | 2.4 | 13.7 | 40.0 | | 12.2 | 9.3 |
| Congenital anomalies | 5.3 | | | 3.1 | 1.4 | NA | | | | | | |
| Alzheimer's disease | | | | | | | | | 31.1 | 12.3 | | |
| Kidney failure | | | | | | | | 4.1 | 35.7 | 10.4 | | 10.2 |
| Septicemia | | | | NA | | | | | | 10.0 | | |
| Homicide and legal intervention | | 18.6 | 11.1 | 2.3 | NA | 4.8 | 4.5 | | | | 10.8 | |
| Suicide | | 9.8 | | NA | NA | 2.2 | | | | | 19.7 | 12.0 |
| Benign neoplasms and carcinoma in situ | | | | | NA | NA | | | | | | |
| Human immunodeficiency virus infection | | 12.3 | 7.8 | NA | NA | NA | 6.7 | 5.3 | | | | |

aRates are not available.

*Source:* National Center for Health Statistics. (1999, June 30). *Deaths: Final data for 1997, 47,* 19. Adapted from Table 9, pp. 39–43.

TABLE 5.3. AGE-SPECIFIC LEADING CAUSES OF DEATH BY TOTAL LATINO AND BY LATINO WOMEN'S AGE GROUPS COMPARED TO THOSE OF WHITES: 1997. (RATES PER 100,000)

| Causes of Death | Total Latino | Latino Women's Age | | | | | | White | | |
| --- | --- | --- | --- | --- | --- | --- | --- | --- | --- | --- |
| | | 1–4 | 5–14 | 15–24 | 25–44 | 45–64 | 65+ | Total Female | Total Male | Total |
| Diseases of the heart | 81.2 | NA[a] | NA | 1.2 | 5.2 | 68.6 | 975.2 | 292.5 | 295.3 | 293.8 |
| Cancer | 63.5 | 2.2 | 2.9 | 3.5 | 19.8 | 128.9 | 513.7 | 203.4 | 233.2 | 217.9 |
| Cerebrovascular diseases | 18.1 | NA | NA | NA | 3.0 | 20.1 | 228.4 | 76.9 | 51.6 | 64.6 |
| Diabetes mellitus | 15.5 | | | | 1.6 | 28.6 | 184.0 | 26.1 | 22.4 | 24.3 |
| Injury or accidents | 27.0 | 10.4 | 4.9 | 14.9 | 12.5 | 15.5 | 41.0 | 26.0 | 47.9 | 36.6 |
| Pneumonia and influenza | 10.6 | NA | NA | NA | 1.2 | 6.5 | 129.3 | 37.2 | 32.3 | 34.8 |
| Chronic obstructive pulmonary diseases | 8.4 | | NA | NA | | 7.2 | 94.1 | 42.3 | 46.9 | 44.6 |
| Conditions related to the perinatal period | | NA | NA | | | | | | | |
| Liver diseases and cirrhosis | 9.5 | | | NA | 2.4 | 13.7 | 40.0 | | 12.2 | 9.3 |
| Congenital anomalies | | 3.1 | 1.4 | | | | | | | |
| Alzheimer's disease | | | | | | | 31.1 | 12.3 | | |
| Kidney failure | | | | | | 4.1 | 35.7 | 10.4 | | 10.2 |
| Septicemia | | NA | | | | | | 10.0 | | |
| Homicide and legal intervention | 11.1 | 2.3 | NA | 4.8 | 4.5 | | | | 10.8 | |
| Suicide | | NA | NA | NA | 2.2 | | | | 19.7 | 12.0 |
| Benign neoplasms and carcinoma in situ | | | NA | NA | | | | | | |
| Human immunodeficiency virus infection | 7.8 | NA | NA | NA | 6.7 | 5.3 | | | | |

[a]Rates are not available.

Source: National Center for Health Statistics. (1999, June 30). Deaths: Final data for 1997, 47, 19. Adapted from Table 9, pp. 39–43.

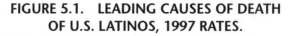

## FIGURE 5.1.   LEADING CAUSES OF DEATH
## OF U.S. LATINOS, 1997 RATES.

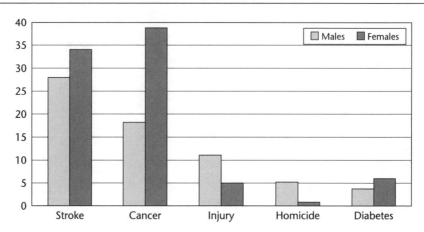

*Source:* Hoyert, D. L., Kochanek, K. D., & Murphy, S. L. (1999). *Deaths: final data for 1997.*
National vital statistics reports, 47, 19. Hyattsville, MD: National Center for Health Statistics.

Latino women, compared to Latino men, are more likely to die of cere-brovascular diseases and diabetes. The age-specific mortality data shown in Tables 5.2 and 5.3 indicate that cancer (for instance, cervical, breast, or lung cancers) for women aged twenty-five to forty-four emerged as the leading cause of death in 1997 (19.8 per 100,000) (Hoyert, Kochanek, & Murphy, 1999). Increased smoking among women in the United States, in Latin America, and in Spain has been the result of heavy marketing by the tobacco industry (Centers for Disease Control and Prevention, 1999). This may explain the increase in cancer rates for lung and other pulmonary conditions. On the other hand, infection with human papillomavirus (HPV), a sexually transmitted disease (STD), may well explain the high incidence of cervical cancer and mortality due to it among Latino women (Centers for Disease Control and Prevention, 1998b; Napoles-Springer & Pérez-Stable, 1996).

Latino women aged twenty-five to forty-four are also more likely to die of injuries, representing the second leading cause of death (12.5 per 100,000); injuries are the number-one cause of death among young women between the ages of fifteen and twenty-four (14.9 per 100,000) (Hoyert, Kochanek, & Murphy, 1999). Motor vehicle accidents accounted in 1997 for most of these types of deaths (see Tables 5.2 and 5.3). Homicide emerged as the second cause of death among young Latino women (fifteen to twenty-four years). HIV/AIDS emerged as the third-leading cause of death for Latino women between the ages of twenty-five and forty-four, despite the fact that this condition has been declining in the past five years or so for the population as a whole (Centers for Disease

Control and Prevention, 1998b). Due to the long period of infection, this means that women of reproductive age become infected in their late teens and early twenties.

## Characteristics of Latino Mothers

Latino women have the highest fertility rates and birth percentages in the United States (Ventura, Martin, Curtin, Mathews, & Park, 2000) (see Table 5.4). About 18.6 percent of the total U.S. births in 1998 were to Latino women. Most of the Latino births were to Mexican American mothers, representing 70.2 percent of the total Latino births. In 1998 the estimated birthrate (number of live births per 1,000 population) for the total Latino population was 24.3, compared to 12.1 for the White population (Ventura, Martin, Curtin, Mathews, & Park, 2000) (see Table 5.4). Birthrates by Latino origin were as follows: 26.4 for Mexican Americans, 19.0 for Puerto Ricans, 10.0 for Cubans, and 23.2 for Central and South American women in the United States. (Figure 5.2). The birthrate for Mexican Americans has increased slightly in the past decade (from 25.7 in 1989 to 26.4 in 1998), while it dropped for Puerto Ricans (from 23.7 to 19.0) and for women of Central and South American origins and for other unidentified Latino women in the United States (from 28.3 to 23.2) (Ventura, Martin, Curtin, Mathews, & Park, 2000; National Center for Health Statistics, 1999).

Data on age-specific fertility rates (number of births per 1,000 women aged fifteen to forty-four) indicate that Mexican American mothers between the ages of twenty and twenty-four in 1998 had the highest fertility rate (197.6) among all women, regardless of race or ethnicity. The fertility rate for this age group is more than twice the rate of White women (90.7). In 1998, Cuban women had the lowest fertility rate (50.1) of all racial and ethnic groups in the United States. Cuban women are also most likely to have their children between the ages of twenty-five and twenty-nine (data not shown). This can be partly explained by their older median age (see Table 5.1) (Ventura, Martin, Curtin, Mathews, & Park, 2000).

In examining selected characteristics of Latino women giving birth in the United States in 1998, we find that Latino mothers were considerably less likely to have completed twelve or more years of education (50.7 percent) than were White and African American mothers (87.2 percent and 73.3 percent, respectively) (Ventura, Martin, Curtin, Mathews, & Park, 2000) (see Table 5.4). Specifically, Mexican American mothers had the lowest levels of schooling of all racial and ethnic groups, with only 44.8 percent reporting twelve or more years of school completed. In 1998, the percentage of Cuban mothers who completed twelve or more years of schooling (87 percent) was the highest, compared to Latino mothers of other nationalities (see Table 5.4) and to African American mothers (73.3 percent). This percentage was similar to that of White women (87.2 percent).

## TABLE 5.4. TOTAL BIRTHRATES AND PERCENTAGE OF BIRTHS BY SELECTED DEMOGRAPHIC CHARACTERISTICS, BY LATINO ORIGIN OF MOTHERS, BY NON-LATINO MOTHERS, AND BY PLACE OF BIRTH OF MOTHERS: UNITED STATES, 1998.

| Characteristics | All Origins[a] | Latino | | | | | | Non-Latino | | |
| --- | --- | --- | --- | --- | --- | --- | --- | --- | --- | --- |
| | | Total Latino | Mexican American | Puerto Rican | Cuban | Central and South American | Other | Total Non-Latino[b] | White | African American |
| Births | 3,941,553 | 734,661 | 516,011 | 57,349 | 13,226 | 98,226 | 49,849 | 3,158,975 | 2,361,462 | 593,127 |
| **Rate** | | | | | | | | | | |
| Birthrate[c] | 14.6 | 24.3 | 26.4 | 19.0 | 10.0 | 23.2 | 20.2 | 13.2 | 12.1 | 18.1 |
| Fertility rate[d] | 65.6 | 101.1 | 112.1 | 75.5 | 50.1 | 90.2 | 11.0 | 59.8 | 56.7 | 72.6 |
| Total fertility rate[e] | 2,058.5 | 2,947.5 | 3,198.0 | 2,268.0 | 1,560.0 | 2,719.0[g] | | 1,919.5 | 1,837.0 | 2,235.5 |
| Sex ratio[f] | 1,047 | 1,040 | 1,037 | 1,044 | 1,105 | 1,042 | 1,050 | 1,049 | 1,052 | 1,034 |
| **Percentage** | | | | | | | | | | |
| **All births** | | | | | | | | | | |
| Births to mothers under 20 years | 12.5 | 16.9 | 17.5 | 21.9 | 6.9 | 10.3 | 20.2 | 11.6 | 9.4 | 21.6 |
| 4th and higher-order births | 10.5 | 13.6 | 14.7 | 12.3 | 5.7 | 11.1 | 11.0 | 9.8 | 8.5 | 15.0 |
| Unmarried mothers | 32.8 | 41.6 | 39.6 | 59.5 | 24.8 | 42.0 | 45.3 | 30.9 | 21.9 | 69.3 |
| Mothers completed 12 years or more of school | 78.1 | 50.7 | 44.8 | 64.1 | 87.0 | 61.5 | 66.4 | 84.4 | 87.2 | 73.3 |
| Mothers born in the United States | 80.5 | 39.9 | 39.7 | 63.8 | 39.7 | 10.1 | 73.3 | 89.9 | 94.9 | 90.3 |

*Percentage*

**Mothers born in the United States**

Births to mothers

| | | | | | | | | | | |
|---|---|---|---|---|---|---|---|---|---|---|
| under 20 years | 13.6 | 25.4 | 26.4 | 23.7 | 12.1 | 21.8 | 24.0 | 12.4 | 9.7 | 23.3 |
| 4th and higher-order births | 9.9 | 11.2 | 11.8 | 11.1 | 4.9 | 5.0 | 10.8 | 9.8 | 8.4 | 15.1 |
| Unmarried mothers | 33.8 | 48.0 | 46.3 | 61.8 | 25.5 | 45.8 | 47.5 | 32.4 | 22.5 | 72.3 |
| Mothers completed 12 years or more of school | 82.2 | 64.5 | 62.7 | 64.3 | 86.1 | 78.4 | 67.9 | 84.0 | 87.0 | 72.2 |

*Percentage*

**Mothers born outside the United States**

Births to mother under

| | | | | | | | | | | |
|---|---|---|---|---|---|---|---|---|---|---|
| 20 years | 8.1 | 11.2 | 11.6 | 18.7 | 3.5 | 9.0 | 9.8 | 3.9 | 3.5 | 6.3 |
| 4th and higher-order births | 12.8 | 15.2 | 16.6 | 14.5 | 6.2 | 11.8 | 11.5 | 9.5 | 9.7 | 13.7 |
| Unmarried mothers | 28.5 | 37.2 | 35.1 | 55.2 | 24.4 | 41.6 | 37.3 | 16.6 | 10.7 | 40.7 |
| Mothers completed 12 years or more of school | 61.0 | 41.4 | 32.7 | 63.6 | 87.6 | 59.5 | 62.2 | 87.6 | 90.2 | 83.5 |

[a]Includes "origin noted stated."

[b]Includes races other than White and African American.

[c]Rate per 1,000 population.

[d]Rate per 1,000 women aged fifteen to forty-four years.

[e]Rates are sums of birthrates for five-year age groups multiplied by five.

[f]Male live births per 1,000 female live births.

[g]Includes Central and South American women and other and unknown Latinas.

*Note:* Race and Latino origin are reported separately on birth certificates. Persons of Latino origin may be of any race. In this table, Latino women are classified only by place of origin; non-Latino women are classified by race.

*Source:* National Center for Health Statistic. (2000, March 28). *National Vital Statistics Report, 48, 3,* Table 14.

### FIGURE 5.2.   LATINO BIRTH RATES, 1998.

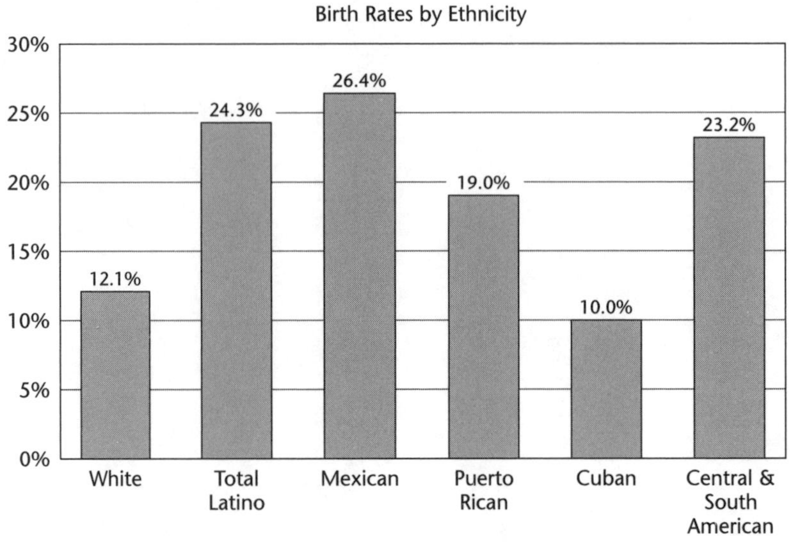

Birth Rates by Ethnicity

*Source:* Ventura, S. J., Martin, J. A., Curtin, S. C., Mathews, T. J., & Park, M. M. (2000). *Births: Final data for 1998.* National vital statistics reports. (DHHS Publication no. [PHS 00-1120] 0-0215 [3/00]). Hyattsville, MD: National Centers for Health Statistics.

Data by place of birth of mothers shown in Figure 5.3 indicate that Latino women born outside of the fifty states and the District of Columbia who gave birth in 1998 were least likely to complete twelve or more years of education (41.4 percent). This was true for women born in Mexico (32.7 percent) and for those born in Central or South America (59.5 percent). No clear pattern emerged in reference to Puerto Rican and Cuban mothers born on either island (see Table 5.4).

The age distribution of Latino women that gave birth in the United States in 1998 indicates that they begin having children at a young age and continue until their older years, with variations by national origin (Ventura, Martin, Curtin, Mathews, & Park, 2000). In addition, Latino mothers were more likely than White mothers to give birth to their fourth- or higher-order child (13.6 percent versus 8.5 percent) (see Table 5.4) (Ventura, Martin, Curtin, Mathews, & Park, 2000). Mexican American and African American mothers were most likely to have larger families (based on their percentages of fourth- and higher-order births: 14.7 percent and 15 percent, respectively; see Table 5.4). The percentages of fourth- and higher-order births for other Latino groups were as follows: Puerto Ricans, 12.3 percent; Cuban Americans, 5.7 percent; Central or South American mothers, 11.1 percent; and "other and unknown Latinas," 9.8 percent (Ventura, Martin, Curtin, Mathews, & Park, 2000).

### FIGURE 5.3. LATINO MOTHERS' LEVELS OF EDUCATION BY PLACE OF BIRTH, 1998.

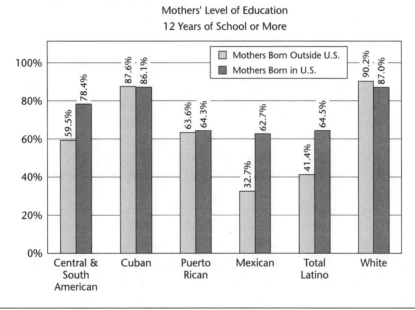

Mothers' Level of Education
12 Years of School or More

Source: Ventura, S. J., Martin, J. A., Curtin, S. C., Mathews, T. J., & Park, M. M. (2000). *Births: Final data for 1998.* National vital statistics reports. (DHHS Publication no. [PHS 00-1120] 0-0215 [3/00]). Hyattsville, MD: National Centers for Health Statistics.

An area of social concern is the increased number of births to unmarried women. Regardless of ethnicity, the proportion of births to unmarried women has been rising steadily in the United States in recent years (Ventura, Martin, Curtin, Mathews, & Park, 2000). Data on marital status shown in Table 5.4 indicate that in 1998 approximately one-third (32.8 percent) of all Latino infants had an unmarried mother, compared to one-fifth (21.9 percent) of White infants and more than two-thirds (69.3 percent) of African American infants (Ventura, Martin, Curtin, Mathews, & Park, 2000). African American and Puerto Rican mothers were the groups most likely to give birth out of wedlock (69.3 percent and 59.5 percent, respectively), whereas Cuban mothers were least likely to do so (24.8 percent). The percentages of births to unmarried women for other Latino groups were as follows: Mexican American mothers, 39.6 percent, Central or South Americans, 42 percent; and "other and unknown Latinas," 45.3 percent (Ventura, Martin, Curtin, Mathews, & Park, 2000). Having children out of wedlock leads to sustained poverty not only for women but also for their children and a stressful life often due to limited financial support of the family from the children's father(s), with consequent severe financial problems and strained family relations (Sherraden & Barrera, 1996; Zambrana, Scrimshaw, & Dunkel, 1996).

## Impact of Acculturation

Acculturation is the process of incorporating aspects of the mainstream (host) culture into each individual's repertoire of behaviors. External acculturation such as changing food habits and styles of clothing, as well as learning and/or adapting to the majority language, tend to take place first, followed by internal acculturation, or the adoption of cultural beliefs, values, and more complex patterns of behavior (Giachello, 1995). All immigrants confront the process of acculturation upon arriving in the United States. Initial studies in the mid-1980s showed that the Mexican immigrant population, which generally had lower socioeconomic status (SES) than that of Whites, had health indicators similar to those of Whites. This relationship has been referred to in the literature as the "Hispanic paradox" (Hayes-Bautista, 1992; Markides & Coreil, 1986; Scribner, 1996). Further research on the Mexican immigrant population has demonstrated that the effect of SES on health indicators is modified by the acculturation status of the individual (Scribner, 1996). English language fluency and place of birth are usually used as principal markers of acculturation. Other indicators often used are length of time in the community, age at time of immigration, language spoken at home and in the community, celebration of certain cultural events (for instance, *Cinco de Mayo*), and contact with ethnic groups and institutions. Acculturation and its measurement are poorly understood (Zambrana & Ellis, 1995). It has been often said that acculturation or adopting behaviors of the mainstream White culture may lead to negative health outcomes among Latinos (Scribner & Dwyer, 1989; Balcazar & Krull, 1999) and, most recently, among other racial and ethnic groups (for example, Asian immigrants) (Ventura, Martin, Curtin, Mathews, & Park, 2000). It has been argued that health status for Latino women deteriorates over time with increasing acculturation to high-risk behaviors such as smoking, alcohol and substance abuse, poor nutrition, and the increased stress of living in U.S. communities (Black and Markides, 1993; Guendelman & Abrams, 1994; Wolf & Portis, 1996).

Lamberty (1994) has summarized some of the "cultural" or "acculturation" explanations in the research literature about the beneficial effect of foreign-born status in reference to Latino pregnancy outcomes:

- Persons with low levels of acculturation maintain indigenous cultural dietary practices, which lead to better nutrition (less sodium, less fat, more fruits and vegetables, and so on).
- Value systems of the indigenous culture promote healthy lifestyles. For example, migrants bring with them or join extended family support networks that buffer the stress generated by the host culture. Apparently, the longer the migrants live in the United States, the more their family and social support networks appear to weaken. Newcomers tend to be healthier, as are their young children (although this may not necessarily be the case for those Latino immigrant groups who have come to the United States as refugees, escaping from violence and political persecution).

The effect of acculturation, measured by place of birth, is clearly seen by the percentage of mothers who give birth out of wedlock (see Figure 5.4). Women, regardless of ethnicity, born in the United States (not including Puerto Rico) were considerably more likely to give birth out of wedlock. The percentages doubled for Whites and almost doubled for African Americans when we examined those born in the United States as opposed to those born in the their countries of origin (Whites, 22.5 percent versus 10.7 percent; African Americans, 72.3 percent versus 40.7 percent; see Table 5.4). This pattern is similar for mothers of other racial groups (for example, various Asian and Pacific islanders (Ventura, Martin, Curtin, Mathews, & Park, 2000). Similar patterns emerged regarding adolescent pregnancy and having births of low birth weight, as we will see in the next section.

## Employment Status and Child Care Arrangements

The 1995 National Survey of Family Growth (NSFG) (Abma, Chandra, Mosher, Peterson, & Piccinino, 1997) found that 57.8 percent of Latino women aged fifteen to forty-four were not employed at the time of their most recent childbirth. This

### FIGURE 5.4.   BIRTHS TO UNMARRIED MOTHERS BY PLACE OF BIRTH, 1998.

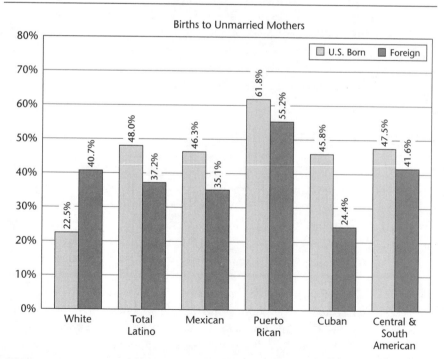

*Sources:* Ventura, S. J., Martin, J. A., Curtin, S. C., Mathews, T. J., & Park, M. M. (2000). *Births: Final data for 1998.* National vital statistics reports. (DHHS Publication no. [PHS 00-1120] 0-0215 [3/00]). Hyattsville, MD: National Centers for Health Statistics.

percentage was much higher than the 44.7 percent for White women and 53.5 percent for African American women. Latino women aged twenty-two to forty-four who were employed at the time of the pregnancy were also most likely not to have taken maternity leave (28.9 percent), compared to 39.6 percent and 34.5 percent for White and African American women, respectively (Abma, Chandra, Mosher, Peterson, & Piccinino, 1997).

In the NSFG, of Latino women who were working most of the time and had at least one child under five years of age, 37.3 percent received help in child care from one of the child's grandparents or from another relative, compared to 28.6 percent and 36.3 percent for White and African American mothers, respectively (Abma, Chandra, Mosher, Peterson, & Piccinino, 1997). This pattern also emerged for Latino women who had children between five and twelve years old (Abma, Chandra, Mosher, Peterson, & Piccinino, 1997), except that White and African American mothers with older children relied less (18.9 percent and 27.9 percent, respectively) on grandparents' support than did Latino women (32.6 percent). Regardless of children's age, Latino mothers depend less on day-care centers or preschool (Abma, Chandra, Mosher, Peterson, & Piccinino, 1997).

In summary, Latino mothers—particularly the Mexican cohort—constitute the most prolific ethnic group in the United States. In 1998, they had the highest birth and fertility rates of all racial and ethnic groups. This was particularly true for women born outside the United States. Latino women were also most likely to have the lowest level of education and to have given birth to four or more children. The impact of acculturation, measured by mothers' place of birth, indicate that Latino women born in the United States are most likely to have children out of wedlock and high levels of adolescent pregnancy, as we will see in the following section.

## Adolescent Pregnancy

Almost 17 percent of the total live births to Latino mothers were to adolescents under the age of twenty, which is almost twice as high as those of White teen mothers (9.4 percent) but lower than those of African American teen mothers (21.6 percent; see Table 5.4 and Figure 5.5) (Ventura, Martin, Curtin, Mathews, & Park, 2000). Puerto Ricans had the highest teen births (21.9 percent) of all racial or ethnic groups. Teen births were also quite high among mothers of "other and unknown" Latino origins (20.2 percent).

Most of the literature indicates that adolescent pregnancy is related to increased sexual activity at an earlier age. Fifty percent of Latino women between the ages of fifteen and seventeen (1) are sexually active, compared to 34.9 percent and 48.2 percent for White and African American teens, respectively (Abma, Chandra, Mosher, Peterson, & Piccinino, 1997), and (2) engage in unprotected sex. Other factors that are related to adolescent pregnancy among Latinas are low use of contraceptive (United States Department of Health and Human

## FIGURE 5.5.    LATINO TEEN BIRTHS BY PLACE OF BIRTH AND NATIONALITY, 1998.

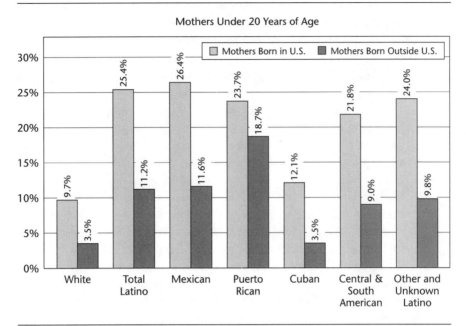

Mothers Under 20 Years of Age

*Source:* Ventura, S. J., Martin, J. A., Curtin, S. C., Mathews, T. J., & Park, M. M. (2000). *Births: Final data for 1998*. National vital statistics reports. (DHHS Publication no. [PHS 00-1120] 0-0215 [3/00]). Hyattsville, MD: National Centers for Health Statistics.

Services, 1999; Piccinino & Mosher, 1998; Abma, Chandra, Mosher, Peterson, & Piccinino, 1997; Darroch-Forrest & Frost, 1996) and low knowledge about sexuality issues and birth control methods (Abma, Chandra, Mosher, Peterson, & Piccinino, 1997). Latino women, including teens, are less likely to have received formal health education (35.2 percent) on birth control methods, STDs, or how to say no to sex, compared to 26 percent and 36 percent for White and African American women, respectively. Others are subjected to involuntary sexual intercourse (including rape) that may result in unwanted pregnancy. Approximately 18 percent of Latino women under the age of sixteen reported that their first intercourse was not voluntary, compared to 15 percent for Whites and African Americans of the same age group. Another factor that influences adolescent pregnancy rates is the lower abortion rates (Alan Guttmacher Institute [AGI], 1999). The AGI estimated that the abortion ratio (abortions per 100 pregnancies of Latino women aged fifteen to nineteen) for Latina teens was 27.5 percent. This is lower than the abortion ratio for White adolescents (32 percent) and considerably lower that the abortion ratio for African American teens (40.8 percent) (AGI, 1999). Obviously, differences prevail by levels of acculturation and assimilation of Latino youth into the mainstream culture or place of origin (for example, urban

versus rural) if those teenagers were born outside the United States (Figure 5.5).
More acculturated adolescents are most likely to be at risk for unwanted pregnancies and to become single mothers. This may be due to conflicts between the
value system of the mainstream culture and that of the parents' country of origin, or to barriers to accessing the medical care system for contraceptive services
and education.

Giachello (1994a) suggests that the high rate of teen pregnancy among Latino
women is also related to the fact that Latino adolescents are least likely to use family planning services (Abma, Chandra, Mosher, Peterson, & Piccinino, 1997). Often
teens have no financial resources or health insurance coverage to pay for family
planning services and/or they feel embarrassed to approach health clinics for family planning services or to go to the drugstore to purchase contraceptives that do
not require prescriptions (for instance, condoms). In addition, family planning services may not be accessible to teens because of distance, inconvenience of clinic
hours, and the high cost of care. When teens visit a clinic they have to complete
complicated intake forms and then often there are long waiting periods before
they are seen. Awkwardness in using the English language as well as low literacy
are additional barriers for many Spanish-speaking teens who may have limited
formal education and who go to clinics where there are no bilingual and/or bicultural staffs. If the clinic is in their neighborhood, teens may be worried that
community workers or other patients may recognize them and find out the purpose
of their visits.

Teen pregnancy is associated with a series of negative social and economic
consequences to the mother and to her child. Teen pregnancy is the most reported
cause of school dropouts among young women. Early childbearing leads to overall lower levels of education, as teen mothers have fewer opportunities to return
to school and limited opportunities to enroll in training programs or to go to
college (United States Department of Health and Human Services, 1999). For
married young Latino women, the possibility of going back to school is even lower
than for single parents. Married women have the responsibility of not only raising a child but also taking care of a home and a husband or partner (Giachello,
1994a) or going to work. Those adolescents that marry or live with the father of
their child are also more likely to become pregnant again, resulting in larger family size with close spacing of children. This leads to the phenomenon often called
"excess fertility." Teenaged mothers are also least likely to marry or stay married, resulting in a higher incidence of female-headed households and to an increase of what sociologists often call the "feminization of poverty." They are more
likely to need public assistance than their peers who are not mothers (United States
Department of Health and Human Services, 1999). Again, caution is needed
as this pattern may vary depending on adolescents' levels of acculturation, parents'
emotional and financial support and involvement, and youth academic or career
aspirations and goals.

With regard to the medical consequences of teen pregnancy, studies on the entire population indicate that such pregnancy may lead to complications during

both gestation and delivery. Their age per se is a medical risk factor. For example, young women's bodies are not prepared for prolonged labor and safe delivery (Giachello, 1994a). The current literature on adolescent pregnancy medical risk factors states that dietary and nutritional patterns of teens before and during the pregnancy (for example, adequacy of the diet, amount of folic acid intake, anemia, obesity, or anorexia), social and cultural factors (notably, support from the family and from the baby's father) (Sherraden & Barrera, 1996), and the use of prenatal care are highly important determinants of complications during and after the pregnancy. In reference to nutrition, Gutierrez (1999) found that the most powerful factors contributing to good food practices among pregnant Mexican immigrant teens were maternal concern about the well-being of the offspring and the role of motherhood, as well as family support. For U.S.-born Mexican teens these concerns were not as strong (Gutierrez, 1999).

Studies also indicate that teen pregnancy, especially of mothers under the age of fifteen, is associated with low birth weight, neonatal death, high infant mortality, and sudden infant death syndrome (SIDS) (United States Department of Health and Human Services, 1999). Some of these consequences are related to a teen's low SES and behaviors before and during the pregnancy. Again, they include poor nutrition; lack of knowledge of proper health care during pregnancy; poor personal health habits or lifestyle practices such as smoking and use of alcohol and illicit drugs (Ventura, Martin, Curtin, Mathews, & Parks, 2000; United States Department of Health and Human Services, 1999; Abma, Chandra, Mosher, Peterson, & Piccinino, 1997; Substance Abuse and Mental Health Services Administration, 1998); young women's and/or parents' financial problems; and delays in obtaining prenatal care, or not getting medical care at all. Furthermore, the infants may be at greater risk of child abuse, neglect, and behavioral and educational problems at later stages (United States Department of Health and Human Services, 1999).

# Smoking Behavior

Scientific evidence indicates that women who smoke during pregnancy have a higher risk of miscarriages, stillbirths, and premature and low-birth-weight babies than do nonsmokers (Giachello, 2000; Floyd, Zahniser, Gunter, & Kendrick, 1991; Center for the Future of Children, 1991). On average, in 1998, 4 percent of Latino mothers reported smoking during the pregnancy, compared with 16.2 percent of White mothers and 9 percent of African American mothers (Ventura, Martin, Curtin, Mathews, & Parks, 2000). Within the Latino population, tobacco use during pregnancy was especially high for Puerto Rican mothers (10.3 percent), particularly those between the ages of eighteen and twenty-four (11.2 percent), while considerably lower for mothers of Central or South American origins (1.5 percent), followed by mothers of Mexican (3.8 percent) and Cuban origins (3.7 percent) (see Table 5.5). Differences by place of birth of the mother (as a marker of acculturation) shown in Table 5.5 indicate that mothers born outside

**TABLE 5.5. PERCENTAGE OF BIRTHS WITH SELECTED MEDICAL OR HEALTH CHARACTERISTICS BY LATINO ORIGIN OF MOTHERS, BY RACE FOR MOTHERS OF NON-LATINO ORIGIN, AND BY PLACE OF BIRTH OF MOTHERS: UNITED STATES, 1998.**

| Characteristics of Mothers | Latino | | | | | | Non-Latino | | |
|---|---|---|---|---|---|---|---|---|---|
| | Total | Mexican American | Puerto Rican | Cuban | Central and South American | Other | Total[a] | White | African American |
| **All births** | | | | | | | | | |
| Prenatal care beginning in the first trimester | 74.3 | 72.8 | 76.9 | 91.8 | 78.0 | 74.8 | 84.8 | 87.9 | 73.3 |
| Late or no prenatal care | 6.3 | 6.8 | 5.1 | 1.2 | 4.9 | 6.0 | 3.4 | 2.4 | 7.0 |
| Smoker[b] | 4.0 | 2.8 | 10.7 | 3.7 | 1.5 | 8.0 | 14.4 | 16.2 | 9.6 |
| Drinker[c] | 0.0 | 0.5 | 0.9 | 0.5 | 0.4 | 1.3 | 1.2 | 1.1 | 1.4 |
| Weight gain of less than 16 lbs[d] | 13.4 | 14.7 | 12.7 | 7.8 | 11.1 | 12.0 | 11.0 | 9.6 | 16.8 |
| Median weight gain[d] | 30.0 | 28.6 | 30.5 | 32.2 | 30.3 | 30.4 | 30.6 | 30.8 | 29.8 |
| Cesarean delivery rate | 20.6 | 20.0 | 21.1 | 31.0 | 22.2 | 18.8 | 21.3 | 21.2 | 22.4 |
| **Births to mothers born in the United States** | | | | | | | | | |
| Prenatal care beginning in the first trimester | 76.4 | 76.0 | 76.8 | 91.5 | 81.7 | 75.0 | 85.0 | 88.1 | 73.0 |
| Late or no prenatal care | 5.1 | 5.2 | 5.0 | 1.4 | 3.5 | 5.9 | 3.3 | 2.3 | 7.0 |
| Smoker[b] | 7.1 | 5.4 | 12.1 | 5.1 | 4.7 | 10.0 | 15.5 | 16.7 | 10.4 |
| Drinker[c] | 1.0 | 0.9 | 0.9 | 0.7 | 0.7 | 1.6 | 1.2 | 1.1 | 1.5 |
| Weight gain of less than 16 lbs[d] | 12.4 | 12.9 | 12.1 | 7.8 | 8.2 | 12.3 | 11.0 | 9.6 | 17.1 |
| Median weight gain[d] | 30.0 | 28.6 | 30.5 | 32.2 | 30.3 | 30.4 | 30.6 | 30.8 | 29.8 |
| Cesarean delivery rate | 20.7 | 20.7 | 20.8 | 27.0 | 20.5 | 19.6 | 21.4 | 21.3 | 22.2 |

**Births to mothers born outside the United States**

| | | | | | | | | | |
|---|---|---|---|---|---|---|---|---|---|
| Prenatal care beginning in the first trimester | 77.1 | 72.9 | 77.2 | 92.0 | 77.6 | 74.7 | 83.0 | 85.5 | 76.6 |
| Late or no prenatal care | 5.8 | 7.0 | 5.1 | 1.2 | 5.0 | 5.9 | 4.0 | 3.5 | 6.4 |
| Smoker[b] | 2.6 | 1.6 | 8.3 | 2.8 | 1.2 | 1.9 | 3.8 | 6.9 | 1.6 |
| Drinker[c] | 0.5 | 0.3 | 0.9 | 0.3 | 0.3 | 0.5 | 0.6 | 1.0 | 0.4 |
| Weight gain of less than 16 lbs[d] | 12.2 | 14.3 | 13.7 | 7.8 | 11.5 | 11.0 | 10.1 | 8.5 | 13.9 |
| Median weight gain[d] | 30.0 | 28.5 | 30.2 | 32.2 | 30.2 | 30.2 | 30.3 | 30.7 | 29.8 |
| Cesarean delivery rate | 20.6 | 20.5 | 21.8 | 33.7 | 22.4 | 20.5 | 20.7 | 19.7 | 24.6 |

[a]Includes races other than White and African American.

[b]Excludes data for California, Indiana, New York State (except for New York City), and South Dakota, which did not report mother's tobacco use on the birth certificate.

[c]Excludes data for California and South Dakota, which did not report mother's alcohol use on the birth certificate.

[d]Excludes data for California, which did not report weight gain on the birth certificate. Median weight gain is shown in pounds.

*Note:* Race and Latino origin are reported separately on birth certificates. Persons of Latino origin may be of any race. In this table, Latino women are classified only by place of origin; non-Latino women are classified by race.

*Source:* National Center for Health Statistic. (2000, March 28). *National Vital Statistics Report, 48,* 3, Table 25.

the United States and Puerto Rico reported considerably less smoking behavior during the pregnancy, regardless of race or ethnicity (Ventura, Martin, Curtin, Mathews, & Parks, 2000). Studies indicate that, also regardless of race or ethnicity, pregnant women reduce their smoking behavior during pregnancy but resume it after the birth of the child (Substance Abuse and Mental Health Services Administration, 1998). This means that more aggressive interventions should be implemented to assist and support mothers to abstain from smoking after they have given birth as well as during pregnancy.

## Alcohol Use

Alcohol use during pregnancy can cause a series of adverse effects such as fetal alcohol syndrome (FAS), which is characterized by growth retardation, facial malformations, dysfunctions of the central nervous system, including mental retardation and low birth weight (Center for the Future of Children, 1991). Data available on FAS indicate that Latino infants' rates of FAS are comparable to those of Whites (0.8 and 0.9 per 10,000 total births, respectively). The 1997 National Household Survey on Drug Abuse (Substance Abuse and Mental Health Services Administration, 1998) found that 14.1 percent of all pregnant women in childbearing years (fifteen to forty-four years) at the time of the survey reported having used alcohol in the past month. In this age group, those most likely to report this behavior were Whites (15.5 percent) and African Americans (16.7 percent), compared to Latino pregnant women (7.1 percent). Binge drinking in the past month during the pregnancy was considerably low for all women: Whites (1.3 percent), African Americans (1.5 percent), and Latino women (1.0 percent) (Substance Abuse and Mental Health Services Administration, 1998). Furthermore, 0.6 percent of pregnant Latino women reported heavy drinking during pregnancy in the past month, compared to 0.3 percent for the total sample (Substance Abuse and Mental Health Services Administration, 1998). No data were available for White or African American pregnant women or for Latino women of different national origins.

Drinking behavior during pregnancy seems to be associated with marital status and with cultural and social factors. One study examined the alcohol behaviors of White, African American, and Latino women and found that women who are most likely to be heavier drinkers before, during, or after the pregnancy were those who were never married, divorced, or separated (Stroup, Trevino, & Trevino, 1988; Zambrana & Scrimshaw, 1997). Cultural factors (such as Latino women's self-sacrificing role), multiple and conflicting roles, and other psychosocial stressors (unplanned pregnancy, not having the partner's financial or emotional support and/or not living with the newborn's father) may lead to higher levels of stress and subsequent heavier drinking (Stoup, Trevino, & Trevino, 1988).

Based on the 1998 national birth data, alcohol consumption during the pregnancy was considerably lower for all women. About 1.1 percent of White mothers and 1.4 percent of African American mothers giving birth in that year reported alcohol use during pregnancy (Ventura, Martin, Curtin, Mathews, & Park, 2000) (see Table 5.5). The percentage for Latino mothers was even lower (0.6 percent) (Ventura, Martin, Curtin, Mathews, & Park, 2000). This behavior increased slightly to 1.3 percent among "other and unknown" Latino women (Ventura, Martin, Curtin, Mathews, & Park, 2000). This behavior was slightly less for all women born outside the fifty states and the District of Columbia. Alcohol consumption during the pregnancy is either substantially underreported on the birth certificates for all women or alcohol use is declining among women during pregnancy. The under-reporting of alcohol use might be the result of stigma associated with alcohol consumption, especially during pregnancy, or the potential negative consequences (such as removal of the infant from the mothers' home if reported to a child welfare agency). Another explanation for the low percentage of reported alcohol use on the birth certificate might be related to the fact that the national birth data exclude California (a state in which one-third of its population is Latino) (Ventura, Martin, Curtin, Mathews, & Park, 2000). The National Household Survey on Drug Abuse (Substance Abuse and Mental Health Services Administration, 1998) found that 16.7 percent of women between fifteen and forty-four years of age drank alcohol in the previous month of the survey. However, the percentage that reported alcohol consumption during the pregnancy dropped to 1.3 percent, which is consistent with the 1998 national birth data (Ventura, Martin, Curtin, Mathews, & Park, 2000). The SAMHSA survey also found that the percentage of women of childbearing age who reported binge drinking in the past month and who had a child under the age of two was 9.2 percent. This could mean that women resume their alcohol use after the birth of the child (Substance Abuse and Mental Health Services Administration, 1998) or that they increase their drinking due to the additional tension of raising a child.

## Nutrition and Maternal Weight Gain During Pregnancy

Overweight is more common in minority populations, particularly women. Combined findings from 1988–1994 (Third National Health and Nutrition Examination Survey [NHANES III]) for adults aged twenty to seventy-four indicate that African American women have the highest prevalence of overweight (53 percent), followed closely by Mexican American women (51.8 percent), compared to 33.9 percent for White women (American Heart Association, 1999). Overweight varies by levels of education and family income, with those having the lowest levels of education and poor or near-poor family income reporting the highest percentages of overweight. This is particularly true among Latinos, regardless of gender. The lack of sustained physical exercise is the main factor for increased overweight among the entire U.S. population, including communities of color. For example, 1988–1991 data from NHANES III indicate that Latino women were least likely to report engaging in physical activity for leisure (43.9 percent), compared to African American women (38.1 percent) or White women (23.1 percent) (American Heart Association, 1999).

Research in the area of pregnancy and nutrition is limited. The number of pregnant women included in most national sample surveys of the general U.S. population is usually too small for analyses that take into account the nutrition-related physiological changes that occur over the nine months of pregnancy (United States Department of Health and Human Services, 1999). Data on maternal weight gain during the pregnancy is one of the key components in the complex relationship between lifestyle characteristics of the mother and the development of the fetus (Chomitz, Cheung, & Lieberman, 1995). In 1990 the National Academy of Science published weight-gain guidelines that varied according to the mother's body-mass index (BMI) calculated from women's prepregnancy weight and height. The guidelines recommend that women who are underweight (low BMI) gain twenty-eight to forty pounds during pregnancy; those who are of normal weight should gain twenty-five to thirty-five pounds; those that are overweight (25 percent and above BMI) should gain fifteen to twenty-five pounds; and obese women should gain no more than fifteen pounds (Institute of Medicine, 1990). The data in Table 5.5 indicate that Puerto Rican women were most likely among Latino mothers to have gained less weight during pregnancy. The relatively low maternal weight gained by Puerto Rican mothers was associated with having infants of low birth weight (see the section to follow on birth weight) (Ventura, Martin, Curtin, Mathews, & Park, 2000).

## Use of Prenatal Care

In 1998, 74.3 percent of Latino mothers of all ages who gave birth began prenatal care in their first three months of pregnancy (see Table 5.5). This percentage was considerably lower than that of White mothers (87.9 percent) but was quite similar to that of African American mothers (73.3 percent) (Ventura, Martin, Curtin, Mathews, & Park, 2000). Among Latinas by nationalities, Mexican mothers reported the lowest use of early prenatal care (72.8 percent), whereas Cuban mothers reported higher use than White mothers during their first trimester (91.8 percent). In the past ten years there has been a remarkable increase of use of prenatal services by Latino women (see Figure 5.6) (Ventura, Martin, Curtin, Mathews, & Park, 2000; National Center for Health Statistics, 1991).

The effects of prenatal care are difficult to measure (Huntington & Connell, 1994; Fiscella, 1995). Early competent care, however, can promote healthier pregnancies by detecting and managing preexisting medical conditions, providing medical advice, and assessing the risk of poor pregnancy outcome. It can, according to Ventura, Martin, Curtin, Mathews, & Park (2000), be vital to maternal health and can serve as a gateway into the health care system, especially for socially disadvantaged women.

In 1998, about 6.3 percent of all Latino mothers had late or no prenatal care at all, compared to 2.4 percent and 7 percent of White and African American mothers, respectively. Within the Latino population, Mexican American mothers

## FIGURE 5.6.    FIRST TRIMESTER PRENATAL CARE: TEN-YEAR TREND.

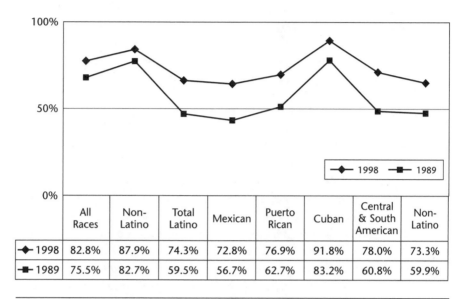

| | All Races | Non-Latino | Total Latino | Mexican | Puerto Rican | Cuban | Central & South American | Non-Latino |
|---|---|---|---|---|---|---|---|---|
| ◆ 1998 | 82.8% | 87.9% | 74.3% | 72.8% | 76.9% | 91.8% | 78.0% | 73.3% |
| ■ 1989 | 75.5% | 82.7% | 59.5% | 56.7% | 62.7% | 83.2% | 60.8% | 59.9% |

*Source:* Ventura, S. J., Martin, J. A., Curtin, S. C., Mathews, T. J., & Park, M. M. (2000). *Births: Final data for 1998.* National vital statistics reports. (DHHS Publication no. [PHS 00-1120] 0-0215 [3/00]). Hyattsville, MD: National Centers for Health Statistics.

(6.8 percent), those from Central and South America (4.9 percent), and Puerto Ricans (5.1 percent) were most likely to delay or not to go for prenatal care at all (Ventura, Martin, Curtin, Mathews, & Park, 2000). The percentage for Cuban mothers was the lowest of any other racial and ethnic group (1.2 percent) (Ventura, Martin, Curtin, Mathews, & Park, 2000). The 1998 birth data shown in Table 5.5 indicate that the percent of prenatal care received varies by mothers' place of birth. Latino mothers born in the United States were more likely to go for prenatal care in their first trimester (76.4 percent) than Latino women born outside the fifty states or the District of Columbia (72.9 percent). The only exception is the Puerto Rican mothers. Those born on the island of Puerto Rico were slightly more likely to go for prenatal care in the first trimester of pregnancy (77.2 percent) than those born on the mainland (76.8 percent) (Ventura, Martin, Curtin, Mathews, & Park, 2000).

## Barriers to Accessing Prenatal Care and Other Services

Latino women confront a series of problems in accessing the health care system either for preventive and maintenance health care or for the treatment of illness (Giachello, 1994b, 1995). The high cost of care and the lack of health insurance make it difficult for Latino women to have access to a broad array of preventive health services, including prenatal care. In the 1995 National Survey of Family Growth (NSFG) (Abma, Chandra, Mosher, Peterson, & Piccinino, 1997), 21 percent of Latino women aged fifteen to forty-four reported no health insurance coverage, compared to 7.5 percent for Whites and 9.3 percent for African Americans of that age group. Latino women were less likely to be covered by their employers (31.5 percent) or by their husbands' employment insurance (28.3 percent), compared to Whites (38.9 percent and 49.9 percent, respectively) and African American women (42.3 percent and 41.1 percent, respectively) (Abma, Chandra, Mosher, Peterson, & Piccinino, 1997). The same survey found that the most often used method of payment for recent delivery for Latino women aged fifteen to forty-four was Medicaid (56.3 percent). The percentage for Medicaid coverage for recent delivery for White women was 23 percent and for African American women, 62 percent (Abma, Chandra, Mosher, Peterson, & Piccinino, 1997). However, having health insurance coverage does not ensure equal access to prenatal care for Latino women, because of inequalities in benefits packages, providers' discretion in deciding which health insurance company to accept, increased search costs due to private cost-containment efforts (for example, deductibles and copayments), and poor quality of care (Raube, Handler, & Giachello, 1995; Oakley, 1990).

Other factors affecting prenatal care use among Latino women are the levels of satisfaction that Latino women experience during such care (Handler, Raube, Kelley, & Giachello, 1996; Brown & Lumley, 1993). In Chicago, Latino women mentioned not minding waiting longer periods of time to see the doctor if their physicians devoted their complete attention to them and answered all the questions they might have about the pregnancy (Handler, Raube, Kelley, & Giachello, 1996).

## Anemia

Anemia is a condition that occurs often during pregnancy, representing the third most frequently reported complication with a rate in 1998 of 21.8 per 1,000 for all mothers (Ventura, Martin, Curtin, Mathews, & Park, 2000). Anemia is more common among mothers under age twenty (30.6 per 1,000), compared with 17.6 for mothers forty years of age and over (Ventura, Martin, Curtin, Mathews, & Park, 2000). In 1998, the rate of anemia per 1,000 live births for Latino mothers was 21.7, compared to 18.4 for Whites. The rate was the highest among African American women (34.6). Among Latino mothers, the rate was almost three times higher among Latino mothers of the "other and unknown" category (44.4), followed by Puerto Rican mothers (32.2), while only 13.9 per 1,000 Cuban mothers reported anemia (see Table 5.6).

## Gestational Diabetes Mellitus (GDM)

This is a condition of insulin resistance that develops during pregnancy or is first recognized during pregnancy; it may lead to respiratory distress syndrome, congenital abnormalities, infant mortality, and heavier-birth-weight babies (a condition known as macrosomia or abnormal largeness: BW > 4,000 grams) (American Diabetes Association, 2000; Pierce, Hayworth, Warburth, Keen, & Bradley, 1999; Illinois Diabetes Control Program, 1999; Glasgow & Eakin, 1998; Smits, Paulk, & Kee, 1995; United States Department of Health and Human Services, 1998). Having large babies may result in early delivery or harm to the baby or mother during delivery. GDM may also lead to increased incidence of preeclampsia, cesarean delivery, and a longer length of maternal hospitalization. Fetal and perinatal deaths are three to eight times greater in pregnancies of mothers with diabetes than in pregnancies of nondiabetic mothers, as well as congenital malformations in children (American Diabetes Association, 2000). The infant may be born with glycemia or hypoglycemia (high or low levels of glucose in the blood) and may be at higher risk of becoming obese and developing diabetes as a child or during adolescence, particularly in children or youth who do not have proper nutrition and do not engage in regular exercise. Latinos have twice the risk of developing diabetes than do Whites. Puerto Rican women have the highest rate of GDM (34.7 per 1,000), compared to Mexicans (25.4), African Americans (24.9), and Whites (25.6) (American Diabetes Association, 2000) (see Table 5.6). High-risk women are those over the age of twenty-five who are overweight, who have family histories of diabetes and/or are Latinas, African Americans, Native Americans, or Asian Americans (American Diabetes Association, 2000; Illinois Diabetes Control Program, 1999), and who have a sedentary lifestyle. Latino women who experience diabetes complications during pregnancy are at much higher risk of developing type 2 diabetes within five years after the pregnancy.

# Hypertension

Hypertension during pregnancy is self-reported in the birth certificates and is usually classified as chronic or pregnancy-related hypertension (Ventura, Martin, Curtin, Mathews, & Park, 2000). Hypertension can lead to preeclampsia or eclampsia complications, a condition during the pregnancy marked by high blood pressure, proteinuria (presence of protein in the urine), and edema (retention of body fluid). If seizures occur, the condition is known as eclampsia or toxemia, which can be fatal for the mother and/or the offspring. Most recent research is associating maternal hypertension and low birth weight among racial and ethnic groups (Fang, Madhavan, & Alderman, 1999).

In 1998, the prevalence of chronic hypertension among mothers of all races was 7.1 per 1,000 live births. This rate doubles among women between the ages of thirty-five and thirty-nine (13.6) and triples among women between the ages of forty and forty-five (24.8) (see Table 5.6) (Ventura, Martin, Curtin, Mathews, & Park, 2000). The rate of pregnancy-associated hypertension in 1998 was considerably higher for mothers of all groups, with a rate of 37.6 per 1,000 live births and increasing to 43.4 for women under twenty and to 48.0 for women between forty and fifty-four (Ventura, Martin, Curtin, Mathews, & Park, 2000). The rate

**TABLE 5.6. NUMBER AND RATE OF LIVE BIRTHS TO MOTHERS WITH SELECTED MEDICAL RISK FACTORS, COMPLICATIONS OF LABOR, AND OBSTETRIC PROCEDURES, BY LATINO ORIGIN OF MOTHERS AND BY RACE OF MOTHERS OF NON-LATINO ORIGIN: UNITED STATES, 1998 (×1,000 LIVE BIRTHS).**

| Medical Risk Factor, Complication, and Obstetric Procedure | Latino | | | | | | Non-Latino | | |
|---|---|---|---|---|---|---|---|---|---|
| | Total | Mexican American | Puerto Rican | Cuban | Central and South American | Other | Total[a] | White | African American |
| **Medical risk factors** | | | | | | | | | |
| Anemia | 22 | 20 | 32 | 14 | 15 | 44 | 22 | 18 | 35 |
| Diabetes | 27 | 25 | 35 | 21 | 29 | 28 | 27 | 26 | 25 |
| Hypertension, pregnancy-associated | 28 | 27 | 32 | 29 | 28 | 37 | 40 | 41 | 41 |
| Uterine bleeding[b] | 5 | 4 | 7 | 4 | 5 | 5 | 7 | 8 | 5 |
| **Complications of labor and/or delivery** | | | | | | | | | |
| Meconium, moderate-to-heavy | 57 | 55 | 62 | 37 | 65 | 58 | 55 | 49 | 77 |
| Premature rupture of membrane | 19 | 17 | 30 | 21 | 20 | 29 | 28 | 28 | 31 |
| Dysfunctional labor | 22 | 18 | 34 | 41 | 28 | 36 | 28 | 29 | 26 |
| Breech/malpresentation | 30 | 28 | 36 | 38 | 32 | 37 | 41 | 44 | 30 |
| Cephalopelvic disproportion | 15 | 15 | 14 | 14 | 15 | 16 | 21 | 22 | 15 |
| Fetal distress[b] | 32 | 30 | 41 | 24 | 34 | 38 | 41 | 39 | 52 |

**Obstetric procedures**

| | | | | | | | | | |
|---|---|---|---|---|---|---|---|---|---|
| Amniocentesis | 13 | 9 | 23 | 28 | 24 | 22 | 32 | 36 | 16 |
| Electronic fetal monitoring | 791 | 773 | 877 | 887 | 799 | 831 | 852 | 859 | 840 |
| Induction of labor | 129 | 122 | 154 | 182 | 122 | 178 | 207 | 226 | 151 |
| Ultrasound | 549 | 527 | 651 | 582 | 559 | 636 | 673 | 699 | 592 |
| Simulation of labor | 163 | 156 | 212 | 166 | 171 | 174 | 181 | 187 | 161 |

[a]Includes races other than White and African American.

[b]Texas does not report this risk factor or complications on the birth certificate.

*Note:* Race and Latino origin are reported separately on birth certificates. Persons of Latino origin may be of any race. In this table, Latino women are classified only by place of origin; non-Latino women are classified by race.

*Source:* National Center for Health Statistics (2000, March 28). *National Vital Statistics Report, 48,* 3.

was lower for Latino mothers as a whole (27.7), compared to White mothers (41.0) and African American mothers (40.8) (see Table 5.6). The rate was the highest among "other and unknown" Latinas (36.6), followed by Puerto Ricans (31.9). For all women, the rate of eclampsia was considerably lower (3.2), increasing slightly among women under twenty (4.4) and among older women between forty and fifty-four (4.3). No data on the rate of eclampsia was available for Latino women (see Table 5.6) (Ventura, Martin, Curtin, Mathews, & Park, 2000).

# Asthma

Asthma is one of the most common illnesses that complicates pregnancy. Approximately 4 percent of pregnancies are complicated by bronchial asthma (National Heart, Lung, and Blood Institute, 1992). The exact incidence of asthma varies by region. For example, among pregnant Latino women in East Boston, Massachusetts, the prevalence of chronic wheeze syndromes were lower in Latino women than in White women. The asthma condition, in this study, appears to be strongly associated with women who are active smokers and have a parental history of asthma. Little research, however, has been conducted among pregnant Latino women with asthma to better understand its causes and its impact on women and fetuses during pregnancy.

# Dysfunctional Labor

This situation occurs when women in active labor suddenly stop making progress without any clear reason or explanation. It can also occur when the head of the newborn is too big in proportion to the mother's cervix. This often occurs when the mother has GDM, as discussed previously. In 1998, Latino mothers as a whole and Mexican American mothers in particular were less likely to have had a dysfunctional labor (22.3 and 18.1 per 1,000), compared to White (29.1) and African American mothers (25.8) (Ventura, Martin, Curtin, Mathews, & Park, 2000). However, Puerto Rican and Cuban mothers were considerably more likely to have had a dysfunctional labor (34.4 and 41.4, respectively) (Ventura, Martin, Curtin, Mathews, & Park, 2000). This can be explained by the fact that Puerto Rican women usually have poorer health prior to pregnancy and a higher tendency to develop GDM, and Cuban women tend to experience higher pregnancy-related complications because of age and/or genetics. More research is needed in this area to better understand ethnic differences.

## Cesarean Section

The rate of primary cesarean section has declined over the last decade from 16.1 per 1,000 to 14.9 per 1,000 (Ventura, Martin, Curtin, Mathews, & Park, 2000).

Vaginal births after previous cesarean delivery rates have increased from 18.9 per 1,000 to 26.3 per 1,000 (Ventura, Martin, Curtin, Mathews, & Park, 2000). In 1998, 20.6 percent of Latino mothers' live births were by cesarean delivery. This rate is slightly lower than those for White and African American mothers (21.2 and 22.4, respectively) (see Table 5.5). However, the rate of cesarean procedures was the highest among Cuban mothers (31.0), regardless of place of birth of the mother, although Cuban mothers born outside the United States had relatively lower rates (27.0) than did Cuban mothers born in the United States (33.7) (Ventura, Martin, Curtin, Mathews, & Park, 2000). Older age places Cuban women at higher risk for pregnancy related complications and therefore for the need to have this procedure done. In addition, in Cuba, cesarean section was fashionable among upper class Cubans. Also, area variation studies (Goldfard, 1984) have found an association between cesarean procedures performed and mothers having health insurance coverage.

# Latino Infants' Overall Physical Health at Birth

The Apgar score is a measure used to evaluate the newborn infant's overall physical condition at birth. This measure consists of five factors: infant heart rate, respiratory effort, muscle tone, irritability, and color. Each component is assigned a value, which ranges from 0 to 2. The overall score is the sum of the five values, with the score of 10 being optimum (Ventura, Martin, Curtin, Mathews, & Park, 2000). Scores are reported at one and five minutes after birth. Data for Latino mothers based on this measure for 1998 indicate that the percentage of Latino babies evaluated as low (a score of less than 7) in the five-minute Apgar score was close to those for White mothers (1.2 and 1.3, respectively), compared to 2.4 for African American mothers. No clear difference emerged regarding the Apgar score and the mother's place of birth (see Table 5.7). The five-minute Apgar score is considered to have better long-term predictive value concerning the infant's health status and survival chances.

## Birth Weight

This is considered to be one of the most critical measures of pregnancy outcomes. There is a well-established association between low birth weight and a greatly elevated risk of infant mortality, congenital malformation, mental retardation, and other physical and neurological impairments. The birth certificate collects data on "very low birth weight" (VLBW; those infants born weighing less than 1,500 grams or 3 lb., 4 oz.) and "low birth weight" (LBW; those infants born weighing 2,500 grams, or 5 lb., 8 oz. or less). These measures are generally used as proxies for the adjective "premature." Latino mothers have rates of VLBW and LBW comparable to those of White mothers (VLBW, 1.1 for each group; Latinos' LBW, 6.4, and Whites' LBW, 6.6). VLBW for Latino mothers slightly increased for those born

**TABLE 5.7.  INFANT HEALTH, PERCENTAGE OF SELECTED MEDICAL OR HEALTH CHARACTERISTICS, BY HISPANIC ORIGIN OF MOTHERS, BY RACE OF MOTHERS OF NON-LATINO ORIGIN, AND BY PLACE OF BIRTH OF MOTHERS: UNITED STATES, 1998.**

| | *Latino* | | | | | | | *Non-Latino* | |
| Characteristics | Total | Mexican American | Puerto Rican | Cuban | Central and South American | Other | Total[a] | White | African American |
|---|---|---|---|---|---|---|---|---|---|
| **Infant health/all births** | | | | | | | | | |
| Preterm births[b] | 11.4 | 11.0 | 13.9 | 11.4 | 11.6 | 12.1 | 11.6 | 10.2 | 17.6 |
| Birth weight | | | | | | | | | |
| Very low birth weight[c] | 1.1 | 1.0 | 1.9 | 1.3 | 1.2 | 1.4 | 1.5 | 1.1 | 3.1 |
| Low birth weight[d] | 6.4 | 6.0 | 9.7 | 6.5 | 6.5 | 7.6 | 7.8 | 6.6 | 13.2 |
| 4,000 grams or more[e] | 9.0 | 9.3 | 7.1 | 10.0 | 9.1 | 7.7 | 10.3 | 11.8 | 5.3 |
| Five-minute Apgar score of less than 7[f] | 1.2 | 1.2 | 1.4 | 0.7 | 1.0 | 1.2 | 1.5 | 1.3 | 2.4 |
| **Infant health/births to mothers born in the United States** | | | | | | | | | |
| Preterm births[b] | 12.1 | 11.7 | 13.6 | 11.3 | 11.4 | 12.6 | 11.7 | 10.3 | 17.9 |
| Birth weight | | | | | | | | | |
| Very low birth weight[c] | 1.3 | 1.2 | 1.8 | 1.3 | 1.4 | 1.4 | 1.5 | 1.1 | 3.1 |
| Low birth weight[d] | 7.2 | 6.7 | 9.7 | 7.0 | 7.1 | 8.1 | 7.9 | 6.6 | 13.5 |
| 4,000 grams or more[e] | 8.1 | 8.4 | 7.2 | 8.9 | 8.4 | 7.1 | 10.5 | 11.9 | 5.0 |
| Five-minute Apgar score of less than 7[f] | 1.3 | 1.2 | 1.4 | 0.8 | 1.1 | 1.3 | 1.5 | 1.3 | 2.4 |

**Infant health/mothers born outside the United States**

| | | | | | | | | | |
|---|---|---|---|---|---|---|---|---|---|
| Preterm births[b] | 11.0 | 10.6 | 14.5 | 11.5 | 11.7 | 10.3 | 10.5 | 9.2 | 14.2 |
| Birth weight | | | | | | | | | |
| Very low birth weight[c] | 1.0 | 0.9 | 1.9 | 1.3 | 1.2 | 1.0 | 1.4 | 1.1 | 2.8 |
| Low birth weight[d] | 5.9 | 5.5 | 9.6 | 6.1 | 6.4 | 5.9 | 7.3 | 6.0 | 9.9 |
| 4,000 grams or more[e] | 9.7 | 10.0 | 6.9 | 10.8 | 9.2 | 9.4 | 8.1 | 11.2 | 8.2 |
| Five-minute Apgar score of less than 7[f] | 1.1 | 1.1 | 1.5 | 0.7 | 1.0 | 0.8 | 1.2 | 1.0 | 2.0 |

[a]Includes races other than White and African American.

[b]Born prior to thirty-seven completed weeks of gestation.

[c]Birth weight of less than 1,500 grams (3 lb., 4 oz.).

[d]Birth weight of less than 2,500 grams (5 lb., 8 oz.).

[e]Equivalent to 8 lb., 14 oz.

[f]Excludes data for California and Texas, which did not report five-minute Apgar score on the birth certificate.

*Note:* Race and Latino origin are reported separately on birth certificates. Persons of Latino origin may be of any race. In this table Latino women are classified only by place of origin; non-Latino women are classified by race.

*Source:* National Center for Health Statistics (2000, March 28). *National Vital Statistics Report, 48,* 3.

in the United States, with a rate of 1.3, compared to 1.0 for foreign-born Latino mothers. Puerto Rican mothers, both in Puerto Rico and on the U.S. mainland, were most likely to have higher rates of VLBW babies (1.9 for mainland-born mothers versus 1.8 for those born on the island; see Table 5.7).

Puerto Rican mothers also were most likely to have LBW infants (9.7), as compared to 6.0 for Mexican mothers. LBW is associated with maternal weight gained during the pregnancy. Puerto Rican women were most likely among Latino mothers to have gained less mean weight during the pregnancy. The rate of LBW varies by the mother's place of birth, with Latino mothers born in the United States having a slightly higher rate of LBW (6.4 versus 5.9). Again, regardless of place of birth, Puerto Rican mothers were most likely to have babies of LBW (mainland born, 9.7; island born, 9.6; see Table 5.7) (Ventura, Martin, Curtin, Mathews, & Park, 2000).

In 1998, 9 percent of all infants born to Latino mothers weighed 4,000 grams (8 lb., 14 oz. or more), compared to 11.8 percent for White mothers. The percentage for African American mothers was the lowest (5.3 percent). This percentage varies by Latino mothers of different origins, with Cuban mothers experiencing the highest percentage (10 percent) and Puerto Rican mothers the lowest (7.1 percent). This percentage slightly increased for Latino mothers born outside the United States (9.7 percent versus 9 percent), with the exception of mothers born in Puerto Rico. For Latino mothers born in the United States the difference is most pronounced among Mexican mothers (U.S.-born, 8.4 percent; Mexico-born, 10 percent) and Cuban mothers (U.S.-born, 8.9 percent; Cuba-born, 10.8 percent) (Ventura, Martin, Curtin, Mathews, & Park, 2000). A number of studies (Zambrana, Scrimshaw, & Dunkel, 1996; Hayes-Bautista, 1992; Guendelman, Gould, Hudes, & Eskenazi, 1990; Sherraden & Barrera, 1996, among others) have demonstrated reduced rates of LBW infants among less acculturated Mexican American women. While LBW rates among Latinos as a group are not among the highest, second-generation Mexican American women are almost twice as likely to experience an LBW outcome than first-generation Mexican immigrants. Zambrana, Scrimshaw, Collins, & Dunkel-Schetter (1997), in a comparative study of Mexican Americans and Mexican-born women, found that Mexican Americans were at higher medical risk during pregnancy but found no significant differences between the two groups in infant gestational age and birth weight. However, the same study did provide evidence that higher acculturation was associated with higher prenatal stress, which was correlated with preterm delivery, substance use, and low social support.

Babies born with LBW vary by the mothers' age. In 1998, 6.4 percent of all Latino births were babies born weighing 2,500 grams (5 lb., 8 oz.) or less. This percentage of LBW infants was close to the percentage of LBW babies born to White mothers (6.6 percent) but considerably less than LBW babies born to African American women (13.2 percent; see Table 5.7) (Ventura, Martin, Curtin, Mathews, & Park, 2000). The percentage of Latino LBW babies was highest among older Latino mothers aged forty-five to fifty-four) (17.4 percent) and among Latino mothers under the age of 15 (10.5 percent; data not shown on the table) (Ventura, Martin, Curtin, Mathews, & Park, 2000). Latino mothers between the ages of twenty-five and twenty-nine were the least likely to have had LBW babies (5.7 percent) (Ventura, Martin, Curtin, Mathews, & Park, 2000). Again, infants born to U.S.-born Latino mothers were at the highest risk.

# Breastfeeding

There are numerous advantages to breastfeeding children, including reduced illness to both the mother and the child after birth, and a more rapid postpartum recuperation period. According to the American Academy of Pediatrics (AAP), breastfeeding (Pickering, et al., 1998) provides the child with numerous advantages, among which are protection against infections, iron deficiency, asthma and other respiratory illnesses, ear infections, bacterial and intestinal disorders, juvenile onset diabetes, and childhood cancer (Wright et al., 1998; Davis, Savitz, & Graubard, 1998). It also reduces the risk of sudden infant death syndrome (SIDS) and Hodgkin's disease, and contributes to decreased infant mortality rates (McKenna, Mosko, Richard, & Christopher, 1997).

Although Latinas are viewed as coming from a breastfeeding culture, nursing rates begin to decline when immigrants settle in the United States. By the third generation, Latinas breastfeed at the same rate as other women in the same socioeconomic group. However, according to the 1995 NSFG (Abma, Chandra, Mosher, Peterson, & Piccinino, 1997), of the Latino babies born in the combined years of 1990–1993, some 62.2 percent were breastfed by their Latino mothers, compared to 59.1 percent of babies breastfed by Whites mothers. Slightly more White women breastfed their infants for five or more months than Latino mothers (53.3 percent and 50.2 percent, respectively). African American babies were the least likely of the three groups to be breastfed by their mothers (25.1 percent); when they were, the duration of breastfeeding was relatively short (Abma, Chandra, Mosher, Peterson, & Piccinino, 1997). Factors that may impact the likelihood of breastfeeding include the mother's age, education, marital status, level of acculturation, employment, perceived benefits of bottle-feeding as opposed to breastfeeding for both the mother's and the child's health, the nature of the interaction with the physician, and the structural characteristics of the health delivery system (Wright et al. 1988; Stern & Giachello, 1977).

Another important factor that affects breastfeeding rates among Latino women is the successful penetration of the baby formula industry into the markets of developing countries such as those in Latin America. Bottle-feeding campaigns attempted to convey the message that utilizing baby formula is healthier for infants than breastfeeding, without consideration of sanitation measures such as access to potable water and proper education regarding the preparation and use of the formula. This trend, in conjunction with a series of myths regarding mothers' inadequacies in their physiological capacity to breastfeed, may explain the decline in breastfeeding rates in Puerto Rico and among groups of Latinas in the United States (Giachello, 1994b). Other factors that affect breastfeeding behaviors are the following: (1) myths such as that it will cause cancer or that thin women and those with small breasts do not produce enough milk to satisfy the new infant; (2) the increased participation of mothers in the labor force; and (3) women's concerns with physical appearance.

## Infant Mortality

The infant mortality rate is generally considered a good index of the standard of living of any population group: the lower the infant mortality rate, the better the standard of living. The rate of infant mortality is also a good indicator of the general health status prevailing in a population.

The infant mortality rate (per 1,000 live births) for Latinos in 1997 was lower than that for non-Latinos (6.0 versus 7.5) (Hoyert, Kochanek, & Murphy, 1999); the rate for African Americans was twice as high (14.2). Among Latino women by nationalities, the infant mortality rate was the lowest among the Mexican American population and the highest among Puerto Ricans. The ten major causes of infant mortality in 1997 for Latino infants as a whole per 100,000 live births were as follows: congenital anomalies (161.3); disorders relating to short gestation and unspecified LBW (73.7); SIDS (47.6); respiratory distress syndrome (26.5); the newborn affected by maternal complications of pregnancy (20.6); the newborn affected by complications of the placenta, cord, and membranes (17.8); injuries and accidents (17.5); infections specific to the perinatal period (16.6); pneumonia and influenza (10.7); and intrauterine hypoxia and birth asphyxia (8.3) (Hoyert, Kochanek, & Murphy, 1999). Studies indicate that infant mortality rates tend to be higher for infants whose mothers began prenatal care after the first trimester, were adolescents or older than forty, did not complete a high school degree, were unmarried, or smoked during pregnancy (MacDorman & Atkinson, 1998). Infant mortality also has been found to be higher among male infants, multiple births, and infants born preterm or of LBW (Hoyert, Kochanek, & Murphy, 1999). In addition, studies document that infant mortality increases by mothers' levels of acculturation, with U.S.-born mothers most likely to have an infant death compared to those born outside the United States. Also, Puerto Rican mothers (both born on the U.S. mainland and in Puerto Rico) are most likely to experience an infant death (Becerra, Hague, Atrash, & Perez, 1991).

## Maternal Deaths

In 1997, Latino women experienced higher maternal deaths than did Whites. The crude rate of Latino maternal mortality due to complications of pregnancy, childbirth, and the puerperium for all age groups was lower, 8.0 per 100,000, than that of White women (5.8). The age-adjusted rate of maternal mortality for Latino women was less (7.6), but still almost twice as high as that for White women (4.4) (National Center for Health Statistics unpublished data for 1997). African American women have a substantially higher risk of maternal death than do

Latinas or Whites; the crude rate for 1997 was 20.8 per 100,000 live births (Hoyert, Kochanek, & Murphy, 1999).

In summary, Latino mothers' pregnancy outcomes are overall quite similar to that of Whites or have outcomes that are in between those obtained by White mothers and African American mothers. Pregnancy outcomes overall were more positive for Mexican mothers and relatively less positive for Puerto Rican women. The impact of acculturation, measured by place of birth, indicate that pregnancy outcomes deteriorate among U.S.-born Latino mothers.

## Role of Family Planning Services

About three-fourths (74.4 percent) of young Latino women between the ages of fifteen and twenty-four reported receiving help from a family planning service at some point in their lives; this compares to 79.9 percent of White women and 83.1 percent of African American women (Abma, Chandra, Mosher, Peterson, & Piccinino, 1997). More than one-third of Latinas (36.9 percent) had their family planning visit at a clinic and an additional 30 percent had it at a private doctor or health maintenance organization (HMO) (Abma, Chandra, Mosher, Peterson, & Piccinino, 1997). All young women reported receiving help with a birth control method, birth control counseling, or a birth control checkup. Consistently, Latino women were least likely to have received any of those services (Abma, Chandra, Mosher, Peterson, & Piccinino, 1997).

In 1995, about one-third (32.7 percent) of Latino women (as well as White and African American women) between the ages of fifteen and forty-four reported receiving family planning services from a medical provider in the twelve-month period prior to the survey (Abma, Chandra, Mosher, Peterson, & Piccinino, 1997). About one-fourth of Latino women received a birth control method, 15 percent received birth control counseling, 20 percent received a birth control checkup or test, and 3.9 percent received sterilization counseling. The percentages of types of services received by White and African American women were quite close to those of Latinas.

In another national survey among 1,852 women whose incomes were below 200 percent of the poverty level and who were sexually active and between the ages of eighteen and thirty-four, Darroch-Forest and Frost (1996) found that Latino women reported that what they liked the most in their last gynecological visit were the cleanliness of the facility, respectful and courteous treatment by staff, and the good quality of care. However, the vast majority of Spanish-speaking Latino women (96 percent) in the survey would have liked to have received their services in Spanish (Darroch-Forest & Frost, 1996).

In the 1995 NSFG, 59 percent of Latino women between the ages of twenty-two and forty-four reported using a method of contraception at the time of the study. This percentage was lower than that of White (66.1 percent) and African American women (62.1) (Abma, Chandra, Mosher, Peterson, & Piccinino, 1997). The methods that these women most often reported using were female sterilization (Latino women, 36.6 percent; Whites, 24.6 percent, and

African Americans, 40.1 percent), the pill (Latino and White women, 23 percent; African Americans, 28.5 percent), and a condom (about 20 percent each) (Abma, Chandra, Mosher, Peterson, & Piccinino, 1997). The most common form of sterilization reported by all women was tubal ligation, ranging from 20.9 percent among Latinas, 16.3 percent among Whites, and 24.6 percent among African Americans (Abma, Chandra, Mosher, Peterson, & Piccinino, 1997). Married women of all racial and ethnic backgrounds reported much higher percentages of sterilization. The percentages were higher among White and African American married women (42 percent and 46.2 percent, respectively), compared to Latino women (36.7 percent) (Abma, Chandra, Mosher, Peterson, & Piccinino, 1997). Also, African American married women reported a much higher percentage of hysterectomies (11.3 percent) than Latino and White women (5 percent and 6.8 percent, respectively) (Abma, Chandra, Mosher, Peterson, & Piccinino, 1997).

Another study conducted by the Alan Guttmacher Institute (1998), which examined trend data on contraceptive use by women between the ages of fifteen and forty-four from the National Survey of Family Growth, found that the percentage of Latino women relying on female sterilization increased from 23 percent in 1982 to 37 percent in 1995 (see Table 5.8). On the other hand, there was a drastic reduction in the use of the IUD (intrauterine device) and the pill. There was has also been an increase in male condom use, reflecting an acceptance of this method as a result of the increased awareness of HIV/AIDS and other sexually transmitted diseases (see Table 5.8).

Finally, about 13 percent of Latino and African American women between the ages of fifteen and forty-four reported in 1995 receiving infertility services to

### TABLE 5.8.   PERCENTAGE OF DISTRIBUTION OF CONTRACEPTIVE USERS AGED 15–44, BY CURRENT METHOD, ACCORDING TO RACE AND ETHNICITY: 1995.

| Method | Latino | White | African American |
|---|---|---|---|
| Female sterilization | 37 | 25 | 40 |
| Male sterilization | 4 | 14 | 2 |
| Pill | 23 | 29 | 24 |
| Implant | 2 | 1 | 2 |
| Injectable | 5 | 2 | 5 |
| IUD | 2 | 1 | 1 |
| Diaphragm | 1 | 2 | 1 |
| Male condom | 21 | 20 | 20 |
| Other | 6 | 7 | 5 |
| Total | 100 | 100 | 100 |
| No. (in thousands) | 3,957 | 28,120 | 5,098 |

*Source:* Henshaw, S. (1998). Unintended Pregnancy in the United States. *Family Planning Perspectives, 30,* 1, 24–29, 46.

help them get pregnant or to prevent a miscarriage, compared to 16.3 percent for Whites (Alan Guttmacher Institute, 1998). The services most often received were advice (with percentages for all women ranging between 4 percent and 7 percent) or tests on women or men (percentages ranging between 2 percent and 5 percent) (Alan Guttmacher Institute, 1998).

## Unintended Pregnancy and Abortion

Data from the 1982, 1988, and 1995 cycles of the National Survey of Family Growth, as well as other supplementary data sets, were used to estimate the 1994 unintended births and abortions among the U.S. population (Henshaw, 1998). The study found that 49 percent of all the pregnancies reported in these surveys in the United States were unintended and that 54 percent of these unintended pregnancies ended in abortion. Among Latino women the study found that about half of all pregnancies were also unintended, that is, that the women did not want to have a child at that time or wanted no more births. Of the total unwanted pregnancies, about half (26 percent) ended in abortion.

The acceptance of abortion seems to be increasing among Latino women, particularly younger ones, with higher levels of acculturation. A mail survey conducted by the National Latino Institute for Reproductive Health (NLIRH) (1999) found that 37 percent of the respondents said that women should have unrestricted access to abortion and another 31 percent stated that access to abortion should be granted under almost all circumstances. Furthermore, 55 percent of the mail respondents identified themselves as "prochoice" and a majority (68 percent) said women should have easy access to abortion. Most of the Latino women who supported a prochoice view were Mexican Americans or women of South American origins, were between the ages of thirty-six and fifty and spoke English fluently. In addition, most of them relied on doctors, Planned Parenthood, and community health clinics for information about birth control. Most of those Latinas who were not prochoice or did not strongly support the prochoice movement were Puerto Ricans, Central Americans, or Cubans, persons whose language was primarily Spanish, or persons between the ages of sixteen and twenty-five (National Latino Institute for Reproductive Health, 1999). Few Latinas said that they rely on the church or school advisers for birth control information, but dependence on the church, according to the NLIRH survey, increased with age (1999). Surprisingly, reliance on family and on friends was relatively low in this study.

# HIV/AIDS and Other Sexually Transmitted Diseases

Through December 1998, women as a group represented 19.1 percent (or 131,446) of all the U.S. adult or adolescent accumulated AIDS cases (688,200) (Centers for Disease Control and Prevention, 1999a, 1999b). Latinas represented 20.2 percent of the total AIDS cases among women. The main modes of transmission for Latino women are heterosexual contact (47 percent) and the use of infected needles (41 percent) during intravenous drug use (IVDU) (Centers for Disease Control and Prevention, 1999a). Prior to the use of a combination of drug therapies to treat HIV infections, AIDS incidence was increasing at rates of 15 percent to 30 percent each year among African American and Latino women (National Institutes of Health, 1998). Despite a decline of HIV/AIDS among the U.S. population as a whole, the number of new infections continues to increase among women of color. African American and Latino women represent less than one-fourth of the total U.S. female population, but they account for more than three-fourths (82 percent) of new infections between 1995 and 1998 among all infected women (African American women, 64 percent; Latino women, 18 percent) (Centers for Disease Control and Prevention, 1998b) (see Chapter Eleven for more information).

Most of the public response in reference to women has been on how to prevent pregnancies among infected women and, if the woman is pregnant, on how to minimize the risk of perinatal transmission and its potential impact on the newborn. Among all the pediatric AIDS cases recorded until December 1998, Latino children under the age of thirteen represented 11.5 percent. Perinatal transmission was the main mode of infection for this population (Centers for Disease Control and Prevention, 1999a). In 1994, research showed that Zidovudine (called AZT in the United States) therapy given to HIV-infected pregnant women from the fourteenth to thirty-fourth week, continuing throughout the pregnancy and during labor and delivery, and then administered to the child for six weeks after birth, could significantly reduce perinatal HIV transmission (Centers for Disease Control and Prevention, 1999a). Antiretroviral therapy has helped to reduce the number of U.S. infants who acquire HIV by 73 percent from 1992 through 1998 (Centers for Disease Control and Prevention, 1999a).

Unfortunately, lack of access to medical care due to financial, cultural, and institutional barriers and lack of knowledge about HIV/AIDS prevention—combined with cultural norms and gender roles, fear of deportation (among undocumented women), and lack of culturally and linguistically competent HIV/AIDS counseling services—are some of the major obstacles that confront poor Latino women who need HIV counseling, testing, and therapy (Kaiser Family Foundation, 1998).

There are more than twenty diseases (including chlamydia, gonorrhea, syphilis, genital herpes [HSV-2], human papillomavirus infection [HPV], hepatitis B, trichomoniasis, bacterial vaginosis, chancroid, and others) that are sexually transmitted, and the trend for each disease varies considerably (Centers for Disease Control and Prevention, 1998b). The latest estimate indicates that there are fifteen million new cases of STDs in the United States each year, and while syphilis and gonorrhea have been brought to all-time lows, others, such as herpes and chlamydia, continue to spread widely throughout the population (Centers for Disease Control and Prevention, 1998a, 1998b).

By far, women bear the greatest burden of STDs. The most serious STDs among women are chlamydia (with one out of ten young women infected), followed by gonorrhea and HPV. The prevalence of chlamydia in 1998 was higher among African American, White, and Mexican American women (7 percent, 5 percent, and 2 percent, respectively) than men (6 percent, 2 percent, and 1 percent, respectively). Among teen women aged fifteen to nineteen, the prevalence was more than 12 percent for African Americans, 6 percent for Mexican Americans, and close to 4 percent for Whites (Centers for Disease Control and Prevention, 1999). The prevalence in Puerto Rico in 1997 was much higher, ranging from 5 percent to 10 percent. No data is available for other Latino groups.

The rate of gonorrhea among all women in 1998 was 119.3 per 100,000 (Centers for Disease Control and Prevention, 1998b). It remained almost three times greater for Latinas (69.4 per 100,000) than for Whites (26.0 per 100,000) of all age groups (Centers for Disease Control and Prevention, 1998b); the rate is substantially higher among African Americans (807.9 per100,000). This condition dramatically affects teen women and young adult women, reaching the rate of 327 per 100,000 among Latino women between the ages of fifteen and nineteen and 251.6 per 100,000 among Latino women between the ages of twenty and twenty-five. Untreated, both chlamydia and gonorrhea can lead to infertility, potentially fatal ectopic pregnancies, and chronic pelvic pain and scarring; they can also increase an individual's risk of becoming infected with HIV if exposed. If not diagnosed and treated in time during pregnancy, women are at risk for spontaneous abortion and stillbirth; moreover, gonorrhea and chlamydia can result in serious health problems for newborn infants. For example, chlamydia can cause conjunctivitis in infants born to infected mothers. In general, infants born to mothers with certain STDs are at risk of blindness, mental retardation, and death.

The rate of congenital syphilis is nine times higher among Latino infants than among White infants. Syphilis elimination efforts are critical to improving infant health, slowing the spread of HIV infection, and reducing racial disparities in health. Untreated syphilis during pregnancy can result in infant death in up to 40 percent of cases (Centers for Disease Control and Prevention, 1998b). Syphilis can be a major cause of cardiovascular disease, neurological disease, and blindness for the mother (Centers for Disease Control and Prevention, 1998b). The incidence is higher among men than women, although the rates of primary and secondary syphilis among Latino women is twice the rate of non-Latino women (Centers for Disease Control and Prevention, 1998b).

Human Papilloma Virus (HPV) infection is the most common STD, affecting 75 percent of the reproductive-age population (Koutsky, 1997). The prevalence among all Mexican Americans is 5.4 per 100,000, and it triples to 14.8 for Mexican Americans between the ages of twenty and twenty-nine (Koutsky, 1997). The rates for African Americans of the same categories are 8.8 and 33.3 per 100,000, respectively; and for Whites, 4.5 and 14.7 per 100,000 (Koutsky, 1997). Herpes is more common among women than men, affecting one out of four women (Centers for Disease Control and Prevention, 1998b).

In summary, health disparities exist among Latinas reflected in the highest rates of HIV/AIDS, chlamydia, gonorrhea, and HPV (Centers for Disease Control and Prevention, 1999b), among other types of STDs. Although, most of these conditions have declined for the U.S. population as a whole and for the White population, for African Americans and Latinos they have either remained stable or have increased in the past decade. A Centers for Disease Control and Prevention study (1999b) demonstrates that many young people at risk lack even basic information about how to protect themselves from infection with STDs. Anecdotal information from health providers suggests that Latinos deny the possibility of having any of the STD conditions and that they are not likely to seek health care for STDs unless symptoms are noticeable or are accompanied by pain. However, perhaps the lack of STD knowledge, lack of basic knowledge about how to protect themselves from infection, combined with lack of health insurance and cultural and linguistic barriers to accessing the health care system, might be better explanations for the lack of early screening, diagnosis, and treatment of STDs.

## Mental Health and Stressful Life Events

In a 1993 national survey, more than one-half of Latino women (53 percent) reported severe chronic depression, compared to Whites (37 percent), and African Americans (47 percent) (Louis Harris and Associates, 1993). This study found that Mexican American women between the ages of twenty and seventy-four were more than twice as likely as Mexican American men to exhibit high levels of depressive symptoms (18.7 percent versus 8.0 percent). It has been argued that Latino women are exposed to a number of psychosocial and environmental stressors that may lead them to mental illness. These include high poverty, stress associated with single parenting, gender roles, low educational achievement, the effects of migration, the process associated with acculturation and adaptation, domestic violence, and social discrimination (see Chapter Seven for more information).

A study investigating the psychosocial factors related to pre- and postnatal anxiety among primiparous Mexican American women in Los Angeles found that high prenatal anxiety was significantly associated with high postnatal anxiety. High postnatal anxiety, in turn, may negatively affect parenting behavior (Engle, Scrimshaw, Zambrana, & Dunkel-Schetter, 1990). High prenatal anxiety was also associated with a lower desire for an active role during labor, lower assertiveness, higher pain expectation, and a lack of support from family members other than the husband. This study, however, did not find any significant correlations of the baby's condition or of complications in labor and delivery with prenatal anxiety (Engle, Scrimshaw, Zambrana, & Dunkel-Schetter, 1990).

## Use of Illicit Drugs

The 1997 National Household Survey on Drug Abuse (Substance Abuse and Mental Health Services Administration, 1998) found that Latinos are less likely than Whites or African Americans to report ever having tried illicit drugs, although they were most likely to report being current users of diverse substances (for example, heroin, cocaine, crack, PCP [phencyclidnine, or "angel dust"], sedatives, tranquilizers, stimulants, or analgesics). These types of drugs are usually associated with physical addiction, with excess mortality and with other negative social consequences for the individual, for his or her family, and for the community. These problems are expected to increase as the percentage of Latinos reporting ever having used cocaine increases, particularly among young adults of both sexes between the ages of eighteen and twenty-five (Substance Abuse and Mental Health Services Administration, 1998). It has been suggested in the literature that Whites may be more likely to experiment with illicit drugs, whereas African Americans and Latinos are more likely to use them regularly (National Council of La Raza, 1990). A series of legal and ethical controversies have emerged regarding substance use during pregnancy. The National Association for Perinatal Addiction Research and Education (NAPARE, 1991) found that an increased number of women have been charged nationwide with felony crimes ranging from delivery of a drug to a minor to use or possession of a controlled substance, based on their prenatal drug use. It has been argued that criminalization of prenatal drug use may lead pregnant drug users to either delay their entry into the medical care system or not to use the medical system at all for prenatal care because of fears of prosecution. This may have particularly negative consequences for Latino women who already delay seeing a health care provider for prenatal care or just do not see one at all (Giachello, 1991). The patterns of illicit drug use among Latino women require attention and monitoring because pregnant addicted women require special intervention and attention. Despite recent increases in drug treatment rehabilitation programs for women, as yet few have the capacity to treat pregnant women with addiction.

## Summary and Conclusions

This chapter has attempted to summarize current knowledge of reproductive health, maternal risk factors and behaviors, and complications regarding pregnancy, labor, and delivery, as well as health problems and illnesses that impact them the most. Most of the information described indicates that Latino women continue having the highest birth and fertility rates of any other racial and ethnic minority group in the United States. The incidence of teen births and births out of wedlock continues to increase among the different Latino groups, particularly to those mothers who have been born in the United States. Latino mothers, as a group, are least likely to benefit from state-of-the-art medical techniques during prenatal care (such as ultrasound diagnosis) and during labor (fetal monitoring). Although most Latinas are not likely to experience complications during delivery, a substantial number may develop gestational diabetes with its associated risks (such as large babies requiring delivery by cesarean section). Finally, the health of Latino infants is comparable to those of White infants, although exceptions in Puerto Rican babies occur (like low birth weight). A series of challenges remain, and they must be addressed to improve the health and well-being of Latino mothers and children.

## Recommendations

- *Diversity of Latino Women*  Currently, we know very little about the health and social needs of women from Central or South America. We know little about posttraumatic stress disorders that many of them might be experiencing as a result of their personal and family experiences related to political persecution or wars in their countries of origin. Also, we know little about the diverse health beliefs and behaviors of Mexican American and Puerto Rican populations. From the research perspective and for effective program development and planning, we need to examine such differences as they reflect specific places of origin (for example, rural villages versus small towns versus big cities).
- *Financial Investment in Public Health*  About 70 percent of premature deaths and illnesses are preventable. They are related to environmental health factors and to individual behaviors and lifestyles. However, 90 percent of U.S. health care resources go to cover medical treatment of conditions once they have occurred. This must change.
- *Race and Sex Bias*  There is a need to reduce institutional racism and sexism, which deprive Latino communities of socioeconomic opportunities, negatively impact the quality of life of communities by producing low self-esteem, and cause a series of psychosocial stresses which increase the risk factors for a number of health and mental illnesses. A recent study on race, ethnicity, and medical care commissioned by the Kaiser Family Foundation (1999), found that 13 percent of Latinos reported that either they themselves had directly experienced unfair treatment in seeking medical care or a family member had done so (25 percent) or a friend or someone else they knew (25 percent).
- *Increase Access to Health and Medical Care*  Recent research and data indicate that 35 percent of Latinos are not linked to a regular source of health care (Kaiser Family Foundation, 1999) and about 35.3 percent do not have health insurance (Giachello, 2000). The lack of health insurance goes up to 44 percent for poor Latinos, compared to 28.5 percent for poor Whites (United States Bureau of the Census, 1999). Furthermore, half of the poor foreign residents in the United States and half of those who are not citizens do not have health insurance (53.3 percent and 58.6 percent, respectively). Therefore, strong policies need to be developed at the national level that clearly convey the message that access to health care is a fundamental human right and not a privilege. Sooner or later the United States must recognize this essential self-evident truth: that without health, "we the people" cannot work, nor take care of our families, nor be productive members of society.
- *Culturally Appropriate Programs*  There must be a strong commitment to developing, implementing, and institutionalizing culturally appropriate programs and approaches in the delivery of health care, as well as in reducing linguistic barriers to medical services.

- *Monitor Accessibility to Health and Medical Services Under Managed Care* A number of concerns have been raised about marketing strategies of HMOs directed to Latinos and other communities and the poor quality of care provided to individuals and families enrolled in these plans. The mainstream media, through cases that have come to public attention or to the courts, have documented the barriers to accessing specialists and hospitals or even emergency rooms; the limited support and follow-up services that these HMOs have in place; and the consequences in terms of premature deaths and/or serious disabilities. There is a need to scrutinize these practices as well as the types of incentives provided by HMOs to health care providers to limit services to patients, including the amount of time spent with each patient, and other possible violations of patients rights.
- *Improve the Quality of Health and Medical Care* Studies have documented variations in the quality of medical care in relation to certain medical procedures used (such as cesareans) and certain patient characteristics (notably having or not having health insurance) (see Lawlor & Raube, 1995). Part of the problem is that physicians and other health care providers have limited familiarity with clinical guidelines and appropriate protocols for the management and treatment of certain conditions such as asthma, diabetes, and cancer (McDermott, Silva, Giachello, & Rydman, 1996; Lipton, Losey, & Giachello, 1996; Raube, Handler, & Giachello, 1995).
- *Innovative Interventions* The federal government's *Racial and Ethnic Approaches to Community Health (REACH) 2010* initiative to eliminate health disparities is a clear example of needed interventions in communities of color. This initiative is aimed at impacting the community as a whole by creating coalitions with health and human services organizations aimed at changing community norms, as well as the development of culturally appropriate and gender-appropriate interventions and the supportive environment for sustaining behavioral changes. Part of this effort is to study the impact of Medicaid and Medicare managed care plans—how they have been implemented, how they have been accepted by poor communities of color and by elderly Latinos, and what is the quality of care that Latinos enrolled in those plans are receiving from them. There is also a need to get managed care organizations to collect data on demographic and socioeconomic characteristics of enrollees to determine the impact of these systems on the health of Latinos, in general, and of Latino women, in particular.
- *Improve Data Systems* Tremendous progress has occurred in the past decade in generating more and better data and research on Latinos (including Latinas), yet more progress is needed in collecting information pertaining to diverse Latino groups. For example, the fastest growing Latino populations are those coming from Central and South America, but data on them are categorized (that is, grouped together) as "Central and South American" and details are practically nonexistent. This category does not provide the needed information that would enable us to understand the health profile of each population in particular and to develop the necessary individual interventions. Local data are very limited even for the larger Latino populations such as recent Mexican immigrants and Mexican Americans. Many public health departments do not

have the financial resources or staffing to develop or support an infrastructure for the gathering, analyses, and dissemination of data; or the data systems do not have the ethnic identifiers to produce detailed information. At the national level, there are also a number of deficiencies: (1) the National Health and Nutritional Examination Survey includes samples of Mexican Americans, yet no information is included for Puerto Ricans or for any other Latino groups; and (2) the national data system does not include the data from the island of Puerto Rico, making it difficult to assess the health of Puerto Ricans who come back and forth from the island. This information could be valuable in understanding the health problems and patterns of health services utilization, as well as risk factors.

- *Assessment of Public Policy Impact* There is also a great need to investigate the performance and impact of public policies such as welfare reform, immigration reform, Medicaid and Medicare managed care plans, child care legislation, and health insurance for children on the life of Latino men, women, and children.

- *Increase the Number of Latinos in Health Professions and Workforce* To increase the representation of Latinos in the health fields in proportion to their total U.S. population, an additional 225,000 Latinos are needed (Gray and Puente, 1996). To accomplish this goal at present seems almost impossible, as Latinos are increasingly going to public or private segregated schools located in areas where those schools have limited financial resources to provide them with the technology for top scientific education and with the resources (financial and human) to teach them well. Moreover, nationally it is estimated that only 3 percent of teachers are Latinos; therefore, the lack of mentorship and role models makes it more difficult to encourage Latino students to enter and finish courses of study at health professional school.

## Specific Recommendations for Latino Women's Health

1. There is a need to educate and support immigrants' families about their daughters (born or raised in the United States) and about their increased risks of unwanted pregnancies, injuries, homicide, HIV/AIDS and other STDs, and tobacco, alcohol, and other drug use.

2. There is a need to study effective ways to engage Latino communities in risk reduction behaviors to delay the development of diabetes and other chronic conditions before, during, and after pregnancy, such as supporting exercise, healthy eating, and/or developing or maintaining other healthy behaviors.

3. There is a need to study biological, behavioral, environmental, and social processes, including community norms, that determine the physical, emotional, and cognitive growth of Latinas from the moment of inception and through transitions of infancy, childhood, and adolescence, which set the foundation for conditions, diseases, and behaviors that impact human reproduction and ultimately lead to health disparities.

4. There is a need to study the quality of prenatal care and Latino women's access to available and new technology during labor and delivery. The information

provided in this chapter indicates that Latino women are least likely to receive the benefits of the available technology in the area of perinatal health.

5. There is little or no research in the area of eating disorders (for example, obesity and anorexia) or estimates about the prevalence of eating disorders in Latino communities.

# References

Abma, J., Chandra, A., Mosher, W., Peterson, L., & Piccinino, L. (1997). Fertility, family planning and women's health: New data from the 1995 National Survey of Family Growth. National Center for Health Statistics. *Vital and Health Statistics, 23,* 19.

Alan Guttmacher Institute. (1999, April). *Teenage pregnancy: Overall trends and state-by-state information.* Washington, D.C.: AGI.

American Diabetes Association. (2000). *Clinical guidelines on diabetes care.* Washington, D.C.: Author.

American Heart Association. (1999). *2000 heart and stroke statistical update.* Dallas, TX: Author.

Balcazar, H., & Krull, J. (1999). Determinants of birth-weight outcomes among Mexican-American women: Examining conflicting results about acculturation. *Ethnicity and Disease, 9,* 3, 410–422.

Becerra, J. E., Hague, C. J., Atrash, H., & Perez, N. (1991). Infant mortality among Hispanics: Portrait of heterogeneity. *Journal of the American Medical Association, 265,* 217–221.

Black, S. A., & Markides, K. S. (1993). Acculturation and alcohol consumption in Puerto Rican, Cuban-American, and Mexican-American women in the United States. *American Journal of Public Health, 83,* 6, 890–893.

Brown, S., & Lumley, J. (1993). Antenatal care: A case of inverse care law? *American Journal of Public Health, 17,* 19–103.

Center for the Future of Children. (1991). *The future of children: Drug-exposed infants.* Los Altos, CA: The David and Lucile Packard Foundation.

Centers for Disease Control and Prevention. (1998a, December 6–9). *National STD Prevention in the New Millennium Conference.* Dallas, TX.

Centers for Disease Control and Prevention. (1998b). *Tracking the hidden epidemics trends in STDs in the United States.* Atlanta, GA: Author.

Centers for Disease Control and Prevention. (1999a). *HIV/AIDS Surveillance Report: U.S. HIV/AIDS cases reported through December 1998.* USDHHS, PHS, CDC, Center for Infectious Diseases, Division of HIV/AIDS. Atlanta, GA: Author.

Centers for Disease Control and Prevention. (1999b). *National HIV Seroprevalence Surveys: Summary of results. Data from serosurveillance activities through 1998.* USDHHS, PHS, CDC, Center for Infectious Diseases, Division of HIV/AIDS. Atlanta, GA: Author.

Centers for Disease Control and Prevention. (1999). Tobacco use in the U.S.: *Report from the U.S. Surgeon General.* Washington, D.C.: Government Printing Office.

Chomitz, V. R., Cheung, L.W.Y., & Lieberman, E. (1995). The role of the lifestyle in preventing low birth weight. *The future of the children: Low birth weight, 5,* 1. Los Altos, CA: Center for the Children, The David and Lucile Packard Foundation, pp. 121–138.

Darroch-Forrest, J., & Frost, J. (1996). The family planning attitudes and experiences of low-income women. *Family Planning Perspectives, 28,* 246–255, 277.

Davis, M. K., Savitz, D. A., & Graubard, B. (1998). Infant feeding and childhood cancer. *Lancet, 2,* 8607, 365–368.

Engle, P., Scrimshaw, S., Zambrana, R. E., & Dunkel-Schetter, C. (1990). Prenatal and postnatal anxiety in Mexican women giving birth in Los Angeles. *Health Psychology, 9,* 3, 285–299.

Fang, J., Madhavan, S., & Alderman, M. H. (1999). The influence of maternal hypertension on low birth weight: Differences among ethnic populations. *Ethnicity and Disease, 9,* 3, 369–376.

Fiscella, K. (1995). Does prenatal improve birth outcomes? A critical review. *Obstetrical and Gynecology, 85,* 3, 46–79.

Floyd, R. L., Zahniser, S. C., Gunter, E. P., & Kendrick, J. S. (1991). Smoking during pregnancy: Prevalence, effects, and intervention strategies. *Birth, 18,* 1, 48–53.

Giachello, A. L. (1991). Issues of substance abuse and AIDS among women, infant and children. In *Common ground: HIV/AIDS, alcoholism and illicit drug use.* Chicago: Illinois Prevention Resource Center.

Giachello, A. L. (1994a). Issues of access and use. In C. W. Molina & M. Aguirre-Molina (Eds.), *Latino health in the U.S.: A growing challenge.* Washington, D.C.: American Public Health Association.

Giachello, A. L. (1994b). Maternal/perinatal health issues. In C. W. Molina & M. Aguirre-Molina (Eds.), *Latino health in the U.S.: A growing challenge.* Washington, D.C.: American Public Health Association.

Giachello, A. L. (1995). Cultural diversity and institutional inequality. In D. L. Adams (Ed.), *Health issues for women of color: Cultural diversity perspective.* Thousand Oaks, CA: Sage.

Giachello, A. L. (2000). Issues and challenges in eliminating health disparities among Hispanics/Latinos in the U.S. [Presentation at a televised meeting]. North Carolina: Chapel Hill School of Public Health.

Glasgow, R. E., & Eakin, E. G. (1998). Issues in diabetes self-management. In S. A. Schumaker et al. (Eds.), *The handbook of health behavior change.* New York: Springer.

Goldfard, M. G. (1984). *Who receives cesareans: Patient and hospital characteristics.* Hospital Cost and Utilization Project Research Note 4. (DHHS Publication PHS 84-3345). Washington, D.C.: National Center for Health Services Research.

Gray, J., & Puente, S. (1996). Overview of Hispanic/Latinos. *Journal of Medical Systems, 20,* 5, 229–233.

Guendelman, S., & Abrams, B. (1994). Dietary, alcohol and tobacco intake among Mexican-American women of childbearing age. Results from NHANES data. *American Journal of Health Promotion, 8,* 5, 363–372.

Guendelman, S., Gould, J. B., Hudes, M., & Eskenazi, B. (1990). Generational differences in prenatal health among the Mexican American population. Findings from NHANES, 1982–1984. *American Journal of Public Health, 80,* Dec Suppl.

Gutierrez, Y. M. (1999). Cultural factors affecting diet and pregnancy outcome of Mexican American adolescents. *Journal of Adolescent Health, 25,* 3, 227–237.

Hajat, A., Lucas, J., & Kington, K. (2000, February 25). *Health outcomes among Hispanic subgroups: Data from the national health interview survey, 1992–95.* (Advance data, No. 310). Atlanta, GA: Centers for Disease Control and Prevention.

Handler, A., Raube, K., Kelley, M., & Giachello, A. (1996, March). Women's satisfaction with prenatal care settings: A focus group study. *Birth, 23,* 1.

Hayes-Bautista, D. E. (1992). Latino health indicators and the underclass model: From paradox to new policy models. In A. Furino (Ed.), *Health policy and the Hispanic.* Boulder, CO: Westview Press.

Henshaw, S. (1998). Unintended pregnancy in the United States. *Family Planning Perspectives, 30,* 1, 24–29, 46.

Hoyert, D. L., Kochanek, K. D., & Murphy, S. L. (1999). Deaths: Final data for 1997. *National Vital Statistics Reports, 47,* 19. Hyattsville, MD: National Center for Health Statistics.

Huntington, J., & Connell, F. A. (1994). For every dollar spent. The cost-savings arguments for prenatal care. *NES.M, 33,* 19, 1303–1307.

Illinois Diabetes Control Program. (1999). *Diabetes clinical practice recommendations.* Springfield: Illinois Department of Health and Human Services.

Institute of Medicine. (1990). Subcommittee on nutritional status and weight gain during pregnancy-nutrition during pregnancy. *National academy of sciences.* Washington, D.C.: National Academy Press.

Kaiser Family Foundation. (1998, Spring). *National Survey of Latinos on HIV/AIDS.* Menlo Park, CA: Author.

Kaiser Family Foundation. (1999). *Medicare and minorities.* Menlo Park, CA: Author.

Koutsky, J. L. (1997). Epidemiology of genital human papillomavirus infection. *American Journal of Medicine, 102,* 5A, 3–8.

Lamberty, G. (1994). *Infant mortality: Experience of Hispanics.* Paper presented to the 1994 National Advisory Committee on Infant Mortality, Washington, D.C.

Lawlor, E., & Raube, K. (1995). Social interventions and outcomes in medical effectiveness research. *Social Science Review, 69,* 383–403.

Lipton, R., Losey, L., & Giachello, A. (1996). Factors affecting diabetes treatment and patient education among Latinos: Results of a preliminary study in Chicago. *Journal of Medical Systems, 20,* 5, 267–276.

Louis Harris and Associates. (1993, July). *The Commonwealth Fund Study of Women's Health.* New York: The Common Wealth Fund.

MacDorman, M. F., & Atkinson, J. O. (1998). Infant mortality statistics from the 1996 period linked birth/infant death data set. *Monthly Vital Statistics Report, 46,* 12, Suppl. Hyattsville, MD: National Center for Health Statistics.

Markides, K. S., Coreil, J. (1986). The health of Hispanics in the Southwestern United States: An epidemiologic paradox. *Public Health Reports, 101,* 3, 253–265.

McDermott, M., Silva, J., Giachello, A. L., & Rydman, R. (1996). Practice variations in treating urban minority asthmatics in Chicago. *Journal of Medical Systems, 20,* 5, 255–266.

McKenna, J. J., Mosko, S. S., Richard, C. A., and Christopher. (1997). Bedsharing promotes breast feeding. *Pediatrics, 100,* 214–219.

Napoles-Springer, A., & Pérez-Stable, E. (1996). Risk factors for invasive cervical cancer in Latino women. *Journal of Medical Systems, 20,* 5, 277–294.

National Association for Perinatal Addiction Research and Education. (1991). *Criminalization of prenatal drug use: Punitive measures will be counterproductive.* Chicago, Illinois.

National Center for Health Statistics. (1999). Hoyert, DL, Kochanek, KD, Murphy, SL. Death: Final data for 1997. *National Vital Statistics Reports, 47,* 19.

National Council of La Raza. (1990, November 17–20). *Hispanic consultation on alcohol and substance abuse: A community network response.* Washington, D.C.: Author.

National Heart, Lung, and Blood Institute. (1992). *Executive summary: Management of asthma during pregnancy. Report of the working group on asthma and pregnancy.* Bethesda, MD: NIH Publication 93-3279a.

National Institutes of Health. (1992). Office of Women's Health Research. *Summary report of women's health.* Bethesda, MD: Author.

National Institutes of Health. (1998). Office of Women's Health Research. *Women of color health data book.* Bethesda, MD: Author.

National Latino Institute for Reproductive Health. (1999, Winter). Latina abortion survey. In *Instantes.* Washington, D.C.

Oakley, A. (1990). Using medical care: The views and experiences of high-risk mothers. *Health Services Research, 26,* 5, 651–669.

Piccinino, L. J., & Mosher, W. D. (1998). Trends in contraceptive use in the United States: 1982–1995. *Family Planning Perspectives, 30,* 1, 4–10, 46.

Pickering, L. et al. (1998). Modulation of the immune system by human milk and infant formula containing nucleotides. *Pediatrics, 101,* 242–249.

Pierce, M., Hayworth, J., Warburth, F., Keen, H., & Bradley, C. (1999). Diabetes mellitus in the family: Perceptions of offspring's risk. *Diabetics Medicine, 16,* 5, 431–436.

Raube, K., Handler, A., & Giachello, A. L. (1995). *Quality of prenatal care of Latinas in the Midwest.* Paper presented at the 123rd American Public Health Association annual meeting, Washington, D.C.

Scribner, R. (1996). Paradox as paradigm: The health outcomes of Mexican Americans [Editorial]. *American Journal of Public Health, 86,* 3, 303–305.

Scribner, R., & Dwyer, J. (1989). Acculturation and low birthweight among Latinos in the Hispanic HANES. *American Journal of Public Health, 79,* 9, 1263–1267.

Sherraden, M., & Barrera, R. (1996). Prenatal care experiences and birth weight among Mexican immigrant women. *Journal of Medical Systems, 20,* 5, 329–350.

Smits, W., Paulk, T., & Kee, C. (1995). *Diabetes Educator, 21,* 2, 129–134.

Stern, G., & Giachello, A. L. (1977). *Applied research: The Latino mother-infant project.* Paper presented at the annual meeting of the American Anthropology Association, New York, NY.

Stroup, M., Trevino, F. M., & Trevino, D. (1988). Alcohol consumption patterns among Mexican-American mothers and children from single- and dual-headed households. *American Journal of Public Health, 80,* Suppl., 36–41.

Substance Abuse and Mental Health Services Administration. (1998). *Preliminary results from the 1997 National Household Survey on Drug Abuse.* NHSDAS Series H-6. (DHHS Publication 98-3251). Bethesda, MD: Author.

United States Bureau of the Census. (1999, December). The Hispanic population in the United States, population characteristics, March 1998. *Publication #P20-525.* Washington, D.C.: U.S. Department of Commerce.

United States Bureau of the Census. (2000, February). The Hispanic population in the United States: March, 1999. *Current Population Reports, Series P20, No. 527.* Washington, D.C.: U.S. Government Printing Office.

United States Department of Health and Human Services. (1999). *Healthy People 2010—Conference Edition* [Family Planning]. Washington, D.C.: U.S. Government Printing Office.

United States Department of Health and Human Services. (1998). *Tobacco use among U.S. racial/ethnic minority groups: A report of the Surgeon General.* Office of the Surgeon General. Washington, D.C.: U.S. Government Printing Office.

Ventura, S. J., Martin, J. A., Curtin, S. C., Mathews, T. J., & Park, M. M. (2000). Births: Final data for 1998. *National Vital Statistics Reports, 48*(3) (DHHS Publication No. [PHS] 00-1120, 0-0215). Hyattsville, MD: National Center for Health Statistics.

Wolf, C. B., & Portis, M. (1996). Smoking, acculturation, and pregnancy outcome among Mexican Americans. *Health Care for Women International, 17,* 6, 563–573.

Wright, A. L. et al. (1988). Infant feeding practices among middle-class Anglos and Hispanics (Pt. 2). *Pediatrics, 82,* 496–503.

Wright, A. L. et al. (1998). Increasing breastfeeding rates to reduce infant illness at the community level. *Pediatrics, 101,* 837–844.

Zambrana, R. E., & Ellis, B. K. (1995). Contemporary research issues in Hispanic/Latino women's health. In D. Adams (Ed.), *Health issues for women of color: A cultural diversity perspective.* Thousand Oaks, CA: Sage.

Zambrana, R. E., & Scrimshaw, S. C. (1997, May–June). Maternal psychosocial factors associated with substance use in Mexican-origin African American low-income pregnant women. *Pediatric Nursing, 23,* 3, 253–259.

Zambrana, R. E., Scrimshaw, S., Collins, N., & Dunkel-Schetter, C. (1997). Prenatal health behaviors and psychosocial risk factors in pregnant women of Mexican origin: The role of acculturation. *American Journal of Public Health, 87,* 6, 1022–1026.

Zambrana, R. E., Scrimshaw, S., & Dunkel, C. (1996). Prenatal care and medical risk in low-income, primiparous, Mexican-origin and African American women. *Families, Systems and Health, 14,* 3, 349–359.

CHAPTER SIX

# THE LATER YEARS

## The Health of Elderly Latinos

Valentine M. Villa, Fernando M. Torres-Gil

The aging of the U.S. population, also referred to as the demographic imperative, has been widely documented and is well known. Less well known is the rapid aging occurring in the Latino population. While the population aged sixty-five and over in the United States is expected to increase 93 percent over the next three decades, the U.S. Latino elderly population will increase by 555 percent. This rapid growth in the Latino elderly population, coupled with the fact that many members of the population are in poor health and economically disadvantaged, often reliant on publicly funded programs that are at risk of cutbacks and restructuring, may well result in this population's access to health and long-term care services being limited and an increasing amount of the financial burden being shifted to the Latino family. Designing programs and policies that will decrease vulnerabilities and dependency among Latinos and better mesh with human need requires an investigation of the health status of the population, and an examination of the economic and social factors that negate as well as protect health. In this chapter we review the health data on Latino elders in the United States, examine economic and social correlates of older Latinos' health status, discuss current and proposed changes in Medicare and Medicaid policy, and address the implications of policy changes for Latino elders and their families. We conclude with policy recommendations that will move us closer to meeting the health and long-term care needs of older Latinos as well as empower the Latino family.

## The Minority Demographic Imperative: The Growth and Graying of the Latino Population

Heretofore, the bulk of research on the health status of the older population has been based on the experience of White males largely because of the small numbers of older minorities represented in the population over age sixty-five (Markides & Black, 1996). As we continue into the twenty-first century, however, the number of ethnic minority elders in the United States will increase drastically (Angel & Hogan, 1994). In 1990, 13 percent of the thirty-two million Americans aged sixty-five and over were members of a minority group. By the year 2030, United States Bureau of the Census projections indicate that 25 percent of the elderly population will be members of a minority group (American Association of Retired Persons, 1994). Between 1990 and 2030, the White population aged sixty-five and over is expected to increase 93 percent, whereas the older minority population over sixty-five is expected to increase by 328 percent, with the number of African American elders tripling, and Asian, Latino, and Native American elders increasing by 693 percent, 555 percent, and 231 percent, respectively (American Association of Retired Persons, 1994; Angel & Hogan, 1994).

Data specific to the elderly Latino population, while not disaggregated by ethnic subgroups, indicate that Latinos are also aging rapidly. The number of elderly Latinos will quadruple between 1990 and 2020 (1.1 million to 4.7 million) and will nearly triple again by 2050, reaching 12.5 million that year (Angel & Hogan, 1994). In terms of composition of the Latino elderly population, the largest percentage are Mexican American (50 percent), followed by Cubans (17 percent), Puerto Ricans (11 percent), and South and Central Americans (22 percent) (United States Bureau of the Census, 1998). Currently, elderly Latinos compose 6 percent of the U.S. elderly population. By 2050, elderly Latinos will represent 15.5 percent of the total U.S. elderly population compared to 7 percent of elderly Asians, 10.4 percent of elderly African Americans, and 67 percent of elderly Whites (United States Bureau of the Census, 1996a). Not only will the proportion of Latinos among the general population aged sixty-five and older increase, but the proportion of the elderly within the Latino population also will increase. Latinos aged sixty-five and older currently represent 5.3 percent of the total Latino population and will grow to 13 percent by 2030 (United States Bureau of the Census, Census 2000 Redistricting Data [P.L. 94-171] Summary Files for states).

Examination of the elderly dependency ratio (the ratio of the number of elderly persons to the number of working-age persons) reveals a sharp rise in that ratio among the Latino population. In 1995 there were 9.5 persons aged sixty-five and older for every 100 persons aged eighteen to sixty-four; by 2030 there will be 21.1 persons aged sixty-five and older for every 100 persons aged eighteen to sixty-four (United States Bureau of the Census, 1996b). The growth in the Latino population aged sixty-five and over is due primarily to improvements in mortality, which for many conditions is equivalent to and in some cases more favorable than that for Whites (Markides & Rudkin, 1995). The bulk of improvement in mortality has occurred among Latinos aged eighty-five and over. Consequently, the largest growth in the Latino elderly population, as with other populations, will be among those aged eighty-five and older. Hispanics aged eighty-five and older tripled between 1980 and 1995 from 50,000 to 139,000 and are expected to increase to one million by 2030 and to 3.2 million by 2050 (United States Bureau of the Census, 1996b). According to Siegel (1999), the average rate of increase for Latinos aged eighty-five and older will be larger than for those aged sixty-five and older. Clearly, the aging of the Latino population suggests that issues relative to health and long-term care will become of increasing importance.

Moreover, the unprecedented increase in the number and proportion of minority elderly should lead to increased emphasis in gerontological research, especially on learning more about the health and well-being of minority elders, and therefore inclusion of these populations in empirical analyses. Indeed, according to Markides and Black (1996), increased attention to diversity and issues of race and ethnicity and minority group membership in aging research is highlighted by the recent adoption of a policy by the National Institutes of Health (NIH) requiring the inclusion of women and minorities in all funded research.

In addition to the "minority demographic imperative," proposed cutbacks at the federal and state levels in health and social services programs that many minority older adults are dependent upon to help maintain health and functioning further underscore the need for a greater understanding of the health status of minority populations (Kiyak & Hooyman, 1994). Investigation of the health of older minorities can help improve their health and decrease health differentials by providing critical information that can be used to design more effective and efficient programs for the elderly and reveal critical points of intervention for policy. In short, designing policies that are more responsive to the needs of a growing, diverse older adult population, increasingly composed of members of minority populations in the midst of growing fiscal constraints, will require that we move beyond current assumptions regarding the older population and investigate how race, ethnicity, immigration, language, economic status, gender, and historical experiences influence the aging process (Stanford & Torres-Gil, 1991).

## Older Minority Health Status

While there has been a general improvement in the health status of Americans aged sixty-five and over, the health of minority elders has not kept pace (Gerontological Society of America, 1994). Empirical evidence reveals that older minorities, in particular Latinos and African Americans, have higher rates of diabetes and hypertension than White elders, and are at increased risk for several acute and chronic conditions including stroke, obesity, and some heart diseases (Markides & Black, 1996; Pérez-Stable, McMillan, & Harris, 1989; Waller, 1989;

Mutchler & Burr, 1991; Jackson, 1988). In addition, older minority group members report more difficulty with functioning and limitations in activity than do Whites (Johnson & Wolinsky, 1994; Wykle & Kaskel, 1994). Still lacking, however, in health research on older minority populations is a comprehensive assessment of health status, in particular investigation of why health differences exist between minority and White populations (Gerontological Society of America, 1994). According to Jackson, Lockery, and Juster (1996), while research continues to demonstrate that racial and ethnic minorities suffer poorer health status and are more likely to develop chronic conditions, the differences in the structure of health, the processes of health, and influence of health problems experienced by older minorities is unclear. The Gerontological Society of America task force on minority issues maintains that exploration of the role that discrimination, socio-economic status, ethnicity, and health practices play in determining health and health differences between majority and minority populations are much needed areas of inquiry in health research (1994). The following sections describe the health status of the Latino population and examine the impact that economic and cultural factors play in determining the health status of this population.

## The Health Status of Older Latinos: A Mixed Picture of Advantages and Disadvantages

Despite their large and growing numbers, Latinos remain "poorly understood and somewhat mysterious to the larger society" (Markides & Rudkin, 1995). While there is a tradition of research on health service usage among the Hispanic population, less is known about the health status of this population, in particular the elderly Latino population (Markides & Rudkin, 1995). What we do know about older Latino's health is based to a large extent on descriptive analyses that explore differences in self-reported health among Latinos, African Americans, and Whites. From these studies we can conclude that African American and Latino elders are more likely to report being in poor health, experience more restricted activity days and bed disability days, and have more difficulty performing activity of daily living (ADL) and instrumental activity of daily living (IADL) tasks than do White elders (Becerra, 1984; Markides, Coreil, & Rogers, 1989; Markides & Mindel, 1987; Markides & Martin, 1983; Markides & Lee, 1990; O'Donnel, 1989; Commonwealth Fund Commission, 1989; National Center for Health Statistics, 1984; Cantor & Mayer, 1976; Newquist, 1976). This conclusion is consistent across both national and local studies, including those of Latinos who primarily self-identify as Mexican Americans.

Data on the health status of older Latinos further reveal that while mortality for certain conditions, for example, heart disease, is equivalent to and in some cases better than that of Whites (Markides & Rudkin, 1995), Latinos are disadvantaged for certain chronic conditions and have higher rates of disability. The majority of elderly Latinos, approximately 85 percent, report having at least one chronic condition (Cuellar, 1990). Major medical problems reported by elderly Latinos include arthritis, cognitive impairment, diabetes, cardiovascular disease, depression, hypertension, and cerebrovascular problems (Espino, 1990). Latinos, when compared to Whites, have a higher prevalence of influenza, pneumonia, gallbladder disease, and infectious and parasitic diseases than the general population (Vega & Amaro, 1994). Studies focusing on cancer by specific cite indicate that Latinos are more likely to have cancer of the cervix, stomach, liver, esophagus, pancreas, and gallbladder (Espino, Burge, & Moreno, 1991; Markides, Coreil, & Rogers, 1989; Rosenwaike, 1988; Bradshaw & Foner, 1978; McDonald & Heinz, 1978). Latino women are especially disadvantaged in cardiovascular and cerebrovascular conditions and have higher levels of obesity than the general population (Sotomayor, 1994).

One of the most consistent findings relative to disease is the excessive prevalence of diabetes found in the Latino population, particularly among Mexican Americans (Hazuda and Espino, 1997). Rates for noninsulin-dependent diabetes are two to five times greater for Latinos than among the general U.S. population, in both sexes and at every age (Pérez-Stable, MacMillan, & Harris, 1989; Hanis et al., 1983; Stern, Gaskill, Hazuda, Gardner, & Haffner, 1983). And there is a much higher mortality from diabetes among Latinos compared to African Americans and Whites, regardless of gender or age (Angel & Angel, 1997; Young, 1982; Bradshaw & Foner, 1978). Not only do they have rates of diabetes that are two to five times greater than the general population and higher mortality from the disease, but Latinos have earlier onset and more severe forms of the disease. They also experience higher rates of diabetes-related complications, including kidney failure, loss of limbs, and blindness (Stern & Haffner, 1990; United States House Select Committee on Aging, 1992).

These health conditions often result in long-term disability and are associated with difficulties in performing daily activities, as well as higher levels of dependency or need for assistance with daily activities (Wallace, Campbell, & Lew-Ting, 1994; Markides, Stroup-Benham, Goodwin, Perkowski, Lichtenstein, & Ray, 1996; Hazuda & Espino, 1997). It is estimated that nationally 45 percent of elderly Latinos have some limitation in activities of daily living (Espino, 1993). Accordingly, Hooyman and Kiyak (1996) maintain that among Latinos physiological aging tends to precede chronological aging, with those individuals in their late forties experiencing health and disability levels similar to those of sixty-five-year-old Whites. Indeed, empirical evidence suggests that while mortality rates for several diseases have improved among Latinos, and mortality for certain disease conditions are equivalent if not more favorable for Latino elders than for White elders, elderly Latinos on average experience earlier and more functional declines than the rest of the older population (Angel & Angel, 1997).

Specific examination of levels of functioning and disability among Latinos emanating from national data sets including the Medicare Current Beneficiary Survey, the National Health Interview Survey, and the United States Bureau of the Census finds evidence of a Latino disadvantage relative to Whites. For example, data from the Current Medicare Beneficiary Survey reveal that while 35 percent of Whites report having difficulty with at least one ADL or IADL, 46 percent of African Americans and 40 percent of Latinos report such limitations (Olin & Liu, 1998). Similarly, Hazuda and Espino (1997), utilizing data from the National Health Interview Survey 1996 and the Latino EPESES ([Mexican American] Establishing Populations for Epidemiological Studies of the Elderly Survey) found that while as many as 5.6 percent of Whites reported difficulty with ADLs, 11.7 percent of Mexican Americans did so. Further, while 11.4 percent of Whites reported IADL difficulty, as many as 22.3 percent of Mexican Americans did. One of the few studies that has looked at functional difficulty and disability across Latinos by ethnic subgroup was done by Trevino and Moss (1984). Utilizing data from the National Health Interview Survey 1978–1980, they examined limitation in major activity and prevalence of limitation in any activity across Mexican Americans, Puerto Ricans, and other Latinos (South and Central Americans). They found that among Latinos with incomes less that $10,000, 48 percent of Mexican Americans, 58 percent of Puerto Ricans, 43 percent of Cubans, and 38 percent of other Latinos had limitation in major activity, compared to 42 percent of Whites. Moreover, examination of the prevalence of limitation of any kind of activity finds that 55 percent of Mexican Americans, 58 percent of Puerto Ricans, 47 percent of Cubans, and 43 percent of other Latinos report limitation in some activity, whereas 49 percent of Whites reported such difficulty. While these data demonstrate that there are differences in these domains of health across Latino ethnic subgroups, Latinos on the whole are disadvantaged relative to Whites.

One of the few studies that has examined functional difficulty among Latinos nationally by gender was also done by Trevino and Moss (1984), utilizing data from the National Health Interview Survey 1978–1980. They found that Latino women were disadvantaged relative to Latino men and relative to White women for prevalence of limitation across major activity as well as limitation of any kind of activity. They found that among women aged sixty-five and older, 44 percent of Mexican Americans, 50 percent of Puerto Ricans, 37 percent of Cubans, and 34 percent of other Latinos had limitation in major activity. Prevalence of limitation in any activity across groups found a similar pattern with prevalence rates ranging from 43 percent among Cuban women to 51 percent among Mexican American women. Prevalence rates of major activity limitation and of limitations of any kind among White women in the same study were 34 percent and 41 percent, respectively.

While it is clear that Latinos are disadvantaged for certain chronic conditions and functional difficulties/disability, they at the same time have an advantage relative to Whites for mortality from both heart disease and cancer (Markides & Black, 1995). Data from the Current Medicare Beneficiary Survey, 1994, finds that prevalence for heart disease, skin cancer, and other cancers is lower among Latinos than Whites. Similarly, an analysis of the National Longitudinal Mortality Study that included 40,000 Latinos found lower death rates in middle age and old age among Latinos of both sexes across all major ethnic subgroups including Mexican Americans, Puerto Ricans, Cubans, and other Latinos origin (Sorlie, Backlund, Johnson, & Rogat, 1993). This advantage has been attributed to certain protective aspects of culture and selective migration; that is, immigrants are healthier than the native-born population, regardless of age (Stephen, Foote, Hendershot, & Schoenborn, 1994), and high rates of immigration therefore contribute to this more favorable mortality profile (Markides & Black, 1995). However, given the data on prevalence of chronic conditions that are associated with higher levels of functional difficulty or disability found among Latinos, better mortality may not mean better health. Put simply, living longer may not mean a better quality of life for Latinos but may instead indicate more years of living with chronic or disabling conditions (Crimmins, Hayward, & Saito, 1994; Angel & Angel, 1997).

# Economic and Social Correlates of Elderly Latino Health Status

Explorations of possible reasons for the observed differences in health status between White and Latino elders has generally followed two paths of inquiry: socioeconomic status and culture. The theoretical perspective often guiding these inquiries is the double jeopardy hypothesis, which predicts an interaction effect between two stratified systems, one based on race or ethnicity and one based on age. It simply predicts that being old and a member of an ethnic minority group is different (worse) than being old and White. The double jeopardy hypothesis can be subsumed under a larger multiple-hierarchy stratification model, where in addition to ethnicity and age, sex and social class are important aspects of inequality. Relative to health the latter model maintains that the accumulated disadvantage suffered by older minorities over a lifetime may adversely affect their health in later life (Markides, Liang, & Jackson, 1990; Dowd & Bengtson, 1978).

## Socioeconomic Status

Socioeconomic status (SES) is a powerful predictor of health status (Olin & Liu, 1994). Poverty, low income, and low education have all been found to be associated with higher mortality, greater morbidity, and greater levels of disability (House, Kessler, Herzog, Mero, Kinney, & Breslow, 1992). According to Kington and Smith (1997), while the exact causal pathways producing racial and ethnic differences in health status have not been clearly delineated, racial and ethnic groups that experience worse health also have lower SES, which these authors maintain may be the underlying cause of the observed differences in health. Indeed, it has been argued that Latino elders are generally in worse health than White elders because they spend the better part of their lives in occupations that are physically taxing and involve debilitating work conditions that impinge upon their health (Lacayo, 1980; Becerra, 1984).

Examination of the SES of elderly Latinos finds clear evidence of vulnerability. Older Latinos are disproportionately disadvantaged in terms of poverty and income levels relative to Whites. Nationally 12 percent of the elderly population are in poverty, whereas 22.5 percent of Latino elders are poor (United States Bureau of the Census, 1993). Statistics as to those in near poverty are equally compelling: 16.7 percent of Whites compared to 36.3 percent of Latinos live in near poverty (United States Bureau of the Census, 1997). Desegregating the data by gender reveals that the most vulnerable group among this population are unmarried Latina older women. In 1990, some 50 percent of this population was in poverty (United States Bureau of the Census, 1991a). While there is evidence of differences among Latino ethnic subgroups, poverty levels for each subgroup are still higher than those of Whites. In 1990, poverty levels for older Mexican Americans were 28 percent; for older Cubans, 17 percent; for older Puerto Ricans, 40 percent; and for older South and Central Americans, 25 percent (United States Bureau of the Census, 1992a). Data on income levels further reflect the Latino elderly's economic disadvantage relative to White seniors. The overall mean annual income for Latino seniors in 1990 was $14,237 compared to $19,816 for those who are White (United States Bureau of the Census, 1996a). Gender differences again reveal the relative disadvantage of Latinas. The median incomes for elderly White men in 1992 was almost triple the income of Latinas aged sixty-five and older ($14,760 versus $4,632) (United States Bureau of the Census, 1992a).

Part of the disparities in poverty and income among older Latinos and Whites can be understood by examining sources of income across the populations. Latinos are highly reliant upon Social Security and not as likely as Whites to have income from pensions or assets. It is estimated that many more Latino elders would be in poverty if it were not for Social Security, which accounts for more than half of their income (52.9 percent). Part of this heavy reliance on Social Security is related to the lack of pension coverage found among Latinos. While 31 percent of older Whites have income from private pensions, only 15 percent of Latino elders have such resources. Moreover, whereas pensions account for 10 percent of older Whites' income, they account for only 6 percent of that of Latino elders (Chen, 1999). Marginal wages across the life course experienced by many Latinos are reflected in Social Security benefit levels. In 1996, the average annual Social Security income for Latino seniors was $6,690, compared to $8,065 for their White counterparts (United States Bureau of the Census, 1996a).

There also are significant disparities between Latinos and Whites in income from assets: 67 percent of White elders as compared to only 27 percent of older Latinos in 1996. Wealth also varies between Whites and Latinos. For those aged seventy in 1995, the median wealth for Whites was $103,000, whereas that for Latino elders was $16,000 (Smith, 1997). The lag in income, assets, and wealth for Latinos and their disproportionately high poverty levels render them economically vulnerable, which carries with it serious implications for health status.

One of the many consequences of poverty and low income is lack of access to medical care. Accordingly, it has been argued that lack of economic resources can influence the severity of onset of a disease and accelerate its onset (Binstock, 1998; Smith & Kington, 1997), as well as exacerbate the burden of disease management (Miles, 1999). Angel and Angel (1992) maintain that the evidence on differential health levels can be summarized as showing that poor minority group members are at elevated risk of the diseases associated with poverty, and that at every age poor African Americans and Latinos suffer more illness and death than do Whites or minority group individuals with higher incomes. Additional support for the link between SES and poor health among Latinos is provided by Markides and Lee (1990, 1991), who found in their exploration of predictors of health status among Mexican Americans in the southwest that low SES defined by household income and education was predictive of poor health.

Moreover, the effects of SES on health have been found to be stronger for those at the bottom of the economic strata than for those at the top. Kington and Smith (1997), utilizing national data emanating from the Health and Retirement Survey (HRS), which included as part of the sample nearly 900 Latinos aged fifty-one to sixty-one (60 percent of whom were Mexican Americans), found that income and wealth were predictive of the probability of having a chronic condition or difficulty in functioning. Specifically, Latinos and African Americans with lower levels of income and wealth reported higher levels of chronicity and difficulty in functioning. Similar findings were evident among the Medicare population. Data from the Current Medicare Beneficiary Survey found that beneficiaries in the lowest income quartiles reported significantly worse health and greater amount of difficulty with ADL than those in the upper income quartile.

## Social and Cultural Correlates

Studies focusing on culture as a possible explanation for health differences between Latino and White elders have for the most part examined the effects of acculturation, concluding that less-acculturated Latinos, that is, those who primarily speak Spanish and were older when they migrated to the United States, in general report poor health (Angel & Guranacia, 1989; Angel & Angel, 1992; Markides & Lee, 1991). The role of ethnicity (being Latino) in explaining health differences has been studied to a lesser extent. One exception is a study conducted by Markides and Lee (1990) in which ethnicity was not found to be significant in predicting health status; however, only Mexican American elders were included in the analysis. Given research concluding that Latinos might have a biological or genetic makeup that predisposes them to certain health conditions, namely, some cancers and diabetes (Sievers & Fisher, 1983; Devor & Buechley, 1980; Morris, Buechley, Key, & Morgan, 1978; Markides, Coreil, & Rogers, 1989; Brosseau,

Eelkema, Gawford, & Abe, 1979), and given the possible link between minority group membership and poor health (Angel & Angel, 1992), it seems pertinent to further test the effect of ethnicity on health status. Williams, Mourey, and Warren (1994) argue that we must broaden our conception of minority group membership and its impact on health status and look at the multiple vulnerabilities associated with race and ethnicity in U.S. society.

Conversely, there has been some discourse relative to the importance of understanding the protective aspects of Latino culture that might explain in part the Latino advantage relative to Whites for mortality caused by certain conditions. Accordingly, Angel and Angel (1997) argue that health is not simply a function of either biology or SES but that there is "something" about culture that mediates the impact of biological and social risk factors on health. Therefore, they maintain we must not only focus our attention on the health risks associated with greater chronicity and disability but must also examine the "health-protective" aspects of Latino culture that translate into better mortality. These may include the impact of *familialism*—the influence of strong family networks on a person's behavior and thus health status—as well as those good health practices associated with Latino culture generally. Similarly, Williams, Mourey, and Warren (1994) argue that it is "imperative" that we devote more attention to the direct assessment of the specific cultural beliefs and behaviors that impact health. An understanding of the impact, both good and bad, that Latino culture has on health status is important for designing effective health promotion and disease prevention programs for the elderly Latino population.

Taken together, this examination of health status and its correlates among Latinos finds evidence of worse health in the areas of functioning and higher prevalence of certain chronic diseases. Explanations for these differences have for the most part looked at SES and to a lesser extent at culture. Clearly, the foregoing explorations of health status and its relationship to SES and culture add to our understanding of Latino health status and offer possible reasons for the differences in health status that we observe between Latinos and Whites. However, the bulk of the mentioned analyses are based on the experience of Mexican Americans of the southwest, making it difficult to extrapolate the results to the rest of the Latino population. Where other ethnic subgroups are included, they are not disaggregated but rather lumped into one category. The diversity of the Latino population with regard to social, economic, and cultural indicators has been widely documented (Council on Scientific Affairs, 1991). Therefore, extrapolation of research findings from one group to the entire Latino population is unwise and can result in what Wolinsky and Arnold (1988) refer to as a homogeneity trap. Therefore, analyses of health status differentials and predictors of such differentials between Latinos and Whites where possible should disaggregate Latinos into ethnic subgroups.

What is clear is that elderly Latinos "on the whole" experience health and economic vulnerabilities to a greater extent than do their White counterparts. Given proposed cutbacks and changes in Medicare and Medicaid, can we expect this vulnerability to persist? In the following section we address some of the current and proposed changes under these two programs and the potential impact they may have on the health status of elderly Latinos.

## Medicare and Medicaid Policy: Implications for Older Latinos and Their Families

Medicare is the United States' version of national health care for the elderly. Medicare was enacted in 1965 and provides benefits to nearly thirty-nine million Americans, including thirty-five million elderly and five million disabled individuals (Kaiser Family Foundation, 1998). The current and expected mounting pressure to curb federal spending will likely lead to major changes in Medicare. This has the potential to significantly impact Latino elders and their families because of their heavy reliance on the program to meet their basic medical needs. Nearly one-third of Latino elders rely on Medicare as their sole source of insurance, compared to 13 percent of Whites. Furthermore, while only 38 percent of Latinos have private medical insurance to supplement their Medicare coverage, 75 percent of Whites have such private coverage (National Center for Health Statistics, 1996).

Projected shortfalls, threats of insolvency, and concerns frequently expressed during the 1990s, coupled with recent dire warnings that the program might be bankrupt as early as 2002, has opened the door for "cost-saving" mechanisms including increasing the age of eligibility for benefits, raising out-of-pocket costs to consumers, and shifting more recipients into managed care arrangements. These proposals were part of the Balanced Budget Act (BBA) of 1997 (Wallace, Enriquez-Haass, & Markides, 1998). In addition to calling for more costs for beneficiaries and increasing the age of eligibility for services, the BBA paved the way for partial (and perhaps eventual total) privatization of the Medicare program. These changes have the potential to limit elderly Latinos' access to medical services, increase their economic vulnerability, and shift an increasing amount of responsibility for meeting their health and economic needs to their families.

The shift to managed care under Medicare is particularly troubling for elderly Latinos who have high levels of chronic and disabling conditions. While managed care systems have been effective at containing costs and reducing out-of-pocket expenses for older persons, there is an incentive to undertreat patients in order to maximize profits, because each managed care program receives a fixed premium per enrollee. One of the biggest problems is that managed care systems do not guarantee universal access as does traditional Medicare, and some of these programs have had a tendency toward "skimming," attracting the healthiest patients who will be the lowest users of services, but avoiding the chronically ill and disabled. This represents a disadvantage relative to access for Latinos and other minority and low-income individuals, who are more likely to be in poor health, have multiple chronic conditions (Wallace & Villa, 1997), and have higher prevalence of diseases that require ongoing medical care (such as diabetes). Managed care programs may also not have expertise, or even interest, in serving culturally diverse groups (Torres-Gil & Villa, in press).

Increasing the age of eligibility under Medicare will also carry serious consequences for elderly Latinos. Raising the eligibility from age sixty-five to sixty-seven will increase the number of Latinos who are uninsured. It will also mean that many older Latinos will have to wait longer for health insurance coverage, a particularly ominous development for a population with high disability levels at all ages and inadequate private health insurance (Torres-Gil & Villa, in press). Among the older population, 11.7 percent of Whites aged sixty-three to sixty-four are uninsured, compared to 33 percent of Latinos. Moreover, data on work-based insurance shows that while two-thirds of the White population aged fifty-three to sixty-four have coverage, nearly two-thirds of Latinos aged sixty-three to sixty-four do not (Wallace, Enriquez-Haass, & Markides, 1998). Raising the age of eligibility for Medicare to sixty-seven will reduce the access of Latinos to needed health care and/or force many low-income Latinos who lack private insurance to pay for their own services, such as the ongoing management of diabetes.

Also troubling is the impact that increased out-of-pocket costs will have on older Latinos' access to medical care and economic security. It is estimated that low-income Latinos with Medicare coverage already spend 30 percent of their own income on health care (Wallace, Enriquez-Haass, & Markides, 1998). As mentioned previously, older Latinos are more likely than Whites to have Medicare as their only source of insurance. The gap in supplemental coverage is in part due to the fact that many minorities have spent their lifetime in jobs that offered no retiree health benefits. Increasing out-of-pocket costs under Medicare will mean that older Latinos will have even less disposable income for other uncovered medical services such as prescription drugs, eyeglasses, or the copayment for doctor visits (Wallace, Enriquez-Haass, & Markides, 1998). This would have a particularly adverse impact on economically vulnerable older Latinos, especially women, and drive many further into poverty and/or decrease their access to health services.

Unlike Medicare, Medicaid is not a universal entitlement program. Medicaid provides health and long-term care services for certain low-income, blind, and disabled individuals. The program is state operated and administered but has federal financial participation. Within broadly defined federal guidelines, states determine eligibility, the duration, amount, and scope of services, rates of payments for providers, and methods for administering the program. Medicaid covers approximately thirty-two million beneficiaries. It categorically covers participants in the Temporary Assistance for Needy Families (TANF; formerly Aid to Families with Dependent Children, AFDC) and persons eligible for Supplemental Security Income, or SSI (Ammons, 1997). While the elderly represent about 12 percent of Medicaid recipients, about one-third of the Medicaid dollars are spent on them. Spending for older people is costly because Medicaid is the single-largest funder of long-term care, covering about 50 percent of all nursing home expenditures in the United States (National Academy on Aging, 1995). Absent a national, comprehensive plan, many low-income and middle-class older people rely on the program to meet their long-term care needs. Spending under Medicaid has grown rapidly over the past two decades and is expected to increase even further. Between 1989 and 1993, expenditures rose an average of 13.2 percent per year, more than twice the inflation rate (Wallace, Enriquez-Haass, & Markides, 1998). As with the Medicare program, political and budgetary pressures, coupled with the fear of possible insolvency, have opened the door for reforming and restructuring the Medicaid program.

One proposal for reform includes funding Medicaid through block grants, instead of as an entitlement program where the federal government underwrites a portion of what a state spends on its recipients. Under such a change, we can expect a wide array of reductions in services, decreases in benefits, and tightening of eligibility requirements (Wallace, Enriquez-Haass, & Markides, 1998). According to Wiener and Stevenson (1998), lowering eligibility and benefits would have a negative impact on quality of and access to care. Indeed, Medicaid has been an important safety net for older Americans who require long-term care. It also supplements expenses under Medicare for the elderly poor, ensuring access to basic medical care for older persons living below the poverty line (Angel & Angel, 1997). Nearly one-third of older Latinos rely on Medicaid to cover the out-of-pocket costs under Medicare (National Center for Health Statistics, 1996). With states under increased financial pressures, it is likely that, if allowed, they would eliminate the payment of these supplements to the elderly poor (Riley, 1995). Older Latinos living in poverty would have to forego medical care, or count on hospital emergency room services, or rely on their families to pay the out-of-pocket costs for their medical care (to the extent that their families can do so).

Policies under Medicare and Medicaid that decrease eligibility, services, and benefits and present increased costs to beneficiaries will not only limit older Latino's access to health and long-term care and increase their economic vulnerability but will also shift even greater responsibility for caregiving to the Latino family. While Latino families tend to have a preference for caring for elders at home rather than putting them into institutions, doing so without some formal assistance is unrealistic (Villa, 1998). Younger members of the Latino population, like their older family members, experience economic and health vulnerabilities (Villa, 1998; Wallace & Villa, 1997) that will impact their ability to provide informal care. For example, the median income for Latino families in 1990 was $22,330, or 70 percent of that for Whites (United States Bureau of the Census, 1991b). The percentage of Latinos living in poverty that same year (28 percent) was more than double that of the general population (12.8 percent) (United States Bureau of the Census, 1992b). According to the Center on Budget and Policy Priorities (1989), about one in four Latino workers paid by the hour does not earn enough to keep a family of three out of poverty. Indeed, Latino families have an SES that is among the lowest of any racial or ethnic group in the United States (less than 51 percent of Latinos completed high school compared to 65 percent of African Americans and 70 percent of Whites) (Flack et al., 1995; United States Bureau of the Census 1991b). Even when education levels are the same, Latinos often earn less than their White counterparts (Council of Economic Advisers, 1998), evidence that occupational segregation and glass ceilings experienced by older family members are still in place. Continued low SES and high poverty levels will make it difficult for Latino families to provide support for their elderly family members (Angel & Angel, 1997; Garcia, 1993). Conversely, increased demand for caregiving will mean that younger members who have opportunities for educational and economic advancement may have to sacrifice those opportunities that might otherwise provide a higher level of economic security (Purdy & Arguello, 1992).

Moreover, Latino families increasingly are faced with the dilemma of deciding how to allocate limited resources for medical care among themselves, their children, and older family members. While only 43 percent of Latinos under age sixty-five have employer-provided health insurance, 70 percent of Whites are covered (Angel & Angel, 1996). Lower rates of insurance persist among younger Latinos even when occupational status and other sociodemographic variables are held constant (Angel & Angel, 1997). Moreover, many Latinos lack coverage even when their employers offer it because they often cannot afford the required employee contributions. Consequently, younger Latinos, too, suffer from lack of access to services, poor health, and/or high out-of-pocket medical costs (Levan, Brown, Hays, & Wyn, 1999), which often means they have to forego other goods such as housing and education (Council of Economic Advisers, 1998). Thus future generations of older Latinos, absent support and assistance in caring for *their* elders in the coming years, will most likely experience the same vulnerabilities as their predecessors.

# Recommendations for Health Policies and Programs: Empowering Older Latinos and Their Families

There are no clear-cut or easy answers for dealing with the fiscal pressures facing Medicare and Medicaid. However, there are other options that minimize risk and reduce costs but also continue the insurance approach to providing for the health needs of our older population. Social insurance programs ensure basic welfare, some reduction of inequality, protection against catastrophic events (Binstock, 1998), and access to routine as well as specialized medical care. Adopting a national health system that would operate according to such an approach and include long-term care as one of the many health services individuals require as they move through their life course is one way that would guarantee all members of society access to basic health and long-term care services.

Another option that is less radical but would improve access to medical care and long-term care for older Latinos and therefore benefit their families is the expansion of community-based managed care systems. These systems (funded in part by Medicare and Medicaid) enable the elderly to remain in the community, as well as give families the support to supplement the care they are already providing, including respite care, adult day care, and home health. They often involve multidisciplinary medical teams (including, for example, a geriatrician, a social worker, a nurse, a physical therapist, and an occupational therapist) that provide services in the community as well as the home setting. There is growing evidence that such community-based managed care arrangements are cost effective and dovetail with consumer needs and preferences (Mollica, 1998; Wiener & Stevenson, 1998).

Moreover, health programs and services to be effective in improving health and, perhaps most importantly, preventing disease must be informed by empirical evidence of the health status of the Latino population. Evidence of the emphasis currently placed on health promotion and disease prevention by the federal government is found in a report that outlines the official U.S. government policy relative to health entitled *Healthy People 2010*. The report delineates more than 300 quantifiable goals relative to older persons. Additionally, there is scientific evidence that reveals that interventions, specifically reducing risk factors and risk behaviors, can reduce mortality, morbidity, and disability.

## Directions for Further Research

Designing health promotion and disease prevention programs that are effective and responsive to health needs requires an understanding of the level of disease that exists among the population, as well as the prevalence of social and health risk behaviors and their relationship to disease conditions. Specifically, Myers, Kagawa-Singer, Kumanyika, Lex, and Markides (1995) argue that improving the health of older Latinos requires an examination of the prevalence and extent of behavioral risk factors and the contribution of these factors to chronic disease among *each ethnic group* within the Latino population. Therefore, future studies should examine the impact that behaviors such as diet, exercise, and alcohol and tobacco use have across each of the ethnic groups that constitute the population.

In addition, while we have some understanding of the impact that SES has on the health status of older Latinos, a deeper, more comprehensive understanding would require that we disentangle the pathways through which SES and race and ethnicity impact health (see Figure 6.1). We must therefore move beyond gross measure of SES such as poverty and income to look at the impact that more specific aspects of occupation and income have on health, including working conditions, physical and psychological demands of work, lack of health insurance, marital stress associated with low income, and availability or lack of pensions and savings. Education should be broadened to examine the impact that not only

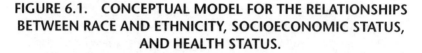

# FIGURE 6.1.   CONCEPTUAL MODEL FOR THE RELATIONSHIPS BETWEEN RACE AND ETHNICITY, SOCIOECONOMIC STATUS, AND HEALTH STATUS.

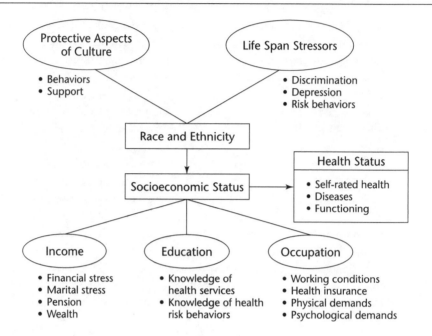

number of years of education have on health, but also the impact that knowledge of health services as well as health risk behaviors have on health status or outcome.

Furthermore, our conceptualization of race and ethnicity and its impact on health should be broadened to examine the protective aspects of culture as well as the life span stressors associated with minority group membership in the United States that impact health. The Latino advantage relative to heart disease and some cancers that persists even when SES is held constant suggests that there are either health-protective behaviors or perhaps family support measures that protect Latinos from these conditions. Conversely, for empirical data to impact policies aimed at the amelioration of institutional racism, segregation, and glass ceilings, we must document the impact that negative stressors such as discrimination and ensuing depression, as well as the use of "bad" health practices (sometimes used as coping with overt racism), have on the health of the Latino population.

Finally, as evidenced here, most of what we know about elderly Latino health is based on the experience of Mexican Americans. For programs, policies, and services to target the health needs of individual groups within the population, data must be disaggregated by ethnic group. Therefore, national surveys of health status must garner large enough samples of Puerto Ricans, Cubans, Dominicans, and South and Central Americans such that multivariate analyses of the predictors of health status among each population can be conducted. This can provide the evidentiary base on which programs and services can be built that better mesh with the needs of each of the ethnic groups constituting the Latino population.

# Conclusion

Clearly, the health and economic profile of our current cohort of older Latinos suggests that they are a vulnerable population, reliant on programs that are subject to changes that have the potential to limit access, increase economic insecurity, and place further pressure on the Latino family. It is also clear that Latino families have accepted the responsibility and have a preference for providing care for their older members in the home rather than in institutions. At the same time, many Latino families are themselves economically and socially vulnerable. This already affects and will continue to limit their ability to provide care without some formal assistance. As such, absent a national health care system inclusive of long-term care services that would guarantee access to all citizens, community-based systems that supplement the care provided by family members must be expanded. These options will empower younger members of the Latino population by providing them the freedom to explore opportunities for educational and economic advancement. At the same time, we must consider the health of future generations of Latinos and create programs and services aimed at health promotion and disease prevention that can improve health among younger members of the Latino population and therefore reverse the current pattern of health vulnerability in old age.

# References

American Association of Retired Persons (1994). *A profile of older Americans*. Washington, D.C.: AARP Fulfillment.

Ammons, L. (1997). Demographic profile of health care coverage in America in 1993. *Journal of the National Medical Association, 89,* 11, 737–744.

Angel, J. L., & Angel, R. (1992). Age at migration, social connections, and well-being among elderly Hispanics. *Journal of Aging and Health, 4,* 4, 480–497.

Angel, J. L., & Hogan, D. P. (1994). Demography of minority populations. In J. S. Jackson (Ed.), *Minority elders: Five goals toward building a public policy base* (2nd ed.). Washington, D.C.: Gerontological Society of America, pp. 9–21.

Angel, R., & Angel, J. (1996). The extent of private and public health insurance coverage among adult Hispanics. *The Gerontologist, 36,* 3, 332–340.

Angel, R., & Angel, J. (1997). *Who will care for us? Aging and long-term care in multicultural America.* New York: New York University Press.

Angel, R., & Guarnacia, P. (1989). Mind, body, and culture: Somatization among Hispanics. *Social Science Medicine, 28,* 12, 1229–1238.

Becerra, R. (1984). *The Hispanic elderly.* New York: University Press of America.

Binstock, R. B. (1998). Public vs. private: Successes and failures. *The Public Policy and Aging Report: National Academy on Aging, 9,* 2, 1–15.

Bradshaw, B., & Foner, E. (1978). The mortality of Spanish-surnamed persons in Texas. In F. Bean & W. Frisbie (Eds.), *The demography of ethnic and racial groups.* New York: Academic Press, 261–282.

Brosseau, J., Eelkema, R., Crawford, A., & Abe, C. (1979). Diabetes among the three affiliated tribes: Correlation with degree of Indian inheritance. *American Journal of Public Health, 69,* 1277–1278.

Cantor, M., & Mayer, M. (1976). Health and the inner-city elderly. *The Gerontologist, 17,* 17–24.

Center on Budget and Policy Priorities. (1989). Minimum wage veto hurts Latinos and Blacks. *Hispanic Link Weekly Reports, 26,* 2–4.

Chen, Y. P. (1999). Racial disparity in retirement income security: Directions for policy reform. In T. P. Miles (Ed.). *Full color aging: Facts, goals, and recommendations for America's diverse elders.* Washington, D.C.: Gerontological Society of America, 21–31.

Commonwealth Fund Commission. (1989). *Poverty and poor health among elderly Hispanic Americans.* [Report]. Baltimore: Author.

Council of Economic Advisers. (1998). *Changing America: Indicators of economic well-being by race and Hispanic origin.* Washington, D.C.: The White House.

Council on Scientific Affairs. (1991). *Journal of the American Medical Association, 265,* 2, 248–252.

Crimmins, E. M., Hayward, M. D., & Saito, Y. (1994). Changing mortality and morbidity rates and the health status and life expectancy of the older population. *Demography, 31,* 159–175.

Cuellar, J. (1990). Hispanic American aging: Geriatric educational curriculum for selected health professionals. In M. S. Harper (Ed.), *Minority Aging* (DHHS Publication No. HRS [P-DV-90-4], pp. 17–24). Washington, D.C.: U.S. Government Printing Office.

Devor, E., & Buechley, R. (1980). Gallbladder cancer in Hispanic New Mexicans. *Cancer, 45,* 1705–1712.

Dowd, J., & Bengtson, V. (1978). Aging in minority populations: An examination of the double jeopardy hypothesis. *Journal of Gerontology, 33,* 427–436.

Espino, D. V. (1990). Mexican-American elderly: Problems in evaluation, diagnosis, and treatment. In M. S. Harper (Ed.), *Minority aging: Essential curricula content for selected health and allied health professions* (DHHS Publication No. HRS (P-DV-90-4), pp. 33–41). Washington, D.C.: U.S. Government Printing Office.

Espino, D. (1993). Hispanic elderly and long-term care: Implications for ethnically sensitive services. In C. Barresi & D. Stull (Eds.), *Ethnic elderly and long-term care.* New York: Springer, 101–112.

Espino, D. V., Burge, S. K., & Moreno, C. (1991). The prevalence of selected chronic diseases among the Mexican American elderly: Data from the 1982–1984 Hispanic Health and Nutrition Examination Survey. *Journal of the American Board of Family Practice, 4,* 217–222.

Flack, J. et al. (1995). Epidemiology of minority health. *Health Psychology, 14,* 7, 592–600.

Garcia, A. (1993). Income security and elderly Latinos. In M. Sotomayor & A. Garcia (Eds.), *Elderly Latinos: Issues and solutions for the 21st century.* Washington, D.C.: National Hispanic Council on Aging, 17–28.

Gerontological Society of America. (1994). Introduction. In J. S. Jackson (Ed.), *Minority elders: Five goals towards building a public policy base* (2nd ed.). Washington, D.C.: Gerontological Society of America, pp. 1–8.

Hanis, C. et al. (1983). Diabetes among Mexican Americans in Starr County, Texas. *American Journal of Epidemiology, 118,* 659–672.

Hazuda, H. P., & Espino, D. V. (1997). Aging, chronic disease, and physical disability in Hispanic elderly. In K. S. Markides & M. R. Miranda (Eds.), *Minorities, aging and health.* Thousand Oaks, CA: Sage, 127–148.

Hooyman, N., & Kiyak, H. A. (1996). *Social gerontology: Multidisciplinary perspective.* Boston: Allyn & Bacon, pp. 441–460.

House, J., Kessler, R., Herzog, A., Mero, R., Kinney, A., & Breslow, M. (1992). Social stratification, age and health. In K. Schaie, D. Blazer, & J. House (Eds.), *Aging, health behaviors and health outcomes.* Hillsdale, NJ: Erlbaum, 1–37.

Jackson, J. J. (1988). Social determinants of the health of aging Black populations in the United States. In J. J. Jackson (Ed.), *The Black American elderly: Research on physical and psychosocial health.* New York: Springer, pp. 69–98.

Jackson, J., Lockery, S., & Juster, F. (1996). Introduction: Health and retirement among ethnic and racial minority groups. *The Gerontologist, 36,* 3, 282–284.

Johnson, R. J., & Wolinsky, F. D. (1994). Gender, race, and health: The structure of health status among older adults. *The Gerontologist, 34,* 1, 24–35.

Kaiser Family Foundation. (1998). *Medicare managed care.* Menlo Park, CA: Author.

Kington, R. S., & Smith, J. P. (1997). Socioeconomic status and racial and ethnic differences in functional status associated with chronic disease. *American Journal of Public Health, 87,* 5, 805–810.

Kiyak, H. A., & Hooymann, N. (1994). Minority and socioeconomic status: Impact of quality of life on aging. In R. P. Ables, H. C. Gift, & M. Ory (Eds.), *Aging and quality of life.* New York: Springer, pp. 295–315.

Lacayo, C. (1980). *A national study to assess the service needs of the Hispanic elderly.* Los Angeles: Asociación Nacional por Personas Mayores.

Levan, R., Brown, E. R., Hays, N., & Wyn, R. (1999, April). Disparity in job-bases health coverage places California's Latinos at risk of being uninsured. Policy Brief, University of California, Los Angeles, Center for Health Policy Research, pp. 1–4.

Markides, K., & Black, S. A. (1996). Race, ethnicity, and aging: The impact of inequality. In R. H. Binstock & L. K. George (Eds.), *Handbook of aging and the social sciences* (4th ed.). San Diego, CA: Academic Press, pp. 153–170.

Markides, K., Coreil, J., & Rogers, L. (1989). Aging and health among Southwestern Hispanics. In K. Markides (Ed.), *Aging and health: Perspectives on gender, race, ethnicity, and class.* Newbury Park, CA: Sage, pp. 177–210.

Markides, K., & Lee, D. (1990). Predictions of well-being and functioning in older Mexican Americans and Anglos: An eight year follow-up. *Journal of Gerontology, Social Sciences Edition, 45,* 1, 69–73.

Markides, K., & Lee, D. (1991). Predictors of health status in middle-aged and older Mexican Americans. *Journal of Gerontology,* 6, 45, 243–249.

Markides, K., Liang, J., & Jackson, J. (1990). Race, ethnicity, and aging: Conceptual and methodological issues. In R. H. Binstock & L. K. George (Eds.), *Handbook of aging and the social sciences.* New York: Academic Press, 112–129.

Markides, K., & Martin, H. (1983). *Older Mexican Americans: A study in an urban barrio.* Austin: University of Texas Press.

Markides, K., & Mindel, C. H. (1987). *Aging and ethnicity.* Beverly Hills, CA: Sage.

Markides, K., & Rudkin, L. (1995). *Health status of Hispanic elderly in the United States.* Galveston: University of Texas Medical Branch.

Markides, K., Stroup-Benham, C., Goodwin, J., Perkowski, L., Lichtenstein, M., & Ray, L. (1996). The effect of medical conditions on the functional limitations of Mexican American elderly. *Annals of Epidemiology, 6,* 386–391.

McDonald, E., & Heinz, E. (1978). *Epidemiology of cancer in Texas.* New York: Raven Press.

Miles, T. P. (1999). Living with chronic disease and the ties that bind. In T. P. Miles (Ed.), *Full color aging: Facts, goals, and recommendations for America's diverse elders.* Washington, D.C.: Gerontological Society of America.

Mollica, R. (1998). State innovations in long-term care delivery systems. *The Public Policy and Aging Report: National Academy on Aging, 9,* 3, 10–12.

Morris, D., Buechley, R., Key, C., & Morgan, M. (1978). Gallbladder disease and gallbladder cancer among American Indians in tricultural New Mexico. *Cancer, 42,* 2472–2477.

Mutchler, J. E., & Burr, J. A. (1991). Racial differences in health and health care service utilization in later life: The effect of socioeconomic status. *Journal of Health and Social Behavior, 32,* 342–356.

Myers, H., Kagawa-Singer, M., Kumanyika, S., Lex, B., & Markides, K. (1995). Behavioral risk factors related to chronic disease in ethnic minorities. *Health Psychology, 14,* 7, 613–621.

National Academy on Aging. (1995). Fast facts on Medicaid. *The Public Policy and Aging Report: National Academy on Aging, 7,* 1, 13.

National Center for Health Statistics. (1984). Health indicators for Hispanic, Black, and White Americans. *Vital and health statistics, 10,* 148, (DHHS Publication No. 84 1576). Washington, D.C.: U.S. Government Printing Office.

National Center for Health Statistics. (1996). *Health in the United States, 1995.* Hyattsville, MD: U.S. Public Health Service.

Newquist, D. (1976). *Prescriptions for neglect: Experiences of older Blacks and Mexican Americans with the American health care system.* Los Angeles: University of Southern California, Andrus Gerontology Center.

O'Donnel, R. (1989). Functional disability among the Puerto Rican elderly. *Journal of Aging and Health, 1,* 2, 244–264.

Olin, G., & Liu, H. (1998). *Health and health care of the Medicare population.* Rockville, MD: U.S. Department of Health and Human Services.

Pérez-Stable, E. J., McMillan, M. M., & Harris, M. I. (1989). Self-reported diabetes in Mexican Americans: HHANES 1982–1984. *American Journal of Public Health, 79,* 770–772.

Purdy, J., & Arguello, D. (1992). Hispanic familism in caretaking of older adults: Is it functional? *Journal of Gerontological Social Work, 19,* 2, 29–43.

Riley, P. (1995). Long-term care: The silent target of the federal and state budget debate. *The Public Policy and Aging Report: National Academy on Aging, 7,* 1, 4–15.

Rosenwaike, I. (1988). Cancer mortality among Mexican American immigrants in the United States. *Public Health Reports, 103,* 195–201.

Siegel, J. S. (1999). Demographic introduction to racial/Hispanic elderly populations. In T. P. Miles (Ed.), *Full color aging: Facts, goals, and recommendations for America's diverse elders.* Washington, D.C.: Gerontological Society of America, 1–19.

Sievers, M., & Fisher, J. (1983). Cancer in North American Indians: Environment versus hereditary. *American Journal of Public Health, 73,* 485–487.

Smith, J. P. (1997). *The changing economic circumstances of the elderly: Income wealth and Social Security.* Syracuse, NY: Syracuse University, Center for Policy Research Policy Brief, no. 8, pp. 8–11.

Smith, J. P., & Kington, R. (1997). Demographic and economic correlates of health in old age. *Demography, 34,* 159–170.

Sorlie, P., Backlund, M., Johnson, N., & Rogat, F. (1993). Mortality by Hispanic status in the United States. *Journal of the American Medical Association, 270,* 2646–2668.

Sotomayor, M. (1994). Aged Hispanic women: The external circumstances of their lives. In M. Sotomayor (Ed.). *Triple jeopardy—Aged Hispanic women: Insights and experiences.* Washington, D.C.: National Hispanic Council on Aging, 9–19.

Stanford, E. P., & Torres-Gil, F. M. (1991). Diversity and beyond: A commentary. *Generations,* Fall/Winter, pp. 5–7.

Stephen, E., Foote, K., Hendershot, G., & Schoenborn, C. (1994). Health of the foreign born population: United States, 1989–90. Advanced data from *Vital and Health Statistics,* no. 241. Hyattsville, MD: National Center for Health Statistics.

Stern, M., Gaskill, S., Hazuda, H., Gardner, L., & Haffner, S. (1983). Does obesity explain excess prevalence of diabetes among Mexican Americans? *Diabetologia, 24,* 272–277.

Stern, M. P., & Haffner, S. M. (1990). Type II diabetes and its complications in Mexican Americans. *Diabetes/Metabolism Review, 6,* 29–45.

Torres-Gil, F. M., & Villa, V. M. (in press). Policy issues for an aging Latino population: Long-term care and natural support systems. *Journal of Health and Social Policy.*

Trevino, F., & Moss, A. (1984). Health indicators for Hispanic, Black and White Americans. In *Vital and Health Statistics* (DHHS Publication No. [PHS] 84 1576, Series 10). Hyattsville, MD: National Center for Health Statistics.

United States Bureau of the Census. (1991a). Poverty in the United States: 1990. *Current population reports.* Washington, D.C.: U.S. Government Printing Office.

United States Bureau of the Census. (1991b). The Hispanic population in the U.S.: March 1991. *Current population reports* (Series P-20, No. 455). Washington, D.C.: U.S. Government Printing Office.

United States Bureau of the Census. (1992a). *Money income of households, families, and persons in the United States: 1992.* Washington, D.C.: U.S. Government Printing Office.

United States Bureau of the Census. (1992b). *Statistical abstract of the United States* (12th ed.). Washington, D.C.: U.S. Department of Commerce.

United States Bureau of the Census. (1993). Poverty in the United States: 1992. *Current population reports.* Washington, D.C.: U.S. Government Printing Office.

United States Bureau of the Census. (1996a). 65+ in the United States. *Current population reports* (Special Studies, P23-190). Washington, D.C.: U.S. Government Printing Office.

United States Bureau of the Census. (1996b). Population projections of the United States by age, sex, race, and Hispanic origin: 1995–2050. *Current population reports.* Washington, D.C.: U.S. Government Printing Office.

United States Bureau of the Census. (1997). Poverty in the United States: 1996. *Current population reports.* Washington, D.C.: U.S. Government Printing Office.

United States Bureau of the Census. (1998). *Hispanic population in the United States.* Washington, D.C.: U.S. Bureau of the Census, Population Division.

United States Bureau of the Census. (2000). *Census redistricting data* (P.L. 94-171), Summary File for states.

United States House Select Committee on Aging. (1992). *Diabetes mellitus: An unrelenting threat to the health of minorities.* Hearing before the Select Committee on Aging, House of Representatives, 102d Cong., 2d Ses. (Committee Publication No. 102-864). Washington, D.C.: U.S. Government Printing Office.

Vega, W. A., & Amaro, H. (1994). Latino outlook: Good health, uncertain prognosis. *Annual Review of Public Health, 15,* 39–67.

Villa, V. M. (1998). Aging policy and the experience of older minorities. In J. Steckenrider & T. Parrott (Eds.), *New directions in old-age policy.* New York: SUNY Press, 211–233.

Wallace, S. P., Campbell, K., & Lew-Ting, C. (1994). Structural barriers to the use of formal in-home services by elderly Latinos. *Journal of Gerontology: Social Sciences, 49,* 5, 253–263.

Wallace, S. P., Enriquez-Haass, V., & Markides, K. (1998). The consequences of color-blind health policy for older racial and ethnic minorities. *Stanford Law and Policy Review, 9,* 2, 329–346.

Wallace, S. P., & Villa, V. M. (1997). Caught in hostile cross-fire: Public policy and minority elderly in the United States. In K. Markides & M. Miranda (Eds.), *Aging health, and ethnicity.* Beverly Hills, CA: Sage.

Waller, J. B. (1989, June). *Challenges to the provision of health care to minority aged.* Paper presented at the first annual summer symposium, Geriatric Education Center of Michigan, Ann Arbor.

Wiener, J., & Stevenson, J. (1998). *Long-term care for the elderly and state health policy.* Washington, D.C.: Urban Institute Press.

Williams, D., Mourey, R., & Warren, R. (1994). The concept of race and health status in America. *Public Health Reports, 109,* 1, 26–41.

Wolinsky, F., & Arnold, C. (1988). A different perspective on health and health service utilization. *Annual Review of Gerontology and Geriatrics, 8,* 71–101.

Wykle, M., & Kaskel, B. (1994). Increasing the longevity of minority older adults through improved health status. In J. S. Jackson (Ed.). *Minority elders: Five goals toward building a public policy base* (2nd ed.). Washington, D.C.: Gerontological Society of America, pp. 32–39.

Young, J. (1982). Cancer in minorities. In D. Parron, F. Solomon, & C. Jenkins (Eds.), *Behavior health risks and social disadvantage.* Washington, D.C.: National Academy Press.

# CHAPTER SEVEN

# LATINO MENTAL HEALTH AND TREATMENT IN THE UNITED STATES

William A. Vega, Margarita Alegría

Latinos have very different histories that link them to U.S. society, including patterns of immigration or migration, the political relationship between the United States and the nation of origin, and the personal and environmental conditions that affected and continue to influence the quality of their adaptation to the United States. Some Latino nationality groups are relatively recent arrivals, and others settled in North America or Puerto Rico under Spanish control before the United States established political dominion over them. The wide dispersal of Latinos across the United States and their unique social-political histories have created many variations in adaptation and ethnic enclave development. In the Latino diaspora, highlighted by cultural fusion, fragmentation, and local cultural idiosyncrasies, signs of cultural strengths, attachment to identity, and a robust community cohesiveness are common. Yet there are many destabilizing aspects of social adaptation in the United States for Latinos: they are a rapidly increasing population, with two-fifths of their children living below the poverty line; they are residentially segregated; and they are affected by pervasive shortfalls in educational attainment. Social adaptation of Latinos to American society poses inherent risks to the healthy development of Latino youth and adults.

The Latino population has been characterized as paradoxical because despite low median income and social marginality it remains much healthier than anticipated, given the expected association between poverty and higher rates of illness (Scribner, 1996). However, most of the "ethnic" protective effect is directly attributable to the superior health and mental health status of immigrants rather than to the benefits accruing to increased education and income of successive generations (Escobar, 1998). At this time we do not possess the knowledge or intervention strategies to reverse the deterioration of health and mental health status that occurs intergenerationally among Latinos (or after migration in the instance of Puerto Ricans). Can we avoid the development of minority status, negative self-concept, demoralization, and exposure to escalating risk factors that seem to render Latinos vulnerable to mental health problems? What are these key protective factors and how do we increase the availability of mental health services (Vega, 2000)?

   This chapter provides a concise review of the mental health status of Latino ethnic groups and some possible explanations for them. The chapter summarizes patterns of using services for mental health problems by Latinos and offers some reasons for inequities in the health care delivery system. We also discuss challenges to the healthy development of Latino youth and their mental health status. These challenges include development of a positive self-image, acculturation and cultural conflicts, and successful transitions into adulthood. The chapter concludes with a summary of research and policy implications derived from the information presented.

## Mental Health Status of Latinos in the United States

The 1980s and 1990s were decades of intense productivity in Latino mental health epidemiology and services research. One area that has progressed is the measurement of psychiatric signs, symptoms, and syndromes among adult Latinos. We now can report rates from several diagnostic and nondiagnostic regional and community studies of adult Latinos. However, because these studies vary in design and in the instruments used in the respective studies, caution should be used in interpreting these findings. Space limitations preclude a detailed presentation of all findings. Readers seeking more details about how Latinos compare to other ethnic groups on a number of nondiagnostic symptom measures are referred to other sources (Vega & Rumbaut, 1991; Alderete, Vega, Kolody, & Aguilar-Gaxiola, 1999; Narrow, Rae, Moscicki, Locke, & Regier, 1990; Vera et al., 1998; Jiménez, Alegría, Peña, & Vera, 1997). An additional limitation is that a majority of symptom studies found in the research literature are about Mexican Americans or Puerto Ricans due to the relatively smaller population sizes of other Latino ethnic or nationality groups. Smaller population sizes make epidemiologic studies much more expensive and difficult to conduct, and there is minimal support among funding agencies for these studies.

   The results of symptom studies are inconsistent. The largest and best-controlled studies, such as the Hispanic Health and Nutrition Examination Survey (HHANES), showed that Mexican Americans and Cubans have lower *caseness rates* (see Table 7.1; in these ethnic groups, a sufficient number of symptoms to indicate a need for treatment) compared to non-Latino populations (Moscicki, Rae, Regier, & Locke, 1987). However, small area studies have often reported higher caseness rates for Mexican Americans than are found among non-Latino ethnic groups (Roberts, 1981; Frerichs, Aneshensel, & Clark, 1981; Vernon & Roberts, 1982; Vega, Warheit, Buhl-Auth, & Meinhardt, 1984). The reasons for

### TABLE 7.1. DIS LIFETIME MAJOR DEPRESSION AMONG LATINOS IN THE UNITED STATES: MID-1980s.

| Study Site and Ethnic Origins | Sample | Caseness Rate[a] | Investigator(s) |
|---|---|---|---|
| Los Angeles | 2,552 | | Karno et al. (1987) |
| Whites | 1,309 | 8.4 | |
| Mexican Americans | 1,243 | 4.9 | |
| Immigrants | 707 | 3.3 | Burnam, Hough, Karno, Escobar, & Telles. (1987) |
| U.S. born | 537 | 6.3 | |
| Puerto Rico | 1,551 | 4.6 | Canino et al. (1987) |
| Miami Cubans | 902 | 3.9 | Moscicki, Rae, Regier, & Locke. (1987) |
| New York City | | | |
| Puerto Ricans | 1,343 | 8.9 | Moscicki, Rae, Regier, & Locke. (1987) |
| Southwest | | | |
| Mexican Americans | 3,555 | 4.2 | Moscicki, Rae, Regier, & Locke. (1987) |

[a]*Caseness rate* is defined as the proportion of persons needing treatment.

With permission from the *Annual Review of Sociology,* Volume 17 © 1991 by Annual Reviews, www.Annual Reviews.org.

these discrepancies are not clear. However, symptom measures focus primarily on transient mood disturbances (demoralization) that often result from current negative personal circumstances such as marital conflicts, illness, or job loss (Frank, 1974). Mood reactions and psychological distress are good indicators of seeking professional assistance. However, the personal hardships that produce depressive symptoms often resolve within a few weeks, accompanied by a reduction or cessation of symptoms.

The limitations of symptom measures have given impetus to the development and use of diagnostic measures of psychiatric disorders that can be used in population research. Here, we present findings from population studies in which the goal was to provide true prevalence estimates for major depressive episode (MDE) using diagnostic criteria derived from three editions of the *Diagnostic and Statistical Manual of Mental Disorders* (DSM-III, DSM-III-R, or DSM-IV) (American Psychiatric Association, 1980, 1987, 1994). MDE is a common psychiatric disorder that tends to be chronic, disabling, with a high recurrence rate. The World Health Organization (WHO) indicates that major depression is responsible for the highest burden of disease among all illnesses, physical or mental, in developed nations (Murray & Lopez, 1996). MDE is associated with social dysfunction in several areas of life activity. Major depression has been measured among various Latino and other ethnic groups, thus permitting comparability.

There have been two generations of diagnostic research studies that used different research protocols for estimating rates of disorders including MDE. Results

TABLE 7.2. LIFETIME PREVALENCE OF PSYCHIATRIC DISORDERS AMONG MIGRANT WORKERS AND RESIDENTS IN THE MEXICAN AMERICAN PREVALENCE AND SERVICES SURVEY, AMONG RESIDENTS OF MEXICO CITY, AND AMONG RESPONDENTS TO THE NATIONAL COMORBIDITY SURVEY.[a]

| | Migrant Workers | Mexican American Prevalence and Services Survey Respondents, Percent (SE) | | | Mexico City Respondents, Percent (SE) | Comorbidity Survey Respondents, Percent (SE) | |
| --- | --- | --- | --- | --- | --- | --- | --- |
| | | Immigrants <13 Years in United States | Immigrants >13 Years in United States | U.S. Born | | Hispanic Sample | Total |
| Any mood disorder | 5.9 (0.8) | 5.9 (1.4) | 10.8 (2.0) | 18.5 (1.7) | 9 (0.1) | 20.4 (2.8) | 19.5 (0.6) |
| Any anxiety disorder | 12.1 (1.1) | 7.6 (1.2) | 17.1 (2.1) | 24.1 (2.0) | 8.3 (0.8) | 28.0 (2.5) | 25.0 (0.8) |
| Any drug abuse or dependence | 10.0 (1.1) | 9.7 (2.6) | 14.3 (1.9) | 29.3 (2.0) | 11.8 (0.8) | 24.7 (2.7) | 28.2 (1.0) |
| Any disorder | 21.1 (1.5) | 18.4 (2.7) | 32.3 (2.6) | 48.7 (2.3) | 24.7 (51.4) | 51.4 (2.7) | 48.6 (1.0) |

[a]All prevalence rates are adjusted to NCS total age-sex distribution and are for persons aged eighteen to fifty-four years.

Reproduced, with permission, from Archives of General Psychiatry, 55, pp. 771–778, 1998. Copyright © 1998 American Medical Association.

for both are presented in Tables 7.1 and 7.2, respectively. The first group used the Diagnostic Interview Schedule (DIS) (Robins, Helzer, Croughan, & Ratcliff, 1981) to estimate DMS-III disorders, and the second group used the Composite International Diagnostic Interview (CIDI) (Wittchen, Robins, Cottler, Burke, & Regier, 1991) to estimate DSM-III-R disorders. The DIS studies were conducted in the mid-1980s. There were three major studies. The largest was again part of the HHANES (Narrow, Rae, Moscicki, Locke, & Regier, 1990; Moscicki, Rae, Regier, & Locke, 1987). This study sampled various regions within the continental United States with major residential concentrations of Mexican Americans, Puerto Ricans, and Cubans. Two other studies were conducted: one in Los Angeles with Mexican Americans (Karno et al., 1987; Burnam, Hough, Karno, Escobar, & Telles, 1987), and the other in Puerto Rico (Canino et al., 1987). These studies have clear and provocative implications. Rates of lifetime major depression among Mexican Americans (the southwest and Los Angeles), Puerto Ricans on the island, and Cubans in South Florida are similar, with lifetime estimates ranging from 3.9 percent to 4.9 percent. These rates are lower than those reported for either Whites in Los Angeles (8.4 percent) or Puerto Ricans in the northeast (8.9 percent). Another insightful finding from the Los Angeles study was that Mexican immigrants had only one-half the rate (3.3 percent) of lifetime major depression than did U.S.-born Mexicans (6.3 percent). Recognizing that perhaps 80 percent of the Cubans in the South Florida survey were immigrants, the conclusion is highly tenable that Latinos born outside the continental United States, including Puerto Rico, have consistently lower rates of major depression than their U.S.-born coethnic Latinos or than Whites. This would also explain lower rates in Miami, where about three-quarters of adult Cubans were immigrants at the time of the survey. Age differences did not produce remarkable differences in rates. However, women had higher rates of major depression in all of these studies.

Although not shown in Table 7.1, the Puerto Rico and Los Angeles studies also estimated rates for other major psychiatric disorders, with similar results. Immigrant Mexicans had disorder rates similar to those of Puerto Ricans on the island, and these estimates were lower than those for U.S.-born Mexicans for dysthymia (chronic minor depression), phobia, alcohol abuse or dependence, and drug abuse or dependence. Substance abuse or dependence disorder rates were negligible among women in Puerto Rico and Mexican immigrant women.

A second set of studies (reported in Table 7.2) used the UM–CIDI (University of Michigan version; see Kessler et al., 1994). The UM–CIDI yields higher rate estimates than does the DIS because the former contains a different structure to enable superior recall of distant events by respondents. Nonetheless, the CIDI contains virtually identical diagnostic criteria to those of the DIS. The CIDI was used to make the first national estimates of psychiatric disorders (DSM-III-R) of the U.S. population in the National Comorbidity Survey (NCS) (Kessler et al., 1994). These results are shown in the far right-hand column of Table 7.2, and include both Latino subsample and total sample estimates. However, interviewing was conducted in English only. As a result, many immigrants and other Spanish speakers were excluded from the sample. English-speaking Latinos in the NCS had similar or higher rates of psychiatric disorders, including major depression, compared to those of the general U.S. population. However, detailed analyses of the same data have shown that even among English-speaking Mexican Americans, higher acculturation predicted having more than one disorder (Ortega, Rosenheck, Alegría, & Desai, 2000).

Table 7.2 contains comparisons to recent population survey results from Mexico City, as well as from a large survey of Mexican Americans in Fresno, California (Alderete, Vega, Kolody, & Aguilar-Gaxiola, 2000; Vega et al., 1998). The results highlight several important points. The Fresno survey reported uniformly lower rates for migrants and immigrants than for U.S.-born respondents, replicating key findings from the DIS studies in Los Angeles. Immigrants with less than thirteen years (which was the median) of U.S. residency had lower disorder rates compared to those with thirteen or more years of residency, underscoring the aversive impact of longer U.S. residency. Rates of psychiatric disorders among recent immigrants are similar to those reported in Mexico City, suggesting population differences in psychiatric disorders across nations and weakening the explanation that immigrants have lower rates due to either biological or social self-selection effects (resulting, say, in extraordinary resilience). A different sample of Mexican migrant agricultural workers (see the far left column, Table 7.2) was found to have similar lifetime rates of total psychiatric disorders as newly arrived Mexican immigrants—between 21.1 percent and 18.4 percent, respectively (Alderete, Vega, Kolody, & Aguilar-Gaxiola, 2000). Mexican Americans born in the United States have similar total lifetime disorder rates as the general U.S. population assessed in the NCS (about 49 percent).

In summary, the findings from recent studies suggest that Latinos such as Mexicans, Cubans, and Puerto Ricans generally immigrate or migrate with superior mental health status compared to the that of the population of the United States as a whole. Over time they have increased risk of mental health problems. Even more disturbing, their offspring's major depression rates may increase to or exceed normal population rates for the United States. These results are perplexing because of the perception that most Latino immigrants and migrants arrive with few resources and experience considerable stress and disruption in their lives. Logic would suggest that they should be at higher risk for mental health problems. Immigrants and migrants appear to carry protective cultural factors with them. Rates of divorce for immigrants are considerably lower than those found among U.S. Latinos despite confronting high life stressors, the limitations of lower educational attainment, and low incomes. Research with Mexican Americans indicates that they are likely to form families quickly after resettlement and to rely on family ties for social support with extensive face-to-face contact (Chavez, 1988; Keefe, 1984; Vega, Kolody, Valle, & Weir, 1991). Evidence is mounting that the erosion of social support and traditional values of Latin American culture occurs in tandem with increasing exposure to U.S. society. For women, the higher rates of marital instability, low educational levels, and greatly increased experimentation and abuse with chemical substances are important risk factors. The loss of traditional emotional support structures and the transition in gender roles that occur with American assimilation appears to seriously increase risk of psychiatric disorders among U.S.-born Latinas in spite of corresponding improvements in education and income. In other words, the loss of cultural supports and social solidarity for women accruing to culture change becomes a risk factor for mental health problems that is mitigated only somewhat by improvements in personal power and social position.

Cultural protective factors may reduce rates of many psychiatric disorders by 50 percent among immigrants (Burnam, Hough, Karno, Escobar, & Telles, 1987). It is not clear whether these protective effects extend to disorders that are less common, such as schizophrenia and manic depression (bipolar disorder), which each affect some 0.5 percent to 1.0 percent of human populations. Regrettably, long-term residency and U.S. nativity weaken protective cultural factors (Escobar, 1998). If we want to promote good mental health for Latinos, how do we—or can we—strengthen indigenous cultural protective factors (Gil & Vega, 1996)? A related issue is the need to reduce structural limitations imposed by poverty and low educational achievement that, in turn, increase Latino's vulnerability to racism, exploitation, and inadequate health care. These issues must be included in the health prevention-promotion agenda for Latinos.

# Mental Health and Development of Latino Children

Latino youth come from many different backgrounds and reside in communities with highly varied social, cultural, and physical characteristics. The degree of personal opportunity and risk of illness or injury for a Latino child or adolescent varies greatly between communities and regions. There is a very important interplay between neighborhoods, family, and individual factors that act as determinants of healthy development. In 1997, 40.3 percent of Latino children were in poverty, a higher rate than any non-Latino ethnic group (United States Bureau of the Census, 1998). Poverty decreases the likelihood of successful transitions into adulthood for adolescents. Poverty is accompanied by an array of problems that have negative consequences for quality of life across the life course. Perilous environments deteriorate neighborhood quality and reduce personal safety and a sense of well-being. Bad schools contribute to extraordinary rates of high school non-completion among low-income Latino youth. Inadequate academic preparation reduces occupational opportunities in adulthood and increases exposures to and participation in high-risk behaviors.

In approaching the issue of social adaptation and personal development of Latino youth, the key issue is family viability. The American way of life imposes cultural changes and structural strains on Latino families, and this is reflected in divorce rates (Gil, Vega, & Biafora, 1998). The inevitable resocialization of Latino families in the United States and the selective influences of American culture on parents and children can undermine family cohesiveness. The socialization and stresses of adaptation among families headed by immigrants are quite different from those of U.S.-born parents, especially in their implications for children's adjustment. Immigrant adults enter the United States with established values, worldviews, and cultural practices. They speak Spanish, which helps reinforce and conserve their cultural background. Their children acquire the English language more quickly than the adults do, thereby accelerating the children's intensive social learning about American culture. Initially children are reached by English-language media in their homes, and eventually in school. These differences in acculturation trajectories across generations can become a source of intergenerational problems undermining family relationships and functioning (Gil & Vega, 1996). If this occurs, the most important personal resource for the healthy development of Latino youth is weakened (Vega & Gil, 1998a).

A second explanatory model emphasizes how minority status produces unfavorable influences on the development of Latino youth. This model is relevant when Latino children are born in the United States and even more so if their parents were (Vega & Gil, 1998a, 1998b). Socialization in the United States from birth represents exposure to minority status from birth. Minority status is reinforced by social experiences such as peer socialization, and contacts with social, educational, health, and criminal justice institutions and agencies. The end result is a greater likelihood of Latino youth's perception that the society is hostile to them and disinterested in their personal well-being (Vega, Khoury, Zimmerman, Gil, & Warheit, 1995). The protective Latino cultural factors are much weaker in U.S.-born Latino families, especially among families in poverty. A weaker family system is less able to offset negative environmental influences on Latino youth. One result can be a higher frequency of adolescent conduct problems and experimentation with behavior that increases the likelihood of foreclosing opportunities for optimal adult development. This explanation is most pertinent to "involuntary minority" groups that have experienced a quasicolonial history of discrimination and minority status in the United States, such as African Americans, Mexican Americans, and Puerto Ricans (Fordham & Ogbu, 1987).

Recent research has provided some understanding of the relationship of attitudes, beliefs, and behaviors related to the mental health of Latino youth. Academic performance of Mexican immigrant children was superior to that of U.S.-born Mexican Americans, and the latter had lower expectations about their prospective academic attainments (Rumbaut & Cornelius, 1995). The U.S.-born children did less homework and spent more time watching television than did the immigrant children. Regrettably, the immigrants had declining academic performance with each year they were in school, and they also increased their TV-viewing time. Other research has shown that Mexican immigrants segregate themselves socially within peer groups from Mexican Americans. U.S.-born cliques are more likely to be oppositional and involved in delinquent behavior. Immigrant youth have a different pattern of exposure to acculturative stresses than that of U.S.-born Latinos, since the former are more likely to face language transition problems during adolescence (Gil, Vega, & Dimas, 1994). Latino parents reporting high acculturative stress were more likely to have children who had low self-esteem and problems relating to teachers (Gil & Vega, 1996). This problem was more acute in low-income families. A study of behavior problems showed that problems with low English language proficiency were associated with behavior problems at school and at home among immigrant youth. For U.S. Latinos, perceived discrimination and limited opportunity were highly correlated with teacher-rated behavior problems (Vega, Khoury, Zimmerman, Gil, & Warheit, 1995).

Most studies of suicidal behavior (ideation, planning, and attempts—but not completions), especially the largest of these, have found that Latino adolescents have higher rates than those of other ethnic groups. The Youth Risk Behavior Survey of the Centers for Disease Control and Prevention (1997) reported that 10.7 percent of Latino youth attempted suicide compared to 7.3 percent of African American youth and 6.3 percent of White youth, with reported rates of suicidal planning of 19.6 percent, 14.3 percent, and 14.3 percent, respectively. However, the suicide completion rates of Latino youth are lower than those of other groups (Canino & Roberts, 2000). There is some evidence, albeit limited, that acculturative stress and drug use interact to increase vulnerability to suicidal behavior, perhaps due to ineffective coping strategies, or comorbidity between depressive mood and drug use (Vega, Gil, Warheit, Apospori, & Zimmerman, 1993). Mood and conduct problems vary by nativity and gender. Immigrant youth experience lower self-esteem and higher levels of suicidal ideation than those of U.S.-born Latinos (Khoury, 1998); however, U.S.-born youth exhibit more serious conduct problems, including school misbehavior, delinquency, premarital teen pregnancy, drug use, and truancy. Latina adolescents are much more likely than teenage Latino boys to report low family support, and adolescent girls consistently report higher levels of depressive symptoms and feeling derogated by adult authority figures (Khoury, 1998). U.S.-born Latina adolescents are more likely to report family substance-abuse problems than their male counterparts and greater perceived peer approval of drug use than immigrant Latinas, and these are risk factors for them (Khoury, Warheit, Vega, Zimmerman, & Gil, 1996).

Psychiatric disorders are difficult to assess in children, especially in community studies for establishing population rates. Syndromes marked by mood or cognitive disturbances that are seen in adults are particularly difficult to determine in early childhood. Children are very dynamic, and sometimes it is difficult to ascertain whether their behavior is truly problematic or merely a short-lived manifestation. Ascertaining the mental health status of children usually requires interviewing both children and their parents or guardians, and a heavy reliance is put on conduct such as early behavior problems or academic performance. In the case of Latinos, language and cultural variability produce an even larger gap in assessing normative functioning and emotional development. We are aware that boys and girls tend to have different profiles of developmental problems, as suggested by findings on depression symptoms and body image.

What additional population information do we have about mental health problems among Latino youth? Not nearly as much as needed, and certainly nothing from major national studies. For some time the science of measuring psychiatric disorders has attempted accurate assessment of children in field studies using diagnostic instruments and problem behavior scales. Below we present information from both types of studies. Initially, we present problem behavior rates from surveys of Latino ethnic groups in Dade County (Greater Miami), Florida (Vega, Khoury, Zimmerman, Gil, & Warheit, 1995) and from a second study in Puerto Rico (Bird et al., 1988). These two studies (Table 7.3) used the Child Behavior Checklist (CBCL) (Achenbach & Edelbrock, 1983) and the Teacher Report Form (TRF) (Achenbach & Edelbrock, 1986), which present (respectively) parents' and teachers' ratings in response to questions covering behaviors that are typically seen in youth referred for mental health treatment. These behaviors cover "externalizing" symptoms such as conduct problems and attention deficit disorder, as well as "internalizing" symptoms such as depression, suicidality, and disassociation. Because parents and teachers observe students in very different social environments, they tend to report different rates for the same types of problems in an individual child. For example, teachers may be more likely to report attention deficit problems than will parents, whereas parents may see more signs of depression. These scales have been used in population and clinical studies with Puerto Ricans, and have been validated and normed by sex and age level; therefore, it is possible to estimate *caseness rates*, defined as the proportion of youth needing treat-

## TABLE 7.3.   DADE COUNTY SCHOOLS (MIAMI, FL) AND PUERTO RICO: COMPARISON OF CBCL AND TRF SCORES BY RACE AND ETHNICITY OF STUDENT[a]

|  | *Parent-Rated CBCL Score* | | *Teacher-Rated TRF Score* | |
| --- | --- | --- | --- | --- |
| **Racial/Ethnic Group** | **Mean Total Problem Score** | **Percent in Caseness Range** | **Mean Total Problem Score** | **Percent in Caseness Range** |
| **Dade County** | | | | |
| African Americans (n = 309) | 26.6 | 23.3 | 30.5 | 15.9 |
| Whites (n = 424) | 25.4 | 21.9 | 17.1 | 5.4 |
| Cubans (n = 697) | 22.0 | 14.1 | 21.9 | 7.2 |
| Nicaraguans (n = 203) | 21.3 | 15.3 | 17.0 | 3.9 |
| Colombians (n = 106) | 24.3 | 16.0 | 18.5 | 4.7 |
| Puerto Ricans | 23.7 | 16.5 | 22.1 | 3.1 |
| Other Latinos (n = 524) | 22.3 | 15.1 | 21.4 | 8.0 |
| **Puerto Rico 6–16 years old (n = 352)** | NA | 37.8 | NA | 23.3 |

[a]All Dade County statistical comparisons with Latino groups and African Americans were significant at $p < .01$ to $p < .001$; no between-group differences among Latinos are significant. (NA = not available.)

ment (Bird et al., 1988; Bird, Gould, Rubio-Stipek, Staghezza, & Canino, 1991). Although both presented in Table 7.3 for efficiency, the two studies are not truly comparable because the characteristics of the samples were very different.

The Miami study covered early adolescents (about ten to twelve years old) in the Dade County school system, and the Puerto Rico study used a community sample six to sixteen years old. In the Miami findings, the parents of African American and White children were more likely to rate their children as CBCL cases than were any of the Latino parents (Vega, Khoury, Zimmerman, Gil, & Warheit, 1995). African American youth were also much more likely to be rated by teachers as "cases" (meaning, presumably in need of treatment). The highest CBCL caseness rate among the Latinos was reported by Puerto Rican parents. Cubans have the highest TRF caseness ratings among Latinos in Miami, yet they have the lowest CBCL caseness ratings. As contrasted with African Americans, the behavior of Latino youth seems to be more tolerable to their teachers than to their own parents, as indicated by much higher CBCL caseness rates. The Nicaraguans, a group almost 90 percent immigrant and very low income, had the lowest caseness ratings on the CBCL and TRF. In general, Latinos in Miami (who are disproportionately immigrant) do not have higher levels of behavior problems than observed among non-Latinos, including among the more affluent White youth.

In contrast to the Miami rates, the CBCL and TRF caseness rates in Puerto Rico are high. The authors of this research have acknowledged that there could be a problem in applying the normative standards from the U.S. population to Puerto Rico without adjustments. Why these adjustments might be necessary is an important and unresolved point. It could be that Puerto Rican parents are less tolerant of deviations from cultural expectations about children's behavior and that they are stricter and less ambiguous about acceptable behavior.

Some population diagnostic data are available from Puerto Rico. Rates of behavior disruptive disorders among four- to sixteen-year-olds were as follows: attention deficit disorder, 9.5 percent; oppositional defiant disorder, 9.9 percent; and conduct disorder, 1.5 percent (Bauermeister, Canino, & Bird, 1994). These rates are difficult to compare to other studies due to methodological issues, but it does appear that they are at the higher end of the range compared to U.S. and British studies, except for conduct disorders. Part of the reason for this is because attention deficit disorder rates decline with age and very few studies other than Puerto Rico have reported data for children as young as four years old. In a more recent study from Puerto Rico, youths nine to seventeen years of age were assessed and compared to other ethnic and national samples from the United States and other nations (Shaffer et al., 1996). Unlike children in other sites, Puerto Rican children were less likely to rate themselves as having a psychiatric disorder when compared to their own parents' ratings, except for substance and alcohol abuse problems and anxiety disorders. In fact, the children's self-reported substance and alcohol use problems were much higher than in any comparison site. Otherwise, DSM-IV disorder rates in Puerto Rico for youth were within the range for disorders reported from other U.S. sites. In sum, from this admittedly inadequate database, there does not appear to be great variance in either diagnostic or nondiagnostic levels of mental health problems when we are comparing Latino youth to White youth, or among Latino groups in the instance of similar problem behavior rates. However, at the population level, the most disturbing information is that problem behaviors will increase with the proportion of U.S.-born Latinos in the youth population, and very high rates of suicidal ideation, planning, and attempts are reported among Latino adolescents by the Centers for Disease Control and Prevention's national Youth Risk Behavior Survey (1997). Such reports suggest widespread demoralization among Latino youth that can have many secondary behavioral consequences, such as increased risk behaviors, and can result in suboptimal personal development such as early termination of education.

## Service Utilization Profiles

The role of ethnicity in the utilization of mental health services has received increased attention during the past two decades. The diversity of Latino ethnic groups has important implications for the patterns of using mental health services. Latinos vary by geography, socioeconomic status, their general knowledge and experience with mental health care, and their familiarity with the U.S. health care system. And there are important differences among ethnic groups in legal residency and in rates of health insurance eligibility. Most research reports (Vega, Kolody, Aguilar-Gaxiola, & Catalano, 1999; Gallo, Marino, Ford, & Anthony, 1995; Sue, Fujino, Hu, Takeuchi, & Zane, 1991; Scheffler & Miller, 1989; Wells, Golding, Hough, Burnam, & Karno, 1989; Hough, Landsverk, & Karno, 1987) suggest that Latinos underutilized most types of mental health services, in comparison to clinical standards and in contrast to Whites.

Findings from the Los Angeles Epidemiologic Catchment Area study showed that Mexican Americans who had experienced psychiatric disorders in the past six months were less likely than Whites to have consulted a mental health specialist (Hough, Landsverk, & Karno, 1987). This finding has been corroborated by more recent information that indicates that despite high needs Latinos continue to underutilize mental health services (Padgett, Patrick, Burns, & Schlesinger, 1994b), even in an insured, nonpoor population. Recently, Vega, Kolody, Aguilar-Gaxiola, and Catalano (1999) found that among U.S.-born Mexican American respondents who had DSM-III-R disorders in the past year, only about one-fourth had used one or more services of any type for a mental health problem in the past twelve months. Mexican immigrants had a utilization rate that was only two-fifths that of U.S.-born Mexican Americans. Overall use of mental health care providers by Mexican Americans with diagnosed mental disorders was 8.8 percent. Wells, Golding, Hough, Burnam, and Karno (1988) reported similar underutilization patterns with very low services use by Mexican immigrants in Los Angeles for both general medical providers and mental health specialists.

However, a few studies have reported comparable levels of service use between Latinos and non-Latinos, especially for Puerto Ricans (in Puerto Rico) and Cubans in Miami (Portes, Kyle, & Eaton, 1992; Alegría et al., 1991). Mental health service use rates of Mariel Cubans in South Florida exceeded the rate reported for the general U.S. population (Portes, Kyle, & Eaton, 1992). In 1980, the third wave of Cuban immigrants began to arrive—an estimated 118,000 people, many of whom had initially sought asylum in the Peruvian Embassy and had subsequently left the island by boat from the Port of Mariel. This wave reflected a mix of social and educational class (Molina & Aguirre-Molina, 1994). The Cuban situation is unique, as was the Mariel exodus from Cuba to Miami in the mid-1980s. Due to special historical and political considerations affecting Cuban immigration, both health and mental health services were provided by government subsidy, and a high volume of Spanish-speaking treatment personnel and physicians reside in the Miami Latino enclave to provide care. Alegría and colleagues (1991) reported that Puerto Ricans living in low-income areas of Puerto Rico showed that approximately one-third of individuals who needed treatment received it during the previous twelve months. The overall rate of mental health service use for these Puerto Ricans (13.9 percent) was comparable to the rates reported in the National Comorbidity Survey (NCS) (see Katz, Kessler, Frank, Leaf, Lin, & Edlund, 1997) and considerably higher than the rates reported for Mexican Americans (Hough, Landsverk, & Karno, 1987). More recent comparisons of mental health service use data between the U.S. population and Puerto Ricans on the island, using the same age range (eighteen to fifty-four years) and parallel definitions of service use, again corroborated no significant differences (8.1 percent for the United States and 8.3 percent for Puerto Rico; Alegría et al., 2000).

These results illustrate how inclusion of varied Latino subgroups into an overencompassing Latino category obscures intergroup and interregional patterns and trends for particular subgroups, such as Mexican Americans, Central Americans, Puerto Ricans, or Cubans (Kessler et al., 1994; Padgett, Patrick, Burns, & Schlesinger, 1994b; Snowden and Cheung, 1990; Regier et al., 1984; Eaton et al., 1985). There are also numerous methodological inconsistencies in survey construction and sampling contributing to divergent results (Alegría et al., 2000; Mezzich et al., 1993; Guarnaccia, 1992, 1997).

Investigators have attributed these variations in underutilization to various factors that influence access to services, such as the following: level of psychiatric morbidity (Flaskerud & Hu, 1992); stigma (Gil, 1999); insurance coverage and socioeconomic status (Schulman, Rubenstein, Chesley, & Eisenberg, 1995; Scheffler & Miller, 1989; Wells, Golding, Hough, Burnam, & Karno, 1988); knowledge of available resources (Council of Scientific Affairs, 1991; De La Rosa, 1989); migratory experiences (Gaviria & Arana, 1987); level of acculturation (Vega, Kolody, Aguilar-Gaxiola, & Catalano, 1999); the delivery system's responsiveness (Gil, 1999; Snowden, 1993); high number of life problems (Zambrana, Ell, Dorrington, Wachsman, & Hodge, 1994); and past service experiences in the country of origin that may include positive or negative experiences with psychiatric and health care providers or restricted availability of such care (Portes, Kyle, & Eaton, 1992). It is difficult to make definitive statements about the relative importance of each factor in the absence of factual information (see following section on barriers to mental health care).

Historically, most studies have shown that Latinos report fewer outpatient mental health visits than Whites (Sue, 1977; Scheffler & Miller, 1989). For example, in a study of insured federal employees (Padgett, Patrick, Burns, & Schlesinger, 1994a), Latinos averaged 8.6 mental health visits as compared to 9.7 visits for African Americans and 13.0 visits for Whites. In contrast, a study examining the relationship of ethnic and racial identity (White, African American, Latino, and Asian) to the amount and type of psychiatric treatment received by patients in the Los Angeles County mental health system, found no significant relationship between ethnicity/race and amount of treatment received (Flaskerud & Hu, 1992). However, the public mental health system of California has reported systematic underutilization of outpatient and partial-day mental health services by Latinos for decades. These differences suggest that underutilization is in large part determined by the operational characteristics of the local delivery system, and not by cultural (ethnic group) characteristics alone (Snowden & Cheung, 1990). Other investigators (Hu, Snowden, Jerrell, & Nguyen, 1991; Wells, Golding, Hough, Burnam, & Karno, 1988) report fewer ethnic differences for persistence in treatment (a key indirect indicator of treatment effectiveness) once patients enter care.

Two national studies produced estimates of Latino use of mental health services in the United States, albeit with important limitations; the Hispanic HHANES of the 1980s (Moscicki, Rae, Regier, & Locke, 1987), and more recently the NCS (Kessler et al., 1994) included subsamples of Latinos but used different sampling designs. The NCS Latino subsample sizes for different groups (for example, Mexican Americans, Puerto Ricans, and Cubans) were small and only English-speaking respondents were included. This imposes certain restrictions on the utility of these data. Spanish-speaking Latinos are the least likely to use mental health services, and they were seriously underrepresented in the NCS. The exclusion of Spanish-speaking respondents artificially inflates the estimates of use of services by Latinos because individuals with the lowest levels of insurance coverage, education, and income are removed, as are the least assimilated. This distortion is greatest in nationality groups with high proportions of recent immigrants, such as Mexicans. A detailed analysis of NCS rates for Latino subgroups (Figure 7.1) of any last-year use of services for a mental health problem show that Cubans (and other Latinos) have the highest rates of total service use (12.1 percent), followed by Mexican Americans (11.9 percent), Mexicans (10.15 percent), and Puerto Ricans (8.9 percent). White rates were 12.7 percent. However, Cubans (5.4 percent) and Puerto Ricans (4.9 percent) were more likely to use mental health specialty care, and Mexican Americans (8.5 percent) were more likely to use human services providers. Whites had the highest rates of specialty care (6.8 percent). Some of the cell sizes were too small to permit comparisons, such as human

## FIGURE 7.1. COMPARISON OF RATES OF MENTAL HEALTH SERVICE USE IN THE LAST TWELVE MONTHS FOR LATINO SUBGROUPS AND WHITES.

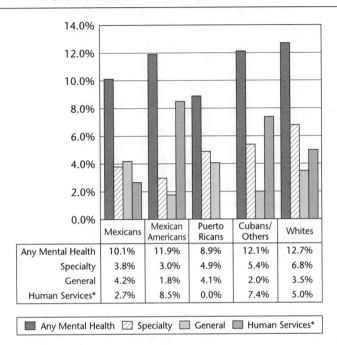

|  | Mexicans | Mexican Americans | Puerto Ricans | Cubans/ Others | Whites |
|---|---|---|---|---|---|
| Any Mental Health | 10.1% | 11.9% | 8.9% | 12.1% | 12.7% |
| Specialty | 3.8% | 3.0% | 4.9% | 5.4% | 6.8% |
| General | 4.2% | 1.8% | 4.1% | 2.0% | 3.5% |
| Human Services* | 2.7% | 8.5% | 0.0% | 7.4% | 5.0% |

■ Any Mental Health ▨ Specialty ▢ General ▩ Human Services*

*Source:* National Comorbidity Survey (Kessler et al., 1994).

\*$\chi^2$ = 11.25; *p* = 0.0306; all others insignificant.

services provider utilization by Puerto Ricans, which points out the need for good comprehensive studies with adequate sample sizes of respective Latino groups.

Large systems of care may also have organizational characteristics, policies, or eligibility criteria that impede or enhance use of inpatient services. For example, only veterans are eligible to receive medical and mental health services from the Veterans Administration (VA), and much more mental health care is available for indigent patients in some states than in others. Furthermore, the most seriously ill Latinos are far more likely to be admitted to hospitals (usually public psychiatric hospitals) involuntarily. Therefore, it is not surprising that a mixed picture of inpatient care emerges. In a rare review of studies of psychiatric hospitalization, López (1981) concluded that Mexican Americans were underrepresented in inpatient psychiatric services. Inspection of 1980 admission rates per 100,000 civilian population revealed that Latinos were admitted to all psychiatric hospitals, public and private, at a rate of 451.4 per 100,000 compared to 550.0 per 100,000 for Whites (Rosenstein, 1980). In contrast, more recent research comparing Latino, African Americans, and Whites in patterns of psychiatric hospitalization in a health-insured population with mental health benefits (Scheffler & Miller, 1989) found that Latinos were 13.5 percent more likely than Whites to be hospitalized. Another study

(Snowden & Cheung, 1990) used a sample of state and county mental health hospitals, VA medical centers with psychiatric inpatient units, private psychiatric hospitals, and psychiatric inpatient services of nonfederal general hospitals. Results showed that Whites were admitted to state and county psychiatric hospitals at a rate lower than that of Latinos (136.8 per 100,000 for Whites in comparison to 146 per 100,000 for Latinos), with the opposite pattern for VA medical centers (64.9 per 100,000 for Latinos and 227 per 100,000 for Whites) and for private psychiatric hospitals (63.4 per 100,000 for Whites and 34.4 per 100,000 Latinos). Unfortunately, the limited number of hospitalization studies makes it difficult to distinguish organizational differences from historical trends in Latino inpatient care.

Little information is available on the patterns of mental health service use for Latino children and adolescents. Studies conducted among the general population of children indicate that Latino youth are underrepresented in mental health services (Bui & Takeuchi, 1992), even after controlling for need (Pumariega, Holzer, & Nguyen, 1993) and socioeconomic status (McCabe et al., 1999). One of the few studies that compared use of mental health services by children and adolescents in four community sites (Atlanta, New Haven, New York, and Puerto Rico), one site having an exclusively Puerto Rican population, was the NIMH Methods for the Epidemiology of Child and Adolescent Mental Disorders (MECA) Study. Mental health service use in children and adolescents varied little in the three continental U.S. sites but was significantly lower for Puerto Ricans on the island (see Figure 7.2). After controlling for having a psychiatric disorder (excluding psychoses

## FIGURE 7.2.   PERCENTAGE OF YOUTHS RECEIVING SPECIFIC MENTAL HEALTH–RELATED SERVICES IN THE PAST YEAR.

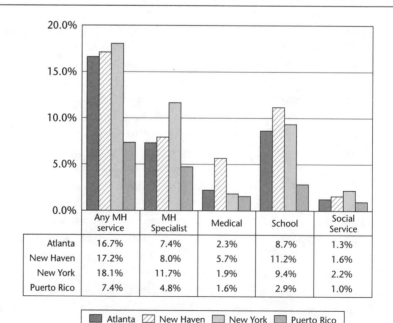

|            | Any MH service | MH Specialist | Medical | School | Social Service |
|------------|---------|---------|---------|--------|---------|
| Atlanta    | 16.7%   | 7.4%    | 2.3%    | 8.7%   | 1.3%    |
| New Haven  | 17.2%   | 8.0%    | 5.7%    | 11.2%  | 1.6%    |
| New York   | 18.1%   | 11.7%   | 1.9%    | 9.4%   | 2.2%    |
| Puerto Rico| 7.4%    | 4.8%    | 1.6%    | 2.9%   | 1.0%    |

■ Atlanta  ▨ New Haven  ▢ New York  ■ Puerto Rico

and phobias), youth of mixed ethnic backgrounds in Atlanta, New Haven, and New York (38.4 percent, 43.5 percent, and 41 percent, respectively) had rates between 38 percent and 44 percent in contrast to youth in Puerto Rico (19.5 percent).

Latino youth are underrepresented in the mental health services sector (Bui & Takeuchi, 1992) but overrepresented in the juvenile social services and justice sectors. Latinos enter child welfare services at rates comparable to that of Whites. After entering the system, they receive fewer therapeutic services compared to Whites (Garland et al., 2000) and remain longer in care (Courtney, Barth, Berrick, Brooks, Needell, & Park, 1996). African American youth have the strongest relationship between need and use of mental health services, whereas Latinos have low service use across all problem severity categories (Garland et al., 2000). A similar finding was observed (McCabe et al., 1999) when patterns of service use of four racial and ethnic groups were compared (African Americans, Latinos, Asians, and Whites) across five public sectors of mental health care (alcohol and drug treatment, child welfare, juvenile justice, mental health, and public school services) for children and youth. San Diego County data reflected Latino's underrepresentation in child welfare and (severe emotionally disturbed) SED programs, overrepresentation in the juvenile justice sector, and representation at the expected rate in the alcohol and drug treatment sector. In the mental health sector, Latinos were at the expected rate when U.S. census data were used but underrepresented when school enrollment data were used.

These findings raise serious concerns about the differential representation of Latinos in mental health services and about the adequacy of the research database to assess deficiencies in services for Latino youth. Less is known about the factors that prevent Latino children from accessing mental health care. Empirical data are crucial to inform public policy on mental health services for Latino children, given widespread concerns about how managed care and welfare reform may affect their access to needed care (Snowden, 1993).

# Barriers to Mental Health Care

A topic of much interest but limited empirical data is the barriers that Latinos experience that impede receiving mental health care. The term "cultural barriers" was coined (Padilla & Keefe, 1984; Ruiz, 1985) to describe how part of Latinos' underutilization of health and mental health services could be attributed to stigma of mental illness or uncertainty about what the established medical system could offer. Some of the barriers mentioned were Latinos' beliefs in spirits or sins as the reason for their illness, which were not understood by health practitioners and much less dealt with in the course of treatment (Ruiz, 1985). Another barrier was the differential expression of mental illness as somatic symptoms (Ruiz, 1985). Latino ethnic groups may also have distinctive expressions for emotional disorders, referred to in psychiatry as "idioms of distress." An example is *ataque de nervios* (Guarnaccia, Rubio-Stipe, & Canino, 1989; Guarnaccia, 1992) among Puerto Ricans, a culture-specific expression of distress that overlaps with core symptoms of anxiety and other categories of disorders. Because such *ataques* are understood by Puerto Ricans as being emotional reactions to difficult life circumstances and events, and as they are considered to be temporary emotional reactions, these beliefs may obstruct an individual and his or her significant others from recognizing symptoms of mental illness or from defining them as appropriate for psychiatric care.

In addition to cultural definitions influencing the recognition of mental disorders, the stigma of mental illness and values of family self-reliance may also influence decisions as to whether to seek mental health care or not. One result may be that Latino communities more readily tolerate and care for the mentally ill outside the treatment sector. The emphasis on family social support in Latin America, and among U.S. Latinos, potentially orients the family toward self-reliance in coping with mental health problems and impairments of family members. Larger social networks composed of family and friends in Puerto Rico (Pescasolido, Wright, Alegría, & Vera, 1998) may keep individuals out of formal mental health treatment, in sharp contrast to the "classic" finding among Whites, where social networks facilitate entry into psychotherapy (Pescasolido, McLeod, & Alegría, 2000; Kadushin, 1969). Other authors (Abad, Ramos, & Boyce, 1974; Rosado, 1980) suggest that indigenous extended networks and informal care providers reduce the need for Latinos to seek formal mental health care. These social resources include the family and the network of friends and godparent relationships, religious denominations, spiritualists and other folk-healing practitioners, and self-help groups (Bird & Canino, 1982; Rosado, 1980). These resources act as alternative therapeutic agents that tend to keep some emotionally distressed Latinos outside the professional health system (Lefley & Bestman, 1984). But several recent studies of service use (Alegría et al., 1991; Vega, Kolody, Aguilar-Gaxiola, & Catalano, 1999) have shown that indigenous social resources are used but not to the degree that they are replacing mental health providers for those who need mental health services. The evidence points to use of both formal and informal services, rather than one excluding the other. Other writers point out how adherence to cultural values such as a collective rather than an individual orientation, self-reliance, fatalism, and avoidance of conflict make Latinos "uncomfortable and even suspicious" of bureaucratic interactions necessary to enter mental health facilities (Rosado, 1980).

Treatment system barriers may also contribute to Latino's low rates of mental health utilization. Low English-language competency and illiteracy among U.S. Latinos is identified as a primary reason for underutilization due to the chronic shortage of Spanish-speaking support personnel and treatment staff, perhaps exacerbated in today's managed care environment (Zambrana, Ell, Dorrington, Wachsman, & Hodge, 1994; Miranda, Andujo, Caballero, Guerrero, & Ramos, 1976). Some researchers (Vega, Kolody, Aguilar-Gaxiola, & Catalano, 1999; Guarnaccia, 1997; Rogler, 1996; Zambrana, Ell, Dorrington, Wachsman, & Hodge, 1994) believe that the main reasons for Latinos' lower rates of use are accessibility factors, such as the affordability of services, the location and knowledge of available services, the lack of confidence in the staff, ineffective and inappropriate therapies, and the inadequacy of the system to attend to Latino clients' needs. Other studies have shown how racism and discrimination are endemic in the delivery, administration, and planning of mental and general health services, obstructing access and use of these services by Latino clients as well as other minorities (Ginzburg, 1991; De la Rosa, 1989; Giachello, 1988; Sue, 1977). For example, when Proposition 187 was passed in California limiting health and educational services to undocumented immigrants, the utilization of outpatient services by Latinos dropped dramatically despite the fact that Proposition 187 was never implemented and was ultimately overturned in court (Fenton, Catalano, & Hargreaves, 1996). Although the mere passage of the proposition succeeded in creating a climate of fear, within weeks emergency room visitation by Latinos increased markedly.

Lack of health insurance (Mueller, Patil, & Boilesen, 1998; Ruiz, 1994; Treviño, Moyer, Valdez, & Stoup-Benham, 1992; Marín, Marín, Padilla, & de la Rocha, 1983) has repeatedly been mentioned as limiting Latinos access to mental and general health services. Recent reports state that of the 44.3 million uninsured in the United States, 35.3 percent (about fourteen million) are of Latino origin (Campbell, 1998) (Figure 7.3). Only about 30 percent of uninsured Latinos rate their health status as being excellent or very good (Ruiz, 1993). Being uninsured makes a considerable difference in people's use of health services and thus often in their mental and physical health status (Aday & Andersen, 1984). This lack of

## FIGURE 7.3.   THE UNINSURED: WHO ARE THEY?

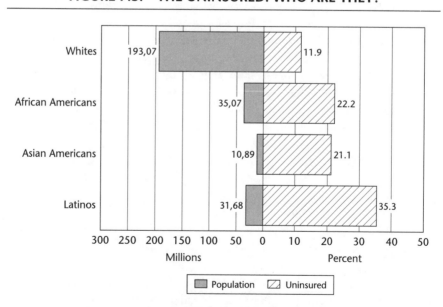

*Source:* United States Bureau of the Census, Current Population Survey, March 1999.

health insurance coverage has been linked to the high use of emergency room visits by Latinos (Marín, Marín, Padilla, & de la Rocha, 1983; Kasper & Barrish, 1982), no routine medical exams (Treviño, Treviño, Stroup & Ray, 1988), limited preventive health care (Cornelius, 1993a, 1993b), no visits to physicians (Short, Cornelius, & Goldstone, 1990), and not having a usual source of care (White-Means, Thornton, & Sung Yeo, 1989). But these ethnic differences in mental health service use are not totally explained by lack of insurance coverage because they are still observed in the insured, nonpoor population (Padgett, Patrick, Burns, & Schlesinger, 1994a).

## Treatment Issues

The accumulated data suggest that services that are responsive to the needs of culturally distinct populations may facilitate use and increase compliance with mental health care (Snowden, Hu, & Jerrel, 1995). Features of ethnic-specific facilities, patient matching on ethnicity or language, and cultural competency are believed to increase the likelihood of establishing good therapeutic rapport, lower dropout rates, improved retention in treatment, and better treatment outcomes (Torres, 1986). For example, Takeuchi, Sue, and Yeh (1995) compared ethnic minorities who entered ethnic-specific programs with their counterparts who entered mainstream programs in terms of return rates, length of treatment, and treatment outcome. Predictor variables for these outcomes included type of program (ethnicity specific versus mainstream), disorder, ethnic match (whether or not the client had a therapist of the same ethnicity), gender, age, and Medicaid eligibility. Results for Latinos show that 68 percent returned to the mainstream programs in comparison to 97 percent who returned to ethnic-specific ones. Latinos were much more likely to return if the program was ethnic-specific. Ethnic programs for the three minority groups (Latinos, African Americans, and Asian Americans) were associated with a significantly greater number of treatment sessions after other variables had been controlled. A similar finding has been reported regarding patient-physician ethnic and racial matching and the perceived quality and satisfaction with health care for Latinos (Saha, Komaromy, Koepsell, & Bindman, 1999). A study found that Latinos with ethnically matched physicians were more likely to be very satisfied with their overall health care than were Latinos with non-Latino physicians. The authors suggest that patient satisfaction is an important aspect of health care quality in that it influences whether the patient continues or drops out of services.

Research addressing Latinos' adherence to treatment and psychotherapy shows a greater dropout rate in comparison to Whites (Ruiz, 1997). The reasons posed for this lower compliance are as follows: poor doctor-patient communication (Ruiz & Ruiz, 1983); lack of cultural sensitivity of the program (Lewis-Fernández & Kleinman, 1995); Latinos' negative attitudes toward health care providers (Rogler, 1996); limited provider responsiveness to familial and cultural concerns of the treatment (Guarnaccia, Parra, Deschamps, Milstein, & Argiles,

1992; Schensul & Schensul, 1982); Latinos' preference for alternative strategies to medication (Lewis-Fernández & Kleinman, 1995); their social isolation and poor transportation (Rogler, 1989); their disappointment at not receiving psychopharmacological treatments (Lawson, Kahn, & Heiman, 1982); and their unfulfilled expectation of the prompt resolution of the problem. How valid and representative are these reasons? Overall, there is a dearth of empirical information about Latinos' adherence to and compliance with mental health treatments, and outcome studies for different treatments. Confirmatory studies are needed that test the significance of these explanatory factors *in the context of consumer interactions with treatment providers* (Hohmann, 1999). This is the essence of the current research agenda for Latino mental health.

## Will Managed Care Increase Services for Latinos?

A compelling group of studies document disparities in access to general health care and use of mental health care by Latinos in the United States. In 1996, for example, $1,428 was spent on the average Latino Medicaid recipient, compared to $4,074 for the average White recipient (Health Care Financing Administration, 1998), reflecting large differences in the per capita volume of services consumed. Under managed care, recent immigrants are especially limited in their ability to obtain care. A recent study compared multiple measures of access and satisfaction of low-income Latinos and African Americans to those of Whites in managed care in Florida, Tennessee, and Texas (Leigh, Lillie-Blanton, Martinez, & Collins, 1999). According to the authors, the ethnic and racial differences in enrollment rates in managed care plans (72 percent of African Americans enrolled in contrast to 63 percent of Whites and 55 percent of Latinos) reflected the diverse patterns of public- and private-sector enrollment in managed care that are mostly driven by state initiatives. Based on the data for these three states, there is no apparent evidence that managed care has resulted in either a substantial improvement or deterioration of health experiences for Latinos and African Americans. Much depends on local policies and regulations controlling eligibility for Medicaid for Latinos. Both Whites and Latinos report more dissatisfaction with managed care plans. Although the authors suggest that language factors may play a role in these findings, the results hold true regardless of whether or not Spanish was the respondent's primary language. Latinos overutilize emergency rooms as the means of access to primary care physicians; as a result, Latinos may be differentially restricted from health care by managed care plans. However, the advent of managed care as a health provider for Medicaid and indigent consumers is so recent that we must await more comprehensive information before drawing conclusions. Nevertheless, an important and contested policy issue is the routine restriction of mental health treatment visits to an average of ten or fewer per annum. This is woefully inadequate for anyone, child or adult, with chronic and persistent mental health problems.

# Conclusion

The mental health of Latinos is similar to their overall health profile. Both are surprisingly good. Latino culture is protective, although we lack an empirically founded explanation about how these protective effects operate. Nevertheless, the demographic expansion of the Latino population will increase the number of individuals at risk for mental health problems—especially among U.S.-born Latinos—and the number requiring treatment. The current profile of low educational and economic attainment must improve to avoid a worsening of population mental health outcomes and a major treatment burden. The importance of early preventive interventions with Latino youth needs greater emphasis, as current epidemiological and biological studies are finding that psychiatric disorders have their origins much earlier in human development, often in childhood and early adolescence. Early detection and intervention with Latino youth is a key research priority. In the near term there will be an escalating need for high-quality services for individuals with serious, disabling mental disorders and co-occurring substance abuse or physical health problems. Untreated mental illness that becomes fully manifested in adulthood is more likely to be accompanied by substance-abuse problems and often result in impaired social functioning, economic losses, and family stresses and care burdens.

Improving the access to care and the quality of care requires significant investment in research. There are no comprehensive national studies about Latino mental health status or services patterns to provide information on discrete Latino nationality groups. There are no major mental health studies that have been conducted on any Latino ethnic groups other than Puerto Ricans and Mexican Americans. Services information derived from administrative data of public providers rarely, if ever, contains immigrant status or nationality group information. Managed care organizations do not regularly collect ethnicity data except for Medicaid patients, and this information is difficult to obtain and use. We have very little information about posttraumatic stress disorder among Latino refugees who have fled political upheaval in their nations of origin. There are no published outcome studies that meet rigorous criteria (including replication) for therapeutic modalities (Miranda, 2000). Research is needed on the impact of welfare reform (Temporary Assistance for Needy Families [TANF]) for mental health services. Preliminary indications are that a reduction of use of services has occurred. TANF provides eligibility for health care for mothers and children, but only until eligibility lapses, which usually occurs after two years. However, the increasing use of managed health plans by TANF-eligible Latinos may eventually increase access. We simply do not know what the patterns will be as TANF and managed care are fully deployed or whether they will vary by ethnicity or region. We do know that the intent of TANF is to bring about women's rapid transition to work, and the types of employment they are likely to be engaged in is least likely to provide health benefits. However, a note of optimism can be sounded.

Virtually every research issue identified in this chapter will be addressed by current research efforts within this decade. Answers to these critical policy questions affecting access and treatment will be available soon.

Better care requires taking into account cultural aspects of mental health including symptom manifestation, recognition, stigma, and help-seeking, as well as myriad issues associated with offering equitable, effective, and accessible services. Most mental health problems of Latinos are not treated; even when they are treated they are most likely to be addressed by primary care physicians, or in emergency rooms in the case of acute episodes, rather than by mental health professionals. We have little knowledge about the adequacy of care because a research literature describing treatment outcomes in these settings is lacking. What is known is that improving aspects of cultural competency, such as language and ethnic matching of Latino clients with providers and therapists, lowers dropout rates (Vega, 2000). There is a serious shortfall in our knowledge of evidenced-based best practices that could be used for training medical and mental health professionals. Future research must move toward improved understanding of which features of the delivery system must change to increase access and quality of care, as well as promote a better understanding of how barriers to improved access or best practices are affected by changing arrangements in the financing and organization of mental health care—especially under managed health plans. There are a few basic steps that critically affect access and quality, and these are insurance availability, knowing where to seek care, and having Spanish-speaking support and treatment staff available.

# References

Abad, V., Ramos, J., & Boyce, E. (1974). A model delivery of mental health services to Spanish-speaking minorities. *American Journal of Orthopsychiatry, 44,* 584–595.

Achenbach, T. M., & Edelbrock, C. (1983). *Manual for the Child Behavior Checklist and Revised Child Behavior Profile.* Burlington, VT: University of Vermont, Department of Psychiatry.

Achenbach, T. M., & Edelbrock, C. (1986). *Manual for the Teacher's Report Form and Teacher Version of the Child Behavior Profile.* Burlington, VT: University of Vermont, Department of Psychiatry.

Aday, L. A., & Andersen, R. M. (1984). The national profile of access to medical care: Where do we stand? *American Journal of Public Health, 74,* 12, 1331–1339.

Aguirre-Molina, M., & Molina, C. (1994). Latino population: Who are they? In C. Molina & M. Aguirre-Molina (Eds.) *Latino Health in the U.S.: A Growing Challenge.* Washington, D.C.: American Public Health Association.

Alderete, E., Vega, W. A., Kolody, B., & Aguilar-Gaxiola, S. (1999). Depressive symtomatology: Prevalence and psychosocial risk factors among Mexican migrant farmworkers in California. *Journal of Community Psychology, 27,* 457–471.

Alderete, E., Vega, W. A., Kolody, B., & Aguilar-Gaxiola, S. (2000). Lifetime prevalence of and risk factors for psychiatric disorders among Mexican migrant farmworkers in California. *American Journal of Public Health, 90,* 608–614.

Alegría, M. et al. (2000). Comparing data on mental health service use between countries. In G. Andrews & S. Henderson (Eds.), *Unmet need for treatment.* New York: Cambridge University Press, pp. 97–118.

Alegría, M. et al. (1991). Patterns of mental health utilization among island Puerto Rican poor. *American Journal of Public Health, 81,* 875–879.

American Psychiatric Association. (1980). *Diagnostic and statistical manual of mental disorders* (3rd ed.). Washington, D.C.: Author.

American Psychiatric Association. (1987). *Diagnostic and statistical manual of mental disorders* (3rd ed., rev.). Washington, D.C.: Author.

American Psychiatric Association. (1994). *Diagnostic and statistical manual of mental disorders* (4th ed.). Washington, D.C.: Author.

Bauermeister, J. J., Canino, G., & Bird, H. (1994). Epidemiology of disruptive behavior disorders. In L. L. Greenhill (Ed.), *Child Adolescent Psychiatric Clinics North America.* Philadelphia: Saunders, 177–194.

Bird, H. R., & Canino, G. (1982). The Puerto Rican family: Cultural factors and family intervention strategies. *Journal of the Academy of Psychoanalysis, 10,* 257–268.

Bird, H. R. et. al. (1988). Estimates of the prevalence of childhood maladjustment in a community sample in Puerto Rico. *Archives of General Psychiatry, 45,* 1120–1126.

Bird, H. R., Gould, M. S., Rubio-Stipek, M., Staghezza, B. M., & Canino, G. (1991). Screening for childhood psychopathology in the community using the Child Behavior Checklist. *Journal of the American Academy of Child and Adolescent Psychiatry, 30,* 116–123.

Bui, K., & Takeuchi, D. T. (1992). Ethnic minority adolescents and the use of community mental health care services. *American Journal of Community Psychology, 20,* 403–417.

Burnam, A., Hough, R., Karno, M., Escobar. J. I., & Telles, C. (1987). Acculturation and lifetime prevalence of psychiatric disorders among Mexican Americans in Los Angeles. *Journal of Health and Social Behavior, 28,* 89–102.

Campbell, J. A. (1998). *Health insurance coverage report.* Suitland, MD: U.S. Bureau of the Census, U.S. Department of Commerce, Economics and Statistics Administration.

Canino, G. J. et al. (1987). The prevalence of specific psychiatric disorders in Puerto Rico. *Archives of General Psychiatry, 44,* 727–735.

Canino, G., & Roberts, R. E. (2000). Suicidal behavior among Latino youth. In L. Davidson & U. Loso (Eds.), *Suicide prevention now: Linking research to practice.* Atlanta, GA: Centers for Disease Control

Centers for Disease Control and Prevention. (1997). *Youth risk behavior survey.* Atlanta, GA: Author.

Chavez, L. R. (1988). Settlers and sojourners: The case of Mexicans in the United States. *Human Organization, 47,* 95–108.

Cornelius, L. (1993a). Barriers to medical care for white, black, and Hispanic children. *Journal of the National Medical Association, 85,* 4, 281–288.

Cornelius, L. (1993b). Ethnic minorities and access to medical care: Where do we stand? *Journal of the Association for Academic Minority Physicians, 4,* 1, 16–25.

Council of Scientific Affairs. (1991). Hispanic health in the United States. *Journal of the American Medical Association, 265,* 248–253.

Courtney, M. E., Barth, R. P., Berrick, J. D., Brooks, D., Needell, B., & Park, L. (1996). Race and welfare services: Past research and future directions. *Child Welfare, 75,* 99–135.

De la Rosa, M. (1989). Health care needs of Hispanic Americans and the responsiveness of the health care system. *Health and Social Work, 14,* 104–113.

Eaton, W. W. et al. (1985). Problems in the definition and measurement of prevalence and incidence of psychiatric disorders. In W. W. Eaton and G. L. Kessler (Eds.). *Epidemiologic field methods in psychiatry: The NIMH Epidemiologic Catchment Area Program.* New York: Academic Press.

Escobar, J. I. (1998). Immigration and mental health: Why are immigrants better off? *Archives of General Psychiatry, 55,* 781–782.

Fenton, J. J., Catalano, R., & Hargreaves, W. A. (1996). Effect of Proposition 187 on mental health service use in California: A case study. *Health Affairs, 15,* 1, 182–190.

Flaskerud, J. H., & Hu, L. (1992). Racial/ethnic identity and amount and type of psychiatric treatment. *American Journal of Psychiatry, 149,* 379–384.

Fordham, S., & Ogbu, J. U. (1987). Black student's school success: Coping with the burden of "acting White." *Urban Review, 18,* 176–206.

Frank, J. (1974). *Persuasion and healing.* New York: Schocken.

Frerichs, P., Aneshensel, C., & Clark, V. (1981). Prevalence of depression in Los Angeles County. *American Journal of Epidemiology, 113,* 691–699.

Gallo, J. J., Marino, S., Ford, D., & Anthony, J. C. (1995). Filters on the pathway to mental health care: II. Sociodemographic factors. *Psychological Medicine, 25,* 1149–1160.

Garland, A. F. et al. (2000). *Racial/ethnic variations in mental health care utilization among children in foster care.* Manuscript submitted for publication.

Gaviria, M., & Arana, J. D. (Eds.), (1987). *Health and behavior: Research agenda for Hispanics* (Monograph 1). Champaign: University of Illinois Press.

Giachello, A. L. (1988). Hispanics and health care. In P. S. Cafferty, S. J. Pastora, & W. C. McCready (Eds.), *Hispanics in the United States: A new social agenda.* New Brunswick, NJ: Transaction Books, pp. 159–194.

Gil, A. G., & Vega, W. A. (1996). Two different worlds: Cuban and Nicaraguan families in Miami. *Journal of Social and Personal Relations, 13,* 437–458.

Gil, A. G., Vega, W. A., & Biafora, F. (1998). Temporal influences of family structure, and family risk factors on drug use initiation in a multiethnic sample of adolescent boys. *Journal of Youth and Adolescence, 23,* 373–393.

Gil, A. G., Vega, W. A., & Dimas, J. (1994). Acculturative stress and personal adjustment among Hispanic adolescent boys. *Journal of Community Psychology, 22,* 43–54.

Gil, R. M. (1999, September 9). Written testimony: Hispanic Health Awareness Week. Congressional Hispanic Caucus, Washington, D.C.

Ginzburg, E. (1991). Access to health care for Hispanics. *Journal of the American Medical Association, 265,* 238–241.

Guarnaccia, P. J. (1992). *Ataques de nervios* in Puerto Rico: Culture-bound syndrome or population illness? *Medical Anthropology, 15,* 1–14.

Guarnaccia, P. J. (1997). Social stress and psychological distress among Latinos in the United States. In I. Al-Issa & M. Tousignant (Eds.), *Ethnicity, immigration and psychopathology.* New York: Plenum.

Guarnaccia, P. J., Parra, P., Deschamps, A., Milstein, G., & Argiles, N. (1992). *Si Dios quiere:* Hispanic families; experiences of caring for seriously mentally ill family members. *Culture, Medicine and Psychiatry, 16,* 2, 187–215.

Guarnaccia, P., Rubio-Stipec, M., & Canino G. (1989). *Ataques de nervios* in the Puerto Rico diagnostic interview schedule: The impact of cultural categories on psychiatric epidemiology. *Culture, Medicine and Psychiatry, 13,* 275–295.

Health Care Financing Administration. (1998). *Medical Recipients and Vendor Payments by Race.* (Table 8). http://www.hcfa.gov/medicaid/2082-8htm

Hohmann, A. A. (1999). A contextual model for clinical mental health effectiveness research. *Mental Health Services Research, 1,* 83–91.

Hough, R. L., Landsverk, J. A., & Karno, M. (1987). Utilization of health and mental health services by Los Angeles Mexican Americans and non-Hispanic Whites. *Archives of General Psychiatry, 44, 702–709.*

Hu, T., Snowden, L. R., Jerrell, J. M., & Nguyen, T. D. (1991). Ethnic populations in public mental health: Services choice and level of use. *American Journal of Public Health, 81,* 1429–1434.*-

Jimenez, A. L., Alegria, M., Peña, M., & Vera, M. (1997). Mental health utilization in women with symptoms of depression. *Women and Health, 25,* 1–21.

Kadushin, C. (1969). *Why people go to psychiatrists.* New York: Atherton.

Karno, M. et al. (1987). Lifetime prevalence of specific psychiatric disorders among Mexican Americans and non-Hispanic whites in Los Angeles. *Archives of General Psychiatry, 44,* 695–701.

Kasper, J., & Barrish, G. (1982). *National health care expenditures' study. Data Preview 12: Usual source of medical care and their characteristics* (DHHS Publication No. [PHS] 83-1572). Washington, D.C.: U.S. Government Printing Office.

Katz, S. J., Kessler, R. C., Frank, R. G., Leaf, P., Lin, E., & Edlund, M. (1997). Utilization of outpatient mental health services in the United States and Ontario: The impact of mental morbidity and perceived need for care. *American Journal of Public Health, 87,* 1136–1143.

Keefe, S. (1984). Real and ideal extended families among Mexican Americans and Anglo Americans: On the meaning of close family ties. *Human Organization, 43,* 65–70.

Kessler, R. C. et al. (1994). Lifetime and 12-month prevalence of DSM-III-R psychiatric disorders in the United States. *Archives of General Psychiatry, 51,* 8–19.

Khoury, E. L., Warheit, G. J. Vega, W. A., Zimmerman, R. S., & Gil, A. G. (1996). Gender and ethnic differences in prevalence of alcohol, cigarette, and illicit drug use among an ethnically diverse sample of Hispanic, African American, and non-Hispanic White adolescents. *Women and Health, 24,* 21–40.

Koury, E. L. (1998). Are girls different? In W. A. Vega & A. G. Gil (Eds.), *Drug use and ethnicity in early adolescence.* New York: Plenum, pp. 95–121.

Lawson, H. E., Kahn, M. W., & Heiman, E. M. (1982). Psychopathology, treatment outcome and attitude toward mental illness in Mexican-American and European patients. *International Journal of Psychiatry, 28,* 20–26.

Lefley, H. P., & Bestman, E. W. (1984). Community mental health and minorities: A multi-ethnic approach. In S. Sue & T. Moore (Eds.), *The pluralistic society: A community mental health perspective.* New York: Human Services Press, pp. 116–148.

Leigh, W. A., Lillie-Blanton, M., Martinez, R. M., & Collins, K. S. (1999). Managed care in three states: Experiences of low-income African-Americans and Hispanics. *Inquiry, 36,* 318–331.

Lewis-Fernández, R., & Kleinman, A. (1995). Cultural psychiatry: Theoretical, clinical, and research issues [Review]. *Psychiatric Clinics of North America, 18,* 3, 433–448.

Lopéz, S. (1981). Mexican-American usage of mental health facilities: Underutilization reconsidered. In A. Barón, Jr. (Ed.), *Explorations in Chicago psychology.* New York: Praeger, pp. 139–164.

Marín, B., Marín, G., Padilla, A., & de la Rocha, C. (1983). Utilization of traditional and nontraditional sources of health care among Hispanics. *Hispanic Journal of Behavioral Sciences, 5,* 65–80.

McCabe, K. et al. (1999). Racial/ethnic representation across five public sectors of care for youth. *Journal of Emotional and Behavioral Disorders, 7,* 2, 72–82.

Mezzich, J. E. et al. (1993). *Cultural proposals and supporting papers for DSM-IV.* Submitted to the DSM-IV task force by the Steering Committee, NIMH-Sponsored Group on Culture and Diagnosis. Unpublished manuscript.

Miranda, J. (2000, May 22–23). *Mental health outcomes for Latinos compared to Anglos: Current knowledge base for improving mental health services.* Unpublished paper presented at the NIMH-sponsored Conference on Disparities in Mental Health Care for Latinos, University of California, Los Angeles.

Miranda, M. R., Andujo, E., Caballero, I. L., Guerrero, C. C., & Ramos, R. A. (1976). Mexican American dropouts in psychological therapy as related to level of acculturation. In M. R. Miranda (Ed.), *Psychotherapy with the Spanish-speaking: Issues in research and service delivery.* (Monograph No. 3, pp. 35–50). Los Angeles: University of California, Spanish-Speaking Mental Health Research Center.

Molina, C., & Aguirre-Molina, M. (1994). Latino populations: Who are they? In Molina & Aguirre-Molina, *Latino Health in the U.S.: A Growing Challenge*. Washington, D.C.: American Public Health Association, pp. 3–22.

Moscicki, E. K., Rae, D., Regier, D. A., & Locke, B. (1987). The Hispanic health and nutrition examination survey: Depression among Mexican-Americans, Cuban-Americans and Puerto Ricans. In M. Gaviria and J. D. Arana (Eds.), *Health and behavior: Research agenda for Hispanics*. (Simón Bolívar Research Monograph Series 1). Chicago: University of Illinois at Chicago, pp. 145–159.

Mueller, K. J., Patil, K., & Boilesen, E. (1998). *The role of uninsurance and race in healthcare utilization by rural minorities*. Omaha: Nebraska Center for Rural Health Research.

Murray, C.J.L., & Lopez, A. D. (1996). *The global burden of disease*. Cambridge, MA: Harvard University Press.

Narrow, W. E., Rae, D. S., Moscicki, E. K., Locke, B. Z., & Regier, D. A. (1990). Depression among Cuban Americans: The Hispanic Health and Nutrition Examination Survey. *Social Psychology and Psychiatric Epidemiology, 25*, 260–268.

Ortega, A. N., Rosenheck, R., Alegría, M., & Desai, R. A. (2000). Acculturation and the lifetime risk of psychiatric and substance use disorders among U.S. Hispanic subgroups. *Journal of Nervous and Mental Disease, 188*, 728–735.

Padgett, D. K., Patrick, C. P., Burns, B. J., & Schlesinger, H. J. (1994a). Ethnicity and the use of outpatient mental health services in a national insured population. *Journal of Public Health, 84*, 2, 222–226.

Padgett, D. K., Patrick, C. P., Burns, B. J., & Schlesinger, H. J. (1994b). Women and outpatient mental health services: Use by Black, Latino, and White women in a national insured population. *Journal of Mental Health Administration, 21*, 347–360.

Padilla, A. M., & Keefe, S. E. (1984). The search for help: Mental health resources for Mexican Americans and Anglo Americans in a plural society. In S. Sue & T. Moore (Eds.), *The pluralistic society: A community mental health perspective*. New York: Human Services Press, pp. 77–115.

Pescasolido, B. A., McLeod, J., & Alegría, M. (2000). Confronting the second contract: The place of Medicaid sociology in research and policy for the 21st century. In C. E. Bird, P. Conrad, & A. M. Fremont (Eds.), *Handbook of medical sociology* (5th ed.). Upper Saddle River, NJ: Prentice-Hall.

Pescasolido, B. A., Wright, E. R., Alegría, M., & Vera, M. (1998). Social networks and patterns of use among the poor with mental health problems in Puerto Rico. *Medical Care, 36*, 7, 1057–1072.

Portes, A., Kyle, D., & Eaton, W. W. (1992). Mental illness and help-seeking behavior among Mariel Cuban and Haitian refugees in South Florida. *Journal of Health and Social Behavior, 33*, 4, 283–298.

Pumariega, A. J., Holzer, C. A., & Nguyen, H. (1993). Utilization of mental health services in a tri-ethnic sample of adolescents. In C. Liberton, K. Kutash, & R. Friedman (Eds.), *The Eighth Annual Research Conference Proceedings—A system of care for children's mental health: Expanding the research base*. Tampa: University of South Florida, pp. 359–364.

Regier, D. A. et. al. (1984). The NIMH Epidemiologic Catchment Area Program: Historical context, major objectives, and study population characteristics. *Archives of General Psychiatry, 41*, 934–941.

Roberts, R. (1981). Prevalence of depressive symptoms among Mexican Americans. *Journal of Nervous Mental Disorders, 169*, 213.

Robins, L. N., Helzer, J. E., Croughan, J. L., & Rattcliff, K. S. (1981). National Institute of Mental Health Diagnostic Interview Schedule: Its history, characteristics and validity. *Archives of General Psychiatry, 38*, 381–389.

Rogler, L. H. (1989). The meaning of culturally sensitive research in mental health. *American Journal of Psychiatry, 146*, 296–303.

Rogler, L. H. (1996). Research on mental health services for Hispanics: Targets of convergence. *Cultural Diversity and Mental Health, 2*, 3, 145–156.

Rosado, J. W. (1980). Important psychocultural factors in the delivery of mental health services to lower class Puerto Rican clients: A review of recent studies. *Journal of Community Psychology, 8*, 215–226.

Rosenstein, M. J. (1980). *Hispanic Americans and mental health services: A comparison of Hispanic, Black, and White admissions to selected mental health facilities.* Washington, D.C.: U.S. Department of Health and Human Services.

Ruiz, P. (1985). Cultural barriers to effective medical care among Hispanic-American Patients. *Annual Review of Medicine, 36*, 63–71.

Ruiz, P. (1993). Access to health care for uninsured Hispanics: Policy recommendations. *Hospital and Community Psychiatry, 44*, 10, 958–962.

Ruiz, P. (1994). Cuban-Americans: Migration, acculturation and mental health. In R. Malgady & O. Rodriguez (Eds.), *Theoretical and conceptual issues in Hispanic mental health.* Malabar FL: Krieger, pp. 70–89.

Ruiz, P. (1997). Issues in the psychiatric care of Hispanics. *Psychiatric Services, 48*, 539–540.

Ruiz, P., & Ruiz, P. P. (1983). Treatment compliance among Hispanics. *Journal of Operational Psychiatry, 14*, 112–114.

Rumbaut, R. G., & Cornelius, W. A. (1995). *California's immigrant children.* San Diego: Center for U.S. Mexican Studies, University of California.

Saha, S., Komaromy, M., Koepsell, T. D. & Bindman, A. B. (1999). Patient-physician concordance and the perceived quality and use of health care. *Archives of Internal Medicine, 159*, 991–1004.

Scheffler, R. M., & Miller, A. B. (1989). Demand analysis of mental health service use among ethnic subpopulations. *Inquiry, 26*, 202–215.

Schensul, S. L., & Schesul, J. J. (1982). Helping resource use in a Puerto Rican community. *Urban Anthropology, 11*, 1, 59–79.

Schulman, K. A., Rubenstein, L. E, Chesley, F. D, & Eisenberg, J. M. (1995). The roles of race and socioeconomic factors in health services research. *Health Services Research, 30*, 1, 179–195.

Scribner, R. (1996). Paradox as a paradigm: The health outcomes of Mexican Americans. *American Journal of Public Health, 86*, 303–305.

Shaffer, D. et al. (1996). The NIMH Diagnostic Interview Schedule for Children (DISC 2.3): Description, acceptability, prevalences, and performance in the MECA study. *Journal of the American Academy of Child and Adolescent Psychiatry, 53*, 865–877.

Short, P. F., Cornelius, L. J., & Goldstone, D. E. (1990). Health insurance of minorities in the United States. *Journal of Health Care for the Poor and Underserved, 1*,1, 9–24.

Snowden, L. (1993). Emerging trends in organizing and financing human services: Unexamined consequences for ethnic minority populations. *American Journal of Community Psychology, 21*, 1–13.

Snowden, L. R., & Cheung, F. K. (1990). Use of inpatient mental health services by members of ethnic minority groups. *American Psychologist, 45*, 347–355.

Snowden, L. R., Hu, T. W., & Jerrel, J. M. (1995). Emergency care avoidance: Ethnic matching and participation in minority-serving programs. *Community Mental Health Journal, 31*, 5, 463–473.

Sue, S. (1977). Community mental health services to minority groups: Some optimism, some pessimism. *American Psychologist, 32*, 616–624.

Sue, S., Fujino, D. C., Hu, I., Takeuchi, D. T., & Zane, N.W.S. (1991). Community mental health services for ethnic minority groups. A test of the cultural responsiveness hypothesis. *Journal of Consulting and Clinical Psychology, 59*, 533–540.

Takeuchi, D. T., Sue, S., & Yeh, M. (1995). Return rates and outcomes from ethnicity-specific mental health programs in Los Angeles. *American Journal of Public Health, 85,* 5, 638–643.

Torres, W. J. (1986). Puerto Rican and Anglo conceptions of appropriate mental health services. *Advances in Descriptive Psychology, 3,* 147–170.

Treviño, F. M., Treviño, D. B., Stroup, C. A., & Ray, L. (1988*). The feminization of poverty among Hispanic households.* San Antonio, TX: National Institute of Policy Studies, Tomas Rivera Center.

Treviño, F. M., Moyer, M. E., Valdez, R. B., & Stoup-Benham, C. A. (1992). Health insurance coverage and utilization of health services by Mexican Americans, Puerto Ricans, and Cuban Americans. In A. Furino (Ed.), *Health policy and the Hispanics.* Boulder, CO: Westview Press, pp. 158–170.

United States Bureau of the Census. (1998). *Current Population Reports, March 1997.* Washington, D.C.: U.S. Government Printing Office.

Vega, W. A. (2000, May 22–23). *Hispanic mental health research and disparities in services.* Unpublished paper presented at the NIMH-sponsored conference on Disparities in Mental Health Care for Latinos, University of California, Los Angeles.

Vega, W. A., & Gil, A. G. (1998a). *Drug use and ethnicity in early adolescence.* New York: Plenum.

Vega, W. A., & Gil, A. G. (1998b). A model of explaining drug use behavior among Hispanic adolescents. *Drugs and Society, 14,* 55–71.

Vega, W. A., Gil, A. G., Warheit, J. G., Apospori, E., & Zimmerman, R. S. (1993). The relationship of drug use to suicide ideation and attempts among African American, Hispanic, and white non-Hispanic male adolescents. *Suicide and Life Threatening Behavior, 23,* 110–120.

Vega, W. A., Khoury, B., Zimmerman, R. S., Gil, A. G., & Warheit, G. (1995). Adolescent problem behaviors in multicultural home and school settings. *Journal of Community Psychology, 23,* 167–179.

Vega, W. A., Kolody, B., Aguilar-Gaxiola, S., & Catalano, R. (1999). Gaps in service utilization by Mexican-Americans with mental health problems. *American Journal of Psychiatry, 156,* 6, 928–934.

Vega, W. A., Kolody, B., Valle, R., & Weir, J. (1991). Social networks, social support, and their relationship to depression among immigrant Mexican women. *Human Organization, 50,* 154–162.

Vega, W. A., & Rumbaut, R. (1991). Ethnic minorities and mental health. *Annual Review of Sociology, 17,* 351–383.

Vega, W. A., Warheit, G., Buhl-Auth, J., & Meinhardt, K. (1984). The prevalence of depressive symptoms among Mexican Americans and Anglos. *American Journal of Epidemiology, 120,* 592–607.

Vera, M. et al. (1998). Help seeking for mental health care among poor Puerto Ricans: Problem recognition, service use, and type of provider. *Medical Care, 36,* 1047–1056.

Vernon, S., & Roberts, R. (1982). Prevalence of treated and untreated psychiatric disorders in three ethnic groups. *Social Science and Medicine, 16,* 1575–1582.

Wells, K. B., Golding, J. M., Hough, R. L., Burnam, M. A., & Karno, M. (1988). Factors affecting the probability of use of general and medical health and social/community services for Mexican Americans and non-Hispanic Whites. *Medical Care, 26,* 441–452.

Wells, K. B., Golding, J. M., Hough, R. L., Burnam, M. A., & Karno, M. (1989). Acculturation and the probability of use of health services by Mexican Americans. *Health Services Research, 24,* 2, 237–257.

White-Means, S. I., Thornton, M. C., & Sung Yeo, J. (1989). Sociodemographic and health factors influencing Black and Hispanic use of the hospital emergency room. *Journal of the National Medical Association, 81,* 1, 72–79.

Wittchen, H. U., Robins, L. N., Cottler, L. B., Burke, J. D., & Regier, D. (1991). Cross-cultural feasibility, reliability, and sources of variance of the Composite International Diagnostic Interview (CIDI). *British Journal of Psychiatry, 159*, 645–653.

Zambrana, R. E., Ell, K., Dorrington, C., Wachsman, L., & Hodge, D. (1994). The relationship between psychosocial status of immigrant latino mothers and use of emergency pediatric services. *Health Social Work, 19*, 2, 93–102.

PART THREE

# PATTERNS OF CHRONIC DISEASES AMONG LATINOS

CHAPTER EIGHT

# THE IMPACT OF CANCER ON LATINO POPULATIONS

Amelie G. Ramirez, Lucina Suarez

The rapid growth of the Latino population in relation to other segments of the American public is cause for a vigorous examination of this population's cancer health status. Unfortunately, such scrutiny has been relatively slow in coming. As a result, our cancer knowledge is still rather imprecise for that portion of the American population that is poised to surpass African Americans as the largest racial or ethnic minority in the country. From registry data we know that Latinos experience lower overall cancer rates than do non-Latinos. Among major cancers—of the prostate, breast, lung, colon, and rectum—the incidence rates are lower as well. However, for some other cancers, most notably cervical and stomach cancers, rates for Latinos are higher than those for Whites. In comparison with rates for African Americans, Latino cervical cancer rates are higher whereas stomach cancer rates are lower. Additionally, it is important to note that cancer mortality rates are disproportionately higher for Latinos than for the general population. Consequently, the impact of cancer on Latinos is considerable and requires increasing attention.

## Cancer Data: Sources and Limitations

Deriving cancer data for Latinos is principally a combined function of the Centers for Disease Control and Prevention (CDC) state cancer registries, funded by the National Program of Cancer Registries (NPCR), and the National Cancer Institute (NCI) Surveillance, Epidemiology, and End Results (SEER) Program. As of 1999, forty-five states, three territories, and the District of Columbia received CDC support for registries. Under the SEER program, coverage provides data for an estimated 14 percent of the total U.S. population. Eleven geographic areas are covered, including the states of Connecticut, Hawaii, Iowa, New Mexico, and Utah, as well as several metropolitan areas in other states. Data are also received from the Alaska Area Native Health Service (Miller et al., 1996) and Native Americans in Arizona.

Cancer surveillance from the registries and SEER represents the cornerstone of our nation's strategy for reducing the cancer burden among all Americans. The information we derive through surveillance is vital for effectively guided research, prevention, and control efforts. Cancer registration data are needed to assess the burden of cancer within the geographic region covered by the registry by monitoring cancer trends among populations (Stiller, 1997). This information is vital in developing cancer control programs targeting those populations.

Although our registry system has expanded and evolved in recent decades, its development is ongoing. As recently as the early 1990s, ten states had yet to establish registries. In many others the resources required to collect adequate population data and to ensure the data that were collected met minimal quality standards were not available (Centers for Disease Control and Prevention, 1999). In 1992, the NPCR was created by Congress to improve existing registries, develop new ones in states where they did not exist, and help states meet quality and timeliness standards. Although the NPCR offers the potential for improvement in collecting Latino cancer data, significantly increased funding would be required to establish quality registries that cover the entire United States and provide adequate, accurate information.

Coverage of Latinos and other minority populations through the SEER program, which began in 1973 with case ascertainment, has expanded in the past decade. Some of the early SEER reporting areas, such as New Mexico and San Francisco–Oakland, included Latinos in the program's coverage. Over the years, other regions have been added and Latino inclusion has increased. The SEER reporting area was significantly expanded in 1992 to cover Los Angeles County and four counties in the San Jose–Monterey area of California, resulting in a 223 percent increase in Latino population coverage (National Cancer Institute, 1999). Recommendations by the NCI Cancer Control Review Group for further expansion to include "Cuba, Puerto Rico, and similar ancestries" are under study by the NCI (Institute of Medicine, 1999).

The U.S. areas covered by SEER include only 25 percent of the Latino population. By comparison, SEER data include 78 percent of the Hawaiian population, 60 percent of the Japanese population, 49 percent of the Filipino population, 43 percent of the Chinese population, 34 percent of the Korean population, 31 percent of the Vietnamese population, 27 percent of the Native American population, and 12 percent of the African American population (Miller et al., 1996).

The distribution of the Latino population covered in these regions also limits how SEER data can be used and applied. Of the total number of Latinos included in SEER areas, 60 percent live in Los Angeles, 10 percent in New Mexico, 9 percent in San Francisco and San Jose–Monterey, and 4 percent in Connecticut. In addition, the majority of Latinos represented in the SEER database are Mexican American. This population accounts for 84 percent of the Latinos living in San Jose–Monterey, 76 percent in Los Angeles, 58 percent in San Francisco–Oakland, and 57 percent in New Mexico. Puerto Ricans comprise more than two-thirds of Connecticut's Latino population and about 4 percent in San Francisco–Oakland (Miller et al., 1996). Although the SEER data on Latinos is far from complete, it should be noted that some of the information the program provides and some state-specific data on distinct Latino populations (for example, in Florida, California, and Texas) have proved useful for planning purposes.

## Identification and Classification Issues

The true measure of the impact of cancer on Latinos can only be as good as the data available. Unfortunately, cancer data are somewhat limited for most racial and ethnic minority populations, including Latinos. For the Latino population, lack of adequate and accurate data can only partially be attributed to insufficient research. Contributing factors include inconsistency in data collection methods, difficulty in interpreting available surveillance information, and the absence of a standard classification system applied to various regions of the country. While reliable and sufficient cancer information is lacking for Latinos in general, the gap is even greater for individual subgroups. This is significant because of the heterogeneity of these populations, which reflect diverse nationalities, backgrounds, origins, cultures, life experiences, lifestyles, and living conditions. For simplicity in discussing Latino cancer issues, overarching generalizations are appealing but are all too often misleading. What is stated as fact for one subgroup may not be applicable to another. Although similarities do exist, particularly with regard to language (Spanish) and religion (Catholic), differences among and within subgroups far outweigh the commonalities. As a result, caution is needed when broad generalizations are applied to the Latino population and its cancer prevention and control knowledge, attitudes, and practices.

Data used to compile cancer statistics for Latinos come from various sources, and fundamental disagreements exist with regard to terminology used to identify and classify Latinos within those sources. For example, references are made to "Hispanics," "Latinos/Latinas," "Latins," and "White Hispanics" in cancer registries. The differences in terminology render determination of cancer rate comparisons more difficult. Inconsistencies in identification and classification of Latinos by the registries, which are a primary source of cancer research data, pose problems for those who depend upon this information for a coherent and effective cancer policy for this population. As a result of these inconsistent standards for classification and substantial misclassification, Latino cancer surveillance data have been negatively impacted, both quantitatively and qualitatively.

Also significant are the various means employed by different entities to identify ethnicity. Cancer registries typically rely on medical records or death certificates. This information is supplied by hospital personnel, whose appraisals are subjective.

Because the quality of registry classification data depends upon the quality of the information provided in the medical records, such subjectivity can and does affect statistical outcomes. For other research purposes, such as population statistics maintained by the U.S. Bureau of the Census, Latino ethnicity is assessed primarily by self-identification (Stewart, Swallen, Glaser, Horn-Ross, & West, 1999). Still other methods of Latino classification include Spanish surname or Spanish-language usage (Giachello, Bell, Aday, & Andersen, 1983).

Cancer rates for Latinos are determined by using a combination of methods: use of medical records and surnames for incidence, death certificates for mortality, and self-identification for population count. Consequently, the systemic differences lead to problems in interpreting and comparing rates. For example, in formulas used to determine rate calculations, designations for cancer cases differ from the designations for population. While the accuracy of each of these classification methods can be questioned, the discrepancies found to exist between them exacerbates the problems. As a result, doubt exists with regard to the accuracy of overall Latino cancer rate determinations and to comparisons between Latinos and other ethnic groups (Stewart, Swallen, Glaser, Horn-Ross, & West, 1999). Moreover, classification discrepancies may be leading to skewed estimates of cancer risk among Latinos. Studies have found lower registry-based cancer incidence rates in this population, which may at least partially result from underestimation of rates derived from ethnic classifications based on medical records alone (Gilliland, Becker, Key, & Samet, 1994; Mallin & Anderson, 1988; Polednak, 1993a, 1993b; Trapido, Chen, Davis, Lewis, & MacKinnon, 1994; Trapido, Chen, Davis, Lewis, MacKinnon, & Strait, 1994; Trapido, McCoy, Stein, Engel, McCoy, & Olejniczak, 1990; Wolfgang, Semeiks, & Burnett, 1991). Augmenting the registry data with classifications based on Spanish surname lists, such as the one developed by Passel and Word for the 1980 U.S. Census (Perkins, 1993), may increase sensitivity and reduce the downward bias in incidence rate comparisons (Stewart, Swallen, Glaser, Horn-Ross, & West, 1999).

The use of different identifying terminology by the numerous registries also negatively impacts our ability to compare cancer rates. Classification term variations, which affect both the number of newly diagnosed cases and the population figures, raise questions about incidence rates, rendering region-to-region comparisons suspect (Trapido, Valdez, Obeso, Strickman-Stein, Rotger, & Pérez-Stable, 1995). Until standards of uniform definitions and consistently applied classification methods are adopted, accurate Latino cancer rate data and comparisons with other ethnic groups, as well as regionally among Latinos, likely will remain elusive.

## Lung Cancer

Lung cancer incidence and mortality rates among Latinos are uniformly lower than among Whites. Among males, the incidence rates are 40 to 50 percent lower in Latinos living in California, New York, Texas, Florida, and New Mexico compared to those of their White counterparts (Table 8.1). Among Latino females, incidence rates of lung cancer are 50 to 70 percent lower than those of non-Latinos living in the same geographic region (Table 8.2). The much lower risk of lung cancer among Latinos is probably due to their historically lower rates of cigarette smoking, since this behavior accounts for nearly 90 percent of all lung cancers.

## Colorectal Cancer

Incidence rates of colorectal cancer also are dramatically lower—by 30 to 40 percent—among Latinos than those among White populations (Table 8.1). This lower risk is seen in both males and females (Table 8.2). The etiology of colorectal cancer has a strong dietary component, and the observed differential may be due to the lower-fat and higher-fiber traditional diet of the various Latino ethnicities as compared to the diets of many Whites (Alaimo et al., 1994; McDowell et al., 1994).

## Breast Cancer

Breast cancer, the leading cause of cancer among Latinas, is nonetheless also lower among Latinas than among Whites. Age-adjusted rates range from sixty-one per 100,000 in New York Latinas to seventy-four per 100,000 in New Mexico Latinas, which are 40 percent lower than those of their White counterparts (Table 8.2). Protective factors that may play a role in the lower risk among Latinas are early and multiple pregnancies, and low dietary fat intake (Henderson, Pike, Bernstein, & Ross, 1996).

## Cervical Cancer

Cervical cancer risk is high among Latinas, with incidence rates that are double those of Whites (Table 8.2). This risk differential has not appreciably improved over the last decades. Cervical cancer mortality is also markedly higher among Latinas. Major risk factors for the development of cervical cancer are early age at initiation of sexual activity, history of multiple sex partners, or promiscuous male sexual partners, factors that are most likely markers for infection with human papilloma virus (Giuliano, Papenfuss, Schneider, Nour, & Hatch, 1999; Schiffman, Brinton, Devesa, & Fraumeni, 1996). Factors related to higher mortality among Latinas are most certainly due to the underutilization of Pap smear screening in this population. Cervical cancers detected at an early stage are 100 percent treatable.

## Prostate Cancer

Incidence rates of prostate cancer among Latino men are lower than those for White males. Age-adjusted rates range from eighty-two per 100,000 in Texas Latinos (predominantly Mexican American) to 108 per 100,000 among California

TABLE 8.1. AGE-ADJUSTED CANCER INCIDENCE RATES PER 100,000 AMONG LATINO
AND WHITE MALES FOR SELECTED REGIONS.[a]

| Cancer | California | | | New York | | | Texas | | | New Mexico | | |
|---|---|---|---|---|---|---|---|---|---|---|---|---|
| | Latino | White | RR | Latino | White | RR | Latino | White | RR | Latino | White | RR |
| Esophagus | 4.3 | 5.6 | 0.8 | 6.9 | 6.4 | 1.1 | 4.4 | 6.1 | 0.7 | 4.2 | 5.2 | 0.8 |
| Stomach | 13.8 | 8.8 | 1.6 | 14.2 | 11.3 | 1.3 | 12.0 | 6.2 | 1.9 | 15.0 | 5.6 | 2.7 |
| Colorectal | 33.8 | 50.7 | 0.7 | 34.6 | 55.0 | 0.6 | 35.4 | 49.4 | 0.7 | 40.3 | 42.1 | 1.0 |
| Liver | 7.4 | 3.6 | 2.1 | 9.4 | 5.5 | 1.7 | 12.6 | 4.5 | 2.8 | 10.1 | 3.8 | 2.7 |
| Gallbladder | 1.1 | 0.5 | 2.2 | NA | NA | NA | 0.9 | 0.5 | 1.8 | 0.9 | 0.5 | 1.8 |
| Lung | 37.9 | 74.0 | 0.5 | 44.0 | 74.7 | 0.6 | 45.7 | 95.5 | 0.5 | 38.8 | 61.7 | 0.6 |
| Prostate | 108.4 | 141.9 | 0.8 | 89.9 | 112.0 | 0.8 | 81.9 | 123.2 | 0.7 | 118.2 | 151.6 | 0.8 |
| Non-Hodgkins | 15.0 | 20.8 | 0.7 | 20.5 | 19.7 | 1.0 | 13.6 | 18.4 | 0.7 | 12.5 | 15.1 | 0.8 |
| Leukemia | 9.5 | 13.1 | 0.7 | 8.5 | 12.2 | 0.7 | 8.7 | 13.0 | 0.7 | 9.5 | 14.0 | 0.7 |

[a]RR, Rate Ratio; NA, not available

## TABLE 8.2. AGE-ADJUSTED CANCER INCIDENCE RATES PER 100,000 AMONG LATINO AND WHITE FEMALES IN SELECTED REGIONS.[a]

| Cancer | California | | | New York | | | Texas | | | New Mexico | | |
|---|---|---|---|---|---|---|---|---|---|---|---|---|
| | Latino | White | RR | Latino | White | RR | Latino | White | RR | Latino | White | RR |
| Esophagus | 0.8 | 1.7 | 0.5 | 2.0 | 1.9 | 1.1 | 1.0 | 1.7 | 0.6 | 0.7 | 1.4 | 0.5 |
| Stomach | 7.5 | 3.4 | 2.2 | 7.8 | 5.1 | 1.5 | 8.1 | 3.2 | 2.5 | 6.4 | 3.2 | 2.0 |
| Colorectal | 22.8 | 35.3 | 0.6 | 25.2 | 39.1 | 0.6 | 20.6 | 33.7 | 0.6 | 27.4 | 28.7 | 1.0 |
| Liver | 2.8 | 1.3 | 2.2 | 3.4 | 2.3 | 1.5 | 5.3 | 1.9 | 2.8 | 4.1 | 1.7 | 2.4 |
| Gallbladder | 3.3 | 0.8 | 4.1 | NA | NA | NA | 3.7 | 0.8 | 4.6 | 3.5 | 1.0 | 3.5 |
| Lung | 19.2 | 50.2 | 0.4 | 16.9 | 44.3 | 0.4 | 16.8 | 49.8 | 0.3 | 20.0 | 36.2 | 0.6 |
| Breast | 68.5 | 119.6 | 0.6 | 61.3 | 104.3 | 0.6 | 63.5 | 104.2 | 0.6 | 79.7 | 108.9 | 0.7 |
| Cervical | 16.3 | 6.9 | 2.4 | 15.4 | 9.1 | 1.7 | 15.9 | 8.8 | 1.8 | 11.3 | 7.2 | 1.6 |
| Non-Hodgkins | 10.2 | 12.1 | 0.8 | 10.8 | 12.6 | 0.9 | 8.6 | 12.8 | 0.7 | 7.7 | 11.0 | 0.7 |
| Leukemia | 6.7 | 7.6 | 0.9 | 5.8 | 7.7 | 0.8 | 6.7 | 7.7 | 0.9 | 7.1 | 7.3 | 1.0 |

[a]RR, Rate Ratio; NA, not available

Latinos (Table 8.1). Overall, prostate cancer incidence rates are about 20 to 30 percent lower among Latinos than among Whites. The causes of prostate cancer are not yet clearly identified but are thought to be related to imbalances in male hormones (Miller et al., 1996). Some research suggests that, as with breast cancer, diets high in fat and low in fiber are a risk factor (Ross & Shottenfeld, 1996). This implies that the traditional diets in various Latino cultures offer some protection against the risk of prostate cancer.

## Stomach Cancer

While rates of stomach cancer have decreased dramatically over the decades among all race and ethnic groups, Latinos still have higher risks than do Whites. Among males, stomach cancer rates are 30 to 90 percent higher than those of Whites in the same geographic area (Table 8.1). Incidence rates are 50 percent to twofold higher among Latinas than those among non-Latina populations (Table 8.2). Although stomach cancer has long been known to be related to socioeconomic status, little is known about the exact causes of the high risk among Latinos. Etiological risk factors related to stomach cancer include high intake of salted, smoked, and pickled foods (Ross & Shottenfeld, 1996). Currently there is interest in infection with *Helicobacter pylori* as a risk factor for stomach cancer (Miller et al., 1996; Nomura, 1996); *H. pylori* is the major cause of chronic gastritis, and studies show that the infection may be more prevalent among Hispanic populations (Everhart, Kruszon-Moran, Perez-Perez, Tralka, & McQuillan, 2000).

## Primary Liver Cancer

Although rare in the United States, primary liver cancer is more frequent in Latino populations than in other groups. For both males and females, incidence of primary liver cancer is about twice as high as that for Whites in the same area (Tables 8.1 and 8.2). Rates of primary liver cancer appear to be particularly high among Mexican Americans in Texas, even when compared to the rates of Latinos in California or other regions (Tables 8.1 and 8.2). Primary liver cancer has several known risk factors: hepatitis B and C viruses, exposure to aflatoxins, cirrhosis, and alcohol use (London & McGlynn, 1996). Which of these risk factors explains the excessive risks observed in Latinos is as yet unknown. Another risk factor suggested but not directly proven is exposure to chemicals or organic solvents via agricultural occupations (London & McGlynn, 1996).

## Gallbladder Cancer

Incidence rates for gallbladder cancer are excessive in Latino populations compared to those of Whites. Although relatively rare, rates are about one per 100,000 in Latino males and about three to four per 100,000 in Latinas (Tables 8.1 and 8.2). Ethnic differentials are particularly pronounced in females, with risks that are four to five times higher than those for Whites in the same region

(Table 8.2). Risk factors related to gallbladder cancer include a history of gallstones and gallbladder disease. In turn, the risk factors associated with gallstones (and therefore gallbladder cancer) are obesity, lipid metabolism, and exogenous estrogens (Fraumeni, Devesa, McLaughlin, & Stanford, 1996).

### Non-Hodgkin's Lymphomas and Leukemia

The frequency of non-Hodgkin's lymphomas is somewhat lower in Latinos than in non-Latino populations. The differentials observed in various regions of the country are 10 to 20 percent lower (Tables 8.1 and 8.2). Leukemia incidence rates are also somewhat lower among Latinos; among Latinas, rates are 10 to 20 percent lower than those among White women.

## Cigarette Smoking

Table 8.3 shows data on current smoking prevalences from the National Health Interview Survey (NHIS) by race and ethnicity (National Center for Health Statistics, 1999). Smoking rates vary by age and gender. In 1993–1995, among males,

**TABLE 8.3. CURRENT CIGARETTE SMOKING BY AGE, ETHNICITY/RACE, AND GENDER, NHIS, 1993–1995.**

|  | Male (Percent) | Female (Percent) |
|---|---|---|
| **18–24 years** |  |  |
| Whites | 31 | 29 |
| African Americans | 17 | 9 |
| Latinos | 24 | 13 |
| **25–34 years** |  |  |
| Whites | 32 | 31 |
| African Americans | 28 | 26 |
| Latinos | 27 | 15 |
| **35–44 years** |  |  |
| Whites | 32 | 28 |
| African Americans | 40 | 31 |
| Latinos | 25 | 20 |
| **45–64 years** |  |  |
| Whites | 27 | 25 |
| African Americans | 39 | 25 |
| Latinos | 24 | 13 |
| **65 and older** |  |  |
| Whites | 13 | 11 |
| African Americans | 28 | 13 |
| Latinos | 12 | 7 |
| **All 18 and older** |  |  |
| Whites | 27 | 24 |
| African Americans | 32 | 22 |
| Latinos | 25 | 14 |

Latinos had slightly lower cigarette smoking rates than those of non-Latinos. This difference in smoking rates is stronger among those younger than forty-five years of age. Among males sixty-five years and older, Latinos had smoking rates similar to those of Whites. Among females, far fewer Latinas smoke than either Whites or African Americans. This holds true for every age group. Overall, only 14 percent of Latinas smoke, compared to 24 percent of White women and 22 percent of African American females. Among males of all ages, 25 percent of Latinos currently smoke, compared to 27 percent of Whites and 32 percent of African Americans.

Current smoking rates vary by Latino ethnic group. Data from the National Hispanic Leadership Initiative on Cancer (NHLIC)–*En Acción* national cancer risk factor surveys showed that Puerto Ricans and Cubans were more likely to be current smokers than were Mexican Americans (Pérez-Stable et al., 2000). Among Latinas, Puerto Rican women were nearly twice as likely to smoke as were Cuban, Mexican American, or Central American women.

## Dietary Factors

For the most part, the traditional diet of Latinos reflects the high-fiber, low-fat diets recommended by the NCI. Data from the Third National Health and Nutrition Examination Survey (NHANES III) show that dietary fiber intake is highest among Mexican Americans, compared to that of Whites and African Americans (Alaimo et al., 1994), and meets NCI recommendations (twenty to thirty grams of fiber daily). The same survey data show that the mean total fat intake was lowest in Mexican Americans compared to that of other groups (McDowell et al., 1994). Although dietary intake data are lacking for other Latino groups, it appears that high-fiber, low-fat diets of Latinos may partially explain their lower risk of colorectal, prostate, and breast cancer.

## Alcohol Consumption

Alcohol consumption is of significant concern to Latino populations because of the increased risk observed for liver cancer. Yet NHIS data indicate that, in general, Latinos are less likely to be current drinkers than Whites (National Center for Health Statistics, 1998). Among males aged eighteen to forty-four years, 80 percent of Whites reported they were current drinkers compared to 71 percent of Latinos. Among those aged forty-five and older, 66 percent of White males reported they were current drinkers compared to 63 percent of Latinos (National Center for Health Statistics, 1998). Far fewer Latinas drink than do White females (age eighteen to forty-four: 42 percent versus 65 percent, respectively; age forty-five and older: 28 percent versus 44 percent, respectively).

# Infectious Agents

Hepatitis B is a major risk factor for primary liver cancer and thus is of major importance to Latinos whose risk is high compared to other populations. Unfortunately, scant data exist on the prevalence of chronic hepatitis B virus infection among different Latino populations. Data from NHANES III covering 1988–1994 on Mexican Americans shows that prevalence of hepatitis B virus infection was similar between Mexican Americans and Whites aged forty-nine and younger (3 percent) (McQuillan, Coleman, Kruszon-Moran, Moyer, Lambert, & Margolis, 1999). However, among Mexican Americans fifty years and older, prevalence of hepatitis B virus infection increased to 11 percent compared to 3 percent among similarly aged Whites. Hepatitis C virus infection also is a major risk factor for primary liver cancer, but little is known about the prevalence and role of that infection. Because of the observed increased risks for primary liver cancer, particularly among Mexican Americans, there is a compelling need to study the prevalence and role of both hepatitis B and hepatitis C virus infections in Latino populations.

As in other populations, human papilloma virus is a very strong risk factor for cervical cancer development in Latinas (Becker et al., 1994) and may explain their higher incidence of cervical cancer. Research suggests that the vehicle by which Latina women are infected with papilloma virus is through the sexual behavior of their male partners, which places Latina women at increased risk for cervical cancer (Giuliano, Papenfuss, Schneider, Nour, & Hatch, 1999; Zunzunegui, King, Coria, & Charlet, 1986). Finally, another important infectious agent that may contribute to the cancer burden in Latinos is *Helicobacter pylori*, a risk factor for gastric ulcers and stomach cancer. The prevalence of *H. pylori* is much higher among Latino populations. National data show that the age-adjusted prevalence is substantially higher among Mexican Americans (62 percent) than among Whites (26 percent) (Everhart, Kruszon-Moran, Perez-Perez, Tralka, & McQuillan, 2000). Infection with *H. pylori* is easily cured with antibiotics and would require relatively simple public health interventions.

# Occupational and Environmental Exposures

The contribution of occupational and environmental toxicant exposures to the development of cancer is still being debated. Yet the strong Latino presence in low-paying occupations (such as farming and industrial work) that frequently subject workers to various chemicals may expose this population to chemical carcinogens more than others. A 1989 study of primary liver cancer death and occupations in Texas suggested increased risks for Mexican American farmworkers possibly exposed to pesticides (Suarez, Weiss, & Martin, 1989). Of all racial and ethnic groups, Latinos were the least likely to reside in counties that met national ambient air quality standards throughout the year (National Center for Health Statistics, 1998). Compared to all persons in 1996 (81 percent), only 56 percent of Latinos in the United States lived in counties that met air quality standards for all pollutants.

## Pap Smear

National surveys consistently demonstrate the low use of Pap smear screening among Latinas. From 1987 to 1992, Latinas were found to have the lowest use of Pap smear screening of all race and ethnic groups in the United States (Anderson & May, 1995; Martin, Calle, Wingo, & Health, 1996). Although risk of cervical cancer is relatively high among Latinas, invasive cervical cancer and death are highly preventable with routine cervical cancer screening.

National data on the Latino population in the United States are misleading because of the variation of screening among Mexican Americans, Puerto Ricans, Cubans, and other subgroups. These subgroups vary considerably by age structure, English-language use, income, education, and nativity—factors that greatly influence participation in Pap smear screening. Data from the NHLIC–*En Acción* surveys show that recent Pap smear use among women aged forty and older vary from under 50 percent among Mexican American women in Laredo, Texas, to 75 percent among Central American women in San Francisco (Figure 8.1).

**FIGURE 8.1.   RECENT PAP SMEAR BY
ETHNO-REGIONAL GROUP.**

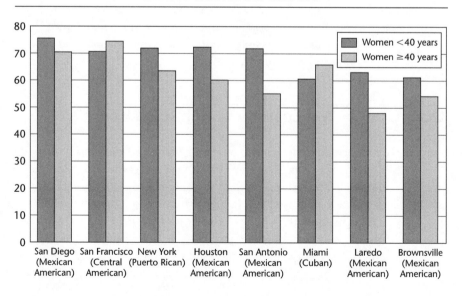

# Mammography

Because Latinas tend to seek health care services less than do women in other ethnic groups, they also are much less likely to participate in mammography screening for early detection of breast cancer. Although mammography participation (use within the past two years) rates among Latinas aged forty and older increased from 18 percent in 1987 to 52 percent in 1994, Latina participation rates are still lower than those for White (61 percent) or African American (64 percent) women (National Center for Health Statistics, 1998).

As with cervical cancer screening, national data fail to reveal the highly variable use of mammography screening among different Latina populations. A recent study based on NHLIC–*En Acción* surveys showed that some Latina groups have met the *Healthy People 2000* cancer objectives for mammogram use (Ramirez et al., 2000): 86 percent of Central Americans in San Francisco and 80 percent of Cuban women aged forty and older in Miami have had at least one mammogram. Data from a study on recent compliance with mammogram guidelines (mammogram within the past two years) show that among women aged forty and older in Texas, Mexican Americans in Laredo (40 percent), Brownsville (50 percent), and Houston (52 percent) were the least likely to report a recent mammogram; recent mammogram use was relatively high among Central American women in San Francisco (82 percent) and in Cuban women in Miami (72 percent) (Figure 8.2). The same study shows that these differences persist even after adjustment for socioeconomic and demographic factors (Ramirez et al., 2000).

## FIGURE 8.2.   RECENT MAMMOGRAPHY BY ETHNO-REGIONAL GROUP.

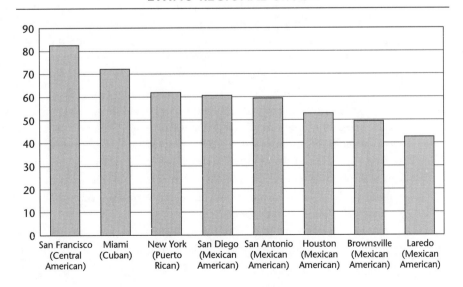

## Digital Rectal Examination

Although Latinos have a lower risk for prostate cancer than do other groups in the United States, prostate cancer is the most frequent cause of cancer death among Latino males. Although the effectiveness of screening for prostate cancer is still under debate, prostate cancer in its early stages can be found through digital rectal examination (DRE), the prostate-specific antigen test, or transrectal ultrasound diagnosis. As a group, Latinos know less about prostate cancer and are less likely to have had a DRE, the least invasive and most common screening modality. Data from the National Center for Health Statistics show that Latino men undergo DREs less often than either Whites or African Americans (39 percent versus 57 percent and 43 percent, respectively, for those ever tested). Data from the NHLIC—*En Acción* study (Talavera et al., 2000) show that among the various Latino groups, Mexican Americans (68 percent) and Central Americans (69 percent) are the least likely to have ever heard of DRE, compared to Cubans (78 percent) or Puerto Ricans (70 percent). Likewise, Mexicans and Central Americans (52 percent combined) are the least likely to ever have had the DRE as compared to Cubans (64 percent) and Puerto Ricans (63 percent).

## Genetic Screening for High-Risk Latinos

In recent decades, there has been an enormous expansion in the knowledge that may be gained from the testing of an individual's genetic material to predict present or future disability or disease, including cancer, that might affect not only the individual but also his or her family. This remarkable progress in knowledge contrasts with the small amount of related information that is available to the public. This is especially true for minority populations, such as Latinos, in which data on the subject and related studies are scarce or nonexistent. In 1990, the National Science Foundation Survey found only 7 percent of Americans to be literate regarding genetics (Miller, 1992). In another survey, the March of Dimes (1992) found that a majority of respondents knew little or nothing about genetic testing or gene therapy. Without some degree of knowledge and a clear understanding of the limitations and the potential risks involved in genetic testing (for example, insurance and employment discrimination, psychological and emotional distress, intrafamilial conflict, and social stigmatization), Latinos and others cannot make truly informed decisions about the use of genetic services. In addition, modern technology is neither accessible nor affordable to all, an issue of particular concern to the Latino population, in which family median income levels are considerably lower than those of Whites.

In the area of cancer genetic research, it is critical to include minority populations, since both the spectrum and the frequency of mutations may vary in different subgroups of the population. In general, women who express interest in genetic testing have been found to be well-educated White women. Extremely little is known about the interest in genetic testing, the need for educational interventions, or the response to genetic information on the part of less-educated or minority groups (Fox Chase Cancer Center, 1995). Information regarding these issues and a clear understanding of concerns related to genetic research and its applications in culturally diverse groups are important in tailoring cancer risk messages to underserved populations. Focus groups conducted with African Americans, Latinos, and low-socioeconomic-status Whites have shown that presentation of cancer genetic risk information to underserved populations can be successfully achieved if done in a linguistically and culturally appropriate manner. Although significant differences exist regarding the importance of religion, the family unit, and the need for privacy versus support groups, African Americans and Latinos expressed similar concerns, especially related to ethical issues, confidentiality, benefits, access to information, and the role of the government. Attitudes of fear and distrust, as well as a general lack of knowledge, were common to all three groups (Fox Chase Cancer Center, 1995; University of Michigan, 1999).

## Impact of Sociocultural Factors Related to Cancer

Culture plays a central role in determining each person's health beliefs, attitudes, and behaviors—and cultural milieu influences health in several ways. Traditions, customs, religious beliefs and practices, and health-related values are all important (Last, 1987). Latinos do not constitute a single population or class, and even though they share a common language, they represent a mosaic of cultural legacies and histories. While similarities exist, Latinos' wide diversity in demographic, cultural characteristics, and other factors can influence cancer screening and related knowledge and attitudes. The lack of well-specified research on individual Latino subgroups in the United States (for example, Mexican Americans, Puerto Ricans, Cubans, and Central and South Americans) has resulted in inadequate data on cancer knowledge, attitudes, and behaviors for these individual populations. Compounding this problem is the scarcity of published data on the sociocultural determinants of the cancer experience among each of these populations (Ramirez, MacKellar, & Gallion, 1988).

Along with culture, socioeconomic status and access to medical care are important mediators of the relationship between ethnicity and cancer outcomes. Compared with Whites, Latinos more frequently are poor, lack health insurance, have fewer years of formal education, and have higher unemployment rates, all of which contribute to inadequate medical care for this population (Hubbel, Waitzkin, Mishra, Dombrink, & Chavez, 1991; Pérez-Stable, Marín, & Marín, 1994). The lack of health insurance is clearly an important influencing factor in the participation of Latinos in screening services, and adequate screening cannot be expected until everyone receives coverage. However, other factors may be responsible for differences among regions and groups. For example, poor physician compliance with screening recommendations and a health care system that has not yet been fully conceptualized and developed in a culturally sensitive and responsive manner to provide Latino users with personal and caring interactions in a familiar language may help account for the underutilization of early detection services by Latinos (Bakemeier, Krebs, Murphy, Shen, & Ryals, 1995; Guerra, Meza, Ho, Casner, & Moldes, 1994; Pérez-Stable, Otero-Sabogal, Sabogal, McPhee, & Hiatt, 1994; Ramirez, Villarreal, Suarez, & Flores, 1995; Vernon, Vogel, Halabi, Jackson, Lundy, & Peters, 1992). In addition, Latinos often experience cultural and language barriers that keep them from seeking health care or cancer-related services, and they have limited knowledge about cancer-related risk factors and cancer screening procedures (Loehrer et al., 1991; Morgan, Park, & Cortes, 1995; Pérez-Stable, Marín, & Marín, 1994; Pérez-Stable, Otero-Sabogal, McPhee, & Hiatt, 1994; Suarez, 1994; Ramirez, Suarez, Laufman, Barroso, & Chalela, 2000). For many, barriers include an inability to speak English, fatalistic beliefs about cancer, and a lack of self-efficacy in reducing individual risks for cancer, all of which may affect the utilization of cancer preventive services (Hubbel, Chavez, Mishra, Magana, & Valdez, 1995; Pérez-Stable, Sabogal, Otero-Sabogal, Hiatt, & McPhee, 1992; Ramirez, MacKeller, & Gallion, 1988). In general, Latinos consider doctors' offices, clinics, and other health care facilities places to go only when one feels ill or when symptoms are present. In other words, they typically believe that the purpose of health professionals and health services is to treat—not to prevent—disease or promote health. This attitude poses an additional obstacle for health-promotion and disease-prevention efforts that seek to achieve widespread participation in cancer screening (Ramirez, Suarez, Laufman, Barroso, & Chalela, 2000).

Conversely, the importance of family and social ties among Latinos is a cultural factor that may be helpful in promoting Latino utilization of cancer screening services. Most Latino groups have strong bonds to community, resulting in a sense of identity and belonging; in many cases the community is considered an extension of the family. This familial and community orientation, in which many functionally connected individuals form a supportive network, can be considered a strength and provides excellent opportunities for cancer-related intervention programs (Ramirez, MacKellar, & Gallion, 1988; Suarez et al., 2000). Several studies, including the *Por La Vida* program and the *A Su Salud* and NHLIC–*En Acción* models, have successfully focused on mobilizing natural social networks to prompt and reinforce improved cancer screening behavior among Latino groups (Navarro, Senn, McNicholas, Kaplan, Roppe, & Campo, 1998; Ramirez et al., 1995; Ramirez et al., 1998).

# Lessons Learned from Cancer Prevention Studies

The past decade has witnessed a substantial growth of research pertaining to cancer prevention and Latinos. Included here is a review of the literature on cancer prevention projects in the Latino community. Projects were identified through a literature search on MEDLINE, ERIC, the Minority Online Services, the Office of Minority Health databases, and reference lists in journal articles. To be included here, a project needed to conduct prevention outreach to a population that was at least 75 percent Latino, and outcome and findings data from the program must have been published in a scientific journal no earlier than 1990. Projects with only baseline survey data were excluded. Tables 8.4 and 8.5 list the seventeen selected projects grouped by cancer risk factor and site. Similarities, innovations, and concepts of the projects are discussed below.

## Theoretical Framework

The majority of the programs are based on behavioral science theory, most often Albert Bandura's social cognitive learning theory (SCLT). SCLT postulates that behavior modification in a given person can be elicited through the use of a role model that the person identifies with who demonstrates the desired behavior. Central tenets to SCLT include social modeling, social reinforcement, and self-efficacy (Bandura, 1986). Other commonly utilized theories include the health belief model, the theory of reasoned action, and Paulo Freire's empowerment pedagogy (Ajzen & Fishbein, 1980; Freire, 1994; Rosenstock, Strecher, & Becker, 1988). To develop a theoretical framework, projects often rely on multiple theories and on theoretical frameworks already established in previous programs. For instance, the original *A Su Salud,* a cancer outreach program developed by Ramirez and colleagues, has not only been replicated but has also served as the basis for the design of other projects and project components (Ramirez, Villarreal, Suarez, & Flores, 1995; Suarez, Nichols, & Brady, 1993; Yancey & Walden, 1994). The *A Su Salud* model incorporates SCLT, the health belief model, and the theory of reasoned action, and its intervention outreach activities were modeled after the Finnish North Karelia Project (McAlister, Ramirez, Amezcua, Pulley, Stern, & Mercado, 1992; Ramirez, Villarreal, Suarez, & Flores, 1995).

## Cultural Appropriateness

In addition to behavioral theories, cancer prevention activities included here must incorporate cultural aspects central to the Latino heritage, such as the Spanish language. Spanish-only or Spanish and English media messages are critical to the acceptance, understanding, retention, and following of the produced messages. This is especially the case with print media, as Latinos rely more heavily on print materials than other media to provide information about cancer detection and treatment (Massett, 1996). An example of a popular smoking cessation guide, *Guia para Dejar de Fumar,* was originally developed for the San Francisco-based *Programa Latino para Dejar de Fumar* (PLDF) (Marín & Pérez-Stable, 1995). The thirty-six-page color booklet presented information on the health risks of smoking and cessation methods and maintenance (Pérez-Stable, Sabogal, Marín, Marín, & Otero-Sabogal, 1991). The *Guia* was initially evaluated through PLDF and later

**TABLE 8.4. SMOKING CESSATION PROGRAMS.**

| Study | Setting | Sample | Risk Factor/ Site | Theory | Intervention Strategies | Findings |
|-------|---------|--------|-------------------|--------|-------------------------|----------|
| **A Su Salud** McAlister et al. (1992) | Eagle Pass, TX (intervention) Del Rio, TX (control) | N = 160 Latinos, predominantly Mexican Americans (N = 160, intervention community; N = 135, comparison community) | Smoking | Social cognitive health belief model | Mass and small media campaigns, varying levels of interpersonal outreach via lay community volunteers | 17 percent self-reported quit rate, 8 percent verified quit rate in intervention community 7 percent self-reported quit rate, 1.5 percent verified in control |
| | | | | Theory of reasoned action | | No differences between differing interpersonal outreach |
| **Guia para Dejar de Fumar** | San Francisco, CA | Less acculturated Spanish speaking Latinos: | Smoking | Transtheoretical model | Distributed Spanish smoking cessation guides as program component of PLDF | Quit rates: |
| Pérez-Stable et al. (1991) | | N = 431 (1991) | | | Compared success of self-administered mood management (1997) | 2.5 months: = 21.1 percent |
| Muñoz et al. 1997 | | N = 136 (1997) | | | | Twelve months: 8.4 percent (validated) fourteenth months = 13.7 percent (1991) Mood management substantially increased abstinence rate (16 of 71 versus 7 of 65) Those previously depressed reported even higher levels of abstinence (31 versus 11 percent) (1997) |

| Program / Study | Location | Population | Topic | Theory | Intervention | Results |
|---|---|---|---|---|---|---|
| **Programa Latino para Dejar de Fumar (PLDF)** | San Francisco, CA | Spanish-speaking less acculturated Latinos | Smoking | Theory of reasoned action | Mass and small media campaign (including *Guia*) | Cigarette-smoking prevalence decreased 1986–1990; stabilized 1991; increased 1993 |
| Marín & Pérez-Stable (1995) | | | | | Personalized consultations | Cessation stable but showed steady increase in less-acculturated Latinos |
| Van Oss et al. (1994) Pérez-Stable et al. (1993) Marín et al. (1990) | | | | | | |
| **Si Puedo** | New York, NY | 93 Latino smokers | Smoking | None | Culturally specific multicomponent behavioral eight-week program | Initial cessation rates higher than in comparison group but month twelve rates: intervention = 8 percent; validated comparison = 7 percent |
| Nevid et al. (1996) | | | | | | Rates and reasons for attrition similar between groups |
| Nevid et al. (1997) | | | | | | |

## TABLE 8.5. WOMEN'S HEALTH ISSUES AND NUTRITION.

| Study | Setting | Sample | Risk Factor/Site | Theory | Intervention Strategies | Findings |
|---|---|---|---|---|---|---|
| **Agricultural Cancer Prevention Project** | California's Central Valley | Hispanic women | Women's health issues focusing on breast and cervical cancers | None | Forty-minute educational sessions led by either health educators or volunteer peer educators | Knowledge increase significant on four of nine test questions |
| Goldsmith and Sisneros (1996) | | | | | One-on-one discussions, informal groups, and formal presentations | Approximately 20.5 percent of 1,732 program participants redeemed cancer screening vouchers |
| **Community Mammography Project** | Los Angeles, CA | Hispanic women, 35+ years | Breast cancer | Health Belief Model | Activities classes, information given in ESL classes, health fairs, pharmacies | Screening rates increased 12–27 percent pre- and postintervention |
| Fox et al. (1998) | | | | | Breast health day at area church | Control community increased only 23–24 percent |
| **Compañeros en la Salud** | Phoenix, AZ | Hispanic women, 18+ years, attending church | Breast, cervical, and diet-related cancers | None | Outreach activities conducted in area churches | Total churches (N) = 14 |
| Castro et al. (1995) | | | | | Lay community health volunteers | Catholic churches tended to be larger |
| | | | | | Education classes led by volunteers and staff | Protestant women tended to be poorer, have lower levels of acculturation, and CBE lifetime levels[a] |
| | | | | | Health promotion activities | Smaller churches tended to have members who lived farther away |
| Fitzgibbon et al. (1996) | Chicago, IL | Low-income Latino families in literacy training program, N = 38 | Nutrition | None | Twelve weekly one-hour family-based classes designed to encourage dietary changes to reduce cancer risk | Intervention group demonstrated dietary behavior change |

| | | | | | |
|---|---|---|---|---|---|
| **Greater Lawrence Family Health Center** | Massachusetts | Hispanic American women, 45–75 years | | Courses activity based and used culturally relevant food | Both experimental and control mothers made dietary changes without related increase of knowledge<br>Parental support of dietary change directly related to number of sessions attended |
| Zapka et al. (1992)<br>Zapka et al. (1993) | | | Breast cancer | None | Client-centered educational strategies<br>Staff training strategies<br>Management strategies | No-show rates for mammography decreased from 27 percent (1987) to 17 percent (1989) |
| **Luces de Salud** | El Paso, TX | Mexican American women, 40+ years | Breast and cervical cancers | Social cognitive learning theory | Media campaign featuring role model stories | 6 percent Pap smear increase and 17 percent mammography increase rates similar to comparision site (7 percent; 19 percent) |
| Suarez et al. (1997) | | | | | Interpersonal communication via community volunteers | 11 percent of surveyed women had heard of program |
| Mishra et al. (1998) | Orange County, CA | Less acculturated Latinas, N = 40 | Breast cancer | Albert Bandura's theory of self-efficacy (empowerment model) | Four two-hour biweekly courses lead by health educator<br>Courses designed to spur thought and discussion about breast cancer and solutions to cancer control | Experiment group more likely to recognize more medically based knowledge, have a greater sense of self-efficacy, and a deeper understanding in conducting BSEs[b] |

*(Continued)*

## TABLE 8.5. WOMEN'S HEALTH ISSUES AND NUTRITION. (*Continued*)

| Study | Setting | Sample | Risk Factor/Site | Theory | Intervention Strategies | Findings |
|-------|---------|--------|------------------|--------|-------------------------|----------|
| **Por la Vida** | San Diego, CA | Low-income Latinas | General women's issues; focus on breast and cervical cancers | Paulo Freire's empowerment pedagogy | Twelve weekly ninty-minute classes led by lay community worker; two postgraduation classes | Intervention group had higher use of cancer screening than did control group (1999) |
| Navarro et al. (1995) | | Thirty-six community workers | | | | |
| Navarro et al. (1998) | | 512 course participants | | | | |
| **Programa a Su Salud** | San Antonio, TX | Latinas | Breast and cervical cancers | Social cognitive learning theory | Mass and small media campaign featuring role model stories | Pap smear use among younger women demonstrated an upward trend, and all age groups yielded a significant growth rate in mammography |
| McAlister et al. (1995) | Houston, TX (control) | | | Health belief model | Interpersonal communication via community volunteers | Eighty-five volunteers conducted outreach to 2,000–3,000 women |
| Ramirez et al. (1995) | | | | Theory of reasoned action | Small group of volunteers provided intensive follow-up assistance to group of community members | |
| **Su Vida, Su Salud** | Corpus Christi, TX | Mexican American women | Breast and cervical cancers | Social cognitive learning theory | Mass and small media featuring role model stories | 57 percent increase in mammography use |
| Suarez et al. (1993) | | | | | Interpersonal communication via lay community volunteers | No substantial Pap smear use increase |
| | | | | | | 365 women contacted program: thirteen received mammograms and 105 received Pap smears; 490 volunteers involved |

| Program/Author | Location | Population | Cancer Focus | Theory | Intervention | Results |
|---|---|---|---|---|---|---|
| **TEL-MED** | Wilmington, DE | Latinas, 40+ years | Breast cancer | None | Media promotion for Spanish TEL-MED message on breast cancer | Peak requests for tape immediately following initial promotional activities |
| Ward et al. (1997) | | | | | | Requested 58 percent times more than English breast cancer tape and 193 percent more than Spanish epilepsy tape |
| Yancey & Walden (1994) | Los Angeles, CA | Latinas | Breast and cervical cancers | None | Played videos on cervical cancer in clinic waiting room | Four-month period following Pap screening video showing demonstrated significantly larger use of Pap smears than in pre-intervention six-month period |
| | | | | | Two developed cervical cancer; one on breast | |
| | | | | | Only cervical cancer results discussed | |
| **Women's Health Loteria** | San Antonio, TX | Adult Latinas (N = 100) | Cervical cancer | Carl Rogers' and Leiniger's theories | Game played where pictures are matched with written messages about cervical cancer | 87 percent of respondents achieved learning objectives |
| Sheridan-Leos (1995) | | | | | Led by health educator | |

[a]Clinical breast exam (CBE).

[b]Breast self exam (BSE).

incorporated in a study with a self-administered mood management intervention (Muñoz, Marín, Posner, & Pérez-Stable, 1997). The *Guia* has been used as a tool for other smoking cessation programs and has been distributed by the American Cancer Society (Nevid, Javier, & Moulton, 1996).

In addition to language, inclusion of and reliance on other cultural factors have greatly enhanced acceptance and success of cancer prevention programs. *Compañeros en la Salud* developed a cancer prevention program in churches in Phoenix, Arizona (Castro et al., 1995). The project compared the differences in accessibility and project implementation in Catholic churches and Protestant churches to determine the most effective methods of working with church communities. The role of the church in Latino culture cannot be overstated and, while many community-based projects rely on the church as a vehicle for distributing information, *Compañeros en la Salud* and Fox and colleagues' Community Mammography Project (Fox, Stein, Gonzalez, Farrenkopf, & Dellinger, 1998) are two of the few projects to examine the logistics and potential of church involvement.

The church is an example of the social support network found in Latino communities. Community-based projects have begun developing programs based on the naturally occurring social networks in Latino communities, relying on existing and natural social networks (Navarro, Senn, McNicholas, Kaplan, Roppe, & Campo, 1998). While the church serves as an example of the institutionalization of social networks (that is, the setting for which these networks may be carried out), the backbone of these networks is the people who constitute them. Lay community volunteers, referred to as *consejeras, promotoras,* or networkers, have assumed an array of duties, including teaching self breast examination, distributing information, and providing emotional support. (Further details regarding these volunteers and their projects are discussed below in the subsection on interpersonal outreach.) Other cultural themes incorporated in projects or, in some cases, combated by the projects were *la familia* (family), *respeto* (respect), *simpatia* (kindness), *fuerza de voluntad* (willpower), and *fatalismo* (fatalism).

Other cultural factors that are particularly useful in project development include religion, games, and music. The Women's Health *Loteria* was based on the traditional Mexican and Mexican American game of the same name and taught women about cervical cancer risk factors and screening guidelines (Sheridan-Leos, 1995).

## Outreach and Education Methods

Health promotion programs employ numerous intervention strategies to deliver health messages to audiences. In Latino cancer prevention programs, the majority of the methods for delivery may be described as media outreach, interpersonal communication, or classroom-based communication. Few of the projects included here relied on just one vehicle of dissemination, preferring to utilize various strategies.

*Media Outreach.* Media activities generally are divided into mass media and small media. Mass media include television, radio, newspapers, and magazines, while small media refer to flyers, newsletters, church bulletins, monthly calendars, recipes, instructional booklets, and video- and audiotapes. Essentially every program incorporates some form of media, and some are solely media-based efforts. For example, TEL–MED produced a Spanish audiotape on breast cancer that was accessed through the telephone (Ward, Bartera, & Hoge, 1997). Yancey and Walden (1994) developed video messages on breast and cervical cancer to be played continuously in a clinic waiting room.

Because presentation of information through a media channel has proven effective, it stands to reason that combining channels increases outreach and education efforts. The *A Su Salud* model requires the use of both small and mass media (McAlister, Ramirez, Amezcua, Pulley, Stern, & Mercado, 1992). In this model the small media, consisting of flyers (calendars, recipes, and so on) distributed by lay community health volunteers, reinforce messages being presented in public service announcements, interviews, and articles aired through mass media venues. The messages are presented through community role model stories to increase community identification with healthy lifestyle behaviors.

*Interpersonal Outreach.* While media outreach can increase knowledge about cancer risks and screening among Latinos, personal contact can enhance and reinforce those messages. SCLT demonstrates that this personal contact is best received when it comes from a person living in the community. Numerous projects have involved lay members of the their target communities. These members often are unpaid volunteers who conduct various outreach activities.

In *Programa a Su Salud,* volunteers distributed monthly calendars with healthy food recipes, role model stories, upcoming events, and scheduling information for mass media segments on breast and cervical cancer (Ramirez et al., 1995). *Luces de Salud* and *Su Vida, Su Salud* are other projects that activated networks of community volunteers (Suarez, Nichols, & Brady, 1993, Suarez, Roche, Pulley, Weiss, Goldman, & Simpson, 1997). These projects were based on the *A Su Salud* model, in which volunteers visit homes and community locations to distribute small media information and initiate personal contact.

*Por la Vida* trained community women called *consejeras* to recruit and lead classes on cancer and women's health issues (Navarro, Senn, McNicholas, Kaplan, Roppe, & Campo, 1998). Though the Agricultural Cancer Prevention Project conducted a range of outreach activities, its health education classes were based on the volunteer network using the *Por la Vida* model (Goldsmith & Sisneros, 1996). *Compañeras en la Salud* recruited women, in this case called *promotoras,* to work as health educators within the church (Castro et al., 1995). In these projects volunteers led education courses in more formalized settings.

*Classroom Education.* More traditional approaches to cancer prevention outreach include education classes. Some programs have built on previous, more general classroom-setting projects and have adapted them to be accessible and relevant to Latino audiences. The programs just discussed in the interpersonal outreach subsection are examples of projects that relied on lay community volunteers to lead the classes. Another project, the Women's Health *Lotería*, was conducted in a clinic setting with a small group of women and led by a health educator (Sheridan-Leos, 1995). A nutrition program conducted by Fitzgibbon and colleagues conducted classes to reduce cancer risk through dietary changes (Fitzgibbon, Stolley, Avellone, Sugerman, & Chavez, 1996). The classes were held at a low-literacy training center in Chicago, and meal and nutritional recommendations were based on the traditional meals of the Mexican and Puerto Rican populations.

***Other Approaches.*** While the majority of the Latino cancer prevention programs conducted outreach to the target community, others have used existing institutions to examine ways to increase screening services within the established infrastructure. For example, the project conducted at the Greater Lawrence Family Health Center in Lawrence, Massachusetts, evaluated the activities and attitudes of both staff and clients to determine an effective multicomponent intervention that would increase breast cancer screening by Latinas (Constanza et al., 1992; Zapka, Harris, Hosmer, Constanza, Mas, & Barth, 1993). The intervention included client education, staff training, and management strategies, and many of these activities continued after the conclusion of the project (Zapka, Harris, Hosmer, Constanza, Mas, & Barth, 1993).

## Effectiveness of the Programs

The previous subsections have demonstrated the setting, frameworks, and outreach methods of Latino cancer prevention projects, and the question remains: Do the programs help in the prevention of cancer in the Latino population? The question is a tricky one, with no single answer.

The projects that have been discussed are by no means an exhaustive listing of all the cancer prevention projects targeting Latinos. Many programs excluded have not included a scientific study design and thus will be unable to produce outcome data. Other projects are in the process of conducting data analysis or have pending publications. For example, the NHLIC–*En Acción* is a nationwide multirisk cancer prevention program for the diverse Hispanic population. Funding for the program recently ended, and its results are eagerly anticipated.

Programs tend to focus on specific research questions and often do not follow a control group, making it difficult to offer sweeping generalizations about project success. From a community involvement standpoint, a number of the projects have had success in obtaining name recognition and community acceptance. Other programs have indeed increased knowledge about cancer risk factors or have been able to recruit large numbers of people to work as volunteers. Some programs have proven successful in increasing smoking cessation rates in their target communities. Other studies have increased our knowledge of effective implementation methods with community-based projects and ways to restructure existing establishments.

Some programs, however, have failed to yield significant results. While much of this may be attributed to study design, we stand to learn as much from the projects that have not worked as from those that have. Additionally, these projects have increased awareness of the difficulties in tracking data in community groups. In short, more research is needed to help us understand the full potential of cancer prevention projects and the most effective manner in which to implement them.

# Recommendations

In recent years the methodology of Latino cancer data collection, including the role of registries, has been examined and analyzed by various researchers, organizations, and groups. As a result, numerous recommendations for improvements in surveillance have been forthcoming. In addition, there are a number of well-defined areas of need in cancer research and care for Latinos. Although far from comprehensive, the following discussion presents some of the recommendations to improve conditions.

## Identification and Classification of Latinos

Upon establishment of the existing federal classification by race and ethnicity, the Office of Management and Budget (OMB) introduced the "Hispanic" category in 1977 with the adoption of Statistical Policy Directive No. 15 (Hayes-Bautista & Chapa, 1987), and United States Bureau of the Census efforts to officially identify persons of "Hispanic" origin have only been forthcoming in recent decades. In the meantime, other identifiers such as "Latino" have gained popularity, and controversy has arisen over which term should be applied. To help develop consistency in data classification, standardization of terminology is needed.

To minimize classification biases in cancer surveillance data and enhance comparability with census data, all persons reported to a registry should be asked to identify their ethnicity and race. Because this approach is not always feasible, the continued use of both medical record reports and surnames will reduce bias in the estimates of disease rates. Bias can be further reduced by training hospital personnel in the use of surname lists and in obtaining information on race and ethnicity from the patient. In addition, descriptive and etiological studies that select subjects based on registry-identified ethnicity may need to adjust for these misclassification errors, either in their design or analysis. For this purpose, a sample of cases should be interviewed periodically to assess the extent of misclassification and the characteristics of those misclassified (Swallen, West, Stewart, Glasser, & Horn-Ross, 1997).

A standard should be developed that incorporates existing data sources (that is, medical records, death certificates, census data, and Spanish surname lists) and describes the appropriate uses for cancer registry data using the standard definition of Latino ethnicity. A standard should be recommended for the future that will include new sources and/or procedures for refining the definition and that will describe the new uses that such an expanded definition would allow (North American Association of Central Cancer Registries Working Group on Methodology, 1996).

The National Center for Health Statistics (NCHS) should continue to conduct studies of the validity of Latino information on death certificates and increase training of individuals who fill out death certificates, with respect to Latino identifiers (North American Association of Central Cancer Registries Working Group on Methodology, 1996).

## Cancer Surveillance and Data Collection

To further enhance the excellent data provided in the SEER program database, adequate resources should be provided to expand SEER program coverage beyond the existing sites to include high-risk populations for which SEER program coverage is lacking. This expansion should address a wider range of demographic and social characteristics by using SEER's consistent nomenclature and uniform data and by reflecting the diverse characteristics of the current U.S. population (Institute of Medicine, 1999).

CDC and NCI should continue to work with the North American Association of Central Cancer Registries (NAACCR) and other organizations to expand the coverage and enhance the quality of the state cancer registries with the intent of ultimately achieving—together with the SEER program state registries—two goals: (1) a truly national data set through a system of longitudinal, population-based cancer registries covering the entire country, and (2) a reliable database for each state to serve as the basis for both the development and evaluation of cancer control efforts in that state (Institute of Medicine, 1999).

Data from the NPCR registry should be assessed to determine the information that could be contributed on Latinos and the level of quality of this information. In the interim, consistent standards should be developed to provide adequate information. In the future this should be monitored to ensure quality data collection.

Annual reporting of cancer surveillance data and population-based research should be expanded to include survival data for all ethnic groups, as well as for medically underserved populations (Institute of Medicine, 1999).

Emphasis should be placed on ethnic groups rather than on race in NIH's cancer surveillance and other population research. This implies a conceptual shift away from the emphasis on fundamental biological differences among "racial" groups to an appreciation of the range of cultural and behavioral attitudes, beliefs, lifestyle patterns, diet, environmental living conditions, and other factors that may affect cancer risk (Institute of Medicine, 1999).

Leadership in Latino and other communities should encourage participation in surveillance and research studies to make sure responses are high and data are complete and representative.

## Cancer Research Issues

To better understand cancer in Latinos and learn why certain forms of the disease are more prevalent in this population than in Whites while others are less prevalent, increased epidemiological and other research is needed. Because incidence of several of the major cancers is lower in Latinos, the opportunity exists for primordial prevention or action to prevent the adoption of lifestyles and other conditions that would likely result in increased incidence of these diseases. Insufficient data are available concerning the effectiveness of cancer treatment in Latinos and how these treatments affect the quality of life. Efforts should be increased to fill these gaps in our knowledge.

More information is also needed about the influence of cultural and demographic considerations on Latino participation in cancer prevention and control efforts. As with other cancer research issues raised here, specific information with regard to the individual Latino subgroups should be pursued. Included in this research should be special efforts to better understand behaviors, risks, and various other influences unique to new immigrants.

## Cancer Care Issues

A major priority should be placed on reducing the many social, financial, institutional, and other barriers facing Latinos with regard to health care in general and cancer care in particular. For example, efforts are needed to reduce the significant number of Latino families who are without health insurance or whose insurance coverage is inadequate. Coverage should be comprehensive, affordable, and culturally responsive.

More equitable distribution of cancer care providers is needed, particularly those who are Latino and/or bilingual, in inner-city and rural areas that are traditionally underserved. For providers in these areas who are not Latino and/or bilingual, increased crosscultural competency should be emphasized.

To increase awareness, encourage positive behaviors, and counter common misconceptions with regard to cancer, increased attention should focus on optimal ways to disseminate information about risk factors and the importance of personal behavior in fighting this disease.

Recommendations such as these require appropriate funding, and the necessary direction and leadership will be required to ensure that positive steps are taken in an effective and efficacious manner. Equally important is the resolution required on the part of national, state, and local health care, research, and education entities to appreciate the need for change and to implement more inclusive policies with regard to Latino cancer issues. Only with due diligence and the involvement of the Latino community can the proper mechanisms and methodology be effected to secure adequate, accurate, and timely cancer information and to provide appropriate attention to all cancer issues for the rapidly growing U.S. Latino population.

## Acknowledgments

The authors would like to thank Patricia Chalela, Dani Presswood, and Marisa Zapata for their assistance with the preparation of this manuscript and its tables and figures.

## References

Ajzen, I., & Fishbein, M. (1980). *Understanding attitudes and predicting social behavior.* Englewood Cliffs, NJ: Prentice Hall.

Alaimo, K. et al. (1994). *Dietary intake of vitamins, minerals, and fiber of persons ages 2 months and over in the United States: Third National Health and Nutrition Examination Survey, Phase I, 1988–91.* Advance data from Vital and Health Statistics; No. 258. Hyattsville, MD: National Center for Health Statistics.

Anderson, L. M., & May, D. S. (1995). Has the use of cervical, breast, and colorectal cancer screening increased in the United States? *American Journal Public Health, 85,* 840–842.

Bakemeier, R. F., Krebs, L. U., Murphy, J. R., Shen, Z., & Ryals, T. (1995). Attitudes of Colorado health professionals toward breast and cervical cancer screening in Hispanic women. *Journal of the National Cancer Institute Monographs, 18,* 95–100.

Bandura, A. (1986). *Social foundations of thought and action: A social cognitive theory.* Englewood Cliffs, NJ: Prentice Hall.

Becker, T. M. et al. (1994). Sexually transmitted diseases and other risk factors for cervical dyplasia among Southwestern Hispanic and non-Hispanic White women. *Journal of the American Medical Association, 271,* 1181–1188.

Castro, F. G. et al. (1995). Mobilizing churches for health promotion in Latino communities: *Compañeros en la Salud. Journal of the National Cancer Institute Monographs, 18,* 127–135.

Centers for Disease Control and Prevention. (1999). *Cancer registries: Foundation for comprehensive cancer control—at a glance.* Retrieved August 24, 1999: http://www.cdc.gov/cancer/npcr/npcrpdfs/npcaag99.pdf

Costanza, M. E. et al. (1992). Impact of a physician intervention program to increase breast cancer screening. *Cancer Epidemiology, Biomarkers and Prevention, 1,* 7, 581–589.

Everhart, J. E., Kruszon-Moran, D., Perez-Perez, G. I., Tralka, T. S., & McQuillan, G. (2000). Seroprevalence and ethnic differences in *Helicobacter pylori* infection among adults in the United States. *Journal of Infectious Diseases, 181,* 4, 1359–1363.

Fitzgibbon, M. L., Stolley, M. R., Avellone, M. E., Sugerman, S., & Chavez, N. (1996). Involving parents in cancer risk reduction: A program for Hispanic American families. *Health Psychology, 15,* 6, 413–422.

Fox Chase Cancer Center. (1995). *Genetic risk for cancer: A model for cancer control.* Report of the Family Risk Assessment Program. Retrieved August 26, 1999: http://www.fccc.edu/research/reports/report95/daly.html

Fox, S. A., Stein, J. A., Gonzalez, R. E., Farrenkopf, M., & Dellinger, A. (1998). A trial to increase mammography utilization among Los Angeles Hispanic women. *Journal of Health Care for the Poor and Underserved, 9,* 3, 309–321.

Fraumeni, J. F., Devesa, S. S., McLaughlin, J. K., & Stanford, J. L. (1996). Biliary tract cancer. In D. Schottenfeld & J. F. Fraumeni (Eds.), *Cancer epidemiology and prevention*. New York: Oxford University Press.

Freire, P. (1994). *Pedagogy of hope: Reliving pedagogy of the oppressed*. New York: Continuum.

Giachello, A. L., Bell, R., Aday, L. A., & Andersen, R. M. (1983). Uses of the 1980 census for Hispanic health services research. *American Journal of Public Health, 73,* 3, 266–274.

Gilliland, F. D., Becker, T. M., Key, C. R., & Samet, J. M. (1994). Contrasting trends of prostate cancer incidence and mortality in New Mexico's Hispanics, non-Hispanic whites, American Indians, and blacks. *Cancer, 73,* 8, 2192–2199.

Giuliano, A. R., Papenfuss, M., Schneider, A., Nour, M., & Hatch, K. (1999). Risk factors for high-risk type human papillomavirus infection among Mexican American women. *Cancer Epidemiology, Biomarkers and Prevention, 8,* 615–620.

Goldsmith, D. F., & Sisneros, G. C. (1996). Cancer prevention strategies among California farmworkers: Preliminary findings. *Journal of Rural Health, 12,* Suppl. 4, 343–348.

Guerra, L. G., Meza, A. D., Ho, H., Casner, P. R., & Moldes, O. (1994). Medicine residents' practices in cancer screening in a Hispanic population. *Southern Medical Journal, 87,* 6, 631–633.

Hayes-Bautista, D. E., & Chapa, J. (1987). Latino terminology: Conceptual bases for standardized terminology. *American Journal of Public Health, 77,* 61–68.

Henderson, B. E., Pike, M. C., Bernstein, L., & Ross, R. K. (1996). Breast cancer. In D. Schottenfeld & J. F. Fraumeni (Eds.), *Cancer epidemiology and prevention*. New York: Oxford University Press.

Hubbel, F. A., Chavez, L. R., Mishra, S. I., Magana, R., & Valdez, R. B. (1995). From ethnography to intervention: Developing a breast cancer control program for Latinas. *Journal of the National Cancer Institute Monographs, 18,* 109–115.

Hubbel, F. A., Waitzkin, H., Mishra, S. I., Dombrink, J., & Chavez, L. R. (1991). Access to medical care for documented and undocumented Latinos in Southern California County. *Western Journal of Medicine, 154,* 4, 415–417.

Institute of Medicine. (1999). *The unequal burden of cancer: An assessment of NIH research and programs for ethnic minorities and medically underserved* (M. A. Haynes & B. D. Smedley, Eds.). Washington, DC: National Academy Press.

Last, J. M. (1987). *Public health and human ecology*. East Norwalk, CT: Appleton & Lange.

Loehrer, P. J. et al. (1991). Knowledge and beliefs about cancer in a socioeconomically disadvantaged population. *Cancer, 68,* 1665–1671.

London, T. W., & McGlynn, K. A. (1996). Liver cancer. In D. Schottenfeld & J. F. Fraumeni (Eds.), *Cancer epidemiology and prevention*. New York: Oxford University Press.

Mallin, K., & Anderson, K. (1988). Cancer mortality in Illinois Mexican and Puerto Rican immigrants, 1979–1984. *International Journal of Cancer, 41,* 5, 670–676.

March of Dimes. (1992, September 29). Birth Defects Foundation News Release. White Plains, NY.

Marín, G., & Pérez-Stable, E. J. (1995). Effectiveness of disseminating culturally appropriate smoking-cessation information: *Programa Latino para Dejar de Fumar. Journal of the National Cancer Institute Monographs, 18,* 155–163.

Martin, L. M., Calle, E. E., Wingo, P. A., & Health, C. W. (1996). Comparison of mammography and Pap test use from the 1987 and 1992 National Health Interview Surveys: Are we closing the gaps? *American Journal of Preventive Medicine, 12,* 82–90.

Massett, H. A. (1996). Appropriateness of Hispanic print materials: A content analysis. *Health Education Research, 11,* 2, 231–242.

McAlister, A. L. et al. (1995). Community level cancer control in a Texas barrio: Part II. Base-line and preliminary outcome findings. *Journal of the National Cancer Institute Monographs, 18,* 123–126.

McAlister, A. L., Ramirez, A. G., Amezcua, C., Pulley, L. V., Stern, M. P., & Mercado, S. (1992). Smoking cessation in Texas–Mexico border communities: A quasi-experimental panel study. *American Journal of Health Promotion, 6,* 4, 274–279.

McDowell, M. A. et al. (1994). *Energy and macronutrient intakes of persons: Ages 2 months and over in the United States. Third National Health and Nutrition Examination Survey, Phase I, 1988–91.* Advance data from vital and health statistics (No. 255). Hyattsville, MD: National Center for Health Statistics.

McQuillan, G. M., Coleman, P. J., Kruszon-Moran, D., Moyer, L. A., Lambert, S. B., & Margolis, H. S. (1999). Prevalence of hepatitis B virus infection in the United States: The National Health and Nutrition Examination Surveys, 1976 through 1994. *American Journal of Public Health, 89,* 14–18.

Miller, B. A. et al. (1996). *Racial/ethnic patterns of cancer in the United States. 1988–1992, National Cancer Institute.* (NIH Publication No. 96-4104). Bethesda, MD. Retrieved August 20, 1999: http://www-seer.ims.nci.nih.gov/Publications/REPoC/

Miller, J. (1992). *The public understanding of science and technology in the United States, 1990.* Report to the National Science Foundation, Washington, D.C.

Morgan, C., Park, E., & Cortes, D. E. (1995). Beliefs, knowledge, and behavior about cancer among urban Hispanic women. *Journal of the National Cancer Institute Monographs, 18,* 57–63.

Muñoz, R. F., Marín, B. V., Posner, S. F., & Pérez-Stable, E. J. (1997). Mood management mail intervention increases abstinence rates for Spanish-speaking Latino smokers. *American Journal of Community Psychology, 25,* 3, 325–343.

National Cancer Institute. (1999, September 13). About SEER: Surveillance, NCI-Surveillance, Epidemiology and End Results Program Web site. Retrieved September 13, 1999: http://www-seer.ims.nci.nih.gov/AboutSEER.html

National Center for Health Statistics. (1998). *Health, United States, 1998 with socioeconomic status and health chartbook.* Hyattsville, MD: Author.

National Center for Health Statistics. (1999). *Health, United States, 1999, with health and aging chartbook.* Hyattsville, MD: Author.

Navarro, A. M., Senn, K. L., McNicholas, L. J., Kaplan, R. M., Roppe, B., & Campo, M. C. (1998). *Por La Vida* model intervention enhances use of cancer screening tests among Latinas. *American Journal of Preventive Medicine, 15,* 1, 32–41.

Nevid, J. S., Javier, R. A., Moulton, J. L. (1996). Factors predicting participant attrition in a community-based, culturally specific smoking-cessation program for Hispanic smokers. *Health Psychology, 15,* 3, 226–229.

Nomura, A. (1996). Stomach cancer. In D. Schottenfeld & J. F. Fraumeni (Eds.), *Cancer epidemiology and prevention.* New York: Oxford University Press.

North American Association of Central Cancer Registries Working Group on Methodology. (1996, January 19–21). *Problems in measuring cancer in Hispanics.* Uniform Data Standards Committee. Subcommittee on Methodologic Issues of Measuring Cancer among Hispanics. Final report of the Atlanta Symposium, Atlanta, GA.

Pérez-Stable, E. J., Marín, G., & Marín, B. V. (1994). Behavioral risk factors: A comparison of Latinos and non-Latino whites in San Francisco. *American Journal of Public Health, 84,* 6, 971–976.

Pérez-Stable, E. J., Otero-Sabogal, R., Sabogal, F., McPhee, S. J., & Hiatt, R. A. (1994). Self-reported use of cancer screening tests among Latinos and Anglos in a prepaid health plan. *Archives of Internal Medicine, 154,* 10, 1073–1080.

Pérez-Stable, E. J. et al. (2000). *Cigarette smoking behavior among U.S. Latinos: A national survey.* Unpublished manuscript.

Pérez-Stable, E. J., Sabogal, F., Marín, G., Marín, B. V., & Otero-Sabogal, R. (1991). Evaluation of *Guia para Dejar de Fumar,* a self-help guide in Spanish to quit smoking. *Public Health Reports, 106,* 5, 564–570.

Pérez-Stable, E. J., Sabogal, F., Otero-Sabogal, R., Hiatt, R. A., & McPhee, S. J. (1992). Misconceptions about cancer among Latinos and Anglos. *Journal of the American Medical Association, 268,* 22, 3219–3223.

Perkins, R. C. (1993, August). *Evaluating the Passel-Word Spanish Surname List: 1990 Decennial Census Post-Enumeration Survey Results.* Washington, D.C.: U.S. Bureau of the Census, Population Division.

Polednak, A. P. (1993a). Estimating cervical cancer incidence in the Hispanic population of Connecticut by use of surnames. *Cancer, 71,* 11, 3560–3564.

Polednak. A. P. (1993b) Lung cancer rates in the Hispanic population of Connecticut, 1980–88. *Public Health Reports, 108,* 4, 471–476.

Ramirez, A. G. MacKellar, D. A., & Gallion, K. J. (1988). Reaching minority audiences: A major challenge in cancer reduction. *The Cancer Bulletin, 40,* 6, 334–343.

Ramirez, A. G. et al. (1995). Community level cancer control in a Texas barrio: Part I. Theoretical basis, implementation and process evaluation. *Journal of the National Cancer Institute Monographs, 18,* 117–122.

Ramirez, A. G. et al. (1998). Prevention and control in diverse Hispanic populations: A national initiative for research and action. *Cancer, 83,* 1825–1829.

Ramirez, A. G., Suarez, L., Laufman, L., Barroso, C., & Chalela, P. (2000). Hispanic women's breast and cervical cancer knowledge, attitudes and screening behaviors. *American Journal of Health Promotion, 14,* 5, 292–300.

Ramirez, A. G., et al. (2000, September). Breast cancer screening in regional Hispanic populations. *Health Education Research, 15,* 5, 559–568.

Ramirez, A. G., Villarreal, R., Suarez, L., & Flores, E. T. (1995). The emerging Hispanic population: A foundation for cancer prevention and control. *Journal of the National Cancer Institute Monographs, 18,* 1–9.

Rosenstock, I. M., Strecher, V. J., & Becker, M. H. (1988). Social learning theory and the health belief model. *Health Education Quarterly, 15,* 2, 175–183.

Ross, R. K., & Shottenfeld, D. (1996). Prostate cancer. In D. Schottenfeld & J. F. Fraumeni (Eds.), *Cancer epidemiology and prevention.* New York: Oxford University Press.

Schiffman, M. H., Brinton, L. A., Devesa, S. S., & Fraumeni, J. F. (1996). Cervical cancer. In D. Schottenfeld & J. F. Fraumeni (Eds.), *Cancer epidemiology and prevention.* New York: Oxford University Press.

Sheridan-Leos, N. (1995). Women's Health *Loteria:* A new cervical cancer education tool for Hispanic females. *Oncology Nursing Forum, 22,* 4, 697–701.

Stewart, S. L., Swallen, K. C., Glaser, S. L., Horn-Ross, P. L., & West, D. W. (1999). Comparison of methods for classifying Hispanic ethnicity in a population-based cancer registry. *American Journal of Epidemiology, 149,* 11, 1063–1071.

Stiller, C. A. (1997). Reliability of cancer registration data. *European Journal of Cancer, 33,* 6, 812–814.

Suarez, L. (1994). Pap smear and mammogram screening in Mexican-American women: The effects of acculturation. *American Journal of Public Health, 84,* 5, 742–746.

Suarez, L., Nichols, D. C., & Brady, C. A. (1993). Use of peer role models to increase Pap smear and mammogram screening in Mexican-American and Black women. *American Journal of Preventive Medicine, 9,* 5, 290–296.

Suarez, L. et al. (2000). Social networks and cancer screening in four U.S. Hispanic groups. *American Journal of Preventive Medicine, 19,* 1, 47–52.

Suarez, L., Roche, R. A., Pulley, L. V., Weiss, N. S., Goldman, D., & Simpson, D. M. (1997). Why a peer intervention program for Mexican-American women failed to modify the secular trend in cancer screening. *American Journal of Preventive Medicine, 13,* 6, 411–417.

Suarez, L., Weiss, N. S., & Martin, J. (1989). Primary liver cancer death and occupation in Texas. *American Journal of Industrial Medicine, 15,* 167–175.

Swallen, K. C., West, D. W., Stewart, S. L., Glasser, S. L., & Horn-Ross, P. L. (1997). Predictors of misclassification of Hispanic ethnicity in a population-based cancer registry. *Annals of Epidemiology, 7,* 3, 200–206.

Talavera, G. A. et al. (2000). *Prostate cancer screening among U.S. Latinos: A national survey.* Unpublished manuscript.

Trapido, E. J., Chen, F., Davis, K., Lewis, N., & MacKinnon, J. A. (1994). Cancer among Hispanic males in South Florida: Nine years of incidence data. *Archives of Internal Medicine, 154,* 2, 177–185.

Trapido, E. J., Chen, F., Davis, K., Lewis, N., MacKinnon, J. A., & Strait, P. M. (1994). Cancer in South Florida Hispanic women: A 9-year assessment. *Archives of Internal Medicine, 154,* 10, 1083–1088.

Trapido, E. J., McCoy, C. B., Stein, N. S., Engel, S., McCoy, H. V., & Olejniczak, S. (1990). The epidemiology of cancer among Hispanic women. The experience in Florida. *Cancer, 66,* 11, 2435–2441.

Trapido, E. J., Valdez, R. B., Obeso, J. L., Strickman-Stein, N., Rotger, A., & Pérez-Stable, E. J. (1995). Epidemiology of cancer among Hispanics in the United States. *Journal of the National Cancer Institute Monographs, 18,* 17–28.

University of Michigan. (1999). *Communities of color and genetics policy project: Focus groups phase report.* Retrieved October 24, 1999: http://www.sph.umich.edu/genpolicy/Focus-Group-Report.htm#Latino Focus Groups

Vernon, S. W., Vogel, V. G., Halabi, S., Jackson, G. L., Lundy, R. O., & Peters, G. N. (1992). Breast cancer screening behaviors and attitudes in three racial/ethnic groups. *Cancer, 69,* 1, 165–174.

Ward, B., Bertera, E. M., & Hoge, P. (1997). Developing and evaluating a Spanish TEL–MED message on breast cancer. *Journal of Community Health, 22,* 2, 127–135.

Wolfgang, P. E., Semeiks, P. A., & Burnett, W. S. (1991). Cancer incidence in New York City Hispanics, 1982 to 1985. *Ethnicity and Disease, 1,* 3, 263–272.

Yancey, A. K., & Walden, L. (1994). Stimulating cancer screening among Latinas and African-American women. A community case study. *Journal of Cancer Education, 9,* 1, 46–52.

Zapka, J. G., Harris, D. R., Hosmer, D., Costanza, M. E., Mas, E., & Barth, R. (1993). Effect of a community health center intervention on breast cancer screening among Hispanic American women. *Health Services Research, 28,* 2, 223–235.

Zunzunegui, M. V., King, M. C., Coria, C. F., & Charlet, J. (1986). Male influences on cervical cancer risk. *American Journal of Epidemiology, 123,* 302–307.

CHAPTER NINE

# CARDIOVASCULAR DISEASE

Eliseo Pérez-Stable, Teresa Juarbe, and Gina Moreno-John

Cardiovascular disease, primarily manifested by coronary heart disease (CHD) and cerebrovascular disease (strokes), is the leading cause of death and disability for all ethnic groups in the United States. Development of cardiovascular disease is related to known major risk factors that increase the likelihood of an event (cardiac death, heart attack, or new onset of angina or chest pain) occurring over time. These risk factors have been evaluated in large epidemiological studies in the United States conducted among mostly White men and women (Gordon & Kannel, 1982; Stamler et al., 1999). However, international epidemiological comparisons and the biological mechanisms underlying atherosclerosis leave little doubt about the importance of these risk factors for all ethnic groups.

The major cardiovascular risk factors for adults are age, premature family history of cardiovascular events, diabetes mellitus, sedentary lifestyle, elevated serum low-density lipoprotein (LDL) cholesterol and low serum high-density lipoprotein (HDL) cholesterol, ten or more cigarettes smoked per day, and hypertension. Although aging and genetics cannot be modified, most other risk factors are amenable to behavioral or medical interventions that can substantially modify the outcome. However, there are unknown factors that contribute to cardiovascular disease, as known risk factors account for only about 60 percent of cardiovascular mortality. The contributing role of new or potential risk factors detected in blood are being evaluated and include homocysteine, lipoprotein A, fibrinogen, C-reactive protein, and prior evidence of specific infections (Visser, Bouter, McQuillan, Werner, & Harris, 1999; Eikelboom, Lonn, Genest, Hankey, & Yusuf, 1999; Harjai, 1999). There is increasing evidence that coronary artery disease outcomes are in part mediated by a systemic inflammatory response in addition to the established role for arterial narrowing, plaque rupture, and thrombus formation (Danesh, 1999).

This chapter examines available epidemiological data for the Latino population on mortality rates and morbidity from cardiovascular disease. Prevalence of high or low lipid levels, hypertension, sedentary lifestyle, and obesity is reviewed for Latinos and compared to that of Whites and African Americans where appropriate. The importance that being overweight and lack of physical activity contribute to the prevalence of risk factors is discussed. Elsewhere in this volume, diabetes mellitus (Chapter Ten) and cigarette smoking (Chapter Fifteen) are examined. When available, specific subgroup data are reviewed and compared, and explanations for observed differences proposed. The role that cultural values play in maintaining specific risk factor profiles is discussed and policy recommendations are made where appropriate. Finally, a summary of interventions to reduce cardiovascular disease risk factors in Latinos is described.

## Mortality Rates

Studies comparing cardiovascular mortality rates by ethnicity in the United States have shown an overall lower rate for Latino men and women as compared to the rates of Whites and African Americans. As early as 1962, Ellis (1962) reported that Spanish-surnamed men in San Antonio had a significantly lower mortality rate than did Whites with non-Spanish surnames, and similar results were observed from 1970 mortality data for Texas (Markides & Coreil, 1986). Studies conducted in New Mexico (1969–1975) (Buechley, Key, Morris, Morton, & Morgan, 1979), Los Angeles (Frerichs, Chapman, & Edmond, 1984), and all of California (1985–1991) (Karter et al., 1998; Wild, Laws, Fortmann, Varady, & Byrne, 1995) have also found lower cardiovascular mortality among Latinos when compared to that of Whites and African Americans. In a recent analysis of data from the National Center for Health Statistics, Gillum (1997) found a lower prevalence of sudden cardiac death among Latinos than among African Americans. Furthermore, national data from the Centers for Disease Control and Prevention (CDC) have shown that Latino men and women on average have a 20 to 30 percent lower death rate from cardiovascular disease when compared to that of Whites (United States Department of Health and Human Services, 1998a).

Some authorities continue to question the accuracy of the mortality data generated for Latinos. However, there is no evidence that misclassification of ethnicity, undercounting of deaths, or other potential explanations account for the lower death rates. As a possible explanation the "salmon" hypothesis was proposed, stating that Latinos, especially Mexican Americans, return to their birthplace to die and thus are missed in U.S. statistics. Alternatively, others have proposed that migrants in general are healthier than their nonmigrant counterparts and this may explain the lower mortality observed among Latinos. Analysis of the National Longitudinal Mortality Study found no support for either the salmon hypothesis or the healthy migrant hypothesis to explain the pattern of overall lower mortality among Latinos (Abraído-Lanza, Dohrenwend, Ng-Mak, & Turner, 1999).

In the 1970s, 1980s, and 1990s, the United States experienced an unprecedented decline in cardiovascular mortality. Although the decrease in stroke mortality accounts for a large proportion of this, coronary heart disease death rates have also decreased substantially. Analyses from Texas from 1970 to 1980 raised concerns that the decline in mortality from CHD was lower for Latinos than for Whites and African Americans of both sexes (Kautz, Bradshaw, & Fonner, 1981; Stern & Gaskill, 1978; Stern et al.,1987). Two recent analyses of CHD mortality from California used death data tapes and classifications from the World Health Organization's (1991) *International Classification of Diseases* to compare CHD mortality by ethnicity between 1985 and 1991. Latino men and women aged twenty-five to eighty-four years had 41 percent and 30 percent lower CHD mortality rates, respectively, when compared to those of White men and women (Wild, Laws, Fortmann, Varady, & Byrne, 1995).

Comparison of 1985 to 1991 showed that Latino men tended to have a less steep annual decline in CHD mortality compared to that of White men ($-2.8$ percent versus $-3.5$ percent), but the rates of decline for men and women for the three ethnic groups were not statistically significantly different within gender (Karter et al.,1998). There is evidence that the overall decline in CHD mortality has flattened considerably in the 1990s (Joint National Committee . . . , 1997), which raises concern that the Latino advantage in cardiovascular disease mortality is also narrowing.

Overall mortality from stroke has declined by more than 40 percent since 1970, but the rate of decline has also flattened considerably. A comparison of stroke mortality data from NCHS for 1989 to 1991 pooled three years of deaths (total $N = 3,655$) from forty-four to forty-seven states; New York was not included due to incomplete assessment of Latino ethnicity (Gillum, 1995). Results indicate that Latino men and women have lower age-adjusted death rates when compared to those of Whites and African Americans. Stroke mortality rates are similar between Latinos and Whites in persons younger than sixty-five years of age, but strokes are relatively uncommon in this age group (Gillum, 1995). Rates are substantially lower for Latinos compared to Whites after age sixty-five years. Latino men have higher rates from age sixty-five to eighty-four years, but Latino women exceed men in age-adjusted rates after age eighty-five years (Gillum, 1995). Analyses from the CDC for 1997 showed that among Latinos there were fifty-five to 100 excess deaths from stroke in persons thirty-five to sixty-four years of age, but the opposite occurred in older groups with nearly 1,400 fewer deaths than expected in persons eighty-five years of age (Centers for Disease Control and Prevention, 2000). Analysis of California data showed that among Latinos compared to Whites age-adjusted stroke mortality rates were 16 percent lower in men and 25 percent lower in women twenty-five to eighty-four years (Wild, Laws, Fortmann, Varady, & Byrne, 1995). Comparison of mortality data for

1985 and 1991 showed a decline in stroke death for Latino men and women ($-1.8$ percent and $-2.4$ percent, respectively) that was steeper than that for Whites and African Americans, although these differences did not reach statistical significance (Karter et al., 1998).

Gender differences may also exist in acute myocardial infarction (AMI) mortality among White, Latina, and African American women. In a retrospective analysis of AMI mortality by race and gender in a County Hospital in Southern California (1966–1980), Norris, deGuzman, Sobel, Brooks, and Haywood (1993) found a higher mortality rate for White (16.9 percent) than for African American (13.8 percent) and Latina women (7 percent). On the other hand, data from the Corpus Christi Heart Project on AMI indicated that case fatality rate twenty-eight days after hospitalization was higher in Mexican American men (1.80 percent) and women (1.49 percent) when compared to that of their White counterparts (Goff, Ramsey, Labarthe, & Nichaman, 1994).

## Latino Subgroup Comparisons

National mortality comparisons for different Latino national groups are limited. Rosenwaike (1987) compared national mortality rates for persons born in Cuba, Mexico, and Puerto Rico who were residing in the United States between 1979 and 1981 to those for all Whites and African Americans. Age-adjusted death rates for diseases of the heart were 15 to 30 percent lower for the aforementioned Latino men compared to the rates for White men, with even greater differentials compared to those for African American men. Women born in Puerto Rico had a 9 percent higher death rate than that for White women, but rates for all three Latina groups were lower than that for African American women. However, women born in Cuba and Mexico had death rates from heart disease that were 15 to 25 percent lower than for White women. Age-adjusted death rates from strokes were lower for men and women born in Cuba, Mexico, and Puerto Rico when compared to those for Whites and African Americans born in the United States (Rosenwaike, 1987).

Data comparing age-adjusted mortality rates among Latino subgroups, Whites, and African Americans were reported by the NCHS (Maurer, Rosenberg, & Keemer, 1990). This report described mortality of Latinos in a fifteen-state reporting area during the three-year period of 1979–1981, thus allowing use of 1980 U.S. Census data for estimating population denominators. Overall, Latinos of the three major subgroups in the U.S. have a lower death rate from heart disease and strokes when compared to that of Whites or African Americans. Compared to Whites, mortality from diseases of the heart was 25 percent lower among Mexican Americans, 12 percent lower among Puerto Ricans, 40 percent lower among Cubans, and 30 percent higher among African Americans. These differences were consistent for each ethnic or sex group except for Puerto Rican women, who had a mortality rate similar to that of White women. Death rates from stroke were also substantially lower among Latinos when compared to that of Whites: 10 percent lower for Mexican Americans, 31 percent lower for Puerto Ricans, and 49 percent lower for Cubans in the United States. This contrasts with a 76 percent higher stroke death rate for African Americans.

Regional studies have also compared cardiovascular mortality by Latino subgroup. Mortality rates of Mexican Americans and Puerto Ricans living in the Chicago area and who were between fifteen and seventy-four years of age were compared to that of Whites (Shai & Rosenwaike, 1987). Compared to White men, Mexican American men had a 67 percent lower death rate for heart disease and a 79 percent lower death rate for stroke. Similarly, Mexican American women had lower mortality from heart disease (42 percent) and for stroke (24 percent) when compared to White women. Adults born in Puerto Rico-born adults had similar mortality from heart disease as Whites, but Puerto Rican women had a 78 percent increase in stroke mortality whereas Puerto Rican men had a 10 percent decrease in stroke deaths compared to Whites (Shai & Rosenwaike, 1987). In an analysis of the influence of birthplace on stroke and coronary heart disease mortality (1988–1992) in New York City, Fan, Madhavan, and Alderman (1997) found that Latinos had a higher mortality rate from stroke and a lower CHD mortality rate when compared to those of Whites and African Americans. Presumably, a majority of the Latinos analyzed in this study were of Puerto Rican origin.

Prospective national data on specific mortality rates from CHD or stroke for U.S.-born and foreign-born Latinos are lacking in the literature. A recent analysis from the Third National Health and Nutrition Examination Survey (NHANES III, 1988–1994) compared risk factor profile, socioeconomic status, acculturation markers, and an estimated ten-year incident CHD mortality for Mexican Americans (Sundquist & Winkleby, 1999). Results indicated that, when data were adjusted for age and education, Mexican-born men had lower estimated incident CHD mortality when compared to U.S.-born, Spanish- or English-speaking Mexican Americans. U.S.-born, Spanish-speaking, Mexican American men had the highest estimated incident CHD mortality rate. Among women, there were significant differences in the estimated incident CHD mortality between U.S.-born, Spanish-speaking but not English-speaking Mexican Americans and those born in Mexico (Sundquist & Winkleby, 1999). Further comparisons to Whites and African Americans would be useful to confirm the above observations and to evaluate possible differences that arise as Latinos adopt more characteristics of the mainstream U.S. culture.

The observation of overall lower mortality seems to be paradoxical in view of the cardiovascular risk factor profile characteristic of Latino populations (Castro, Baezconde-Garbanati, & Beltran, 1985; Markides & Coreil, 1986; Diehl & Stern, 1989). These risk factors include the low HDL cholesterol and high triglyceride levels associated with obesity, a two- to threefold higher prevalence of diabetes mellitus (Stern, Rosenthal, Haffner, Hazuda, & Franco, 1984; Pérez-Stable et al., 1989), and a disadvantaged socioeconomic status of Latinos compared to those of Whites. However, these risk factors of Latinos may be countered by a lower prevalence of smoking (Marcus & Crane, 1985), less hypertension (Franco et al., 1985;

Pappas, Gergen, & Carroll, 1990), and similar total and LDL cholesterol levels (Stern, Rosenthal, Haffner, Hazuda, & Franco, 1984). The best cohort study with a large sample of Latinos is the San Antonio Heart Study. A comparison of cardiovascular risk factors between 3,301 Mexican Americans and 1,877 Whites, ages twenty-five to sixty-five years, showed that cardiovascular risk scores were higher in Mexican Americans of both sexes (Mitchell, Stern, Haffner, Hazuda, & Patterson, 1990). The presence of undetermined protective genetic or lifestyle factors have been proposed as possible explanations for the epidemiological paradox of lower Latino death rates with higher risk factor profiles (Mitchell, Stern, Haffner, Hazuda, & Patterson, 1990).

# Prevalence of Symptomatic Cardiovascular Disease: Morbidity

There are limited data that enable us to derive prevalence estimates of CHD and stroke for Latino populations in the United States. The Hispanic Health and Nutrition Examination Survey (HHANES) conducted between 1982 and 1984 was a cross-sectional survey of Latinos representative of the three major subgroups in the United States. The NHANES III study initiated in 1989 included a large sample of Mexican Americans but not other Latinos. Estimates of symptoms related to cardiovascular disease and self-reported morbidity from CHD and stroke can be derived from these studies. Clinical studies provide data on outcomes and evaluation of persons with established disease.

## Coronary Heart Disease

LaCroix, Haynes, Savage, and Havlik (1989) evaluated the prevalence of Rose Questionnaire angina among a representative sample of Whites and African Americans who participated in the Second Health and Nutrition Examination Survey (NHANES II) and Mexican Americans from Southwestern HHANES. The Rose Questionnaire is a reliable and valid set of questions about the character of chest pain and circumstances in which it occurs that has been used in other epidemiological studies. The aforementioned authors found that age-adjusted prevalence rates of angina for Mexican Americans were 5.4 percent for women and 2.8 percent for men. Comparisons of Mexican American results to those for Whites and African Americans showed similar rates for women (6.3 percent and 6.8 percent, respectively) and a lower rate for men (3.9 percent and 6.2 percent, respectively). Of Mexican American women with angina, 31 percent had two cardiovascular risk factors compared to 47 percent and 39 percent for White and African American women, respectively. These results indicate that Mexican American women are as likely to report angina as are White and African American women even though the Latinas are less likely to have heart disease.

A study of 5,312 men and women with hypertension who entered a union-sponsored treatment program in New York City included 28 percent Latinos who completed a Rose Questionnaire on angina (Madhavan, Cohen, & Alderman, 1995). Results showed that angina was twice as prevalent in women (15 percent) than in men (7 percent), with Latina women showing the highest overall prevalence of angina (20 percent). Over a four-year average follow-up the incidence of AMI was not associated with presence of angina as determined by the Rose Questionnaire in men or women after adjusting for other known risk factors (Madhavan, Cohen, & Alderman, 1995). Latino men were the exception (RR [relative risk] = 3.12; 95 percent CI [confidence interval] = 1.31 − 7.50) for subsequent AMI if the Rose Questionnaire was positive for angina (Madhavan, Cohen, & Alderman, 1995). The Rose Questionnaire appears to lack predictive value of subsequent AMI, especially among women (Madhavan, Cohen, & Alderman, 1995).

In a clinical study where half of the patients were Latinos or African Americans, physicians had a greater tendency to attribute chest pain reported by women to psychiatric and noncardiac causes as compared to men, even in the presence of objective evidence of ischemia (Tobin et al., 1987). Because there are no detectable ethnic differences in reporting of angina by African American or Latino women, these factors should not be considered in the evaluation of chest pain among women.

Based on the HHANES southwestern portion, about 1.8 percent of men and 1 percent of women reported having had a diagnosis of a heart attack (Lecca, Greenstein, & McNeil, 1987). These rates increased markedly after age forty-five years and peaked at about 9.4 percent for men between sixty-five and seventy-four years of age. Available results from the Puerto Rican portion of HHANES show that men reported more heart attacks than women at all age groups. (Muñoz, Lecca, & Goldstein, 1988). Overall rates were approximately 2.5 percent for men and 1.5 percent for women, but peak rates were observed in persons over sixty-five years of age, where about 9 percent of men and women reported having had heart attacks. The use of reliable and valid ethnic identifiers in hospital discharge data and in data from ambulatory care visits will eventually produce more reliable information on the prevalence of heart attacks and strokes among Latino populations.

Clinical studies have reported on outcomes and evaluation of patients with AMI or established CHD. The GUSTO I and III clinical trials and the National Registry on Acute Myocardial Infarction (1994–1996) reported on results in 734 and 6,896 Latinos, respectively (Canto et al., 1998; Cohen et al., 1999). In both studies, Latinos, compared to Whites, were younger and were more likely to be men and to have diabetes (Canto et al., 1998; Cohen et al., 1999). In the GUSTO trials, Latinos began thrombolysis nine minutes later, fewer received angiography (70 percent versus 74 percent) or underwent coronary artery bypass surgery (11 percent versus 13.5 percent) compared to Whites (Canto et al., 1998). In the larger registry study, multivariate analyses showed that Latino ethnicity was not associated with less acute reperfusion therapies (OR [odds ratio] = 0.97;

95 percent CI = 0.86 – 1.09), less angiography (OR = 0.94; 95 percent
CI = 0.82 – 1.08) or revascularization procedures (OR = 0.95; 95 percent CI =
0.82 – 1.16) (Cohen et al., 1999). Although mortality outcomes did not differ at
thirty days, use of angiotensin-converting enzyme inhibitors was higher among
Latinos in both studies, but fewer Latinos received beta-blockers in the registry
study (42 percent versus 46 percent) (Canto et al., 1998; Cohen et al., 1999).

The Stanford Five-City Project (1986–1992) (Oka, Fortmann, & Varady,
1996) established a surveillance system to identify fatal and nonfatal AMI in five
Northern California cities. Of 3,016 participants identified as having definite
AMI, 325 (11 percent) were Mexican Americans. Multivariate analyses showed
that although Latinos were as likely as other participants to undergo angiography
and thrombolytic therapy, they were significantly less likely to have revascularization (OR = 0.45; 95 percent CI = 0.27 – 0.76) (Oka, Fortmann, & Varady,
1996). Although other clinical studies have also found less revascularization procedures in Latinos compared to Whites (Ness & Aronow, 1999), analyses of procedures in hospitalized patients in California also show significant differences by
ethnicity (Carlisle, Leake, & Shapiro, 1995; Rubinstein, Barber, & Jackson, 1994).
Independent of insurance status, Latinos were less likely to receive coronary angiography or revascularization procedures (after investigators adjusted for available confounders; see Carlisle, Leake, & Shapiro, 1995, and Rubinstein et al.,
1994). This differential use of potentially life-saving interventions in Latinos has
not been as well studied as for African Americans, but the current level of evidence indicates that these differences are not due to access or disease severity. Nevertheless, current evidence indicates that Latinos are more likely than others to
delay care after the onset of AMI symptoms (Canto et al., 1998), may receive delayed thrombolytic therapy once hospitalized (Cohen et al., 1999), and are less
likely to receive beta-blocker therapy at discharge (Canto et al., 1998). Socioeconomic issues, including lack of health insurance, have been found to be strong
predictors on delaying access for AMI chest pain (Ell et al., 1995) in Latinos.
Prospective studies are needed to investigate both stroke- and AMI-related mortality and the associated ethnic and gender differences on treatment, behaviors,
and follow-up recommendations.

## Stroke

In the HHANES reports, self-reported strokes among Mexican Americans were
uncommon, with about 0.8 percent of men and 0.7 percent of women having had
a stroke. More women than men reported strokes at ages younger than fifty-four
years and the reverse was true for older age groups. Nearly 4.5 percent of men
and 3.2 percent of women between sixty-five and seventy-four years of age
reported having had a stroke (Lecca, Greenstein, & McNeil, 1987). Among Puerto
Ricans in HHANES, stroke rates were lower but equal for both sexes at about
0.4 percent. Among Puerto Ricans over sixty-five years of age, women were more
likely than men to report having had a stroke (about 3.5 percent versus 2.5 percent, respectively) (Muñoz, Lecca, & Goldstein, 1988).

National data from the NCHS for 1989–1991 compared self-reported cerebrovascular disease by age and ethnicity (Gillum, 1995). Compared to Whites, Latinos had a similar stroke rate per 1,000 persons for those forty-five to sixty-four years of age, but a substantially higher rate for those aged sixty-five years (seventy-three versus fifty-nine) (Gillum, 1995). Unfortunately, the small number of strokes in Latinos results in wide confidence intervals and makes meaningful comparisons to Whites or African Americans difficult. Furthermore, validity of self-reported stroke must be questioned in view of the language barrier and the potential for cultural interpretation of the stroke. Despite this, the observations of higher prevalence and lower mortality presents an opportunity to prevent poor outcomes by a more proactive blood pressure control program.

In an analysis of the Barrow Neurological Institute Stroke Database in Phoenix, Arizona (1990–1996), Frey and colleagues found no significant differences in stroke outcomes among Whites, Latinos, and Native Americans (1998). Nonetheless, Latino patients were more likely to suffer intracerebral hemorrhages, compared to White and Native American patients (48 percent versus 37 percent and 27 percent, respectively) (Frey, Jahnke, & Bulfinch, 1998). In another retrospective analysis of data from Bernalillo County, New Mexico (1993), investigators found that the sex-adjusted incidence of intracerebral hemorrhages was two times higher among Latinos than Whites (RR = 2.10; 95 percent CIs = 1.35 − 3.26) (Bruno, Carter, Qualla, & Nolte, 1996). These observations would support the conclusion that untreated hypertension among Latinos, especially Mexican Americans, may result in a significant increase in the catastrophic consequence of cerebral bleeding.

The Northern Manhattan Stroke Study (1993–1996) is a population-based study designed to determine stroke incidence, risk factors, and outcomes in a multiethnic urban area (Sacco et al., 1998). Latinos, presumably mostly Puerto Ricans and Dominicans, had a twofold increase in stroke prevalence compared to Whites of all age groups older than fifty-five years (Sacco et al., 1998). This was consistent in both men and women, and in fact Latino stroke rates were only about 40 percent less than those for African Americans. The rate of intracerebral hemorrhage was highest among Latinos. In this study, the prevalence of hypertension in patients with stroke was highest among Latinos (79 percent) compared to Whites (63 percent) or African Americans (76 percent) (Sacco, Kargman, & Zamanillo, 1995).

# Lipid Levels

Lipid levels are directly associated with development of CHD. The increment in risk is proportional to the increase in cholesterol, but approximately 36 percent of all U.S. adults aged twenty to seventy-four years are considered to have cholesterol levels in the moderate-risk range (Sempos et al., 1989). A national education campaign to encourage Americans to eat less saturated fats, to have their cholesterol levels checked, and to consult physicians regarding therapy if the level is elevated has been in place for more than two decades. There is compelling evidence that lowering cholesterol prevents deaths from CHD in persons with that disease established. Based on available primary prevention clinical trials, high levels of cholesterol (LDL cholesterol greater than 160 mg/dl) should be treated in men younger than seventy-five years of age and especially if there are additional cardiovascular risk factors. Controversy persists about treatment with medications of elevated serum cholesterol in women or older persons who do not have established CHD or at a minimum another cardiovascular risk factor. Women in primary prevention trials treated with medications or placebo for elevated cholesterol have had very few events, and there is no conclusive evidence that treatment has a mortality benefit. Furthermore, in persons with established CHD the target to lower LDL cholesterol should be set at less than 100 mg/dl, and in general the desirable level is now considered to be less than 130 mg/dl.

## Lipoprotein Fractions

Although total cholesterol is a strong predictor of heart disease morbidity and mortality, lipoprotein subfractions are independently correlated with outcome: LDL cholesterol is the fraction responsible for at least part of the mechanisms by which arterial vessels become diseased with atheroma; on the other hand, HDL cholesterol is protective of arterial vessels and has a strong negative correlation with cardiovascular morbidity and mortality. Women have a biological advantage with regards to cardiovascular disease due to substantially higher HDL cholesterol levels as a result of the estrogen effect.

The independent contribution of serum triglycerides as a risk factor for cardiovascular disease remains controversial. Multivariate analyses from epidemiological studies have shown that when cholesterol levels and other risk factors are evaluated, triglycerides lose their significant influence on cardiovascular mortality. More recent analyses have shown that for an increase of 90 mg/dl of serum triglycerides there is a 14 percent increased risk in men and 32 percent increased risk in women of cardiovascular disease (Harjai, 1999). There is no evidence that isolated treatment of elevated triglycerides decrease risk, and most of the effect seems to be mediated by lowering LDL cholesterol or raising HDL cholesterol. Regardless, a high level of triglycerides in the blood is a marker of obesity and poorly controlled diabetes mellitus, both of which are prevalent among Latinos. Although isolated elevations may not warrant treatment with medications, hypertriglyceridemia can be a sign of other conditions needing intervention.

There is evidence that elevation of lipoprotein(a), or Lp(a), coupled with high concentrations of LDL cholesterol, is an independent risk factor contributing to arteriosclerosis in Whites, African Americans, and (Asian) Indians (Harjai, 1999). However, other studies have found no association between Lp(a) levels and vascular disease. Lp(a) is a cholesterol-carrying plasminogen-like protein that contains apolipoprotein B100 and apolipoprotein A. Levels for Latino populations have not been reported.

# Lipid Profiles Among Latinos

Although total cholesterol levels have tended to be slightly higher among Mexican American men when compared to those of Whites, these differences have not always been statistically or clinically significant (Stern et al., 1981a). The Mexican American cardiovascular risk factor profile has been labeled an "obesity-related" pattern characterized by upper trunk obesity, diabetes, hypertriglyceridemia, and low levels of HDL cholesterol (Stern, Rosenthal, Haffner, Hazuda, & Franco, 1984).

The San Antonio Heart Study is a population-based study of 1288 Mexican Americans and 929 Whites living in three San Antonio neighborhoods: the low-income barrio included only Mexican Americans, and the samples of both ethnic groups were drawn from the middle-income transitional neighborhood and the higher-income suburbs. Mexican American men had an increase in total and LDL cholesterol as affluence increased from the barrio to the suburbs, while their HDL cholesterol did not change. Among Mexican American women, HDL cholesterol increased and triglycerides decreased with increasing affluence, but total and LDL cholesterol did not change. Ethnic comparisons among persons living in the transitional and suburban neighborhoods showed a statistically significant difference only for the higher triglyceride levels of suburban-dwelling Mexican American women. These results led the authors to conclude that cultural factors may exert a stronger influence on cardiovascular risk factors than do purely socioeconomic status (Stern, Rosenthal, Haffner, Hazuda, & Franco, 1984).

Lipid levels from the HHANES showed that the age-adjusted mean serum cholesterol levels for Latino men and women by subgroups were 207 and 207 mg/dl for Mexican Americans, 203 and 209 mg/dl for Puerto Ricans, and 205 and 199 mg/dl for Cuban, respectively (Lecca, Greenstein, & McNeil, 1987; Muñoz, Lecca, & Goldstein, 1988; Carroll et al., 1990). There were no significant sex or Latino subgroup differences in the proportion with elevated total cholesterol levels, and the data compared favorably with data for Whites and African Americans (Carroll et al., 1990). In HHANES, HDL cholesterol levels were consistently lower for Latino men compared to Latina women at all age groups. There were no significant differences in HDL levels among the three Latino subgroups after controlling for sex. Low HDL-cholesterol levels (less than 35 mg/dl) were found in about 10 percent of Mexican Americans, 32 percent of Puerto Ricans, and 12 percent of Cubans. LDL cholesterol levels (calculated for the subsample fasting twelve hours or more) averaged 127 and 129 mg/dl for Mexican American, 145 and 132 mg/dl for Puerto Rican, and 137 and 129 mg/dl for Cuban men and women, respectively. An estimated 17 percent of Mexican Americans, 26 percent of Puerto Ricans, and 21 percent of Cubans had LDL cholesterol levels of 160 mg/dl or more. Poverty status and level of formal education were not significantly associated with total or HDL cholesterol levels among Mexican Americans, but detailed analyses were not possible in Puerto

Ricans and Cubans (Carroll et al., 1990). The Stanford Five-City Project analyzed matched data from 1979 to 1990, comparing cardiovascular risk factors between Latinos and Whites. Although total cholesterol did not differ between the two groups, HDL cholesterol was lower among Latinos (48 versus 50 mg/dl; $p < .03$) (Winkleby, Fortmann, & Rockhill, 1993).

The NHANES III study included representative samples of African Americans, Whites, and Mexican Americans. An analysis has been published comparing cardiovascular risk factors among the three ethnic groups of young adults and of women twenty-five to sixty-four years of age participating in NHANES III. Lipid levels were reported as a single measure of "non-HDL cholesterol," which closely parallels LDL cholesterol and incorporates a contribution of the triglyceride-rich VLDL (very low-density lipoprotein) cholesterol. Mexican American women had a slightly elevated level of non-HDL cholesterol compared to that of Whites (148.2 mg/dl versus 143.1 mg/dl), but this was not significant in the multivariate models after adjusting for age and education (Winkleby, Kraemer, Ahn, & Varady, 1998). There were no significant differences in levels of non-HDL cholesterol among children and young adults (aged six to twenty-four years) of either sex among the three ethnic groups (Winkleby, Robinson, Sundquist, & Kraemer, 1999). However, among Mexican American men twenty-five to thirty-four years of age, non-HDL cholesterol was higher than for White men (150 mg/dl versus 139 mg/dl). The transcultural analysis of cardiovascular risk factors in Mexican Americans participating in NHANES III reported that U.S.-born Spanish-speaking women had significantly higher non-HDL cholesterol compared to White women (after adjustment of data for socioeconomic factors: 154.7 versus 149.0 mg/dl; Sundquist & Winkleby, 1999). These differences were not observed among Mexican Americans who were English-speaking U.S.-born or Mexican-born women. No association with language use or birthplace was found for men (Sundquist & Winkleby, 1999).

## Detection and Treatment of Elevated Cholesterol

Detection, treatment, and control of hypercholesterolemia is a priority of health-promotion campaigns. This emphasis is based on persuasive evidence that screening and treatment of men decreases morbidity and mortality. However, there is no evidence that treatment of elevated cholesterol in women at average risk is of benefit in any ethnic group. Using the National Institutes of Health (NIH) guidelines defining age-related levels of cholesterol that confer a moderate risk for cardiovascular disease in the San Antonio Heart Study, investigators found that only 7 percent of Mexican Americans compared to 24 percent of Whites were aware that their total cholesterol was high (Pugh, Stern, Haffner, Hazuda, & Patterson, 1988). A low proportion of aware subjects in both ethnic groups were being treated and controlled for elevated cholesterol. These results focus attention on the importance of educating the public about health-promotion and disease-prevention interventions as these become available. The observation that Latinos lag behind Whites in awareness is not surprising and emphasizes the need for culturally appropriate information campaigns that include a Spanish-language component.

# Hypertension

Chronic elevation of arterial blood pressure is one of the major risk factors for CHD and is the principal risk factor for the development of strokes. Although the level of systolic and diastolic blood pressure connotes a continuous risk for cardiovascular morbidity and mortality, hypertension is operationally defined at specific levels to facilitate detection and treatment of persons most likely to benefit. Hypertension is defined by the Joint National Committee on Detection, Evaluation, and Treatment of High Blood Pressure as a systolic blood pressure (SBP) of 140 mm Hg or more and a diastolic blood pressure (DBP) of 90 mm Hg or more or a condition that requires taking antihypertensive medication (Joint National Committee . . . , 1997; Burt et al., 1995). Some epidemiological studies have used different definitions that include higher cutoff levels or the presence of either an elevated SBP or DBP to identify hypertension in a population. Stage 1 hypertension is now defined as measurement of SBP greater than or equal to 140 mm Hg or DBP greater than or equal to 90 mm Hg on at least two separate occasions two to four weeks apart under standard conditions (Joint National Committee . . . , 1997). Among Latinos, as in most populations, blood pressure levels increase with age (Burt et al., 1995; Stroup-Benham, Markides, Espino, & Goodwin, 1999).

## Prevalence of Hypertension in Latinos

The prevalence of hypertension in Latinos has now been demonstrated to be no greater than among Whites and age-adjusted rates may actually be somewhat lower (Franco et al., 1985; Pappas, Gergen, & Carroll, 1990; Haffner, Mitchell, Stern, Hazuda, & Patterson, 1990; Stamler, 1991; Rewers, Shetterly, & Hamman, 1996; Juarbe, 1998). Results from the Stanford Five-City Project (Winkleby, Fortmann, & Rockhill, 1993), the HHANES (Pappas, Gergen, & Carroll, 1990) and the NHANES III (Burt et al., 1995) confirm earlier observations that Mexican Americans have a prevalence of hypertension similar to that of Whites (Leonard, Igra, & Felten, 1983). Regarding gender, the prevalence of hypertension for Latino men is higher than for Latino women (Juarbe, 1998). Among Mexican Americans sixty-five years of age and older, the prevalence of hypertension was 62.7 percent in the 1982–1984 HHANES study and 61.4 percent in the 1994 Hispanic EPESE (Established Populations for the Epidemiologic Study of the Elder) investigation. Average population levels of SBP decreased slightly, but the difference is not clinically significant (Stroup-Benham, Markides, Espino, & Goodwin, 1999).

It was reported that the prevalence of hypertension among 1,175 adult Latinos in New Mexico was lower when compared to that of Whites examined in NHANES II. The lower prevalence was consistent for men and women of all age groups and was present despite the observation of a much greater prevalence of obesity among Latinos. In the San Luis Valley Diabetes Study in Colorado, Burchfiel and colleagues (1990) found that Latinos and Whites had similar levels of SBP and DBP when the diagnosis of diabetes or impaired glucose tolerance was controlled. In addition, the prevalence of hypertension did not differ significantly between nondiabetic Latinos and Whites in the San Luis Valley Study (Rewers, Shetterly, & Hamman, 1996; Shetterly, Rewers, Hamman, & Marshall, 1994).

The San Antonio Heart Study reported the investigators' results on prevalence, detection, and control of hypertension among 1,288 Mexican Americans and 929 Whites (Franco et al., 1985). They defined hypertension as either a DBP greater than or equal to 95 mm Hg or the condition of those currently taking antihypertensive medications. The overall age-adjusted prevalence rates of hypertension for Mexican Americans were 10 percent for men and 7.8 percent for women. These were similar to rates for Whites (9.8 percent for men and 9.7 percent for women), but when adjusted for obesity differences Mexican Americans had a lower prevalence of hypertension (Haffner, 1996).

Combining the data from both recruitment phases of the San Antonio Heart Study, Haffner, Mitchell, Stern, Hazuda, and Patterson (1990) compared the prevalence of hypertension in 3,297 Mexican Americans and 1,873 Whites, twenty-five to sixty-five years of age. The investigators used four different definitions of hypertension and found that by all of them the crude prevalence of hypertension in Mexican Americans was similar to or lower than in Whites in both sexes. Defining hypertension as SBP greater than or equal to 140 mm Hg or DBP greater than or equal to 90 mm Hg or the condition of those currently taking antihypertensive medications, prevalence was 17.8 percent for men and 14.6 percent for women among Mexican Americans and 17.5 percent for men and 15.9 percent for women among Whites. After adjustment for age, body mass index (BMI), and prevalence of diabetes, the data showed that Mexican Americans had a statistically lower prevalence of hypertension in both sexes with odds ratio ranging from 0.66 to 0.71 depending on the definition (Haffner, Mitchell, Stern, Hazuda, & Patterson, 1990).

Data from Starr County, Texas, one of several counties on the Mexican border that is overwhelmingly Mexican American, indicate that some subgroups of Mexican Americans may have substantially higher rates of hypertension. Using similar sampling and measurement methodology, Hanis (1996) reported rates of hypertension among men and women eighteen to seventy-four years old that were substantially higher than those found by others. For example, in Starr County the prevalence of hypertension in persons fifty-five to sixty-five years of age was 31.6 percent in men and 21.9 percent in women compared to 17.4 percent and 22.6 percent, respectively, in NHANES III Mexican Americans. These data imply that there may be some heterogeneity of hypertension frequency among Latinos of similar national origin but living under different social conditions (Hanis, 1996).

## HHANES and NHANES III Results

The HHANES is the only study that compares samples from three major Latino subgroups and the results on hypertension prevalence provide convincing evidence that their rates are lower than for Whites (Pappas, Gergen, & Carroll, 1990). Defining hypertension as a DBP greater than or equal to 90 mm Hg, SBP greater than or equal to 140 mm Hg, or the condition of those currently taking antihypertensive medications, age-adjusted hypertension prevalence estimates did not exceed 23 percent for any of the Latino subgroups in either sex. Mexican American men had a rate of 22.9 percent, Puerto Rican men had a rate of 19.7 percent, and Cuban men had a prevalence of 20.5 percent. Among Latino women, rates were lower than those of Latino men, with Mexican American women at 19.7 percent, Puerto Rican women at 18 percent, and Cuban women at 13.8 percent (Pappas, Gergen, & Carroll, 1990). Although a White and African American comparison group was not included in HHANES, these estimates are lower than those reported in NHANES II for Whites (32.6 percent for men and 25.3 percent for women) and for Blacks (37.9 percent for men and 38.6 percent for women) (Pappas, Gergen, & Carroll, 1990). However, Geronimus, Neidert, and Bound (1990) also used the HHANES and NHANES II data and concluded that HHANES may not be a reliable source of information on hypertension among Mexican American women. Comparisons to the small sample of Mexican American women included in NHANES II showed discrepant rates, and these authors questioned specific methods in HHANES. Despite these concerns, most of the published studies indicate that Latinos have a rate of hypertension that is not higher than that of Whites.

NHANES III, conducted from 1988 to 1991, surveyed Mexican Americans aged eighteen to seventy-four years old in the United States. Overall age-adjusted prevalence of hypertension among Mexican Americans was 22.6 percent, which is similar to the HHANES survey of 21.1 percent. This prevalence rate is similar to the NHANES III rate for Whites at 23.3 percent and lower than the prevalence rate among African Americans at 30.2 percent (Burt et al., 1995). Rates of hypertension did not differ substantially by sex among Mexican Americans with the age-adjusted rates of 23.2 percent for men and 21.6 percent for women. This translates into an estimated Mexican American population with hypertension of 604,000 men and 539,000 women. The overall mean SBP and DBP for Mexican Americans in NHANES III was 124/73 mm Hg for all adults (men = 127/76 mm Hg; women = 121/70 mm Hg), and this did not differ from that of Whites (Burt et al., 1995).

Analyses of the NHANES III data for women twenty-five to sixty-four years of age showed that comparison of the three ethnic groups revealed significant differences in SBP (Winkleby, Kraemer, Ahn, & Varady, 1998). After adjusting for education, SBP was significantly higher for Mexican American and African American women compared to that of Whites. Mexican American women had SBP levels intermediate between those of African American and Whites, as was evident in a steeper increase in SBP of the Latinas with increasing age (Winkleby, Kraemer, Ahn, & Varady, 1998). However, in the analysis of younger adults (eighteen to twenty-four years of age) there were no significant differences in adjusted SBP between Mexican Americans and Whites of either sex (Winkleby, Robinson, Sundquist, & Kraemer, 1999). In the NHANES III Mexican American sample, being born in the United States and speaking Spanish was associated with a significantly higher adjusted SBP for both women and men when compared to that of Whites. This difference was not observed for U.S.-born, English-speaking and Mexican-born participants who had SBP levels similar to or lower than those of their White counterparts (Sundquist & Winkleby, 1999).

## Hypertension Awareness, Treatment, and Control

Results from HHANES on awareness, treatment, and control of hypertension are not any better than those reported by Franco and colleagues (1985) in San Antonio. The proportion of controlled hypertension in HHANES Latinos was 34 percent of Mexican Americans, 29 percent of Puerto Ricans, and 27.8 percent of Cubans (Pappas, Gergen, & Carroll, 1990). These rates fell short of the goal set by the U.S. Public Health Service, namely, having 50 percent of all Latinos attain controlled hypertension by the year 2000. Specifically, the proportion of aware, treated, and controlled Latinos was highest for Mexican American and Puerto Rican women (43.6 percent and 41.6 percent, respectively), but less than 30 percent of Latino men and Cuban American women were aware of and had their hypertension controlled (Pappas, Gergen, & Carroll, 1990). Rates of awareness, treatment, and control were consistently lower in Latino men compared to Latino women in the HHANES survey, where less than 10 percent of Latino men had their hypertension controlled (Crespo, Loria, & Burt, 1996).

According to data from NHANES III, 54 percent of Mexican Americans were aware of their hypertension, 35 percent were being treated, and 14 percent were controlled compared to Whites, where 70 percent were aware, 54 percent treated, and 24 percent controlled (Burt et al., 1995). Mexican Americans had lower levels of treated and controlled hypertension compared with those of Whites and African Americans after adjustments for age, gender, and obesity (Centers for Disease Control and Prevention, 1995).

Similar trends were seen in other studies. In the San Antonio Heart Study, Mexican American men were found to be less likely to be treated than Whites (79.1 percent versus 92.2 percent), although ethnicity did not affect the percentage in treatment among women (Haffner, 1996). Remarkably, the Laredo Project

(Stern et al., 1981b) in Texas nearly twenty years ago found that, compared to Whites of the same socioeconomic level, fewer Mexican Americans were aware of their hypertension, fewer were under treatment, and the degree of hypertension control was inferior.

One study of Puerto Ricans in the South Bronx, New York, showed that only 50 percent of persons with hypertension were aware of it. Of those aware of their hypertension, 57.5 percent were taking medication and 22.5 percent attained control (Barrios et al., 1987; Sica & Cangiano, 1999).

Knowledge and behaviors related to the prevention and treatment of coronary heart disease have also been evaluated by the San Antonio Heart Study (Hazuda, Stern, Gaskill, Haffner, & Gardner, 1983). Comparisons of samples from three distinct neighborhoods found that Whites were significantly more informed than Mexican Americans about prevention of heart attacks even when comparisons were limited to within the transitional and suburban neighborhoods. Knowledge items that were significantly different included eating a low-fat diet, not smoking, and exercising, but knowledge that control of high blood pressure was related to prevention of heart attacks was similar in both ethnic groups. Similar to general knowledge, Whites reported engaging in significantly more individual behaviors to prevent heart attacks than did Mexican Americans. For both Whites and Mexican Americans, knowledge about behavior to prevent heart attacks is directly correlated to socioeconomic status.

## Nutritional Factors, Acculturation, and Stress

These results on estimates of hypertension prevalence are contrary to what may have been expected, given the higher prevalence of obesity among Latinos. Additional dietary factors that influence the development of hypertension include high intake of sodium chloride and potassium, factors which have been less well studied among Latinos. Kerr, Amante, Decker, and Callen (1982) reported that salt purchases among four predominantly Latino census tracts were 1.5 to two times that of thirty-seven predominantly White census tracts in Houston, but both were lower than that of predominantly African American census tracts. In the Chicago survey only 26 percent of Latinos between twenty and fifty years of age were aware that lowering salt intake would help prevent high blood pressure (Kumanyika et al., 1989). Bauer and Mayne (1997) found that Mexican Americans and Puerto Ricans showed statistically significantly higher rates of sodium use compared with those of African Americans and Whites. There were also differences in potassium and calcium intake rates, but none of the dietary differences explain difference in hypertension prevalence among the three ethnic groups. Although dietary potassium and calcium have been found to have a significant effect on the prevalence of hypertension, there are few published studies evaluating Latinos in the United States. In addition to these nutrients, consumption of an average of more than two ounces per day of alcohol has been associated with hypertension. Among women and persons of lower weight, the effect of alcohol on blood pressure may be observed at a lower threshold. Alcohol use among Latinos varies substantially by sex, and a significant proportion of persons who abstain from alcohol may mask the consequence of binge drinking in Latino men (see Chapter Fourteen; also Caetano, 1983; Pérez-Stable, Marín, & Marín, 1994).

The presence of a significant African admixture in many Cubans and Puerto Ricans does not seem to confer the greater likelihood of elevated blood pressure seen in African Americans. Possible explanations for these observations include differences in micronutrient content of the diet, genetic differences, and qualitative differences in environmental stress. The association of darker skin color with higher blood pressures among African Americans with fewer years of formal education implies a societal component of discrimination that may promote manifestation of hypertension (Klag, Whelton, Coresh, Grim, & Kuller, 1991). Data from the Puerto Rico Heart Study have reported similar findings. Puerto Rican men with darker skin color had higher SBP after investigators controlled for differences in socioeconomic status (Costas, García-Palmieri, Sorlie, & Hertzmark, 1981). Subsequently, the same group of investigators found that dark-skinned men had approximately twice the prevalence of left ventricular hypertrophy (a result of hypertension) than did lighter-skinned men (Sorlie, García-Palmieri, & Costas, 1988). The significance of these findings is in need of further study.

The stress associated with acculturation to the mainstream English-language culture may promote blood pressure elevation. Using the HHANES data, Espino and Maldonado (1990) found that among Mexican Americans between fifty-five and seventy-four years of age, acculturation and age were stronger predictors of hypertension than was poverty status. Analyses of the San Antonio Heart Study showed that poor blood pressure control was significantly associated with low sociocultural status and low levels of assimilation among Mexican Americans (Hazuda, 1996). Among Mexican American women, studies show that the prevalence of hypertension decreases with higher socioeconomic status (Juarbe, 1998). One hypothesis is that modernization and acculturation have a harmful effect on health until a particular threshold is reached whereupon assimilation becomes protective (Franco et al., 1985). The possible contribution of acculturation-derived stress to the presence of hypertension in Latinos is in need of further study (Martinez-Maldonado, 1995). The transcultural analysis of the NHANES III data showing association of elevated SBP in Mexican Americans who were born in the United States but preferred to respond to the questionnaire in Spanish is intriguing. Perhaps the burden of sustaining a bicultural identity represents an additional factor to be considered in the acculturation process. The role of stress in development of hypertension has been much debated in the literature but has been hypothesized to contribute to the greater prevalence of hypertension among African Americans (Marmot, 1985). Although intuitively the role of stress is recognized by all, operationally stress is difficult to ascertain. Regardless, stress does not appear to have the same effect on Latinos in the United States or is manifested differently in African Americans. The fact that Latinos are of a less privileged socioeconomic status, endure language barriers, and to a great extent are subject to overt pressures to assimilate to the mainstream culture has not resulted in a higher prevalence of hypertension among Latinos than among Whites.

## Treatment and Control of Hypertension

Untreated mild hypertension (DBP between 90 and 104 mm Hg) progresses to more severe levels in approximately 12 percent of untreated adults (Joint National Committee . . . , 1988). In New York City, of 100 patients presenting in hypertensive crisis, 39 percent were Latinos and 26 percent of the group spoke no English (Bennett & Shea, 1988). This severe form of hypertension should be a rare event in the United States, and the relatively high proportion of Latinos indicates that access barriers may be worsening detection and early treatment of hypertension. These data emphasize the importance of adequate access to preventive health care for poor persons of all backgrounds—and with special emphasis on those who speak little or no English.

Treating hypertension reduces the risk of stroke incidence, coronary artery disease, congestive heart failure, and cardiovascular death (Joint National Committee . . . , 1997). Hypertension control can be readily achieved in most persons with simple medication regimens. Mild elevations in DBP or SBP should be initially managed with nonpharmacological methods that address weight loss, alcohol restriction, and modification of intake of dietary micronutrients such as sodium and potassium, especially when the patient has no other cardiovascular risk factors (Joint National Committee . . . , 1997). Structured instruction in relaxation techniques and sustained increases in physical activity have also been found to decrease blood pressure in some populations. In the presence of other major cardiovascular risk factors (cigarette smoking, hyperlipidemia, or diabetes) or evidence for end-organ damage from hypertension (the heart, kidneys, eyes, or brain), pharmacological approaches for control of blood pressure are indicated. Treatment with a recommended single agent is successful in about half of all patients with hypertension. Combinations of small doses of two types of medication and maintenance of nonpharmacological approaches to treatment should be sufficient to control hypertension in the majority of patients. Latinos have not been reported to have differential response to medications, but clinical trials have often included only small samples of Latinos.

Hypertension is a risk factor that is usually "silent" or without any symptoms until there is an event such as a heart attack or stroke. In order to maximize adherence to treatment of hypertension, regimens need to be simple and have as little effect as possible on quality of life. Adherence to nonpharmacological regimens requires high motivation and the ability to initiate major lifestyle behavioral changes. Adherence to medication regimens will be promoted by once-a-day dosing of an affordable agent, anticipating adverse effects and changing the drug dose appropriately, and forging a strong therapeutic alliance between the health care provider and the patient.

# Obesity

Increasing evidence has established the association of adverse outcomes with a higher body-mass index (BMI). For epidemiological studies the prevalence of overweight is usually defined in terms of BMI, or the weight in kilograms divided by the height in meters squared. A large cohort study with over a million White and African American participants found that the association between increased BMI and mortality was confirmed (Calle, Thun, Petrelli, Rodriguez, & Heath, 1999). However, the association of being overweight and mortality was substantially modified by smoking and the presence of disease. Although heavier men and women in all age groups had an increased risk of death, the magnitude of the association was decreased among African Americans and among persons older than seventy-five years of age (Calle, Thun, Petrelli, Rodriguez, & Heath, 1999). There are no similar studies that include Latinos.

These data must be viewed with greater concern when we consider that the epidemic of obesity is uncontrolled in the United States. Based on the 1998 Behavioral Risk Factor Surveillance Survey, 20.8 percent of Latino adults are obese defined by a BMI of greater than 30. Compared to data from 1991, this represents a relative increase of 80 percent and an absolute increase of 9.2 percent, and this is larger than for Whites or African Americans (Mokdad et al., 1999). The disease burden represented by obesity is striking. In the NHANES III analysis, men and women from the three ethnic groups included who had a BMI of greater than 30 were more likely to have gallbladder disease, CHD, hypertension, and diabetes (Must et al., 1999). The likelihood of having two or more health conditions increased with weight status across all ethnic groups (Must et al., 1999).

There is considerably higher prevalence of obesity among Latinos than among Whites (Diehl & Stern, 1989; Igra, Stavig, & Leonard, 1979; United States Department of Health and Human Services, 1985; Stern, Gaskill, Hazuda, Gardner, & Haffner, 1983; Centers for Disease Control and Prevention, 1989).

Among HHANES participants, BMI cutoff points for defining overweight and severely overweight were greater than 27.8 and greater than 31.1, respectively, for men, and greater than 27.3 and greater than 32.2, respectively, for women. Results showed that prevalence of overweight among men was 30 percent for Mexican Americans, 29 percent for Cubans, and 25 percent for Puerto Ricans. This compares to a prevalence of overweight of 24 percent in White men and 26 percent in African American men in 1976–1980. Among HHANES women, 39 percent of Mexican Americans, 34 percent of Cubans, and 37 percent of Puerto Ricans were overweight. This compares to an overweight prevalence of 25 percent for White women and 44 percent for African American women.

In addition, 15.6 percent of Mexican American, 7.7 percent of Cuban, and 14.4 percent of Puerto Rican women are severely overweight. African American women had an even greater prevalence of severe overweight at 19 percent (Centers for Disease Control and Prevention, 1989). A population-based survey of cardiovascular disease risk factors in Chicago found that only 10 percent of 391 African Americans and 20 percent of 396 Latinos thought that maintaining ideal body weight would help prevent high blood pressure (Kumanyika et al., 1989).

In the San Antonio Heart Study, Mexican Americans and Whites living in the transitional and suburban neighborhoods were interviewed regarding knowledge, attitudes, and behavior related to obesity and dieting after completing an examination (Stern, Pugh, Gaskill, & Hazuda, 1982). For each of the four sex and neighborhood categories, Mexican Americans were significantly heavier than their White counterparts. Mexican Americans residing in the suburban neighborhood were leaner than those in the transitional neighborhood, but they were still more overweight than Whites living in the suburbs. Knowledge about the health consequences of obesity seemed to have little influence on the prevalence of the condition itself in either ethnic group. However, Mexican American men—but not women—in the transitional neighborhood were more likely to believe than the other three groups that an increase in body weight as one grew older was all right. More important, Mexican American men and women of both neighborhoods were significantly more likely to agree that "Americans" are too concerned about losing weight. This finding indicates that despite the prevailing cultural attitudes about the desirability of leanness, Mexican Americans are skeptical about this societal ideal. This may in part account for the markedly higher prevalence of overweight in Latinos than in their White counterparts and suggests that an important barrier will have to be overcome in developing and implementing dietary interventions for Latino populations.

Other epidemiological studies consistently find higher rates of obesity among Latinos, and women are disproportionately affected. In the NHANES III analyses of children and young adults, BMI was not significantly different in males among the three ethnic groups. Among females, there was a consistent difference, with Mexican American and African American girls and young women having significantly higher BMI than Whites after adjusting for other factors (Winkleby, Robinson, Sundquist, & Kraemer, 1999). The differences became more evident among women twenty-five to thirty-four years of age. In the Stanford-Five-City Project the average BMI for Latinos was 27.5 compared to 25.6 for a White matched sample ($p < .001$) (Winkleby, Fortmann, & Rockhill, 1993). In NHANES III Mexican American women had a significantly higher adjusted BMI than White women (28.6 versus 26.3), although somewhat lower than was observed for African American women (29.7) (Winkleby, Kraemer, Ahn, & Varady, 1998). These differences were sustained with increasing education even though the average BMI decreased slightly for each group. For example, among women with more than high school education, Mexican Americans' average BMI was 27.5 compared to 25.4 for Whites and 28.3 for African Americans (Winkleby, Kraemer, Ahn, &

Varady, 1998). Finally, the NHANES transcultural analysis showed again that U.S.-born, Spanish-speaking women had significantly higher average BMI compared to that of their U.S.-born, English-speaking, Mexican-born, and White counterparts (Sundquist & Winkleby, 1999). Mexican American men born in the United States had higher average BMI regardless of their language preference when compared to Mexican born or White study participants (Sundquist & Winkleby, 1999).

Comparisons of dietary nutrients between Whites and Mexican Americans were also conducted in the San Antonio Heart Study from 1979 to 1982 (Haffner, Knapp, Hazuda, Stern, & Young, 1985). Based on a twenty-four-hour dietary recall, Mexican Americans had a greater proportion of total calories from carbohydrates compared to Whites for both men (42.4 percent versus 39.2 percent) and women (43.7 percent versus 41.5 percent). However, Mexican American men ate more saturated fat and less polyunsaturated fatty acids than did White men. Using a saturated fat and cholesterol avoidance scale, the San Antonio group of investigators found that independent of socioeconomic status Mexican Americans were less likely than Whites to recognize and avoid whole milk, visible fat on meats, and eggs as sources of fat in their diet (Knapp, Hazuda, Haffner, Young, & Stern, 1988). The Stanford Five-City Project found that even though Latinos had higher BMI than Whites, the percentage of calories from fat (35.1 percent versus 37.6 percent) and from saturated fat (12.3 percent versus 13.6 percent) was significantly lower than for Whites (Winkleby, Fortmann, & Rockhill, 1993). In the NHANES III report of children and young adults aged six to twenty-four years, Mexican American females but not males were more likely to derive energy from fat than were Whites (Winkleby, Robinson, Sundquist, & Kraemer, 1999). This difference was not observed in young adults aged twenty-five to thirty-four years (Winkleby, Robinson, Sundquist, & Kraemer, 1999). Simple and practical information on the nutritional changes needed to lower the intake of calories from saturated fat and cholesterol in Latino populations should begin in all health-promotion and disease-prevention community activities.

## Physical Activity

Absence of leisure-time physical activity is an independent risk factor for adverse cardiovascular outcomes. Based on self-reported behavior from regional and national surveys, Latinos may be less likely to participate in leisure-time physical activity. In San Francisco, this was observed among women but not among men after investigators adjusted data for confounding factors (Pérez-Stable, Marín, & Marín, 1994). In the Stanford Five-City Project, there was no difference between Latinos and Whites in physical activity measured as kilocalories per kilogram per day (Winkleby, Fortmann, & Rockhill, 1993). NHANES III data indicate that Mexican American women had the highest rate of absence of leisure-time physical activity compared to that of Whites and African Americans (43.5 percent versus

20.5 percent and 39.7 percent, respectively) (Winkleby, Kraemer, Ahn, & Varady, 1998). There were independent effects of ethnicity, socioeconomic status, and age on the lack of leisure-time activity. These data are consistent with previous studies that Latina women are less active that Whites, although "leisure time" may be an inappropriate measure for Latinas (Juarbe, 1998). For example, vigorous physical activity during work may be discounted and not properly adjusted for with socioeconomic variables.

A report from the National Health Interview Survey found that physicians only counsel about a third of adults about the benefits of physical activity (Wee, McCarthy, Davis, & Phillips, 1999). Persons with diabetes, those with cardiovascular disease, those older than age forty years, those with more education, and those who have a BMI of greater than 25 were more likely to be counseled. Younger adults are the least likely to be counseled. There were no differences in physician counseling practices across ethnic groups (8 percent of the respondents were Latinos) (Wee, McCarthy, Davis, & Phillips, 1999).

## Interventions to Lower Cardiovascular Risks Among Latinos

During the 1990s, social and behavioral scientists have argued that effective interventions to improve health behaviors must be tailored to age, gender, and sociocultural conditions. Several interventions have been developed to lower cardiovascular risk factors in Latinos. Individual, family, and community interventions have emerged in an effort to develop culturally sensitive approaches to promote behavioral changes, in particular for smoking, physical activity, and weight management. Clinicians, community health workers, family members, peers, support groups, and significant others have been used as an avenue for interventions to reduce cardiovascular disease risk factors.

There are few organized programs with strict evaluation components to lower cardiovascular risks that specifically target Latino populations in the United States. The Stanford Heart Disease Prevention Program has conducted community interventions in medium-size urban areas with a substantial proportion of Latinos (Farquhar et al., 1990). In 1994, the National Heart, Lung, and Blood Institute developed a guide entitled *Salud Para Su Corazón*—Bringing Heart Health to Latinos (United States Department of Health and Human Services, 1998a). Preparation of this guide involved health educators, community and business leaders, media experts, and many other representatives of the Latino community, who developed recommendations for programs to reduce cardiovascular disease risk factors. Focus-group analyses were primarily used to develop a complex and effective community intervention for the promotion of heart health and the prevention of cardiovascular disease (Moreno et al., 1997). Information obtained from these analyses was used to develop and implement a program that included culturally and linguistically relevant written community and family education materials, music, recipe books, contests, personal guides to heart health, audiotapes, and videotapes. A comprehensive conceptual framework was developed for this multilevel community intervention program, which focuses on behavioral changes as outcomes. A pre- and posttest program evaluation was designed and used to measure the impact of the program. The program was effective as an information source and in increasing awareness of cardiovascular disease risk factors as well as the importance of preventive behaviors (United States Department of Health and Human Services, 1998b). Differences in the sources of information were found between men and women and between the young and the elderly, indicating that a variety of strategies are needed to reach all groups in a community.

A multidisciplinary research team in San Diego developed a community-based intervention called Project Salsa to alter nutritional habits among low-income Mexican Americans (Elder et al., 1998). This program was successful at increasing cardiovascular disease knowledge and screening behaviors. A salient outcome of this program was the ability to institutionalize the screening of risk factors and school health education in the community. Community coalitions and organizations were found to be effective in implementing and preserving educational programs.

Nader and colleagues (1989) conducted a family-based intervention to reduce cardiovascular risk factors among healthy Mexican Americans and Whites. Findings from the baseline evaluation showed that in Mexican American families the mother's diet but not the father's was highly correlated with the children's diet regardless of age. In White families, both parents' diets correlated with the diets of younger but not older children (Patterson, Rupp, Sallis, Atkins, & Nader, 1988). Significant correlation of blood pressure was found between Mexican American fathers and their children, compared to father and son and mother and daughter correlations among White families (Patterson, Kaplan, Sallis, & Nader, 1987). Preliminary results after one year showed that families of both ethnic groups receiving the intervention reported improved eating habits on a food frequency index compared to control families (Nader et al., 1989). Although reported changes are modest, this innovative approach to cardiovascular risk reduction may be potentially applicable to all Latinos, with special emphasis on reaching Latino families through schools (Nader et al., 1986; Nader et al., 1989) and persons at highest risk. This project provided critical information related to recruitment issues, decisions to participate (Atkins et al., 1987), and potential predictors for the attendance to and outcomes of community interventions to reduce cardiovascular disease risk factors (Atkins et al., 1990).

The Rio Grande Valley Community Diabetes Education Program was part of a longitudinal study designed to conduct diabetes research with a rural Texas–Mexico border community (Brown & Hanis, 1995). The program consisted of a culturally tailored educational program based on group support and used culturally tailored support groups, educational materials, and research-based videotapes (Brown, Duchin, & Villagomez, 1992). This community program was successful at achieving statistically significant changes in people's understanding of the symptoms of diabetes and its consequences; overall, it focused the community's attention on diabetes-related health matters, especially the need to determine fasting blood sugar levels.

"On the Move!" is a California physical activity initiative for multiethnic community-based approaches (Cassady, Jang, Park-Tanjasiri, & Morrison, 1999) and two Latino community programs were developed as part of this initiative. *La Vida Caminando* (Grassi, Gonzalez, Tello, & He, 1999) was a program based on a rural Latino community in San Joaquín, California. Four communities were included with the aim of increasing moderate physical activity for Latino family members. Walking clubs were developed in each community to involve individuals and families. Overall, the participants were more likely to be younger women (thirty-five to fifty-seven years of age) who spoke mostly Spanish. While this program was successful at increasing physical activity awareness, the results are conflicting. Rather than an increase in total mean hours of physical activity among program participants, there was a statistically significant difference in all four communities in decreased weekly walking activity from baseline to six months. In particular, in one community the mean hours decreased from 12.9 to 5.9 from baseline to six months. There were no changes from six months to a year. The second "On The Move!" project, La Vida Buena's Salsa Aerobics (Evernham-Whitehorse, Manzano, Baezconde-Garbanati, & Hahn, 1999), was a culturally tailored physical activity program for Latina women in Escondido, California. This program trained and collaborated with promoters of health to implement the intervention. A final evaluation of outcomes from this project is not available at this time; however, this program is ongoing and has been successful at using promoters of health in recruiting and enrolling Latino women in a community-wide program.

Other interventions have been developed to reduce cardiovascular risk factors such as overweight and obesity (Foreyt, Ramirez, & Cousins, 1991; Cousins et al., 1992) and physical inactivity (Avila & Hovell, 1994). Overall, these and the community-based projects have shown that for interventions to be effective they must be tailored to gender and particular culture. Young Latina women are more likely than older Latinas to participate in these interventions. Support or self-help groups may have some effectiveness in increasing self-esteem and/or self-efficacy for cardiovascular disease-related behaviors, but due to family and individual Latina characteristics, they are less likely to be as effective as family interventions. In addition, family rather than individual approaches may guarantee long-term outcomes. Peer models are effective with young Latino and Latina populations, but their effectiveness in adult and older groups needs further research.

# Conclusions

The major risk factors for cardiovascular disease can be modified by behavioral lifestyle changes that present a unique challenge for Latino health care. Promotion of smoking prevention and cessation, altering the fat consumption of Latino diets in favor of traditional complex carbohydrates, promotion of increased physical activity, and facilitation of access to health care in order to improve hypertension control are priorities to be met in the control of cardiovascular disease in Latinos.

It is essential to develop educational materials that are culturally appropriate using Latino models and Latino examples. The health-promotion and disease-prevention materials should be written in Spanish first, then translated into English, back-translated into Spanish, and finally the two versions should be reconciled. By first developing educational materials in Spanish, awkward translations from English-language materials are avoided. Materials that are to be used by more than one Latino subgroup need to use universal (or "broadcast") Spanish in order to avoid strictly regional preferences for idiomatic expressions. In addition, specific approaches that are more effective with Latinos may become evident during the development and pretesting process. In general, the less acculturated Latinos are less knowledgeable about risk factors and how to initiate behavioral changes to prevent cardiovascular disease (Vega et al.,1987), and thus they have the most to gain from culturally appropriate interventions. Improvement in risk factor profiles among Latinos will require leadership from the Latino community. Scientists, policy makers, community activists, and health care professionals need to collaborate, and Latinos must have a prominent role in the process.

# References

Abraído-Lanza, A. F., Dohrenwend, B. P., Ng-Mak, D. S., & Turner, J. B. (1999). The Latino mortality paradox: A test of the "salmon bias" and healthy migrant hypothesis. *American Journal of Public Health, 89,* 1543–1548.

Atkins, C. J. et al. (1987). Recruitment issues, health habits, and the decision to participate in a health promotion program. *American Journal of Preventive Medicine, 3,* 2, 87–94.

Atkins, C. J. et al. (1990). Attendance at health promotion programs: Baseline predictors and program outcomes. *Health Education Quarterly, 17,* 4, 417–428.

Avila, P., & Hovell, M. F. (1994). Physical activity training for weight loss in Latinas. *International Journal of Obesity and Related Metabolic Disorders, 18,* 7, 476–481.

Barrios, E. et al. (1987). Hypertension in the Hispanic and Black population in New York City. *Journal of the National Medical Association, 79,* 749–752.

Bauer, U. E., & Mayne, S. T. (1997). Do ethnic differences in dietary cation intake explain ethnic differences in hypertension prevalence? Results from a cross-sectional analysis. *Annals of Epidemiology, 7,* 479–485.

Bennett, N. M., & Shea, S. (1988). Hypertensive emergency: Case criteria, sociodemographic profile, and previous care of 100 cases. *American Journal of Public Health, 78,* 6, 636–640.

Brown, S. A., Duchin, S. P., & Villagomez, E. T. (1992). Diabetes education in a Mexican-American population: Pilot testing of a research-based videotape. *Diabetes Education, 18,* 1, 47–51.

Brown, S. A., & Hanis, C. L. (1995). A community-based, culturally sensitive education and group-support intervention for Mexican Americans with NIDDM: A pilot study of efficacy. *Diabetes Education, 21,* 3, 203–210.

Bruno, A., Carter, S., Qualla, C., & Nolte, K. B. (1996). Incidence of spontaneous intracerebral hemorrhage among Hispanics and non-Hispanic Whites in New Mexico. *Neurology, 47,* 2, 405–408.

Buechley, R. W., Key, C. R., Morris, D. L., Morton, W. E., & Morgan, M. V. (1979). Altitude and ischemic heart disease in tricultural New Mexico: An example of confounding. *American Journal of Epidemiology, 109,* 6, 663–666.

Burchfiel, C. M. et al. (1990). Cardiovascular risk factors and impaired glucose tolerance: The San Luis Valley Diabetes Study. *American Journal of Epidemiology, 131,* 1, 57–70.

Burt, V. et al. (1995). Prevalence of hypertension in the U.S. adult population. *Hypertension, 25,* 305–313.

Caetano, R. (1983). Drinking patterns and alcohol problems among Hispanics in the U.S.: A review. *Drug and Alcohol Dependence, 18,* 1–15.

Calle, E. E., Thun, M. J., Petrelli, J. M., Rodriguez, C., & Heath, C. W. (1999). Body-mass index and mortality in a prospective cohort of U.S. adults. *New England Journal of Medicine, 341,* 1097–1105.

Canto, J. G. et al. (1998). Presenting characteristics, treatment patters, and clinical outcomes of non-Black minorities in the National Registry of Myocardial Infarction 2. *American Journal of Cardiology, 82,* 9, 1013–1018.

Carlisle, D. M. Leake, B. D., & Shapiro, M. F. (1995). Racial and ethnic differences in the use of invasive cardiac procedures among cardiac patients in Los Angeles County, 1986 through 1988. *American Journal of Public Health, 85,* 3, 352–356.

Carroll, M. et al. (1990). Serum lipids and lipoproteins of Hispanics, 1982–1984. *Vital and Health Statistics, 11,* 240, 1–65.

Cassady, D., Jang, V. L., Park-Tanjasiri, S., & Morrison, C. M. (1999). California gets "on the move." *Journal of Health Education, S30,* 2, S6–S12.

Castro, F. G., Baezconde-Garbanati, L., & Beltran, H. (1985). Risk factors for coronary heart disease in Hispanic populations: A review. *Hispanic Journal of Behavioral Sciences, 7,* 2, 153–175.

Centers for Disease Control and Prevention. (1989). Prevalence of overweight for Hispanics: United States, 1982–1984. *MMWR [Morbidity and Mortality Weekly Report], 38,* 838–842.

Centers for Disease Control and Prevention. (1995). Hypertension among Mexican Americans: United States, 1982–1984 and 1988–1991. *MMWR [Morbidity and Mortality Weekly Report], 44,* 34, 635–639.

Centers for Disease Control and Prevention. (2000). Age-specific excess deaths associated with stroke among racial/ethnic minority populations: United States, 1997. *MMWR [Morbidity and Mortality Weekly Report], 49,* 94–97.

Cohen, M. G. et al. (1999). Outcome of Hispanic patients treated with thrombolitic therapy for acute myocardial infarction: Results from the GUSTO I and III trials. Global utilization of streptokinase and TPA for occluded coronary arteries. *Journal of the American College of Cardiology, 34,* 6, 1729–1737.

Costas, R., García-Palmieri, M. R., Sorlie, P., & Hertzmark, E. (1981). Coronary heart disease risk factors in men with light and dark skin in Puerto Rico. *American Journal of Public Health, 71,* 6, 614–619.

Cousins, J. H. et al. (1992). Family versus individually oriented intervention for weight loss in Mexican American women. *Public Health Reports, 107,* 5, 549–555.

Crespo, C. J., Loria, C. M., & Burt, V. L. (1996). Hypertension and other cardiovascular disease risk factors among Mexican Americans, Cuban Americans, and Puerto Ricans from the Hispanic Health and Nutrition Examination Survey. *Public Health Reports, 111,* 7–10.

Danesh, J. (1999). Smoldering arteries?: Low grade inflammation and coronary artery disease. *Journal of the American Medical Association, 282,* 2169–2171.

Diehl, A. K., & Stern, M. P. (1989). Special health problems of Mexican-Americans: Obesity, gallbladder disease, diabetes mellitus, and cardiovascular disease. *Advances in Internal Medicine, 34,* 73–96.

Eikelboom, J. W., Lonn, E., Genest, J., Hankey, G., & Yusuf, S. (1999). Homocyt(e)ine and cardiovascular disease: A critical review of the epidemiologic evidence. *Annals of Internal Medicine, 131,* 363–375.

Elder, J. P. et al. (1998). Project Salsa: Development and institutionalization of a nutritional health promotion project in a Latino community. *American Journal of Health Promotion, 12,* 6, 391–401.

Ell, K. et al. (1995). Differential perceptions, behaviors, and motivations among African Americans, Latinos, and Whites suspected of heart attacks in two hospital populations. *Journal of the Association of Academic Minority Physicians, 6,* 2, 60–69.

Ellis, J. M. (1962). Spanish surname mortality differences in San Antonio, TX. *Journal of Health and Human Behavior, 3,* 125–127.

Espino, D. V., & Maldonado, D. (1990). Hypertension and acculturation in elderly Mexican Americans: Results from 1982–84 Hispanic HANES. *Journal of Gerontology, 45,* 6, M209–M213.

Evernham-Whitehorse, L., Manzano, R., Baezconde-Garbanati, L., & Hahn, G. (1999). Culturally tailoring a physical activity program for Hispanic women: Recruitment successes of La Vida Buena's Salsa Aerobics. *Journal of Health Education, S30,* 2, S18–S24.

Fan, J., Madhavan, S., & Alderman, M. H. (1997). The influence of birthplace on mortality among Hispanic residents of New York City. *Ethnicity and Disease, 7,* 1, 55–64.

Farquhar, J. W. et al. (1990). Effects of communitywide education on cardiovascular disease risk factors: The Stanford Five-City Project. *Journal of the American Medical Association, 264,* 3, 359–365.

Foreyt, J. P., Ramirez, A. G., & Cousins, J. H. (1991). *Cuidando el Corazón:* A weight-reduction intervention for Mexican Americans. *American Journal of Clinical Nutrition, 53,* 1639S–1641S.

Franco, L. J. et al. (1985). Prevalence, detection, and control of hypertension in a biethnic community. *American Journal of Epidemiology, 121,* 5, 684–695.

Frerichs, R. R., Chapman, J. M., & Edmond, F. M. (1984). Mortality due to all causes and to cardiovascular diseases among seven race ethnic populations in Los Angeles County, 1980. *International Journal of Epidemiology, 13,* 291–298.

Frey, J. L., Jahnke, H. K., & Bulfinch, E. W. (1998). Differences in stroke between White, Hispanic, and Native American patients: The Barrow Neurological Institute Stroke Database. *Stroke, 29,* 1, 29–33.

Geronimus, A. T., Neidert, L. J., & Bound, J. (1990). A note on the measurement of hypertension in HHANES. *American Journal of Public Health, 80,* 12, 1437–1442.

Gillum, R. F. (1995). Epidemiology of stroke in Hispanic Americans. *Stroke, 26,* 9, 1707–1712.

Gillum, R. F. (1997). Sudden cardiac death in Hispanic Americans and African Americans. *American Journal of Public Health, 87,* 9, 1461–1466.

Goff, D. C., Ramsey, D. J., Labarthe, D. R., & Nichaman, M. Z. (1994). Greater case-fatality after myocardial infarction among Mexican Americans and women than among non-Hispanic Whites and men. *American Journal of Epidemiology, 139,* 5, 474–483.

Gordon, T., & Kannel, W. B. (1982). Multiple risk functions and predicting coronary heart disease: The concept, accuracy, and application. *American Heart Journal, 102,* 1031–1039.

Grassi, K., Gonzalez, M. G., Tello, P., & He, G. (1999). *La Vida Caminando:* A community-based physical activity program designed by and for rural Latino families. *Journal of Health Education, S30,* 2, S13–S17.

Haffner, S. M. (1996). Hypertension in the San Antonio Heart Study: Clinical and metabolic correlates. *Public Health Reports, 111,* Suppl. 2, 11–14.

Haffner, S. M., Knapp, J. A., Hazuda, H. P., Stern, M. P., & Young, E. A. (1985). Dietary intakes of macronutrients among Mexican Americans and Anglo Americans: The San Antonio heart study. *American Journal of Clinical Nutrition, 42,* 1266–1275.

Haffner, S. M., Mitchell, B. D., Stern, M. P., Hazuda, H. P., & Patterson, J. K. (1990). Decreased prevalence of hypertension in Mexican-Americans. *Hypertension, 16,* 3, 225–232.

Hanis, C. L. (1996). Hypertension among Mexican Americans in Starr County, Texas. *Public Health Reports, 111,* Suppl. 2, 15–17.

Harjai, K. J. (1999). Potential new cardiovascular risk factors: Left ventricular hypertrophy, homocysteine, lipoprotein(a), triglycerides, oxidative stress, and fibrinogen. *Annals of Internal Medicine, 131,* 376–386.

Hazuda, H. P. (1996). Hypertension in the San Antonio Heart Study and the Mexico City Diabetes Study: Sociocultural correlates. *Public Health Reports, 111,* Suppl. 2, 18–21.

Hazuda, J. P., Stern, M. P., Gaskill, S. P., Haffner, S. M., & Gardner, L. I. (1983). Ethnic differences in health knowledge and behaviors related to the prevention and treatment of coronary heart disease: The San Antonio Heart Study. *American Journal of Epidemiology, 117,* 6, 717–728.

Igra, A., Stavig, G. R., & Leonard, A. (1979). *Hypertension and related health problems in California: Results from the 1979 California hypertension survey.* Sacramento: California Department of Health Services.

Joint National Committee . . . (1988). The 1988 Report of the Joint National Committee on Detection, Evaluation and Treatment of High Blood Pressure. *Archives of Internal Medicine, 148,* 1023–1038.

Joint National Committee . . . (1997). The Sixth Report of the Joint National Committee on Prevention, Detection, Evaluation and Treatment of High Blood Pressure. *Archives of Internal Medicine, 157,* 2413–2446.

Juarbe, T. C. (1998). Risk factors for cardiovascular disease in Latina women. *Progress in Cardiovascular Nursing, 13,* 17–27.

Karter, A. J. et al. (1998). Ischemic heart disease and stroke mortality in African American, Hispanic, and non-Hispanic White men and women. *Western Journal of Medicine, 169,* 3, 139–145.

Kautz, J. A., Bradshaw, B. S., & Fonner, E. (1981). Trends in cardiovascular mortality in Spanish surnamed, other White and Black persons in Texas, 1970–75. *Circulation, 64,* 730–735.

Kerr, G. R., Amante, P., Decker, M., & Callen, P. W. (1982). Ethnic patterns of salt purchase in Houston, Texas. *American Journal of Epidemiology, 115,* 6, 906–916.

Klag, M. J., Whelton, P. K., Coresh, J., Grim, C. E., & Kuller, L. H. (1991). The association of skin color with blood pressure in U.S. Blacks with low socioeconomic status. *Journal of the American Medical Association, 265,* 5, 599–602.

Knapp, J. A., Hazuda, H. P., Haffner, S. M., Young, E. A., & Stern, M. P. (1988). A saturated fat/cholesterol avoidance scale: Sex and ethnic differences in a biethnic population. *Journal of the American Dietetic Association, 2,* 172–177.

Kumanyika, S. et al. (1989). Beliefs about high blood pressure prevention in a survey of Blacks and Hispanics. *American Journal of Preventive Medicine, 5,* 1, 21–26.

LaCroix, A. Z., Haynes, S. G., Savage, D. D., & Havlik, R. L. (1989). Rose Questionnaire angina among United States Black, White, and Mexican American women and men: Prevalence and correlates from the Second National and Hispanic Health and Nutrition Examination Surveys. *American Journal of Epidemiology, 129,* 4, 669–686.

Lecca, P. J., Greenstein T. N., & McNeil, J. S. (1987). *A profile of Mexican American health: Data from the Hispanic Health and Nutrition Examination Survey 1982–84.* Arlington, TX: Health Services Research, pp. 1–93.

Leonard, A. R., Igra, A., & Felten, P. G. (1983). California's approach to hypertension control: An overview. *Western Journal of Medicine, 139,* 388–394.

Madhavan, S., Cohen, H., & Alderman, M. H. (1995). Angina pectoris by Rose Questionnaire does not predict cardiovascular disease in treated hypertensive patients. *Journal of Hypertension, 13,* 11, 1307–1212.

Marcus, A. C., & Crane, L. A. (1985). Smoking behavior among U.S. Latinos: An emerging challenge for public health. *American Journal of Public Health, 75,* 169–172.

Markides, K. S., & Coreil, J. (1986). The health of Hispanics in the Southwestern United States: An epidemiologic paradox. *Public Health Reports, 101,* 3, 253–265.

Marmot, M. G. (1985). Psychosocial factors and blood pressure. *Preventive Medicine, 14,* 451–465.

Martinez-Maldonado, M. (1995). Hypertension in Hispanics. Comments on a major disease in a mix of ethnic groups. *American Journal of Hypertension, 8,* 120S–123S.

Maurer, J. D., Rosenberg, H. M., & Keemer, J. B. (1990). Deaths of Hispanic Origin, 15 Reporting States, 1971–1981. NCHS. *Vital & Health Statistics,* Series 20, #18: 1–73.

Mitchell, B. D., Stern, M. P., Haffner, S. M., Hazuda, H. P., & Patterson, J. K. (1990). Risk factors for cardiovascular mortality in Mexican Americans and non-Hispanic Whites. *American Journal of Epidemiology, 131,* 3, 423–433.

Mokdad, A. H. et al. (1999). The spread of the obesity epidemic in the United States, 1991–1998. *Journal of the American Medical Association, 282,* 1519–1522.

Moreno, C. et al. (1997). Heart disease education and prevention program targeting immigrant Latinos: Using focus group responses to develop effective interventions. *Journal of Community Health, 22,* 6, 435–450.

Muñoz, E., Lecca, P. J., & Goldstein, J. D. (1988). *A profile of Puerto Rican health in the United States: Data from the Hispanic Health and Nutrition Examination Survey 1982–84.* New Hyde Park, NY: Long Island Jewish Medical Center; Arlington, TX: Health Services Research, pp. 1–93.

Must, A. et al. (1999). The disease burden associated with overweight and obesity. *Journal of the American Medical Association, 282,* 1523–1529.

Nader, P. R. et al. (1989). A family approach to cardiovascular risk reduction: Results from the San Diego Family Health Project. *Health Education Quarterly, 16,* 2, 229–244.

Nader, P. R. et al. (1986). San Diego Family Health Project: Reaching families through the schools. *Journal of School Health, 56,* 6, 227–231.

Ness, J., & Aronow, W. S. (1999). Prevalence of coronary artery disease, ischemic stroke, peripheral arterial disease, and coronary revascularization in older African Americans, Asians, Hispanics, Whites, men and women. *American Journal of Cardiology, 84,* 9, 932–933.

Norris, S. L., deGuzman, M., Sobel, E., Brooks, S., & Haywood, J. (1993). Risk factors and mortality among Black, Caucasian, and Latina women with acute myocardial infarction. *American Heart Journal, 126,* 6, 1312–1319.

Oka, R. K., Fortmann, S. P., & Varady, A. N. (1996). Differences in treatment of acute myocardial infarction by sex, age, and other factors (the Stanford Five-City Project). *American Journal of Cardiology, 78,* 8, 861–865.

Pappas, G., Gergen, P. J., & Carroll, M. (1990). Hypertension prevalence and the status of awareness, treatment, and control in the Hispanic Health and Nutrition Examination Survey (HHANES), 1982–84. *American Journal of Public Health, 80,* 12, 1431–1436.

Patterson, T. L., Kaplan, R. M., Sallis, J. F., & Nader, P. R. (1987). Aggregation of blood pressure in Anglo-American and Mexican-American families. *Preventive Medicine, 16,* 616–625.

Patterson, T. L., Rupp, J. W., Sallis, J. F., Atkins, C. J., & Nader, P. R. (1988). Aggregation of dietary calories, fats, and sodium in Mexican-American and Anglo families. *American Journal of Preventive Medicine, 4,* 75–82.

Pérez-Stable, E. J., Marín, G., & Marín, B. V. (1994). Behavioral risk factors: A comparison of Latinos and non-Latino Whites in San Francisco. *American Journal of Public Health, 84,* 971–976.

Pérez-Stable, E. J. et al. (1989). Self-reported diabetes in Mexican Americans: HHANES 1982–84. *American Journal of Public Health, 79,* 6, 770–772.

Pugh, J. A., Stern, M. P., Haffner, S. M., Hazuda, H. P., & Patterson, J. (1988). Detection and treatment of hypercholesterolemia in a biethnic community, 1979–1985. *Journal of General Internal Medicine, 3,* 331–336.

Rewers, M., Shetterly, S. M., & Hamman, R. F. (1996). Hypertension among rural Hispanics and non-Hispanic Whites: The San Luis Valley Diabetes Study. *Public Health Reports, 111,* Suppl. 2, 27–29.

Rosenwaike, I. (1987). Mortality differentials among persons born in Cuba, Mexico, and Puerto Rico residing in the United States, 1979–81. *American Journal of Public Health, 77,* 5, 603–606.

Rubinstein, F., Barber, E., & Jackson, J. E. (1994). Use of cardiac procedures among Hispanics in California. *Journal of General Internal Medicine, 9,* Suppl. 2, 107.

Sacco, R. L. et al. (1998). Stroke incidence among White, Black, and Hispanic residents of an urban community: The Northern Manhattan Stroke Study. *American Journal of Epidemiology, 147,* 3, 259–268.

Sacco, R. L., Kargman, D. E., & Zamanillo, M. C. (1995). Race–ethnic differences in stroke risk factors among hospitalized patients with cerebral infarction: The Northern Manhattan Stroke Study. *Neurology, 45,* 659–663.

Samet, J. M., Coultas, D. B., Howard, C. A., Skipper, B. J., & Hanis, C. L. (1988). Diabetes, gallbladder disease, obesity, and hypertension among Hispanics in New Mexico. *American Journal of Epidemiology, 128,* 6, 1302–1311.

Sempos, C. et al. (1989). The prevalence of high blood cholesterol levels among adults in the United States. *Journal of the American Medical Association, 262,* 45–52.

Shai, D., & Rosenwaike, I. (1987). Mortality among Hispanics in metropolitan Chicago: An examination based on vital statistics data. *Journal of Chronic Diseases, 40,* 5, 445–451.

Shetterly, S., Rewers, M., Hamman, R., & Marshall, J. (1994). Patterns and predictors of hypertension incidence among Hispanics and non-Hispanic Whites: The San Luis Valley Diabetes Study. *Journal of Hypertension, 12,* 1095–1102.

Sica, D. A., & Cangiano, J. L. (1999). Hypertension and renal disease in Puerto Ricans. *American Journal of the Medical Sciences, 318,* 369–373.

Sorlie, P. D., García-Palmieri, M. R., & Costas, R., Jr. (1988). Left ventricular hypertrophy among dark- and light-skinned Puerto Rican men: The Puerto Rico Heart Health Program. *American Heart Journal, 116,* 777–783.

Stamler, J. et al. (1999). Low risk-factor profile and long-term cardiovascular and non-cardiovascular mortality and life expectancy. Findings from 5 large cohorts of young adult and middle-aged men and women. *Journal of the American Medical Association, 282,* 2012–2018.

Stamler, R. (1991). Implications of the INTERSALT Study. *Hypertension, 17,* Suppl. 1, 16–20.

Stern, M. P. et al. (1987). Secular decline in death rates due to ischemic heart disease in Mexican American and non-Hispanic Whites in Texas, 1970–1980. *Circulation, 76,* 6, 1245–1250.

Stern, M. P., & Gaskill, S. P. (1978). Secular trends in ischemic heart disease and stroke mortality from 1970–1976 in Spanish-surnamed and other White individuals in Bexar County, Texas. *Circulation, 58,* 3, 537–543.

Stern, M. P. et. al. (1981a). Cardiovascular risk factors in Mexican Americans in Laredo, Texas: I. Prevalence of overweight and distributions of serum lipids. *American Journal of Epidemiology, 113,* 546–555.

Stern, M. P. et al. (1981b). Cardiovascular risk factors in Mexican Americans in Laredo, Texas: II. Prevalence and control of hypertension. *American Journal of Epidemiology, 113,* 556–562.

Stern, M. P., Gaskill, S. P., Hazuda, H. P., Gardner, L. I., & Haffner, S. M. (1983). Does obesity explain excess prevalence of diabetes among Mexican Americans? Results of the San Antonio Heart Study. *Diabetologia, 24,* 272–277.

Stern, M. P., Pugh, J. A., Gaskill, S. P., & Hazuda, H. P. (1982). Knowledge, attitudes, and behavior related to obesity and dieting in Mexican Americans and Anglos: The San Antonio Heart Study. *American Journal of Epidemiology, 115,* 6, 917–928.

Stern, M. P., Rosenthal, M., Haffner, S. M., Hazuda, H. P., & Franco, L. J. (1984). Sex differences in the effects of sociocultural status on diabetes and cardiovascular risk factors in Mexican Americans: The San Antonio Heart Study. *American Journal of Epidemiology, 120,* 6, 834–851.

Stroup-Benham, C. A., Markides, K. S., Espino, D. V., & Goodwin, J. S. (1999). Changes in blood pressure and risk factors for cardiovascular disease among older Mexican-Americans from 1982–1984 to 1993–1994. *Journal of the American Geriatric Society, 47,* 804–810.

Sundquist, J., & Winkleby, M. A. (1999). Cardiovascular risk factors in Mexican American adults: A transcultural analysis of NHANES III, 1988–1994. *American Journal of Public Health, 89,* 5, 723–730.

Tobin, J. N. et. al. (1987). Sex bias in considering coronary bypass surgery. *Annals of Internal Medicine, 107,* 19–25.

United States Department of Health and Human Services. (1985). *Report of the Secretary's Task Force on Black and Minority Health (Vol. 1).* Executive Summary. Washington, D.C.: Author.

United States Department of Health and Human Services. (1998a). *Tobacco use among U.S. racial/ethnic minority groups—African Americans, American Indians and Alaska Natives, Asian Americans and Pacific Islanders, and Hispanics: A report of the Surgeon General.* Atlanta, GA: Centers for Disease Control and Prevention, National Center for Chronic Disease Prevention and Health Promotion, Office on Smoking and Health.

United States Department of Health and Human Services (1998b). *Salud para su corazón— Bringing heart health to Latinos: A guide for building community programs.* Bethesda, MD: Public Health Service, National Institutes of Health, National Heart, Lung, and Blood Institute.

Vega, W. A. et al. (1987). Assessing knowledge of cardiovascular health-related diet and exercise behaviors in Anglo- and Mexican-Americans. *Preventive Medicine, 16,* 696–709.

Visser, M., Bouter, L. M., McQuillan, G. M., Wener, M. H., & Harris, T. B. (1999). Elevated C-reactive protein levels in overweight and obese adults. *Journal of the American Medical Association, 282,* 2131–2135.

Wee, C. C., McCarthy, E. P., Davis, R. B., & Phillips, R. S. (1999). Physician counseling about exercise. *Journal of the American Medical Association, 282,* 1583–1588.

Wild, S. H., Laws, A., Fortmann, S. P., Varady, A. N., & Byrne, C. D. (1995). Mortality from coronary heart disease and stroke for six ethnic groups in California. *Annals of Epidemiology, 5,* 6, 432–439.

Winkleby, M. A., Fortmann, S. P., & Rockhill, B. (1993). Health-related risk factors in a sample of Hispanics and Whites matched on sociodemographic characteristics. *American Journal of Epidemiology, 137,* 1365–1375.

Winkleby, M. A., Kraemer, H. C., Ahn, D. K., & Varady, A. N. (1998). Ethnic and socioeconomic differences in cardiovascular disease risk factors. *Journal of the American Medical Association, 280,* 356–362.

Winkleby, M. A., Robinson, T. N., Sundquist, J., & Kraemer, H. C. (1999). Ethnic variation in cardiovascular disease risk factors among children and young adults: Findings from the Third National Health and Nutrition Examination Survey, 1988–1994. *Journal of the American Medical Association, 281,* 1006–1013.

World Health Organization. (1991). *International classification of diseases, 9th revision (ICD-9).* Geneva: Author.

CHAPTER TEN

# DIABETES

José Alejandro Luchsinger

In 1998, diabetes was one of the most prevalent diseases in the United States, and the proportion of the population with diabetes is rising (Harris, 1998). Diabetes was the seventh cause of death in the United States, accounting for 2.7 percent of total deaths (Centers for Disease Control and Prevention, 1999). It is estimated that approximately 10.5 million people had diabetes in 1998, up from 1.5 million in 1958, when surveys began (Harris, 1998). The cost of general medical care for people with diabetes is $11,000 per capita, compared to $2,600 for people without diabetes (Rubin, Altman, & Mendelson, 1994). Diabetes care accounts for 15 percent of all health care expenses in the United States and for 27 percent of Medicare expenditure (Rubin, Altman, & Mendelson, 1994).

Diabetes is a disease characterized by abnormalities in the metabolism of glucose. There are two types of diabetes: type I and type II (Report of the Expert Committee . . . , 1997). Type I, sometimes referred to as juvenile-onset diabetes or insulin-dependent diabetes, is caused by an absolute deficiency in the pancreatic secretion of insulin; its usual onset is in childhood or early adulthood, and diabetic ketoacidosis (DKA) as a characteristic complication. Type-I diabetes can only be treated with insulin, and it accounts for less than 5 percent of the cases of diabetes in the Unites States. Type-II diabetes, sometimes referred to as non-insulin-dependent diabetes mellitus (NIDDM) or adult-onset diabetes, is characterized by relative insulin deficiency and/or insulin resistance and the absence of DKA as a complication; its usual onset is in adulthood. Type-II diabetes accounts for more than 90 percent of the total cases of diabetes and is the focus of this chapter.

One of the most striking features of type-II diabetes (unlike type-I diabetes) is that it affects ethnic and racial groups differently (Harris, 1998). The prevalence of type-II diabetes in Latinos in the United States is approximately twice that of

Whites (Self-reported prevalence . . . , 1999) and varies among Latino subgroups. Diabetes ranks as the fifth cause of death for Latinos overall, though it ranks as the seventh cause of death for the general U.S. population. It is the fourth cause of death in Latino women and the sixth cause of death in Latino men (National Center of Health Statistics, 2000). This chapter describes the epidemiology of diabetes among Latinos and its subgroups where data are available, and it explores the causes for the increased risk of diabetes among Latinos. In addition, possible avenues for new research and policy are proposed.

## Diagnostic Criteria

The criteria for the diagnosis of type-II diabetes have changed recently and have affected the reporting of the epidemiology of diabetes. The American Diabetes Association (ADA) Expert Committee on the Diagnosis and Classification of Diabetes Mellitus developed new criteria in 1997 for the diagnosis of diabetes. Diabetes is now defined by the presence of a fasting glucose of 126 mg/dl or more, compared with the previous criteria that defined diabetes by a fasting glucose of 140 mg/dl or more (Report of the Expert Committee . . . , 1997). The rationale for this change was to enable the early detection and treatment of cases of asymptomatic diabetes in order to prevent complications that formerly developed before the disease was diagnosed. The World Health Organization (WHO) criteria define diabetes as two-hour postchallenge glucose level of 200 mg/dl or more. The new ADA recommendations for the diagnosis of diabetes did not recommend the two-hour glucose tolerance test for routine clinical use. As a consequence of this change in criteria, individuals previously considered to be at risk for diabetes and classified as having impaired glucose tolerance by the previous fasting glucose criteria (Keen, 1998) are now considered to have the disease. However, epidemiological concerns have arisen about the use of the new criteria. Ideally, the new ADA criteria and the WHO criteria should identify the same individuals with diabetes. The ADA reported that, based on the new criteria, the prevalence of diabetes would fall from 6.4 percent to 4.4 percent in the Third National Health and Nutrition Examination Survey (NHANES III) (Harris, Eastman, Cowie, Flegal, & Eberhardt, 1997), thereby underestimating the prevalence of the disease. Supporting this concern is a study that found the concordance of the two criteria to be only 28 percent (Decode Study Group . . . , 1998). Furthermore, one study found the WHO criteria to predict morbidity and mortality better than the new ADA criteria (Glucose tolerance . . . , 1999). With the new ADA criteria, middle-aged people and overweight people are more likely to be diagnosed (Keen, 1998). The use of different criteria for the diagnosis of diabetes in epidemiological studies has a potential important impact on our understanding of changes in the epidemiology of diabetes generally and in particular on the epidemiology of diabetes in Latinos.

The main sources of epidemiological data of diabetes in Latinos are NHANES III, carried out between 1988 and 1992, and the earlier Hispanic Health and

Nutrition Examination Survey (HHANES), conducted between 1982 and 1984. NHANES III contained a probability sample of 18,825 U.S. adults twenty years of age or older who were interviewed, including an inquiry as to a history of diagnosed diabetes. African Americans and Mexican Americans were oversampled in NHANES III. Other Latino subgroups were not included in this survey. There was a subsample of 6,587 adults for whom fasting plasma glucose values were obtained (2,798 Whites; 1,753 African Americans; 1,771 Mexican Americans; and 265 people of other ethnic and racial groups), according to which diabetes can be diagnosed by ADA criteria. A subsample of adults aged forty to seventy-four years also received an oral glucose tolerance test, with which diabetes can be diagnosed by WHO criteria. The procedures used were similar to those used in HHANES and the Second National Health and Nutrition Examination Survey (NHANES II). The prevalence of diagnosed diabetes in 1988–1994 was estimated to be 5.1 percent for adults older than twenty years based on NHANES III data (10.2 million). Table 10.1 shows the prevalence of diagnosed and undiagnosed diabetes, impaired fasting glucose, and impaired glucose tolerance by ethnic and racial group in adults forty to seventy-four years of age in the three aforementioned surveys, comparing the ADA and WHO criteria. The proportion of the population with diabetes was higher for Mexican Americans compared to African Americans and Whites. The age-standardized ratio of diabetes for African Americans compared to Whites was 1.70, and for Latinos compared to Whites it was 1.92 (Harris, 1998).

The prevalence of diabetes and glucose intolerance was lower in NHANES III when ADA criteria were used than when WHO criteria were used. Almost half of the individuals with diabetes by WHO criteria were normal by the ADA criteria. Moreover, 70 percent of individuals with impaired glucose tolerance by WHO criteria (that is, individuals deemed at risk for developing diabetes) were normal by ADA criteria (Harris et al., 1998). In light of the differences between the criteria used for the diagnosis of diabetes, these must be taken into account when we are interpreting the epidemiology of diabetes and its burden on Latinos, with particular attention to the changes between surveys.

## Differences in the Epidemiology of Diabetes Among Latino Subgroups

There are limited data sources describing the differences in the epidemiology of diabetes across Latino subgroups. Most studies of diabetes in Latinos have been conducted in Mexican Americans (Stern & Mitchell, 1995), who represent 65 percent of the total Latino population of the United States; however, the remaining 35 percent of the Latino population are not as well represented. Other Latino subgroups in the United States as described by the United States Bureau of the Census are Central and South Americans (14.3 percent), Puerto Ricans (9.6 percent), Cubans (4.3 percent), and "other Latinos" (6.6 percent) (Ramirez, 2000). There is a paucity of data particularly concerning the Central and South Americans and the "other Latinos" subgroups. The diversity of groups in the Latino population of the United

## TABLE 10.1.   PERCENTAGE OF THE U.S. POPULATION AGED 40–74 YEARS WITH DIABETES, IMPAIRED FASTING GLUCOSE, AND IMPAIRED GLUCOSE TOLERANCE, BASED ON THREE NATIONAL SURVEYS.

|  | NHANES II (1976–1980) | HHANES (1982–1984) | NHANES III (1988–1994) |
|---|---|---|---|
| **1997 ADA criteria** | | | |
| Diabetes (diagnosed and undiagnosed) | | | |
| All races | 8.9 | — | 12.3 |
| Whites | 8.1 | — | 11.2 |
| African Americans | — | 18.2 | — |
| Mexican Americans | 17.4 | 20.3 | — |
| Impaired fasting glucose | | | |
| All races | 6.5 | — | 9.7 |
| Whites | 6.6 | — | 9.5 |
| African Americans | — | 9.4 | — |
| Mexican Americans | 8.1 | 12.2 | — |
| Total diabetes and impaired fasting glucose | | | |
| All races | 15.4 | — | 22.0 |
| Whites | 14.7 | — | 20.8 |
| African Americans | — | 27.5 | — |
| Mexican Americans | 25.5 | 32.5 | — |
| **1985 WHO criteria** | | | |
| Diabetes (diagnosed and undiagnosed) | | | |
| All races | 11.4 | — | 14.3 |
| Whites | 10.7 | — | 13.4 |
| African Americans | — | — | 19.2 |
| Mexican Americans | — | 21.5 | 23.6 |
| Impaired glucose tolerance | | | |
| All races | 15.6 | — | 15.6 |
| Whites | 14.8 | — | 15.3 |
| African Americans | — | — | 13.1 |
| Mexican Americans | — | 17.7 | 19.4 |
| Total diabetes and impaired glucose tolerance | | | |
| All races | 27.0 | — | 29.9 |
| Whites | 25.6 | — | 28.6 |
| African Americans | — | — | 32.3 |
| Mexican Americans | — | 39.2 | 43.0 |

*Source:* Adapted from Harris et al. (1998, p. 523). Copyright © 1998 by the American Diabetes Association. Used with permission.

States represents a heterogeneous array of genetic admixtures, socioeconomic conditions, and behavioral factors that affect the prevalence of diabetes.

The HHANES was a multipurpose cross-sectional survey of Mexican Americans in the Southwestern United States, Cubans in Florida, and Puerto Ricans in the New York City area conducted between 1982 and 1984. Table 10.2 compares the prevalences of diagnosed diabetes, undiagnosed diabetes, and total diabetes among Latino subgroups in HHANES, and with Whites and African Americans in NHANES II. In summary, the prevalence of diagnosed diabetes in Cubans in Florida was similar to that in Whites, but it was nearly twice as high in Mexican Americans and Puerto Ricans. However, the prevalence of undiagnosed

TABLE 10.2.   PREVALENCE OF SELF-REPORTED DIABETES, UNDIAGNOSED DIABETES (WHO CRITERIA), AND TOTAL DIABETES BY ETHNIC AND RACIAL GROUP AND AGE GROUP IN HHANES AND NHANES II.

| | Prevalence | |
|---|---|---|
| | 20–44 Years Old | 45–74 Years Old |
| **Previously diagnosed diabetes** | | |
| HHANES | | |
| Mexican Americans | 1.9 | 14.3 |
| Cubans (U.S.) | 1.5 | 5.9 |
| Puerto Rican | 2.0 | 14.3 |
| NHANES II | | |
| Whites | 0.9 | 5.9 |
| African Americans | 2.3 | 10.1 |
| **Undiagnosed diabetes** | | |
| HHANES | | |
| Mexican Americans | 1.8 | 9.6 |
| Cubans (U.S.) | 1.0 | 9.9 |
| Puerto Ricans | 2.1 | 11.8 |
| NHANES II | | |
| Whites | 0.7 | 6.1 |
| African Americans | 1.0 | 9.3 |
| **Total diabetes (diagnosed and undiagnosed)** | | |
| HHANES | | |
| Mexican Americans | 3.8 | 23.9 |
| Cubans (U.S.) | 2.4 | 15.8 |
| Puerto Ricans | 4.1 | 26.1 |
| NHANES II | | |
| Whites | 1.6 | 12.0 |
| African Americans | 3.3 | 19.3 |

*Source:* Adapted from Flegal et al. (1991). Copyright © 1991 by the American Diabetes Association. Used with permission.

diabetes was similar in Cubans, Mexican Americans, and Puerto Ricans, but higher than that in Whites. There are no reports with comparisons of Cubans, Puerto Ricans, and Mexican Americans in the 1990s, or among any other Latino subgroups. However, data from NHANES III has demonstrated an increasing trend in the prevalence of diabetes for the population as a whole and for Mexican Americans in particular. There is no reason to believe that this trend is different for Puerto Ricans, Cubans, and other Latinos in the United States. More studies are needed examining the trends in the prevalence of diabetes in all Latino subgroups.

One report based on the Behavioral Risk Factor Surveillance System (BRFSS) indirectly shows the heterogeneity of diabetes prevalence among Latinos in the 1990s. The BRFSS was a state-based household telephone survey performed by random-digit dialing of adults eighteen years of age or older in the community. In this study the prevalence of diabetes and the interviewee's ethnic and racial group were determined by self-report; obviously data on undiagnosed diabetes were not available by this method. In data aggregated for 1994–1997, 6 percent of adults in Puerto Rico and the U.S. mainland reported being told that they had diabetes, which was somewhat higher than the NHANES III estimate. The age-adjusted prevalence of diabetes in Latinos was twice that of Whites (8 percent versus 4 percent). The prevalence of self-reported diabetes did not differ by gender. However, the prevalence of diabetes varied by geographic location: 10.7 percent in Puerto Rico, 5.8 percent in the Western and Southwestern United States, 4.9 percent in the Southern and Southeastern United States, and 4.1 percent in the Northeastern and Midwestern United States. Latino adults in Puerto Rico were almost three times more likely than Whites to have diabetes, whereas Latinos in the West and Southwest were two times as likely, and those in the Northeast and Midwest and South and Southeast were 1.4 times as likely to have the disease. This report had several limitations: only Latinos who had a telephone could be reached, and the survey information depended on self-reports; also, Latinos are more likely to have lower levels of educational attainment and lower socio-economic status compared to Whites (Ramirez, 2000), and so may be less likely to be aware of their diabetes status. This information probably underestimated the true prevalence of diabetes given these limitations, in addition to the fact that information on undiagnosed diabetes was not available. No specific data were available on specific Latino subgroups in this survey, and so these data can only indirectly suggest the prevalence of diabetes by Latino subgroups in the different regions based on our knowledge of the predominant subgroups in each location.

More studies comparing the prevalence of diabetes within Latino subgroups and with other racial and ethnic groups would help to identify the factors related to the increase of diabetes in the general population and contribute to our understanding of the differences in prevalence among different ethnic and racial groups.

## Genetic Factors

There is evidence that insulin metabolism is affected by genetic factors. Insulin metabolism can vary tremendously even among subjects with no diabetes and no impaired glucose tolerance who have a similar body-mass index (BMI) (Hollenbeck & Reaven, 1987). Insulin resistance is a risk factor for diabetes. However, there is great variation in who will develop diabetes even among subjects with insulin resistance, suggesting that there is a genetic basis for such variation (Stern & Mitchell, 1999). Many studies have determined that insulin resistance is higher in nondiabetic relatives of subjects with diabetes. One study showed that in Mexican Americans the concentration of insulin, indicative of risk of diabetes, increases as the number of parents with diabetes increases (Haffner, Stern, Hazuda, Mitchell, & Patterson, 1989). Diabetes varies with the distribution of genes and genetic admixture. Diabetes occurs most frequently among Native Americans (Amerindians) and less frequently among Whites. Mexican Americans, who are genetically heterogeneous, with genes derived from both Amerindians and Whites, show intermediate rates of diabetes, reflecting their genetic admixture (McKeigue, 1999). A study performed in Texas showed substantial genetic heterogeneity among

Mexican Americans, with a mean of 65 percent of genes derived from Whites and 35 percent of genes derived from Amerindians (Hanis, Chakraborty, Ferrell, & Schull, 1986). This study showed the lack of an association between genetic admixture and diabetes. However, in another study the higher White admixture in individuals with higher socioeconomic status is posited as explaining the correlation between lower rates of diabetes and higher socioeconomic status observed in Mexican Americans (Chakraborty, Ferrell, Stern, Haffner, Hazuda, & Rosenthal, 1986). Moreover, differences in diabetes between Mexican Americans and Whites do not seem to be explained solely by differences in obesity. A study comparing the risk of diabetes between Mexican Americans and Whites found that the prevalence of diabetes in Whites was lower, even when comparisons were made within BMI groups: lean Mexican Americans had a higher prevalence of diabetes than lean Whites (Stern, Gaskill, Hazuda, Gardner, & Haffner, 1983). There is evidence that these differences are accounted for by major genes. So far, the search for these genes has been unsuccessful (Stern & Mitchell, 1999). One study conducted among Mexican Americans in Texas estimated that the contributions of the additive effects of genes to the heredity of fasting insulin and two-hour, post-glucose-load insulin results (both indicative of diabetes risk) was 39 percent and 16 percent, respectively, after researchers adjusted for other diabetes risk factors (Mitchell et al., 1996). A separate report from the same population found that a putative major gene in the heritability of insulin resistance accounted for 31 percent in the variance of two-hour, post-glucose-load insulin levels (Mitchell et al., 1995). There are more than fifty mutations of the insulin gene characterized to date. However, they only explain rare causes of insulin resistance (Hone, Accili, Al-Gazali, Lestringant, Orban, & Taylor, 1994), and genes that explain common cases need to be found. One problem with studies of diabetes in families and communities is that genetic traits and environmental factors (including behavior) tend to cluster in families and communities, making it very difficult to separate the effects of shared environment from the effects of genetic traits. The study of genes related to diabetes in Latino subgroups may present a unique opportunity to identify the effects of genes and environmental factors on the prevalence of diabetes.

## Overweight, Obesity, and Insulin Resistance

Overweight and obesity have been shown to be risk factors for diabetes. Overweight and obesity are defined by BMI, which is a measure of body fat tissue derived from height and weight (weight in kilograms divided by the squared value of height in meters). The World Health Organization (1997) defines normal weight as a BMI of 18.5 to 24.9, overweight as a BMI of 25.0 to 29.9, and obesity as a BMI of more than 30.0. These criteria further classify obesity by severity: class I obesity, BMI, 30.0 to 34.9; class II obesity, BMI, 34.9 to 39.9; and class III obesity, BMI, greater than 39.9. The prevalence of type-II diabetes in NHANES III was more than twice as great in overweight men than in normal men (4.93 percent versus 2.03 percent), and more than three times greater in overweight women than normal women (7.12 percent versus 2.38 percent). The prevalence of diabetes in men in the highest obesity category (BMI, greater than 40 kg/dl) was more than fivefold that of normal men (10.65 percent versus 2.03 percent), and was more than eight times greater in the most obese women compared with normal women (19.89 percent versus 2.38 percent) (Must, Spadano, Coakley, Field, Colditz, & Dietz, 1999). The adjusted prevalence of overweight for the population as a whole showed little change between NHANES II and NHANES III. Mexican American men had the highest increase in class-I obesity from HHANES to NHANES III (Flegal, Carroll, Kuczmarzki, & Johnson, 1998). The prevalence of class-II and -III obesity also increased in the general population, with African American women showing the largest increase (Glucose tolerance . . . , 1999). This increase in obesity has paralleled the increase in the prevalence of diabetes. According to NHANES III data, 63 percent of men and 55 percent of women aged twenty-five years or older in the U.S. population were overweight or obese; 42 percent of men and 28 percent of women were overweight, and 21 percent of men and 27 percent of women were obese. These data reflect the fact that more than half of the U.S. population is at risk for developing diabetes. However, it may take some fifteen to twenty years before the increase in body weight is followed by the onset of diabetes (Ravussin, 1993). As seen with diabetes, the prevalence of overweight and obesity vary with ethnicity. For Mexican American men the prevalence of overweight increased from 30.9 percent in HHANES to 39.8 percent in NHANES III, and for Mexican American women from 41 percent in HHANES to 48.1 percent in NHANES III. The increase in overweight for White men was from 24.2 percent in NHANES II to 32 percent in NHANES III (Kuczmarski, Flegal, Campbell, & Johnson, 1994).

The ethnic variation in diabetes mellitus parallels the ethnic variation in insulin resistance. Mean fasting and postprandial plasma insulin levels, which are higher in persons at risk of diabetes, are higher in Mexican Americans compared to people of Northern European heritage (McKeigue, 1999). Post-glucose-load insulin levels are higher in Mexican Americans compared to Whites, even after researchers adjusted for BMI (Stern, Gaskill, Hazuda, Gardner, & Haffner, 1983), suggesting that Mexican Americans respond differently to overweight compared to Whites (Europeans Americans), probably due to genetic differences. The distribution of body fat is more central in Mexican Americans than in Americans of European descent, which is thought to be related to a higher risk of diabetes, and obesity in Mexican Americans is accompanied by a profile of cholesterol and triglycerides that is characteristic of the insulin resistance syndrome and diabetes (Després & Marette, 1999).

## Obesity in Children

Overweight and obesity in children have been determined to be predictors of overweight and obesity in adulthood. Once overweight and obesity are established in childhood, it tends to persist into adulthood (DiPietro, Mossberg, & Stunkard, 1994). Thus, childhood is a critical period in the study of risk factors for diabetes in adulthood. Children who are obese under three years of age are at a low risk to become obese as adults if they have no obese parents. Among children older than three years, childhood obesity predicts adult obesity regardless of parental obesity status. Parental obesity more than doubles the risk of adult obesity among both obese and nonobese children under ten years of age (Whitaker, Wright, Pepe, Seidel, & Dietz, 1997). This underscores the interdependence of childhood and adult obesity, as well as the importance of targeting adults and children together for prevention. Data from NHANES III showed that body circumferences, skinfold thickness, and BMIs, which are higher in obese children, were highest in Mexican American children compared to African American and White children (Gillum, 1999). Overweight and obesity in children aged two months to five years has increased in the last few decades, particularly in Mexican Americans, paralleling the trends in overweight and obesity described in adult Mexican Americans (Ogden, Troiano, Briefel, Kuczmarski, Flegal, & Johnson, 1997). A conventional explanation for this phenomenon is that Latina mothers believe that heavier children are healthier. However, studies have failed to support this (Sherman, Alexander, Dean, & Kim, 1995), and other explanations need to be found.

Childhood is the critical period for prevention of obesity and the development of diabetes. There is a paucity of data on obesity in children belonging to Latino subgroups other than Mexican Americans, and more studies are needed examining potential differences and their causes.

## Dietary Risk Factors

Diet is one of the modifiable risk factors for diabetes (United States Department of Health and Human Services, Public Health Service, 1991), in part through its impact on overweight and obesity, and probably through a direct effect on insulin metabolism. Data from a cross-sectional study in the San Luis Valley diabetes project conducted in a rural Latino and White population showed that the prevalence of type-II diabetes and impaired glucose tolerance increased with an increase of fat intake, as determined by twenty-four-hour diet recall. A 40 g increase in fat intake increased the risk of diabetes by 50 percent and the risk of glucose intolerance by 60 percent (Marshall, Hamman, & Baxter, 1991). Another cross-sectional study from the same population conducted in 1,069 Latinos and Whites without diabetes reported that high insulin concentrations (characteristic of diabetes and the insulin resistance syndrome) were higher in subjects with a high intake of total fats and a low intake of fiber and starch. The risk of high insulin levels with a low intake of fiber and starch was highest in lean subjects (Marshall, Bessesen, & Hamman, 1997), underscoring the importance of diet independent of the presence of overweight and obesity. A study comparing Latino Catholics and Latino Seventh-day Adventists in Colorado found that Seventh-day Adventists had a lower intake of total fat, saturated fat, and cholesterol and a higher relative intake of carbohydrate and dietary fiber, compared to Catholics. This correlated with significantly lower BMI, waist-to-hip ratios, lower fasting insulin and glucose concentrations in Seventh-day Adventists, and a lower risk of type-II diabetes

(Alexander, Lockwood, Harris, & Melby, 1999). A study comparing Latinos and Whites in the San Francisco Bay area found that Latinos were significantly more likely to report eating vegetables and more likely to eat rice, beans, fried foods, and whole milk. Less acculturated Latinos were more likely to eat fruits, rice, beans, meat, fried foods, and whole milk than more acculturated Latinos. Acculturation in this chapter refers to the process by which an individual assimilates the cultural traits of the dominating group in the country and does not include socioeconomic class. Overall, although Latinos reported a high consumption of high-fiber foods, they also reported high use of saturated fat (Otero-Sabogal, Sabogal, Pérez-Stable, & Hiatt, 1995), which is associated with a higher BMI and risk of diabetes.

Data from HHANES and NHANES II comparing caloric intake and the intake of various nutrients among Mexican Americans, Puerto Ricans, Cubans (in the United States), and Whites showed that Mexican Americans had a higher intake of total fat, saturated fat, and monounsaturated fat than Puerto Ricans and Cubans. Cubans and Puerto Ricans had similar intakes, although younger Cubans had a higher intake of total fat and saturated fat and low carbohydrate intake. In general, fat intake was lower in the Latino groups compared to that of Whites (Loria et al., 1995), and this finding is supported by other studies. The dietary patterns seen in adults are also seen in children and parallel the prevalence of obesity, overweight, and diabetes in adults. A study conducted in 3,436 children who participated in the Mexican American portion of HHANES examined the intake of food in Mexican American children with current diet recommendations and found that meat and milk servings were higher than recommended, whereas servings of fruits and vegetables were lower than recommended (Murphy, Castillo, Martorell, & Mendoza, 1990).

There is a paucity of data on diet of children of other Latino subgroups. A study conducted in Southeast Texas compared the intake of different nutrients between Whites, African Americans, and Mexican Americans obtained by twenty-four-hour dietary recall. The mean caloric intake was highest for Whites, followed by Mexican Americans and then African Americans. Mexican Americans had a higher carbohydrate intake than Whites and lower total fat intake (Newell, Borrud, McPherson, Nichaman, & Pillow, 1988). The paradoxical finding of a lower caloric intake in Latinos, who are at a higher risk of diabetes, is probably explained by the influence of genetic factors in the relationship between diet and the risk of diabetes. Although Latinos appear to have a lower intake of total fats and calories than Whites, they are still more prone to having diabetes. Within Latino subgroups, those with lower intakes of fiber and higher fat intakes had a higher risk of diabetes, supporting the idea that the influence of diet in Latinos is modified by specific genetic factors.

## Low Levels of Physical Activity

Data from the San Luis Valley Diabetes Study conducted in a Latino and White population showed that lower levels of physical activity were associated with features of the insulin resistance syndrome and higher risk of diabetes (Regensteiner et al., 1991, 1995). Data from the San Antonio Heart Study failed to confirm that diet and physical activity predict obesity in Mexican Americans, but this was thought to result from the imprecision of the instruments used to measure diet and physical activity (Haffner, Stern, Mitchell, & Hazuda, 1991).

According to NHANES III data, 15.8 percent of men and 27.1 percent of females in the United States reported no participation in leisure time physical activity. Latino males (29.1 percent) and Latino females (43.8 percent) were even less physically active. According to data from the Behavioral Risk Factor Surveillance System (BRFSS), the overall proportion of self-reported physical inactivity was 26.5 percent in U.S. males and 30.7 percent in U.S. females; in Latinos 38.5 percent of men and 42.7 percent of females were inactive, higher than for the U.S. population as a whole (United States Department of Health and Human Services, Public Health Service, 1996). A study looking at 573 Latinas from Los Angeles found that more acculturated women under the age of sixty-five, a critical period when diabetes starts, were less physically active than their less acculturated counterparts. However, acculturation did not affect physical activity in those over the age of sixty-five (Cantero, Richardson, Baezconde-Garbanatti, & Marks, 1999).

The trends in physical activity observed in adults and their consequences are also observed in children. Data from the Framingham Children's Study showed that preschool children with low levels of physical activity gained substantially more subcutaneous fat than did more active children (Moore, Nguyen, Rothman, Cupples, & Ellison, 1995). A study conducted among 351 four-year-olds of different ethnicities and from families of low-to-middle socioeconomic status found that Mexican American children were less active than White children both at home and during school recess (McKenzie, Sallis, Nader, Broyles, & Nelson, 1992). This was influenced by the Mexican American children spending more time in the presence of adults and having less access to toys. Data from 4,063 children surveyed in NHANES III showed that African American and Mexican American girls were less likely to engage in vigorous physical activity (three or more bouts a week) compared to Whites (Andersen, Crespo, Bartlett, Cheskin, & Pratt, 1998).

Latinos have diet and physical activity patterns that increase the risk of diabetes and that are apparently independent of genetic risk factors. Less acculturated Latinos appear to be less aware of healthy patterns of behavior. A higher proportion of Latinos have lower socioeconomic status and lower educational attainment compared to Whites (Ramirez, 2000), which may explain in part the lower awareness of healthy behaviors in Latinos. However, the reasons for such differences seem to be more complex, not simply explained by socioeconomic and educational differences. A telephone survey conducted by the New York State Healthy Heart Program found that ethnicity was related to overweight, less physical activity, and a diet that increased the risk of coronary heart disease—all associated with a higher risk of diabetes. However, this effect was independent of educational attainment, suggesting that factors other than socioeconomic status and education were at play (Shea et al., 1991). Other studies have also found that socioeconomic status does not explain the higher risk of diabetes in Latinos. A study based on HHANES data found that income and education were not associated with obesity in Cubans, Mexican Americans, and Puerto Ricans (Khan, Sobal, & Martorelli, 1997). Data from a survey conducted in five populations of Northern California showed that Mexican American men and women had higher BMIs than Whites, and these differences were not predicted by differences in age, gender, education, the city of residence, or the language spoken (Winkleby, Gardner, & Taylor, 1996).

There is a need to look for risk factors that explain the high prevalence of diabetes in Latinos beyond the conventional ones so far considered in this chapter. Most studies that have examined the risk factors for diabetes among Latinos have focused on the characteristics of individuals and have not looked at the influence of family, neighborhood, community, and the media. Multilevel analysis has been suggested as a method of studying the context of the individual at different levels as a risk factor for disease interaction with individual risk factors (Diez-Roux, 1998). Neighborhood environment has been suggested as one such risk factor (Diez-Roux et al., 1997). There is a paucity of data on this type of risk factor for diabetes, in general, and for diabetes in Latinos, in particular. Studies are needed that explore environmental risk factors that explain the differences in the prevalence of diabetes between Latinos, Latino subgroups, and Whites, beyond what can be explained at the individual level.

## Consequences of Diabetes

The adverse consequences of diabetes are classified as macrovascular and microvascular. Macrovascular consequences are coronary heart disease and cerebrovascular disease, which result in myocardial infarction, congestive heart failure, stroke, and sudden death. Microvascular complications are related to effects on small blood vessels and the organs they perfuse, and are mainly diabetic retinopathy, diabetic nephropathy, and diabetic neuropathy. The available data suggest that non-White ethnic and racial groups have a risk of coronary artery disease similar to that of Whites. Mexican Americans with diabetes have a risk elevation of coronary disease similar to that of Whites with diabetes (Carter, Pugh, & Monterrosa, 1996). End-stage renal disease is more prevalent in African Americans and Latinos than in Whites. In African Americans this is thought to be mostly secondary to the high prevalence of hypertension. There is insufficient information on Latinos in the literature, but data from Texas indicates that end-stage renal disease is higher in Mexican Americans in that state than in Whites and that diabetes is the main cause of end-stage renal disease in the former group (Feldman, Klag, Chiapella, & Whelton, 1992). In a cohort study of end-stage renal disease in Texas, 93 percent of Latinos who had end-stage renal disease had diabetes, compared to 84 percent of African Americans and 60 percent of Whites (Harris, Eastman, Cowie, Flegal, & Eberhardt, 1997). Studies looking at diabetic retinopathy in Latinos have had conflicting results: one study found higher rates than in

Whites, and the other showed lower rates (Haffner, Fong, Stern, Pugh, & Hazuda, 1988; Hamman et al., 1991). Although data on rates of diabetic neuropathy among ethnic and racial groups are scarce, the San Luis Valley Study (Hamman et al., 1991) and the National Health Interview Survey suggest there is no difference between Latinos and Whites in this regard (Harris, Eastman, & Cowie, 1993). One study based on a database from California reported that Latinos had a higher proportion of amputations (82.7 percent) attributable to diabetes than African Americans (61.6 percent) or Whites (56.8 percent) (Lavery, Ashry, Van Houtum, Pugh, Harkless, & Basu, 1996).

Diabetes in Latinos has also been found to be associated with other important diseases that are not traditionally considered as being diabetes related. A case-control study using discharge data from California hospitals found that diabetes was a significant predictor of tuberculosis, particularly in middle-aged Latinos: 25 percent of the cases of tuberculosis were attributable to diabetes in this group, similar to the risk of tuberculosis attributable to HIV infection (Pablos-Mendez, Blustein, & Knirsch, 1997). The risk of dementia associated with stroke (the second-most important cause of dementia after Alzheimer's disease) attributable to diabetes was found to be double in Latinos (33 percent) as in Whites (17 percent) in a cohort of elderly subjects from Upper Manhattan in New York City (Luchsinger, Tang, Stern, Shea, & Mayeux, 2000).

The available data on diabetes complications do not show that Latinos develop complications of diabetes differently than other ethnic and racial groups. However, given the higher prevalence of diabetes in Latinos, it is clear that the burden of these complications attributable to diabetes is higher than in other ethnic and racial groups. The existing data do not provide information on the impact of access to care on the rates of complications from diabetes. It is reasonable to assume, however, that appropriate access to care prevents the development of complications from diabetes and that persons with diabetes without access to proper care will have more complications. Studies are needed that explore the influence of access to care and the differences in diabetes-related complications between Latinos and other groups.

## The *Healthy People 2000* and *Healthy People 2010* Programs

The *Healthy People 2000* program was the prevention agenda for the nation in the decade of the 1990s. It identified the most significant preventable threats to health. Diabetes was one of the main focus areas of *Healthy People 2000*, which made special mention of the problem among Latinos. Although some of the health goals for Latinos in *Healthy People 2000* were met, that was not the case with diabetes (United States Department of Health and Human Services, Public Health Service, 1997). The *Healthy People 2000* program stated as objectives a decrease in the incidence of diabetes to no more than 2.5 per 1,000 people and a decrease in its prevalence to no more than twenty-five per 1,000 people. There were also objectives specific to Latino subgroups: a decrease in the prevalence of diabetes in

Puerto Ricans to no more than forty-nine per 1,000, in Mexican Americans to no more than forty-nine per 1,000, and in Cubans to no more than thirty-two per 1,000 (United States Department of Health and Human Services, Public Health Service, 1988). The prevalence of diabetes in Mexican Americans actually *increased* from fifty-four per 1,000 in 1986 to sixty-six cases per 1,000 in 1994 (United States Department of Health and Human Services, Public Health Service, 1997), but there are no data on Puerto Ricans and Cubans or other Latino subgroups. The *Healthy People 2010* project again includes diabetes as one of its main focus areas (United States Department of Health and Human Services, Public Health Service, 2000).

The logical target for the prevention of diabetes is the reduction of obesity and overweight through the adoption of appropriate dietary habits and physical activities. Current treatments for obesity are limited, and available treatments only produce 10 to 15 percent weight loss (Thomas, 1995), which is most often regained after the treatment stops. New, more effective treatments for obesity may be found in the future after the discovery of leptin (Zhang et al., 1994), which has broadened the understanding of energy balance (Bray & York, 1998) and created new opportunities for the development of new therapeutic agents. In the meantime, most of the efforts for the prevention of diabetes are geared toward the prevention of overweight and obesity themselves. The average dietary fat intake among people two years of age and over has declined slightly, and the percentage of the whole population that meets the dietary guidelines has increased. However, the main objective related to diabetes has not been met: overweight prevalence has increased, and the number of adults who attempt weight loss with diet and exercise has declined (United States Department of Health and Human Services, Public Health Service, 1998/99; National Center for Health Statistics, 1999). As before, *Healthy People 2010* has as one of its objectives the reduction of obesity and overweight as a risk factor for diabetes through a healthy diet and regular physical activity, particularly among Latinos (United States Department of Health and Human Services, Public Health Service, 2000).

The prevalence of light-to-moderate physical activity has remained unchanged for the population as a whole at approximately 23 percent, while it had a modest increase for Latinos, to approximately 22 percent. *Healthy People 2000* included as a physical activity and fitness objective the reduction of overweight to no more than 20 percent among people aged twenty and older, and no more than 15 percent among adolescents aged twelve to nineteen. The specific objectives for Latinos were to reduce overweight to a prevalence of no more than 25 percent in Latino women aged twenty and older, and to reduce overweight to a prevalence of no more than 25 percent among Mexican American men. The proposed way to achieve these goals was by increasing to at least 25 percent the proportion of Latinos who engaged in light-to-moderate physical activity for at least thirty minutes per day, five or more times per week, and by increasing to at least 17 percent the proportion of Latinos who engaged in vigorous physical activity. The combined objective of *Healthy People 2000* for diet and exercise was to increase the proportion of overweight Latinos who adopted sound dietary practices combined with regular physical activity to attain appropriate body weight to at least 24 percent in men and 22 percent in women (United States Department of Health and Human Services, Public Health Service, 1998/99).

The role of education is paramount in the promotion of healthy practices and the achievement of these goals. Several studies have explored the role of education programs in the promotion of health in Latinos. "Jump Into Action," a school-based program for the prevention of NIDDM (type-II diabetes) through the promotion of intake of low-fat foods and regular exercise was found to be effective in increasing knowledge and preventive behavior related to the disease that was sustained for four weeks (Holcomb, Lira, Kingery, Smith, Lane, & Goodway, 1998). The San Diego Family Health Project studied the effectiveness of a family-based cardiovascular risk reduction intervention in 206 White and Mexican Americans families. Families were randomized to a year-long educational intervention geared toward the reduction of high-fat foods and salt, as well as an increase in physical activity. This study showed that both White and Mexican American families changed their behaviors in the desired manner, and the adaptive behavioral changes persisted for one year beyond the completion of the intervention (Nader et al., 1989). A weight reduction program for Mexican Americans that involved information about lifestyle changes and classes for a year was compared to an information-only approach. This study compared three groups: one that received written information only, one geared toward individuals in classes, and another one involving the whole family. The groups of individuals in classes and in families had the greatest weight loss, with subjects in the family group having the best result (Foreyt, Ramirez, & Cousins, 1991). A survey of physical activity in 127 Latinos in California found that the factors predicting vigorous physical activity were self-efficacy, friends' support, childhood physical activity, and eating a healthy diet (Hovell et al., 1991). One study compared family aggregation of physical activity habits in ninety-five White families and 111 Mexican American families, and found a moderate degree of family aggregation of physical activity in both samples, but the intrafamily correlations were higher in Mexican Americans (Sallis, Patterson, Buono, Atkins, & Nader, 1988). Data from the San Diego Family Health Project found in a study examining knowledge of health-related diet and exercise behavior in White and Mexican Americans that marginally acculturated Mexican Americans were least aware of adaptive and productive health behavior. Acculturation was the most important predictor among Mexican Americans of knowing adaptive and productive health behavior (Vega, Sallis, Patterson, Rupp, Atkins, & Nader, 1987), which decreases the risk of diabetes.

The studies cited show several factors that affect the promotion of adaptive and productive health behaviors and the prevention of diabetes in Latinos. Those Latinos who are less acculturated are less aware of these behaviors, and a special effort must be made to reach them in a culturally appropriate manner. The influence of family and support groups is very important in the health practices of Latinos. Programs that promote healthy practices in Latinos must target not only the individual but also the family nucleus, the extended family, and friends.

The programs should also heavily target children. Targeting Latino children through school-based programs may not be enough, and it is important to get Latino parents involved as well.

*Healthy People 2010* has set the agenda for the improvement of health in the United States for the next decade. Diabetes, obesity and overweight, diet, and physical activity again figure as main focus areas, with particular attention to Latinos (United States Department of Health and Human Services, Public Health Service, 2000).

## Screening for Diabetes in High-Risk Persons

The American Diabetes Association (ADA) recommends screening people at high risk for diabetes. These include the following: individuals over the age of forty-five; obese individuals at any age; those who have a first-degree relative (parents or siblings) with diabetes; members of a high-risk ethnic group (African Americans, Latinos, or Native Americans); women diagnosed with gestational diabetes or who have delivered a baby weighing more than 9 lbs. (4.4 kg); those with a high-density-lipoprotein (HDL) cholesterol level less than 35 mg/dl; those with a triglyceride level over 250 mg/dl; and those with impaired glucose regulation (Report of the Expert Committee . . . , 1997). The objective of screening is early diagnosis and intervention of diabetes. The main barrier to screening is access to care. In order for screening to occur, contact with an appropriate health care provider must exist. Latinos are less likely to have health insurance (Ramirez, 2000) and to have access to primary care services. Given the disparities between the ADA criteria and the WHO criteria in diagnosing diabetes and predicting adverse outcomes, the health care provider should consider using a post-glucose-load tolerance test in individuals in whom diabetes is ruled out by ADA criteria but in whom a high degree of suspicion for diabetes remains. This should be particularly true for Latinos, who have a higher prevalence of undiagnosed diabetes.

## Treatment

Until recently, the merit of aggressive treatment of type-II diabetes was questioned. Several studies have shown an increased morbidity and mortality in subjects treated for type-II diabetes (University Group Diabetes Program, 1970; Abraira et al., 1997), and its intensive management was a controversial issue. The Diabetes Control and Complications Trial (DCCT) Research Group (1993) showed that individuals with type-I diabetes treated intensively had better microvascular outcomes, and experts extrapolated this benefit to subjects with type-II diabetes. Recently, the United Kingdom Prospective Diabetes Study (UKPDS) Group (1998) showed decreased rates of macrovascular and microvascular complications related to type-II diabetes with aggressive treatment as compared to conventional treatment. These results are considered the strongest evidence as yet supporting tight control of glucose in subjects with type-II diabetes. In addition to a change in how aggressively diabetes is treated, the 1990s saw the introduction of new medications for diabetes in the U.S. market. Metformin, an oral agent widely used in Europe, was approved in the United States by the Food and Drug Administration (FDA) in 1995 (DeFronzo, 1999). It is an anti-insulin-resistance agent of particular utility in treatment of obese diabetic patients. Another family of anti-insulin-resistance agents, the thiazolidinediones, was also introduced. The first member of this family, troglitazone, was retired from the market after reports of liver toxicity and with the introduction of two new agents of the same family: pioglitazone and rosiglitazone. The introduction of these anti-insulin-resistance agents is having a particular impact in populations with diabetes related to overweight and obesity, and it has broadened what used to be a very limited array of medications against diabetes.

The advances in the treatment of diabetes and the trend for more aggressive control entail more frequent follow-up of treated subjects with physician consultation and laboratory test monitoring. Thus, the prerequisite for proper treatment of diabetes is access to the necessary health care resources. This is a particular issue for Latinos who have less access to health care. Access to appropriate care is not assured by health insurance. For example, are there enough ambulatory facilities that provide appropriate care for diabetes in areas where Latinos are concentrated? Can a working Latino with diabetes access appropriate diabetes care after hours, on weekends, or at work? Given the new emphasis on intensive management of type-II diabetes, these questions are of major importance and need to be addressed.

The conventional wisdom is that Latinos make more use of alternative medicine and are therefore less likely to follow traditional medicine. The data on this issue are conflicting. A recent study conducted in Texas dispels this notion: 84 percent of Mexican American individuals with diabetes that were interviewed in this study mentioned the use of herbs for the treatment of diabetes. However, they viewed herbs as complementary to traditional medicine, not as a substitute (Hunt, Nedal, & Akana, 2000). Another study conducted in Latino populations in Mexico, Guatemala, Texas, and Connecticut found that knowledge about diabetes increased with higher acculturation and higher educational attainment; however, beliefs about diabetes were homogeneous and were concordant with the biomedical model. A survey performed in 100 non–Mexican American Latinos showed quite the contrary results: 78 percent of patients believed they had diabetes due to God's will, and 17 percent reported using herbs to treat diabetes (Zaldivar & Smolowitz, 1994). Given these data, it seems reasonable to suggest that Latinos should be offered standard treatment for diabetes without making assumptions as to issues of compliance or as to preference of traditional versus alternative medicine. However, health practitioners must be sensitive to those cases in whom there may be resistance to traditional treatment. In these cases, a didactic approach to modify beliefs may be needed with sensitivity to the patient's beliefs, and the participation of a culturally concordant practitioner may be warranted.

A new area that is developing in the management of diabetes is the exchange of clinical information from home via computers and telephone networks (Drucker et al., 1998). Given that a substantial proportion of Latinos have low educational attainment and low socioeconomic status, it is reasonable to believe that Latinos have less access to such high-tech information resources than the rest of the population. A telemedicine project on the care of diabetes is currently under way in New York State including Latinos from New York City (Columbia University, Health Sciences Division, Office of External Relations, 2000). This study will help to elucidate the applicability of modern chronic care resources in Latinos and explore barriers to their use.

## Summary and Implications

Diabetes is one of the most prevalent chronic diseases in the United States, affecting more than 10 percent of the population over the age of sixty-five. The prevalence of diabetes in Latinos is almost double that of Whites. Furthermore, four out of ten Latinos are at risk for developing diabetes. Diabetes is more prevalent in Mexican Americans and Puerto Ricans than in Cubans in the United States. Data are lacking on the prevalence of diabetes in other Latino subgroups. More studies are needed comparing the prevalence of diabetes within Latino subgroups and with other racial and ethnic groups. Such studies would help to identify the factors related to the increase of diabetes in the general population and contribute to our understanding of the differences in prevalence among different ethnic and racial groups. Latinos appear to have a genetic makeup that increases the risk of diabetes, but the exact genes involved in this increased risk are yet to be determined. Latinos are more likely than Whites to be physically inactive and to have less than ideal dietary practices. These differences are partially explained by acculturation, and several studies indicate that educational level and socioeconomic status per se do not explain the differences. Overweight and obesity are also more prevalent in Latinos compared to Whites, and this is explained by a combination of genetic predisposition and inadequate diet and physical activity. More data are needed on the influence of the environment at the family, neighborhood, and community level, and the influence of the Latino media on the high prevalence of diabetes in Latinos. The burden of complications of diabetes is higher in Latinos compared to other groups, given the high prevalence of the disease. Access to care may affect the rate of complications from diabetes in Latinos, and there is a lack of studies looking at this issue. The treatment of diabetes is intensive and needs frequent access to appropriate health care resources. Current evidence suggests that Latinos favor conventional medical therapy for diabetes, although the use of alternative therapies is possible and must be taken into account. Beliefs in the causation of diabetes do not appear to be a barrier for diabetes treatment in Latinos. The main obstacle to the treatment of diabetes in Latinos is lack of health insurance and access to the appropriate health care setting.

# Recommendations

From a research standpoint, the study of different Latino subgroups presents a unique opportunity to identify genes that increase the risk of diabetes while teasing out the effects of environment and culture. Latinos comprise a heterogeneous ethnic and racial group that share language and some cultural aspects but who represent diverse genetic admixtures. There is a dearth of data on the epidemiology of diabetes in the United States in Latino subgroups since the 1980s, and more studies should be conducted that include Puerto Ricans, Cubans, Mexican Americans, and other groups previously not studied, such as South and Central Americans and Latinos from the Caribbean. Studies are also needed on the impact of access to care on the prevention, detection, and treatment of diabetes in Latinos. In light of the new tendency for aggressive treatment of diabetes, an assessment is needed of the presence and access to appropriate ambulatory care settings in the areas where Latinos live. The area of research that is perhaps most needed is the exploration of risk factors for diabetes beyond the individual, such as the neighborhoods where Latinos live and the role of Spanish-language and Latino media.

From a health promotion standpoint, the targeting of Latinos by education programs geared toward the prevention of diabetes and adoption of healthy practices must be increased. The higher prevalence of diabetes and its risk factors in Latinos show that education programs need to be more effective. The objectives of the *Healthy People 2000* program for Latinos were to decrease the prevalence of overweight and obesity, promote healthy diet practices, increase physical activity, and decrease the proportion of Latinos with diabetes. However, the targets set by that program in these areas were not met, and they are again priority goals of *Healthy People 2010*. Education is the main conduit to achieve these objectives. Educational programs for Latinos must target the whole family as well as friends and must involve active interaction. Special programs are needed to reach less-acculturated Latinos. The most important group that needs to be targeted is Latino children; prevention at an early age is the most effective way to reduce the prevalence of diabetes in Latinos. A way to achieve this is to expand educational programs to the Latino media and to design education programs with characteristics that are distinctly important for Latinos, such as interactive programs, the participation of the network of family and friends, and special sensitivity to less-acculturated Latinos and those who only speak Spanish. Latino children need a special effort in terms of health promotion.

From the standpoint of medical care, Latinos are a high-risk group for the development of diabetes and should be screened with a fasting glucose measure, complemented with a two-hour post-glucose-load measure when diabetes is suspected despite a normal result with fasting glucose.

From a policy standpoint, the main needs are the increase in insurance coverage for Latinos and their access to appropriate health care settings for the detection and treatment of diabetes. Given the growing proportion of people with diabetes and its high burden on society, this disease should be given special treatment from a policy perspective. Health care agencies must ensure that all geographic areas have ambulatory care settings appropriate for the detection and treatment of diabetes. Access to emergency care services on an as-needed basis is not enough.

# References

Abraira, C. et al. (1997). Cardiovascular events and correlates in the Veterans Affairs Diabetes Feasibility Trial. *Archives of Internal Medicine, 157,* 181–188.

Alexander, H., Lockwood, L. P., Harris, M. A., & Melby, C. L. (1999). Risk factors for cardiovascular disease and diabetes in two groups of Hispanic Americans with differing dietary habits. *Journal of the American College of Nutrition, 18,* 127–136.

Andersen, R. E., Crespo, C. J., Bartlett, S. J., Cheskin, L. J., & Pratt, A. M. (1998). Relationship of physical activity and television watching with body weight and level of fatness among children: Results from the Third National Health and Nutrition Examination Survey. *Journal of the American Medical Association, 279,* 938–942.

Bray, G. A., & York, D. A. (1998). The MONA LISA hypothesis in the time of leptin. *Recent Progress in Hormone Research, 53,* 95–118.

Cantero, P. J., Richardson, J. I., Baezconde-Garbanatti, L., & Marks, G. (1999). The association between acculturation and health practices among middle-aged and elderly Latinas. *Ethnicity and Disease, 9,* 166–180.

Carter, J. S., Pugh, J. A., & Monterrosa, A. (1996). Non-insulin-dependent diabetes mellitus in minorities in the United States. *Annals of Internal Medicine,125,* 221–232.

Centers for Disease Control and Prevention. (1999, June 30). Deaths: Final data for 1997. *National Vital Statistics Reports, 47,* 19, 27–37. Retrieved August 2000 from: http://www.cdc.gov/nchs/data/nvs47_19.pdf

Chakraborty, R., Ferrell, R. E., Stern, M. P., Haffner, S. M., Hazuda, H. P., & Rosenthal, M. (1986). Relationship of prevalence of non-insulin-dependent diabetes mellitus to Amerindian admixture in the Mexican-Americans of San Antonio, Texas. *Genetic Epidemiology, 3,* 435–454.

Columbia University. Health Sciences Division, Office of External Relations. (2000). Doctors reinvent the house call: $28 million telemedicine demonstration project largest ever funded by the federal government's Department of Health and Human Services. Press release. Retrieved September 2000 from: http://informatics.cpmc.columbia.edu/ideatel/news/press.html

Decode Study Group on behalf of the European Diabetes Epidemiology Study Group. (1998). Will new diagnostic criteria for diabetes mellitus change phenotype of patients with diabetes?: Reanalysis of European epidemiological data. *British Medical Journal, 317,* 371–375.

DeFronzo, R. A. (1999). Pharmacologic therapy for type 2 diabetes mellitus. *Annals of Internal Medicine, 131,* 281–303.

Després, J. P., & Marette, A. (1999). Obesity and insulin resistance: Epidemiologic, metabolic, and molecular aspects. In G. M. Reaven & A. Laws (Eds.), *Insulin resistance: The metabolic syndrome X.* Totowa, NJ: Humana Press.

Diabetes Control and Complications Trial Research Group. (1993). The effect of intensive treatment of diabetes on the development and progression of long-term complications in insulin-dependent diabetes mellitus. *New England Journal of Medicine, 329,* 977–986.

Diez-Roux, A. V. (1998). Bringing context into epidemiology: Variables and fallacies in multilevel analysis. *American Journal of Public Health, 88,* 216–222.

Diez-Roux, A. V. et al. (1997). Neighborhood environments and coronary heart disease: A multilevel analysis. *American Journal of Epidemiology, 146,* 48–63.

DiPietro, L., Mossberg, H. O., & Stunkard, A. J. (1994). A 40-year history of overweight children in Stockholm: Life-time overweight, morbidity, and mortality. *International Journal of Obesity and Related Metabolic Disorders, 18,* 585–590.

Drucker, D. et al. (1998). Nationwide telecare for diabetics: A pilot implementation of the HOLON architecture. *Proceedings of the AMIA [American Medical Informatics Association] Annual Symposium,* pp. 346–350.

Feldman, H. I., Klag, M. J., Chiapella, A. P., & Whelton, P. K. (1992). End-stage renal disease in U.S. minority groups. *American Journal of Kidney Diseases, 19,* 397–410.

Flegal, K. M., Carroll, M. D., Kuczmarzki, R. J., & Johnson, C. L. (1998). Overweight and obesity in the United States: Prevalence and trends, 1960–1994. *International Journal of Obesity and Related Disorders, 22,* 39–47.

Flegal, K. M. et al. (1991). Prevalence of diabetes in Mexican Americans, Cubans, and Puerto Ricans from the Hispanic Health and Nutrition Examination Survey, 1982–1984. *Diabetes Care, 14,* 628–638.

Foreyt, J. P., Ramirez, A. G., & Cousins, J. H. (1991). *Cuidado el Corazón:* A weight-reduction intervention for Mexican Americans. *American Journal of Clinical Nutrition, 53,* Suppl. 6, 1369S–1641S.

Gillum, R. F. (1999). Distribution of waist-to-hip ratio, other indices of body fat distribution and obesity and associations with HDL cholesterol in children and young adults aged 4–19 years: The Third National Health and Nutrition Examination Survey. *International Journal of Obesity and Related Metabolic Disorders, 23,* 556–563.

Glucose tolerance and mortality: Comparison of WHO and American Diabetes Association criteria (1999). The Decode Study Group. European Diabetes Epidemiology Group. Diabetes Epidemiology: Collaborative analysis of diagnostic criteria in Europe. *Lancet, 354,* 610–611.

Haffner, S. M., Fong, D., Stern, M. P., Pugh, J. A., & Hazuda, H. P. (1988). Diabetic retinopathy in Mexican Americans and non-Hispanic Whites. *Diabetes, 37,* 878–874.

Haffner, S. M., Stern, M. P., Hazuda, H. P., Mitchell, B. D., & Patterson, J. K. (1989). Increased insulin concentrations in non-diabetic offspring of diabetic siblings. *Diabetes, 319,* 1297–1301.

Haffner, S. M., Stern, M. P., Mitchell, B. D., & Hazuda, H. P. (1991). Predictors of obesity in Mexican Americans. *American Journal of Clinical Nutrition, 53,* Suppl. 6, 1571S–1576S.

Hamman, R. F. et al. (1991). Microvascular complications of NIDDM in Hispanics and non-Hispanic Whites. San Luis Valle Diabetes Study. *Diabetes Care, 18,* 955–961.

Hanis, C. I., Chakraborty, R., Ferrell, R. E., & Schull, W. J. (1986). Individual admixture estimates: Disease associations an individual risk of diabetes and gallbladder disease among Mexican-Americans living in Starr County, Texas. *American Journal of Physical Anthropology, 70,* 433–441.

Harris, M. I. (1998). Diabetes in America: Epidemiology and scope of the problem. *Diabetes Care, 21,* Suppl. 3, C11–C14.

Harris M. I., Eastman, R., & Cowie, C. (1993). Symptoms of sensory neuropathy in adults with NIDDM in the U.S. population. *Diabetes Care, 16,* 1446–1452.

Harris, M. I., Eastman, R. C., Cowie, C. C., Flegal, K. M., & Eberhardt, M. S. (1997). Comparison of diabetes diagnostic categories in the U.S. population according to 1997 American Diabetes Association and 1980–1985 World Health Organization diagnostic criteria. *Diabetes Care, 20,* 1859–1862.

Harris, M. I. et al. (1998). Prevalence of diabetes, impaired fasting glucose, and impaired glucose tolerance in U.S. adults: The Third National Health and Nutrition Examination Survey, 1988–1994. *Diabetes Care, 21,* 518–524.

Holcomb, J. D., Lira, J., Kingery, P. M., Smith, D. W., Lane, D., & Goodway, J. (1998). Evaluation of Jump into Action: A program to reduce the risk of non-insulin dependent diabetes mellitus in school children on the Texas–Mexico Border. *Journal of School Health, 68,* 282–288.

Hollenbeck, C., & Reaven, G. M. (1987). Variations in insulin-stimulated glucose uptake in healthy individuals with normal glucose tolerance. *Journal of Clinical Endocrinology and Metabolism, 64,* 1169–1173.

Hone, J., Accili, D., Al-Gazali, L. I., Lestringant, G., Orban, T., & Taylor, S. I. (1994). Homozygosity for a new mutation (Ile$^{119}$→Met) in the insulin receptor gene in five sibs with familial insulin resistance. *Journal of Medical Genetics, 31,* 715–716.

Hovell, M. et al. (1991). Identification and correlates of physical activity among Latino adults. *Journal of Community Health, 16,* 23–36.

Hunt, L. M., Nedal, H. A., & Akana, L. L. (2000). Herbs, prayer, and insulin: Use of medical and alternative treatments in a group of Mexican American diabetes patients. *Journal of Family Practice, 49,* 216–223.

Keen, H. (1998). Impact of the new criteria for diabetes on pattern of disease. *Lancet, 352,* 1000–1001.

Khan, L. K., Sobal, J., & Martorelli, R. (1997). Acculturation, socioeconomic status, and obesity in Mexican Americans, Cuban Americans, and Puerto Ricans. *International Journal of Obesity and Related Metabolic Disorders, 21,* 91–96.

Kuczmarski, R. J., Flegal, K. M., Campbell, S. M., & Johnson, C. L. (1994). Increasing prevalence of overweight among U.S. adults: The National Health and Nutrition Examination Surveys, 1960 to 1991. *Journal of the American Medical Association, 272,* 205–211.

Lavery, L. A., Ashry, H. R., Van Houtum, W., Pugh, J. A., Harkless, L. B., & Basu, S. (1996). Variation in the incidence and proportion of diabetes-related amputations in minorities. *Diabetes Care, 19,* 48–52.

Loria, C. M. et al. (1995). Macronutrient intakes among adult Hispanics: A comparison of Mexican Americans, Cuban Americans, and Mainland Puerto Ricans. *American Journal of Public Health, 85,* 684–689.

Luchsinger, J. A., Tang, M. X., Stern, Y., Shea, S., & Mayeux, R. (2000). Diabetes and risk of Alzheimer's disease and dementia with stroke in a multiethnic cohort. Manuscript submitted for publication.

Marshall, J. A., Bessesen, D. H., & Hamman, R. F. (1997). High saturated fat and low starch and fibre are associated with hyperinsulinemia in a non-diabetic population: The San Luis Valley Diabetes Study. *Diabetologia, 40,* 430–438.

Marshall, J. A., Hamman, R. F., & Baxter, J. (1991). High-fat, low-carbohydrate diet and the etiology of non-insulin-dependent diabetes mellitus: The San Luis Valley Diabetes Study. *American Journal of Epidemiology, 134,* 590–603.

McKeigue, P. M. (1999). Ethnic variation in insulin resistance and risk of type II diabetes. In G. M. Reaven & A. Laws (Eds.), *Insulin resistance: The metabolic syndrome X.* Totowa, NJ: Humana Press.

McKenzie, T. L., Sallis, J. F., Nader, P. R., Broyles, S. L., & Nelson, J. A. (1992). Anglo and Mexican American preschoolers at home and at recess: Activity patterns and environmental influences. *Journal of Developmental and Behavioral Pediatrics, 13,* 173–180.

Mitchell, B. D. et al. (1996). Genetic and environmental contributions to cardiovascular risk factors in Mexican Americans: The San Antonio Family Heart Study. *Circulation, 94,* 2159–2170.

Mitchell, B. D. et al. (1995). Evidence for a major gene affecting post-challenge insulin levels in Mexican Americans. *Diabetes, 44,* 284–289.

Moore, L. L., Nguyen, U. S., Rothman, K. J., Cupples, L. A., & Ellison, R. C. (1995). Preschool physical activity level and change in body fatness in young children: The Framingham Children's Study. *American Journal of Epidemiology, 142,* 982–988.

Murphy, S. P., Castillo, R. O., Martorell, R., & Mendoza, F. (1990). An evaluation of food group intakes by Mexican-American children. *Journal of the American Dietetic Association, 90,* 388–393.

Must, A., Spadano, J., Coakley, E. H., Field, A. E., Colditz, G., & Dietz, W. H. (1999). The disease burden associated with overweight and obesity. *Journal of the American Medical Association, 282,* 1523–1529.

Nader, P. R. et al. (1989). A family approach to cardiovascular risk reduction: Results from the San Diego Family Health Project. *Health Education Quarterly, 16,* 229–244.

National Center for Health Statistics. (1999). *Healthy People 2000: Review, 1998–99.* Hyattsville, MD: Author. Retrieved August 2000 from: http://www.cdc.gov/nchs/data/hp2k99.pdf

National Center for Health Statistics. (2000). *Health, United States, 2000, with adolescent health chart book.* Hyattsville, MD: Author.

Newell, G. R., Borrud, L. G., McPherson, R. S., Nichaman, M. Z., & Pillow, P. C. (1988). Nutrient intakes of Whites, Blacks, and Mexican Americans in Southeast Texas. *Preventive Medicine, 17,* 622–633.

Ogden, C. L., Troiano, R. P., Briefel, R. R., Kuczmarski, R. J., Flegal, K. M., & Johnson, C. L. (1997). Prevalence of overweight among preschool children in the United States, 1971 through 1994. *Pediatrics, 99,* E1.

Otero-Sabogal, R., Sabogal, F., Pérez-Stable, E. J., & Hiatt, R. A. (1995). Dietary practices, alcohol consumption, and smoking behavior: Ethnic, sex and acculturation differences. *Journal of the National Cancer Institute Monographs, 18,* 73–82.

Pablos-Mendez, A., Blustein, J., & Knirsch, C. A. (1997). The role of diabetes mellitus in the higher prevalence of tuberculosis among Hispanics. *American Journal of Public Health, 87,* 574–579.

Ramirez, R. R. (2000). The Hispanic population of the United States: Population characteristics. *Current population reports.* Suitland, MD: United States Bureau of the Census. pp. 1–5. Retrieved August 2000 from: http://www.census.gov/pub/prod/2000pubs/p20-257.pdf

Ravussin, E. (1993). Energy metabolism in obesity: Studies in the Pima Indians. *Diabetes Care, 16,* 232–238.

Regensteiner, J. G. et al. (1991). Relationship between habitual physical activity and insulin levels among non-diabetic men and women: The San Luis Valley Diabetes Study. *Diabetes Care, 14,* 1066–1074.

Regensteiner, J. G. et al. (1995). Relationship between habitual physical activity an insulin area among individuals with impaired glucose tolerance: The San Luis Valley Diabetes Study. *Diabetes Care, 18,* 490–497.

Report of the Expert Committee on the Diagnosis and Classification of Diabetes Mellitus. (1997). *Diabetes Care, 20,* 1183–1197.

Rubin, R. J., Altman, W. M., & Mendelson, D. N. (1994). Health care expenditures for people with diabetes mellitus. *Journal of Clinical Endocrinology and Metabolism, 78,* 809A–809F.

Sallis, J. F., Patterson, T. L., Bouno, M. J., Atkins, C. J., & Nader, P. R. (1988). Aggregation of physical activity habits in Mexican-American and Anglo families. *Journal of Behavioral Medicine, 11,* 31–41.

Self-reported prevalence of diabetes among Hispanics: United States, 1994–1997, (1999). *MMWR [Morbidity and Mortality Weekly Report], 48,* 8–12.

Shea, S. et al. (1991). Independent associations of educational attainment and ethnicity with behavioral risk factors for cardiovascular disease. *American Journal of Epidemiology, 134,* 567–582.

Sherman, J. B., Alexander, M. A., Dean, A. H., & Kim, M. (1995). Obesity in Mexican-American and Anglo children. *Progress in Cardiovascular Nursing, 10,* 27–34.

Stern, M. P., Gaskill, S. P., Hazuda, H. P., Gardner, L. I., & Haffner, S. M. (1983). Does obesity explain excess prevalence of diabetes among Mexican Americans? *Diabetologia, 24,* 272–277.

Stern, M. P., & Mitchell, B. D. (1995). Diabetes in Hispanic Americans. In M. I. Harris, C. C. Cowie, M. P. Stern, E. J. Boyko, G. E. Reiber, & P. H. Bennett (Eds.), *Diabetes in America* (2nd ed.). Washington, D.C.: U.S. Department of Health and Human Services, National Institutes of Health (DHHS Publication No. [NIH] 95-1468).

Stern, M. P., & Mitchell, B. D. (1999). Genetics of insulin resistance. In G. M. Reaven & A. Laws (Eds.), *Insulin resistance: The metabolic syndrome X.* Totowa, NJ: Humana Press.

Thomas, P. R. (1995). *Weighing the options: Criteria for evaluating weight management programs.* Washington, D.C.: National Academy Press.

United Kingdom Prospective Diabetes Study [UKPDS] Group. (1998). Intensive blood-glucose control with sulphonylureas or insulin compared with conventional treatment and risk of complications in patients with type 2 diabetes (UKPDS 33). *Lancet, 352,* 839–855.

University Group Diabetes Program. (1970). A study of the effects of hypoglycemic agents on vascular complications on patients with adult-onset diabetes II: Mortality results. *Diabetes, 19,* Suppl. 2, 789–830.

United States Department of Health and Human Services, Public Health Service. (1988). *The Surgeon General's report on nutrition and health.* Washington, D.C.: Author.

United States Department of Health and Human Services, Public Health Service. (1991). *Healthy People 2000: National health promotion and disease prevention objectives.* Washington, D.C.: Author.

United States Department of Health and Human Services, Public Health Service. (1996). Patterns and trends in physical activity. In Physical activity and health. A report of the Surgeon General—Executive summary. Washington, D.C.: Author. Retrieved August 2000 from: http://www.cdc.gov.nccdphp/sgr/pdf/chap5.pdf

United States Department of Health and Human Services, Public Health Service. (1997, April 20). *Healthy People 2000: Progress review, Hispanic Americans.* Washington, D.C.: Author. Retrieved August 22, 2000 from: http://odphp.osophs.dhhs.gov/pubs/hp2000/PROG_RVW.HTM

United States Department of Health and Human Services, Public Health Service. (1998/99). Priority area 1: Physical activity and fitness. In *Healthy People 2000: Review,* pp. 29–37.

United States Department of Health and Human Services, Public Health Service. (2000). *Healthy People 2010* (Conference ed., in 2 vols.). Washington, D.C.: Author, pp. 1–3.

Vega, W. A., Sallis, J. F., Patterson, T., Rupp, J., Atkins, C., & Nader, P. R. (1987). Assessing knowledge of cardiovascular health-related diet and exercise behaviors in Anglo- and Mexican-Americans. *Preventive Medicine, 16,* 696–709.

Whitaker, R. C., Wright, J. A., Pepe, M. S., Seidel, K. D., & Dietz, W. H. (1997). Predicting obesity in young adulthood from childhood and parental obesity. *New England Journal of Medicine, 337,* 869–873.

Winkleby, M. A., Gardner, C. D., & Taylor, C. B. (1996). The influence of gender and socioeconomic factors on Hispanic/white differences in body-mass index. *Preventive Medicine, 25,* 203–211.

World Health Organization. (1997, June 3–5). *Obesity: Preventing and managing the global epidemic.* Geneva: Author.

Zaldivar, A., & Smolowitz, J. (1994). Perception of the importance place on religion and folk medicine by non-Mexican-American Hispanic adults with diabetes. *Diabetes Educator, 20,* 303–306.

Zhang, Y. Y. et al. (1994). Positional cloning of the mouse obese gene and its human homolog. *Nature, 372,* 425–432.

CHAPTER ELEVEN

# GENDER, CONTEXT, AND HIV PREVENTION AMONG LATINOS

Hortensia Amaro, Rodolfo R. Vega, and Dellanira Valencia

In order to understand the significant impact of HIV/AIDS among Latinos and approaches to prevention, we need to be cognizant of the context and circumstances in which their lives are embedded in the United States (Amaro, 1995; Sweat & Denison, 1995; Tawil, Verster, & O'Reilly, 1995). Current prevention practices have not been successful in curtailing the rising rates of HIV infection among U.S. Latinos and African Americans.

The number of cumulative AIDS cases among minorities reported since 1981 now exceeds the cumulative total among Whites (Centers for Disease Control and Prevention, 2000). Moreover, while Latinos comprise only 13 percent of the continental U.S. population, they represent 18 percent of cumulative AIDS cases (Centers for Disease Control and Prevention, 1999b). While in the White population, the estimated adult and adolescent AIDS incidence decreased sharply from 1996 to 1998 (from 21,191 to 13,839), the estimated decrease in number of new AIDS cases among Latinos (from 26,479 to 21,065 cases) is much smaller (Centers for Disease Control and Prevention, 1999b). Latinas now represent 20 percent of females ever diagnosed with AIDS and have an AIDS case rate that is strikingly higher (16.6 per 1,000) than that of White females (2.4 per 1,000) (Centers for Disease Control and Prevention, 1999b). Latino males represent 18 percent of males ever diagnosed with AIDS and have a significantly higher case rate (58.2) than that of White males (17.8) (Centers for Disease Control and Prevention, 1999b). Cumulative AIDS cases among Latino children and youth ages zero to nineteen represent 32.2 percent of all cases in this age group (Centers for Disease Control and Prevention, 1999b). Within this younger age group, there is a near 1:1 male-to-female ratio of AIDS cases (1,501 cases in boys and 1,200 cases in girls).

Reported routes of transmission among adult and adolescent women ever diagnosed with AIDS indicate that heterosexual transmission (47 percent) and injection drug use are the primary route of infection (28 percent) (Centers for Disease Control and Prevention, 1999b) for Latinas. Among Latino adolescents and men, male-to-male sexual transmission (41 percent) and injection drug use (12 percent) account for the major routes of transmission, whereas heterosexual contact accounts for a small proportion of cases (6 percent) (Centers for Disease Control and Prevention, 1999b).

AIDS case rates among Latinos are highest in such northeastern states as New York, Connecticut, Pennsylvania, Rhode Island, and Delaware, as well as in Puerto Rico (Centers for Disease Control and Prevention, 1999b). Furthermore, Puerto Rico has a female AIDS case rate (27.6) that is significantly higher than that for the general U.S. population (9.6) (Centers for Disease Control and Prevention, 1999b). While the CDC does not report AIDS case data by Latino subgroups, data on birthplace of persons with AIDS indicate that 71 percent of Latinos with AIDS were born outside the continental United States, with 55 percent of these born in Puerto Rico and 21 percent born in Mexico (Centers for Disease Control and Prevention, 1999b).

In this chapter, we review evidence on risk factor indicators and outcomes of prevention studies among Latinas and Latino men. We discuss implications for HIV prevention among the Latino population.

## HIV-Related Sex and Drug Risk Behaviors

This section reviews existing evidence on risk behaviors among Latinas and factors that seem to influence these behaviors.

General population studies of condom use with primary partners among both female and male respondents have consistently reported low level of use across all race and ethnic groups (Gómez & Marín, 1996; Harrison et al., 1991; Sabogal & Catania, 1996). However, Latinos have the lowest rates (Catania et al., 1994; Marín, Tschann, Gómez, & Kegeles, 1993; He, McCoy, Stevens, & Stark, 1998). Few studies have investigated Latino subgroup differences in condom use.

Even in the face of clear risk, one study found that nearly half of Latina women reported that they would not use condoms with a primary partner who was HIV positive (Harrison et al., 1991). In a study of female partners of male injection and noninjection drug users, He, McCoy, Stevens, and Stark (1998) found that Latinas, especially Mexican American women, had the lowest rates of condom use compared to those of Whites, African Americans, and other races or ethnic groups.

While studies indicate that Latinas have fewer sex partners compared to women in other ethnic groups (Romero, Wyatt, Chin, & Rodriguez, 1998; Flaskerud, Uman, Lara, Romero, & Taka, 1996; Marín, Tschann, Gómez, & Kegeles, 1993), they may be at elevated risk for HIV infection because Latino men are more likely than non-Latino men to have multiple sex partners, both men and women, outside of their primary relationships (Choi, Catania, & Dolcini, 1994; Romero-Daza, Weeks, & Singer, 1998; Peragallo, 1996; Arguelles & Rivero, 1988). While the prevalence is not known, there are indications that at least some Latino men who have sex with men also have sex with women (Doll, Petersen, White, Johnson, Ward, & the Blood Donor Study Group, Centers for Disease Control and Prevention, 1992) and that bisexual men tend to engage in anal sex with their female partners, a behavior with significant risk for transmission (Gavey & McPhillips, 1997). Stigma related to male–male sex further places some women at risk because their partners are unlikely to disclose their sexual behavior (Flaskerud, Uman, Lara, Romero, & Taka, 1996; Peragallo, 1996).

The degree to which Latinas are involved in the commercial sex trade is not well documented. However, Latinas' poverty and socioeconomic stagnation (Romero-Daza, Weeks, & Singer, 1998) may place them at increased risk of prostitution. Vulnerability for HIV and STD infection increases drastically when sex trade occurs in unregulated environments such as street prostitution, or when the trade occurs because of a drug habit (Khabbaz et al., 1990; Albert, Warner, Hatcher, Trussell, & Bennett, 1995) in which the need for drugs may be a stronger immediate motivator than safer sex practices (Romero-Daza, Weeks, & Singer, 1998; Arguelles & Rivero, 1988).

Drug use also increases the risk of infection through sharing unclean needles, a behavior still prominent among the majority of women injection drug users (Stevens, Estrada, & Estrada, 1998). Compared to African American and White injection drug users, Puerto Rican men and women and Mexican American women had the highest levels of drug-related risks due to one or more of the following: they injected drugs at a greater frequency than did the other groups; they attended "shooting galleries" and/or shared needles; and they had male partners who also were drug users (Sufian, Friedman, Neaigus, Stepherson, Rivers-Beckman, & Des Jarlais, 1990).

Furthermore, use of other drugs such as crack cocaine reduces inhibition and has been shown to increase sexual activity (Romero-Daza, Weeks, & Singer, 1998) as well as influence risky sexual behavior (Inciardi, Lockwood, & Pottieger, 1993). Injection and noninjection drug use may impede decision making (whether to use a condom) during sexual intercourse as well as decrease the efficacy of the condom (Stevens, Ruiz, Romero, & Gama, 1995; Marín, Gómez, Tschann, & Gregorich, 1997). Levels of sex-related risk among women drug users do not seem to vary by racial and ethnic groups (Stevens, Ruiz, Romero, & Gama, 1998).

# Factors Associated with Sexual Risk Behaviors Among Latinas

The late Jonathan Mann (1991), past director of the World Health Organization's AIDS Office, observed that "[e]pidemiology has thus far not succeeded in providing sufficiently powerful understanding of the behavioral determinants of high-risk sexual behavior. Behaviors associated with sexual transmission of HIV are now being linked, at least conceptually, with issues of empowerment, social and economic status, education and age and sex roles" (p. 12). His observation reflects what Latino community-based providers have been pointing out for many years—that risk of HIV infection takes place within a larger social context that is shaped by how gender, race and ethnicity, and class are defined, how resources are allocated, and how scientific activities are carried out. Yet, even a decade after Mann's observations, most HIV prevention research does not pay sufficient attention to these contextual factors.

Most research on HIV risk has focused on individual-based factors stemming from the person-centered tenets of learning theory. This framework has greatly favored investigation of cognitive-level factors (that is, knowledge, attitudes, beliefs, and motivations), rather than social and structural influences that shape risk (that is, broader social arrangements related to social, legal, and economic factors; relational aspects of sexuality). While individual level characteristics have been useful in illuminating HIV risk, they are limited in accounting for the strong external forces that determine risk.

For Latinos as well as other groups highly affected by HIV, broader sociostructural factors create a set of life conditions that frame the nature of women's HIV risk. Social inequalities (for example, inequities in pay, discrimination based on gender, and gender role inequalities in relationships) lie at the heart of HIV risks for women, especially poor, Latina, and African American women (Amaro, 1995; Amaro & Raj, in press; Zierler & Krieger, 1997). Racism, sexism, and classism all work in intricate ways to oppress and sustain those who are already marginalized into more extreme conditions.

Poor Latinas who are recent immigrants in particular often face more survival-related issues in their daily lives (namely, unemployment, lack of food or shelter for self or children, living in areas with high crime or violence, or fear of deportation), especially when they are undocumented. Therefore, HIV risk may not be as high priority an issue as other more salient factors (Romero, Wyatt, Chin, & Rodriguez, 1998; Arguelles & Rivero, 1988; Romero & Arguelles, 1993). Their situation is exacerbated further because of inaccurate HIV information, language barriers, new cultural norms, and fear of deportation, all of which decrease a women's chances of seeking health treatment and prevention information (Gómez, Hernández, & Faigeles, 1999). It is important to note that there are very few studies available on this population of Latinas, especially those who are undocumented. Because of their social and economic marginalization, research on their HIV risk is especially needed.

Age has been found to be an important correlate of risk behaviors and associated factors. Younger women tend to show higher rates of condom use, may be more comfortable with sexual communication, show higher levels of HIV/AIDS knowledge, and are less likely to expect negative reactions from partners upon request to use a condom (Moore, Harrison, Kay, Deren, & Doll, 1995; Fleisher, Senie, Minkoff, & Jaccard, 1994; Deren, Shedlin, & Beardsley, 1996; Gómez, Hernández, & Faigeles, 1999; Organista, Organista, Garcia de Alba, Castillo

Moran, & Ureta Carrillo, 1997; Carmona, Romero, & Loeb, 1999). However, age in these studies is often confounded with length of time in the relationship, which has been associated with condom use (Deren, Shedlin, & Beardsley, 1996; Fleisher, Senie, Minkoff, & Jaccard, 1994; Moore, Harrison, Kay, Deren, & Doll, 1995). In a study of sexually active African American and Latina women residing in the Northeast, Fleisher and colleagues (1994) showed that younger women had higher rates of condom use but also had higher rates of infections with sexually transmitted diseases (STDs), suggesting that they may be using condoms incorrectly or not using them for every sexual encounter.

AIDS knowledge alone has not been found to be related to sexual risk behaviors among women (Nyamathi, Bennett, Leake, Lewis, & Flaskerud, 1993; Sikkema et al., 1995; Gil, 1998), although it is an important and necessary precursor to behavior change (Wyatt, Vargas Carmona, Burns Loeb, Guthrie, & Gordon, 2000). While Latinos have evidenced an increase in *knowledge* regarding the known routes of transmission, they continue to have greater misconceptions about HIV transmission compared to other racial and ethnic groups (Aruffo, Coverdale, & Vallabona, 1991; Romero, Wyatt, Chin, & Rodriguez, 1998; Flaskerud, Uman, Lara, Romero, & Taka, 1996; Harrison et al., 1991). Studies have consistently found that other factors beyond knowledge are important predictors of condom use. These are discussed in the rest of this section.

Women's attitudes toward condoms are significant predictors of condom use with their primary and other sex partners (Catania, Kegeles, & Coates, 1992; Gielen, Faden, O'Campo, Kass, & Anderson, 1994; Raj & Pollack, 1995; Sikkema et al., 1995). This is an important finding as positive attitudes toward condoms are not common among Latina women (Marín & Gómez, 1997; Worth, 1989) and these attitudes are related to lower rates of use (Gómez & Marín, 1996; Gil, 1998). Compared to other racial and ethnic groups, Latinos have more negative *attitudes* toward condoms because of their association with illness, prostitution, and emotional distance (Peragallo, 1996; Marín, Tschann, Gómez, & Kegeles, 1993).

Perception of risk has been considered to be an important predictor of condom use. Nyamathi and colleagues (1993) found that Latinas who perceived themselves at high risk for infection were ten times more likely to have multiple partners and approximately seven times more likely to be injection drug users compared to the women who expressed no concerns. Some authors have suggested that compared to other racial and ethnic groups, Latinos are less likely to believe that they could do something to prevent HIV/AIDS (Marín, Tschann, Gómez, & Kegeles, 1993) even when there is clear evidence of risk (Deren, Shedlin, & Beardsley, 1996). Some studies indicate that low-income ethnic minority women who are at high risk for HIV infection due to their behaviors or those of their partners are significantly more likely to engage in condom use and get tested for HIV (Fleisher, Senie, Minkoff, & Jaccard, 1994; Gielen, Faden, O'Campo, Kass, & Anderson, 1994; Heckman et al., 1996; Wagstaff et al., 1995). However, these findings also suggest that women in monogamous relationships report significantly lower HIV risk perceptions and are less likely to engage in safer sex practices.

A woman's perception of risk seems to vary greatly by *type of relationship*, wherein women perceive steady partners as less risky and casual partners or partners of shorter duration as higher risk; therefore, they are less likely to use condoms in longer or more committed relationships (Misovich, Fisher, & Fisher, 1997; Doval, Duran, O'Donnell, & O'Donnell, 1995; Flaskerud, Uman, Lara, Romero, & Taka, 1996; Romero, Wyatt, Chin, & Rodriguez, 1998; Castañeda, 2000; Gutierrez, Oh, & Gillmore, 2000; Deren, Shedlin, & Beardsley, 1996; Moore, Harrison, Kay, Deren, & Doll, 1995). Due to the stigmatization attached to condom use as a tool for casual sex, some Latinas may opt *not* to promote condom use rather than risk conflict with their male partners (Miller, Bettencourt, DeBro, & Hoffman, 1993). Further, a primary goal for women is relationship establishment (Holland, Ramazanoglu, Scott, Sharpe, & Thompson, 1992; Miller, 1986), and they may not want to introduce condom use, which is associated with casual relationships, into their sexual encounters with a potential long-term partner.

Some evidence suggests that Latinas may have low perceived personal risk because they themselves may not be engaging in high-risk behaviors (Harrison et al., 1991; Arguelles & Rivero, 1988). Perceived risk, however, is not always a true reflection of risk; some relationships that women believe to be safe are not, as male partners may be engaging in sex outside the relationship or they may be practicing unsafe injection drug use without the woman's knowledge (Misovich, Fisher, & Fisher, 1997). Other women who suspect or know that sex with their current partner is risky may choose to have unsafe sex because they desire a committed relationship and condoms represent casual sexual encounters to them (Wingood & DiClemente, 1997). However, much of the existing research in this area is not specific to Latinos and is not informative on how Latinos specifically may view issues of intimacy and condom use.

One of the main motivations for condom use among Latinos is pregnancy prevention (Fleisher, Senie, Minkoff, & Jaccard, 1994; Romero, Wyatt, Chin, & Rodriguez, 1998; Flaskerud, Uman, Lara, Romero, & Taka, 1996; Gómez & Marín, 1996), which is a stronger motivator than prevention of sexually transmitted diseases (Fleisher, Senie, Minkoff, & Jaccard, 1994; Gómez & Marín, 1996). Latinas who use condoms to prevent pregnancy may be more likely to use condoms more consistently than those who use condoms for HIV or STD prevention alone; however, a study of low-income Mexican American women found that married women who may not have this motivation feel that they have less control over condom use (Fleisher, Senie, Minkoff, & Jaccard, 1994; Flaskerud, Uman, Lara, Romero, & Taka, 1996). These findings indicate that when women think about sexual protection they think of contraception and not generally of HIV or STD prevention.

Acculturation, the process of adaptation and transition to a host society's norms, beliefs, and behaviors, has been noted to be a difficult and vulnerable period for many poor Latina immigrants (Padilla & Salgado de Snyder, 1992), and a number of studies have explored its relationship to HIV risk behaviors. Highly acculturated Latinas have been found to have more sex partners (Flaskerud,

Uman, Lara, Romero, & Taka, 1996; Sabogal & Catania, 1996; Carmona, Romero, & Loeb, 1999; Hines & Caetano, 1998), but they are also more likely to use and carry condoms (Marín, Tschann, Gómez, & Kegeles, 1993) and use condoms more frequently with primary and nonprimary partners (Sabogal & Catania, 1996). The actual role of acculturation in HIV risk is likely to be complex as other studies indicate that traditional cultural norms may serve as buffers for HIV risk factors.

In recognition that condom use is not under a woman's control, some authors have begun to explore the influence of gender roles in women's HIV risk and condom use. Traditional gender role norms ascribed to Latino cultures present Latina women as submissive, self-sacrificing, dependent, and obedient to husbands and other males, and also dedicated totally to motherhood (Comas-Diaz, 1996; Peragallo, 1996). On the other hand, some authors claim that Latino men have been characterized as dominant, distant, and removed from their roles as fathers despite rather inconclusive data supporting these characterizations (De la Cancela, 1996). Based on these ascriptions, some authors have suggested that these roles may contribute to Latinas' unawareness that their partners may be engaging in high-risk behaviors (Arguelles & Rivero, 1988; Marín, 1989). However, adherence to traditional gender roles may decrease with acculturation, as American culture is more permissive of female sexual attitudes (Sabogal, Faigeles, & Catania, 1993) and may give women more sexual freedom, which may reduce or increase risk. Little empirical research exists on the actual adherence to these cultural characterizations of Latinos and how adherence to such gender role norms may affect HIV risk behavior.

It is clear that the power relationship in Latino couples (Mikawa, Morones, Gómez, Olsen, & Gonzalez-Huss, 1992; Pulerwitz, Gortmaker, & De Jong, 2000; Romero, Wyatt, Chin, & Rodriguez, 1998; Peragallo, 1996) and fear of speaking to a partner affect condom use (Gómez & Marín, 1996). However, it is not clear whether modifications of gender role norms occur among Latinos and whether the distribution of various gender roles differ significantly across racial and ethnic groups once socioeconomic differences are controlled. Support for the idea that gender role norms are not monolithic among Latinos comes from studies that indicate that some Latino men are willing to use condoms but fear that their partners will think they are being unfaithful (Doval, Duran, O'Donnell, & O'Donnell, 1995); others are willing to use condoms when given the opportunity to participate in family planning decisions (Riehman, Sly, Soler, Eberstein, Quadagno, & Harrison, 1998). Existing research demonstrates the great need to examine gender role norms and behaviors among diverse Latino populations and how these affect HIV risk behaviors and risk among Latina women.

Further complications in safer sex negotiation arise for women out of their perceptions of their male partner's views about condoms. Some evidence indicates that men are more likely than women to have negative views about condoms and are more likely to view them as interfering with sexual pleasure (Marín,

Tschann, Gómez, & Kegeles, 1993); it is also known that a partner's willingness to use condoms is a major predictor of condom use reported by women (Fleisher, Senie, Minkoff, & Jaccard, 1994; Amaro et al., 1998; Moore, Harrison, Kay, Deren, & Doll, 1995). Thus, women who accurately or inaccurately perceive their partners as having negative attitudes toward condom use are less likely to discuss or be successful in condom use.

Women who feel able to communicate with their partners about HIV and sexual matters (Catania et al., 1994; Heckman et al., 1996; Quina, Harlow, Morokoff, Burkholder, & Deiter, 2000) and those who believe they could refuse unsafe sex with their partners (Sikkema et al., 1995) are more likely to have engaged in condom use with their partners. For this reason, condom use and communication skills training are commonly used as strategies in HIV prevention (Carey, Maisto, Kalichman, Forsyth, Wright, & Johnson, 1997; DiClemente & Wingood, 1995; Hobfoll, Jackson, Lavin, Britton, & Shepherd, 1994; Kalichman, Rompa, & Coley, 1996; Kelly et al., 1994). Having the power within a relationship to negotiate sexual behaviors is likely to support women's perceived self-efficacy in condom use. However, when cultural norms and social status ascribed to women preempt a woman's power to communicate or negotiate condom use, self-efficacy is more difficult to maintain (Amaro, 1995; Gómez & Marín, 1996; Pulerwitz, Gortmaker, & De Jong, 2000).

Some women may perceive themselves to be at risk but hold little actual control over their ability to engage in risk reduction behaviors. For example, being in an abusive relationship and having a history of victimization have been linked to subsequent HIV risk factors, including involvement in sex trade, multiple partnering, casual sexual encounters, risky sex partners, teen pregnancy, substance use, and low condom use (Zierler, Feingold, Laufer, Velentgas, Kantrowitz-Gordon, & Mayer, 1991; Cunningham, Stiffman, & Dore, 1994; He, McCoy, Stevens, & Stark, 1998; Romero-Daza, Weeks, & Singer, 1998; Kilpatrick, Resnick, Saunders, & Best, 1998; Gómez & Marín, 1996; Pulerwitz, Gortmaker, & De Jong, 2000; Martin, 1997). Clearly, there are many areas of overlap within these risk factors. Women's violent experiences with sex (that is, rape or coerced sexual relations), which may occur within their relationships, often increases the possibility of unsafe sex, and heightens the risk of HIV infection (Zierler & Krieger, 1997). Moreover, because Latinas tend to have low rates of condom use (Marín, Tschann, Gómez, & Kegeles, 1993; Harrison et al., 1991), engaging in other risky sexual behavior exacerbates their risk. Even if Latinas in these relationships manage to communicate HIV-related concerns to partners, that does not indicate an increase in condom use (Deren, Shedlin, & Beardsley, 1996; He, McCoy, Stevens, & Stark, 1998).

In addition, the social and psychological isolation that comes from victimization by male partners may be higher among illegal immigrants. Being undocumented may increase a woman's vulnerability to abuse, as many women face isolation from their families, have language barriers, may stay with males regardless of the way they are treated (Arguelles & Rivero, 1988), and may be afraid of seeking help for fear of deportation.

# Latino Men

Having thus far reviewed important themes related to Latino women, we now turn our attention to salient issues relevant to the lives of Latino men in the United States in relation to the AIDS epidemic. These issues include knowledge of HIV, the roles of acculturation and immigration, cultural values, gender roles, oppression, discrimination, and finally the prevalence of risk factors such as substance abuse and sexually transmitted diseases. Recognition of these important factors will inform the context in which prevention interventions with Latinos are implemented.

## Knowledge of HIV/AIDS

A recent survey on U.S. Latinos and HIV (Kaiser Family Foundation, 1998) revealed that both Latino men and women have knowledge about how HIV is transmitted, yet they also continue to hold misconceptions such as the availability of a vaccine and the existence of a cure for AIDS. Latinos also reported that they would like to receive more information about condom use and HIV testing, and that they want to talk with their partners about sex and about the need for HIV testing.

In a longitudinal study that included a total of 1,290 male participants ages twenty-two to twenty-six, Bradner, Ku, and Duberstein-Lindberg (2000) found that young Latino and African American men tend to receive more HIV/AIDS prevention messages than do young White men. However, the study points out that Latino men receive their HIV/AIDS information mostly from social sources such as the radio rather than from public health interventions or medical providers. This fact confirms what community-based agencies have long acknowledged: the importance of TV and radio outlets as venues of information dissemination for this population. In a social context in which Latinos are isolated from formal structures such as schools, health care providers, and other institutions, the radio becomes the medium of choice for effective outreach.

## Sexual Risk Behavior

National health surveillance reports provide a comprehensive portrayal of Latino men's risk behavior for HIV/AIDS. For example, cumulative estimates from the latest Centers for Disease Control and Prevention HIV/AIDS surveillance report (1999b) reveal that male–male sex is the largest exposure category among Latino men (43 percent), followed by injection drug use (IDU) (36 percent) and heterosexual contact (7 percent). Latinos were similar to African American males but four times more likely than Whites to report IDU as the source of exposure.

The impact of IDU on HIV transmission among members of the Latino community has been corroborated in studies using community cohorts that consistently find that IDU is more frequent among Latino men than among any other ethnic or racial group (Estrada, 1998; Deren et al., 1998; Freeman, Williams, & Saunders, 1999; Singer, 1999). Negative effects of IDU behavior may be augmented by environmental constraints. For example, Puerto Ricans, who inject drugs at higher rates than other Latinos, tend to do so in high-risk settings in which sterile equipment and cleaning materials are scarce (Freeman, Williams, & Saunders, 1999). Data from the National Behavioral Survey showed (Sabogal, Faigeles, & Catania, 1993; Sabogal, Pérez-Stable, Otero-Sabogal, & Hiatt, 1995) that among Latino men, those that were Cuban, unmarried, aged eighteen to nineteen, better educated, and had lower income, reported higher numbers of sexual partners. In comparison to Whites, Latino men generally had a comparable number of sexual partners in a lifetime. However, in the year prior to the survey, Latino men reported higher frequency of sex and that sex was initiated at an earlier age. The National Behavioral Survey, however, also showed that acculturation was related to sexual behavior. Highly acculturated Latinos reported a higher number of sexual partners, more sexual intercourse during the previous year, and sexual intercourse at an earlier age than their less acculturated counterparts (Sabogal, Faigeles, & Catania, 1993; Sabogal, Pérez-Stable, Otero-Sabogal, & Hiatt, 1995). The role of acculturation on sexual behavior changes among Latino males has seldom been empirically examined. The few studies that have examined it have yielded inconclusive results. Some studies have observed a positive relation between acculturation and sexual risk behavior (Peragallo, 1996; Marks, Cantero, & Simoni, 1998), whereas others suggest a negative relation (Marín & Marín, 1992).

Inconsistent findings between acculturation and behavioral indicators are not uncommon and could be attributed to a myriad of methodological and conceptual factors (see Rogler, Cortés, & Malgady, 1991, for an extensive discussion). The inclusion of other contextual factors in the research framework may reveal a more complex relation between acculturation and risk behavior. For example, Marín and colleagues (1997) showed that acculturation is not directly related to condom use. In their study, acculturation was inversely related to traditional gender roles. Latino males upholding traditional gender role beliefs—that is, low-acculturated Latinos—were less comfortable sexually and more sexually coercive. Greater sexual comfort and lower levels of sexual coercion were positively related to self-efficacy, which in turn had a direct influence upon condom use.

## Risk Behaviors Among Latino Male Adolescents

As of June 1999, the CDC reported 19,484 AIDS cases among Latino males ages twenty-two to twenty-nine (Centers for Disease Control and Prevention, 2000). This figure not only represents 18 percent of the AIDS cases among Latino males but is higher than the percentage of AIDS cases of similar ages among African American males (15 percent) and Whites (16 percent). Because of the long incubating period of HIV, a significant portion of the adolescent AIDS cases may have become infected during adolescence.

Substance abuse behavior, alcohol drinking, age of sexual initiation, and condom use may contribute to the high prevalence of AIDS among young Latino men. Moreover, being under the influence of alcohol or drugs may directly affect condom use, making individuals less likely to use a condom and more likely to use them incorrectly (Raj, Silverman, & Amaro, 2000; Inciardi, Lockwood, & Pottieger, 1993).

Data from the Youth Risk Behavior Surveillance (Centers for Disease Control and Prevention, 1999c) show that Latino and White adolescents reported similar rates of current alcohol use, lifetime alcohol use, and episodic heavy drinking than those of their African American counterparts (see Table 11.1). Rates of lifetime and current marijuana use among Latino adolescents were higher than those among White adolescents but lower than those reported for African American adolescents. However, those differences across all three groups were not statistically significant. Current marijuana use was higher for adolescent males across all three ethnic groups. Finally, Latino adolescents were more likely than White and African American adolescents to use cocaine in their lifetime.

Latino adolescents also appeared to initiate alcohol and drug use at a younger age. A higher percentage of Latino adolescents reported drinking alcohol, marijuana use, and cocaine use before age thirteen than of White and African American adolescents.

Regarding sexual initiation, Latino adolescents (7.7 percent) were significantly more likely than White adolescents (4.0 percent) to experience sexual intercourse before age thirteen but significantly less likely than African American adolescents (21.7 percent). About 15.5 percent of Latino adolescents have had four or more partners during their lifetime. This total is significantly lower than the

## TABLE 11.1. ALCOHOL AND DRUG USE AMONG LATINO, AFRICAN AMERICAN, AND WHITE ADOLESCENTS (YOUTH RISK BEHAVIOR SURVEILLANCE).

| Substance Use | Latino (Percent) | African American (Percent) | White (Percent) |
|---|---|---|---|
| Lifetime alcohol use | 83.1 | 73.0 | 81.3 |
| Current alcohol use | 53.9 | 36.9 | 54.0 |
| Episodic heavy drinking | 34.9 | 16.1 | 37.3 |
| Lifetime marijuana use | 49.5 | 52.2 | 45.4 |
| Current marijuana use | 28.6 | 28.2 | 25.0 |
| Lifetime cocaine use | 16.1 | 2.9 | 8.5 |
| Onset of substance use before age 13: | | | |
| Alcohol | 37.9 | 33.1 | 28.8 |
| Marijuana | 13.2 | 11.0 | 7.5 |
| Cocaine | 1.4 | 0.4 | 0.9 |

*Source:* Adapted from Centers for Disease Control and Prevention (1999c).

percentage of African American students reporting four or more partners (38.5 percent) and significantly higher than the percentage of White students (11.6 percent). Similarly, Latino adolescents (52.2 percent) were less likely than African American adolescents (72.7 percent) but significantly more likely than White adolescents (43.6 percent) to report ever having sexual intercourse. It should be noted that with regard to sexual behavior, male and female Latino students reported a similar pattern of behavior (that is, male respondents reported higher rates of sexual behavior than those of female students, and the relation between ethnic groups remained the same).

Latinos (48.3 percent) were less likely than White (55.8 percent) and African American students (64 percent) to have used condoms during their last sexual intercourse. The difference in condom use between Whites and Latinos was not significant. About one in five African Americans and one in four Whites and Latinos reported alcohol or drug use at the last sexual intercourse. No significant differences across all three groups were observed.

## The Role of STD Prevalence Among Latino Males

Sexually transmitted diseases have a strong epidemiological association with the HIV epidemic (Devita, Hellman, & Rosenberg, 1997; Centers for Disease Control and Prevention, 1998a). Individuals with STDs are two to five times more likely to be at risk for HIV infection. Early detection and treatment of non-HIV STDs have been identified as an effective strategy for HIV prevention (Centers for Disease Control and Prevention, 1998a).

The latest STD surveillance report indicates that Latino males have STD rates per 100,000 of 129.6 for chlamydia, of 73.5 for gonorrhea, and of 313 for syphilis (Centers for Disease Control and Prevention, 1998b). These totals are higher than those of their White male counterparts for chlamydia and gonorrhea but not for syphilis. White males reported STD rates per 100,000 of 29.6 for chlamydia, 21.3 for gonorrhea, and 531 for syphilis. African American males had significantly higher prevalence rates per 100,000 than those of Latino or White males: for chlamydia, 403.9; for gonorrhea, 943.9; and for primary and secondary syphilis, 3,001. It should be noted that the CDC obtains surveillance data from state and local health departments. Since Latinos and African Americans tend to use public facilities more often, this reporting bias may increase ethnic and racial differences in STD rates.

## Gender Roles: Machismo

For Latino men in the United States, the idea of the masculine is the by-product of a multitude of social, cultural, economic, and contextual factors (for example, characteristics prescribed by their culture of origin, the context of migration, and the new culture's exemplars of masculinity), as well as the social inequalities the vast majority of Latinos face in the new society.

In the context of the U.S. society, Latinos encounter an ideal of masculinity that promotes aggressiveness, independence, emotional resiliency, achievement, status, and avoidance of the feminine (David & Brannon, 1976). Masculinity and its by-products have important influence on sexual risk behavior. For example, among a representative sample of adolescent boys, which included Latino, African American, and White young men, Pleck, Sonenstein, & Ku (1993) found that scores on a validated scale of masculinity ideology were significantly associated with HIV-risk-related sexual behavior. Young men who held highly traditional attitudes toward the male gender role were significantly more likely than others to have negative attitudes toward condoms and use them less often; have more sexual partners; believe that male–female relationships are adversarial in nature; and believe that getting a girl pregnant is a sign of their masculinity. These findings suggest that male gender role norms and beliefs are relevant risk factors for all groups, not just Latino men.

Another important context that interfaces with the idea of the masculine is the migration process. For many Latinos, the process of migration has the potential for altering basic conceptual and behavioral constructions of masculinity. The process of migration generally involves three major changes: (1) the experience of cultural changes; (2) changes in socioeconomic structures; and (3) disruption of interpersonal networks. All three are potential sources of distress (Rogler, 1994). Upon arriving to the United States, many Latinos are confronted with cultural and behavioral norms different from those in their country of origin; for example, they encounter a social milieu that tends to favor a more egalitarian man–woman relationship.

In the new country, changes in socioeconomic structures usually translate into occupational and social downward mobility (Leslie & Leitch, 1989; Pérez, 1998), particularly when immigrants lack English proficiency and when discriminatory practices impede them from obtaining well-paying jobs. In addition, the migratory move cuts interpersonal relationships that provided social support in the country of origin. The impact of these three migration-related changes upon the Latino masculine ideal can be overwhelmingly detrimental.

Latino men also encounter a sociocultural and legal environment that prescribes equal rights and opportunities for women. They face a milieu in which ethnicity is more salient than gender identity. Therefore, among ethnic minorities, being a "man" does not always translate into social or economic opportunities. These changes set the conditions for the emergence of what Pleck (1995) calls gender role discrepancy conflicts. For example, Latino males find themselves being challenged by a system that does not necessarily recognize the social power they derived in their culture of origin by virtue of their sex. These challenges may lead them to believe that it is not possible to attain their idea of the masculine as they knew it, and their subsequent frustration translates into behaviors that put them at risk for HIV (for example, abuse of alcohol, tobacco, or other drugs [ATOD], promiscuous behavior, or domestic violence).

## Programs That Work

The *Compendium of HIV Prevention Interventions with Evidence of Effectiveness,* developed by the Centers for Disease Control and Prevention (1999a) HIV/AIDS Research Synthesis Project, is one of the most significant efforts in identifying prevention programs, tools, and mechanisms to address the HIV/AIDS epidemic. In developing the *Compendium,* the authors first identified 216 behavioral intervention studies that met relevance criteria such as having a positive behavioral outcome. Of those 216 intervention studies, 126 met methodological criteria that varied by type of intervention. Of these twenty-four intervention studies represent the "best state-of-the-science interventions available as of June 30, 1998" (pp. 4–6).

The *Compendium* is meant to serve as a useful planning guide for institutions and communities that intend to develop and implement HIV intervention activities. However, the *Compendium* has a number of limitations in its use as a guide for prevention with Latinos. Most, if not all, studies selected in the *Compendium* were guided by learning theories, and they tell us that for the most part the interventions were effective in producing behavioral change. The *Compendium,* however, does not report differential effects of ethnicity and gender. Because none of these interventions were provided in Spanish, it is not clear whether they would be effective (even if translated) with monolingual Spanish speakers, recent immigrants, or less acculturated Latinos. The studies highlighted in the *Compendium* represent the "best science" on HIV prevention. It is clear that our "best science" has largely left out Latinos and that it can provide us with little empirical basis for specific HIV prevention with Latinos. Glaring gaps in the literature make evident the need for empirical studies on the effectiveness of HIV prevention strategies that (1) are geared toward Latinos; (2) are contextual in nature; (3) include the contexts of oppression and gender; and (4) incorporate important ingredients of culture and gender role norms and practices in the design, development, and implementation of preventive intervention.

## Summary and Conclusions

Existing evidence reviewed in this chapter demonstrates the clear and disproportionate impact of AIDS among Latino populations. Distinct patterns of populations affected (for instance, women or men, adult or youth) and modes of transmission (for instance, male–male, IDU, and heterosexual contact) exist by gender and Latino group. Yet, the lack of Latino subgroup identifiers in AIDS and HIV data poses a major limitation in the use of these data for targeted prevention planning. The literature also provides some indications of the individual, relationship, and contextual factors that increase risk for HIV infection among Latinos. Factors such as age, misconceptions about AIDS, level of acculturation, attitudes and beliefs about condoms, type of relationship, perceived risk, and relationship power have shown to be critical factors that shape HIV risk among Latinos. Again, however, the lack of systematic study of various Latino subgroups and reporting of such data pose real limitations in what we know about HIV risk factors among Latinos. Finally, a review of the state-of-the-art, evidence-based HIV prevention interventions revealed a dearth of information on their effectiveness in Latino populations. The lack of scientifically based, Latino-specific approaches to HIV prevention in the *Compendium* is especially troubling considering that cultural competency (messages and methods specifically tailored to target audiences) is a generally recognized hallmark of effective programs (Holtgrave, Qualls, Curran, Valdiserri, Guinan, & Parra, 1995). In the context of the lack of systematic study of factors that influence risk behaviors among Latinos, there has been great room for speculation about the role of culture, with resulting broad generalizations and focus on this as a major determining factor. Recent studies with more specific research focus and nuanced understanding of culture have revealed that homophobia and relationship power are important determinants of risk behaviors and that acculturation and socioeconomic status are important mediators of these factors. However, Latinos and Latino culture do not have a sole claim on these oppressive norms, which are evident to various degrees across populations throughout the world. Further comparative research within Latino groups and across Latino and other groups is needed to understand how unique these factors are to Latinos and the factors that mediate their importance among HIV risk in various Latino populations.

There has been even less effort to test HIV prevention strategies that are specific to Latinos and that consider the role of cultural values. For these reasons, the Minority AIDS Council has developed initiatives that advocate specific funding for research and testing of prevention approaches targeted at Latino populations (Salazar, 2000). Three clear target populations emerge as the focus of needed HIV prevention intervention studies:

1. Heterosexual transmission is the primary mode of HIV transmission among Latinas diagnosed with AIDS. Development of effective prevention strategies for this population will need to include individual- and community-based approaches that target women at risk and heterosexual Latino men whose risk behaviors place their female partners at risk. There is an astounding absence of prevention targeted at Latino heterosexual male youth and adults. Such interventions will need to focus on changing community norms regarding the acceptability of condom use among men and identifying effective ways to engage Latino men in prevention efforts.

2. A second area of needed development is prevention targeted at Latino men who have sex with men, both those who identify as gay and those who do not. Considering the high representation of Latino men who have sex with men among identified AIDS cases, this is an alarming deficit in our current public health efforts, which have so effectively reduced risk behaviors among

White gay men. Since community norms stigmatize people based on sexual preference or behaviors and such stigma is likely to inhibit participation and exposure to HIV prevention messages and interventions, these interventions will need to target such norms as well as individuals.

3. Finally, IDU-related risk behaviors and, more broadly, drug use contribute significantly to HIV transmission among Latino men and women. Efforts are needed to increase access to drug treatment as well as harm-reduction interventions to reduce risk in this population. Because sexually transmitted diseases increase the risk of HIV infection, screening and treatment of STDs will also be an important intervention to reduce HIV risk in all Latino groups. Disproportionately high rates of STDs among Latinos (Centers for Disease Control and Prevention, 1998a) make it critical that we find more effective ways to engage people in screening and treatment. In summary, much of what we have learned about effective public health methods of HIV prevention has yet to be tested among Latinos. There is an urgent need for both basic behavioral risk research and applied intervention research that can inform public health practice.

## Policy Recommendations

Throughout the last two decades, HIV/AIDS-related social policies emphasizing person-centered prevention efforts have not served Latinos well. As our review shows, HIV/AIDS health disparities among Latinos remain at unacceptable levels. Current social policy efforts are guided by person-centered paradigms that are not well suited to consider or have an influence on contextual factors that affect risk (for example, gender roles or cultural values) and the socioeconomic factors delineating the life circumstances of Latinos in the United States. Although the main paradigm guiding prevention efforts is based on social learning theory, the person-centered nature of this theoretical approach obviates power inequalities that often exist in female–male sexual relationships, the impact of the immigration process, important values of Latino culture such as collectivism and *familialismo* (influence of relatives on a person's behavior or ideas), and most important, the impact of social injustices in the lives of Latinos. As the findings of this chapter imply, gender and culture need to be part and parcel of social policy formulations addressing the AIDS epidemic among Latinos. Although a significant portion of federal monies is allocated to community-based efforts, the focus of the intervention is primarily on the person—with the emphasis on learning theories—and not on contextual factors. This approach has resulted in a curtailment of the AIDS epidemic among gay White males but not among Latinos and other minorities. Funding agencies such as the National Institutes of Health, Centers for Disease Control and Prevention, Health Resources and Services Administration, and Substance Abuse and Mental Health Services Administration should develop focused initiatives to inform and support a program of HIV prevention research on Latinos that include the study of contextual factors (for example, gender norms, cultural values, discrimination, and socioeconomic indicators) and HIV risk in Latino communities. Common approaches (such as scientific knowledge development conferences and targeted requests for proposals) used by these agencies in the past to move science forward would be productive mechanisms to increase the development of knowledge about HIV risk factors and effective strategies for prevention within Latino communities.

In addressing the shortcomings of Latino HIV/AIDS policies, researchers and policymakers have advocated the implementation of cultural competency strategies. Although these efforts are commendable, they do not fully address the features of Latinos' social realities. The field of cultural competence remains too focused on issues of language, social interaction, and the identification of a menu-like list of values and beliefs of Latino culture. A clear articulation of how cultural competency strategies should be implemented is lacking. The inclusion of gender roles and contextual factors affecting the target population would enhance the specificity of policy formulations regarding Latino prevention strategies. In addition, by elaborating on the interface of culture, gender, and context, policymakers and researchers would be able to acquire the tools necessary to implement effective prevention strategies that are not only culturally competent but also tailored to the specific needs of the diverse Latino population. Federal agencies should develop a mechanism to engage Latino researchers and community service providers in an initiative to clearly articulate definitions of what constitutes cultural competency in HIV prevention and elucidate the social contextual factors that place Latinos at risk for HIV. One possible mechanism for this purpose could be a working group whose work results in the development of a manual that defines cultural and contextual factors and that provides examples of effective strategies for HIV prevention with Latinos.

The aforementioned CDC *Compendium* on effective HIV prevention strategies clearly demonstrates the lack of attention to gender, race, and ethnicity in current intervention research. While many of these studies have included Latinos in their samples, they have not systematically analyzed effectiveness of interventions across ethnic groups. As part of this effort, President Clinton's initiative to eliminate racial disparities in health needs to be embraced by the new administration. In addition, it needs to develop an aggressive federal response to HIV prevention targeted to Latinos. The Office of the President should require federal agencies to clearly articulate current and future efforts to develop the scientific base on HIV prevention among Latinos and initiatives to implement HIV prevention programs in Latino communities. Federal agencies that fund such research should fund initiatives whose *primary* focus is testing the effectiveness of existing HIV prevention strategies across gender, racial, and ethnic populations.

Related to the funding of research on HIV prevention is the issue of representation of Latino researchers on scientific review committees. Funding agencies must ensure that reviewers have demonstrated expertise in conducting research with Latino populations and have knowledge of and familiarity with contextual issues that shape the lives of Latinos and that are related to HIV risk.

Existing methods for collecting race and ethnicity data in the national HIV/AIDS surveillance system do not identify Latino subgroups. This presents a serious problem in the understanding of the epidemiology of HIV and AIDS among Latinos. Studies reviewed in this chapter indicate that the prevalence of HIV and AIDS and the transmission modes vary significantly across Latino subgroups. Yet our national surveillance system does not allow us to track the HIV/AIDS epidemic across these Latino groups. The Centers for Disease Control and Prevention should change Hispanic origin identifiers in HIV and AIDS reporting forms to include information specific to Latino subgroups, and it should utilize these identifiers to report data. Such information would better enable public health prevention efforts to be targeted to specific populations of Latinos in relation to the various transmission modes.

It is clearly evident based on our review that alcohol and drug use and abuse continued to be an important transmission source for Latinos. Yet the scientific literature on addiction treatment provides limited guidance on effective methods of treatment for Latinos. The Substance Abuse and Mental Health Services Administration, the National Institute on Drug Abuse, and the National Institute on Alcohol and Alcohol Abuse should develop meaningful initiatives to fund research on addiction treatment within Latino populations at risk for HIV infection.

Elected officials at the state and federal level have a responsibility to oversee that public dollars are allocated for the purposes identified here. The Hispanic Congressional Caucus should continue to collaborate with the Black Congressional Caucus on ensuring that sufficient funds are allocated to target HIV prevention efforts in Latino and other minority communities. Further, the Hispanic Congressional Caucus should hold yearly hearings to monitor progress in the federal response to the HIV epidemic in Latino communities.

Finally, in order to hold federal agencies responsible for developing and contiuing initiatives to improve the scientific and practice base of HIV prevention in Latino communities, these communities, as well as Latino service providers and researchers, must continue to organize and make these issues visible to the public and to elected officials.

# References

Albert, A. E., Warner, D. L., Hatcher, R. A., Trussell, J., & Bennett, C. (1995). Condom use among female commercial sex workers in Nevada's legal brothels. *American Journal of Public Health, 85,* 1514–1520.

Amaro, H. (1995). Love, sex, and power: Considering women's realities in HIV prevention. *American Psychologist, 50,* 437–447.

Amaro, H., & Raj, A. (in press). On the margin: The realities of power and women's HIV risk reduction strategies. *Journal of Sex Roles.*

Amaro, H. et al. (1998, June). *Study report: Clients presenting for HIV counseling and testing at MDPH-funded agencies.* Report prepared for the Massachusetts Department of Public Health. Boston: Boston University School of Public Health.

Arguelles, L., & Rivero, A. M. (1988). HIV infection/AIDS and Latinas in the Los Angeles County: Considerations for prevention treatment and research practice. *California Sociologist, 11,* 1–2, 69–89.

Aruffo, J. F., Coverdale, J. H., & Vallbona, C. (1991). AIDS knowledge in low-income and minority populations. *Public Health Reports, 106,* 115–119.

Bradner, C. H., Ku, L., & Duberstein-Lindbergh, B. (2000). Older, but not wiser: How men get information about AIDS and sexually transmitted diseases after high school. *Family Planning Perspectives, 32,* 33–38.

Carey, M. P., Maisto, S. A., Kalichman, S. C., Forsyth, A. D., Wright, E. M., & Johnson, B. T. (1997). Enhancing motivation to reduce the risk of HIV infection for economically disadvantaged urban women. *Journal of Consulting and Clinical Psychology, 65,* 4, 531–541.

Carmona, J. V., Romero, G. J., & Loeb, T. B. (1999). The impact of HIV status and acculturation on Latinas' sexual risk taking. *Cultural Diversity and Ethnic Minority Psychology, 5,* 209–221.

Castañeda, D. (2000). The close relationship context and HIV/AIDS risk reduction among Latinas/os. *Sex Roles, 42,* 7–8, 551–580.

Catania, J. A. et al. (1994). Correlates of condom use among black, Hispanic, and white heterosexuals in San Francisco: The Amen Longitudinal Survey. *AIDS Education and Prevention, 6,* 1, 12–26.

Catania, J. A., Kegeles, S. M., & Coates, T. (1992). Towards an understanding of risk behavior: An AIDS risk reduction model (ARRM). *Health Education Quarterly, 17,* 53–72.

Centers for Disease Control and Prevention. (1998a). HIV prevention through early interventions and treatment of other sexually transmitted diseases, United States. *MMWR [Morbidity and Mortality Weekly Report], 47,* No. RR-12.

Centers for Disease Control and Prevention. (1998b). *Sexually transmitted disease surveillance 1997.* Atlanta, GA: U.S. Department of Health and Human Services.

Centers for Disease Control and Prevention. (1999a). *HIV/AIDS Research Synthesis Project: Compendium of HIV prevention interventions with evidence of effectiveness.* Atlanta, GA: U.S. Department of Health and Human Services.

Centers for Disease Control and Prevention. (1999b). *HIV/AIDS surveillance report: U.S. HIV and AIDS cases reported through June 1999.* Atlanta, GA: U.S. Department of Health and Human Services.

Centers for Disease Control and Prevention. (1999c). *Youth risk behavior surveillance: National Alternative High School Youth Risk Behavior Survey, United States, 1998.* Vol. 48, No. SS-7. Atlanta, GA: U.S. Department of Health and Human Services.

Centers for Disease Control and Prevention. (2000). HIV/AIDS among racial/ethnic minority men who have sex with men—United States, 1989–1998. *MMWR [Morbidity and Mortality Weekly Report], 49,* 4–11.

Choi, K., Catania, J. A., & Dolcini, P. (1994). Extramarital sex and HIV risk behavior among U.S. adults: Results from the National AIDS Behavioral Survey. *American Journal of Public Health, 84,* 2003–2007.

Comas-Diaz, L. (1996). Feminist therapy with Hispanic/Latin women: Myth or reality? *Women and Therapy, 6,* 4, 39–61.

Cunningham, R. M., Stiffman, A. R., & Dore, P. (1994). The association of physical and sexual abuse with HIV risk behaviors in adolescence and young adulthood: Implications for public health. *Child Abuse and Neglect, 18,* 3, 233–245.

David, D., & Brannon, R. (1976). *The forty-nine percent majority: The male sex role.* Reading, MA: Addison-Wesley.

De la Cancela, V. (1996). A critical analysis of Puerto Rican machismo: Implications for clinical practice. *Psychotherapy, 23,* 2, 291–296.

Deren, S. et al. (1998, June 28–July 3). *Issues in studying high risk populations in diverse locations: Puerto Ricans in New York and Puerto Rico.* Paper presented at the 12th World AIDS Conference, Geneva, Switzerland, 242, p. 14,297.

Deren, S., Shedlin, M., & Beardsley, M. (1996). HIV-related concerns and behaviors among Hispanic women. *AIDS Education and Prevention, 8,* 335–342.

Devita, D. V., Hellman, S., & Rosenberg, S. A. (1997). *AIDS: Etiology, diagnosis, treatment and prevention* (4th ed.). Philadelphia: Lippincott-Raven.

Diaz, T., & Klevens, M. (1997). Differences by ancestry in sociodemographics and risk behaviors among Latinos with AIDS: The supplement to HIV and AIDS Surveillance Project Group. *Ethnicity and Disease, 7,* 200–206.

DiClemente, R. J., & Wingood, G. M. (1995). A randomized controlled trial of an HIV sexual risk-reduction intervention for young African-American women. *Journal of the American Medical Association, 274,* 16, 1271–1276.

Doll, L. S., Petersen, L. R., White, C. R., Johnson, E. S., Ward, J. W., & the Blood Donor Study Group, Centers for Disease Control and Prevention. (1992). Homosexually and nonhomosexually identified men who have sex with men: A behavioral comparison. *Journal of Sex Research, 29,* 1–14.

Doval, A. S., Duran, R., O'Donnell, L., & O'Donnell, C. R. (1995). Barriers to condom use in primary and nonprimary relationships among Hispanic STD clinic patients. *Hispanic Journal of Behavioral Sciences, 17,* 3, 385–397.

Estrada, A. L. (1998). Drug use and HIV risks among African-American and Puerto Rican drug injectors. *Journal of Psychoactive Drugs, 30,* 247–253.

Flaskerud, J. H., Uman, G., Lara, R., Romero, L., & Taka, K. (1996). Sexual practices, attitudes, and knowledge related to HIV transmission in low income Los Angeles Hispanic women. *Journal of Sex Research, 33,* 343–353.

Fleisher, J. M., Senie, R. T., Minkoff, H., & Jaccard, J. (1994). Condom use relative to knowledge of sexually transmitted disease prevention, method of birth control, and past or present infection. *Journal of Community Health, 19,* 6, 395–407.

Freeman, R. C., Williams, M. L., & Saunders, L. A. (1999). Drug use, AIDS knowledge and HIV risk behaviors of Cuban-, Mexican-, and Puerto Rican-born drug injectors who are recent entrants into the United States. *Substance Use and Misuse, 34,* 13, 1765–1793.

Gavey, N., & McPhillips, K. (1997). Women and the heterosexual transmission of HIV: Risks and prevention strategies. *Women and Health, 25,* 2, 41–64.

Gielen, A. C., Faden, R. R., O'Campo, P., Kass, N., & Anderson, J. (1994). Women's protective sexual behaviors: A test of the health belief model. *AIDS Education and Prevention, 6,* 1, 1–11.

Gil, V. E. (1998). Empowerment rhetoric, sexual negotiation, and Latinas' AIDS risk: Research implications for prevention health education. *International Quarterly of Community Health Education, 18,* 9–27.

Gómez, C. A., Hernández, M., & Faigeles, B. (1999). Sex in the New World: An empowerment model for HIV prevention in Latina immigrant women. *Health Education and Behavior, 26,* 200–212.

Gómez, C. A., & Marín, B. V. (1996). Gender, culture, and power: Barriers to HIV-prevention strategies for women. *Journal of Sex Research, 33,* 355–362.

Gutierrez, L. M., Oh, H. J., Gillmore, M. R. (2000). Toward an understanding of (em)power(ment) for HIV/AIDS prevention with adolescent women. *Sex Roles, 42,* 7–8, 581–611.

Harrison, D. F. et al. (1991). AIDS knowledge and risk behaviors among culturally diverse women. *AIDS Education and Prevention, 3,* 79–89.

He, H., McCoy, H. V., Stevens, S. J., & Stark, M. J. (1998). Violence and HIV sexual risk behaviors among female sex partners of male drug users. *Women and Health, 27,* 161–175.

Heckman, T. G. et al. (1996). Predictors of condom use and human immunodeficiency virus test seeking among women living in inner-city public housing developments. *Sexually Transmitted Diseases, 23*, 5, 357–365.

Hines, A. M., & Caetano, R. (1998). Alcohol and AIDS-related sexual behavior among Hispanics: Acculturation and gender differences. *AIDS Education and Prevention, 10*, 533–547.

Hobfoll, S. E., Jackson, A. P., Lavin, J., Britton, P. J., & Shepherd, J. B. (1994). Reducing inner-city women's AIDS risk activities: A study of single, pregnant women. *Health Psychology, 13*, 5, 397–403.

Holland, J., Ramazanoglu, C., Scott, S., Sharpe, S., & Thompson, R. (1992). Risk, power, and the possibility of pleasure: Young women and safer sex. *AIDS Care, 4*, 3, 273–283.

Holtgrave, D. R., Qualls, N. L., Curran, J. W., Valdiserri, R. O., Guinan, M. E., & Parra, W. C. (1995). An overview of the effectiveness and efficiency of HIV prevention programs. *Public Health Reports, 110*, 2, 134–146.

Inciardi, J. A., Lockwood, D., & Pottieger, A. E. (1993). *Women and crack cocaine.* New York: Macmillan.

Kaiser Family Foundation. (1998). *Latinos and AIDS.* Retrieved March 10, 2000, from: http://www.kff.org

Kalichman, S. C., Rompa, D., & Coley, B. (1996). Experimental component analysis of a behavioral HIV-AIDS prevention intervention for inner-city women. *Journal of Consulting and Clinical Psychology, 64*, 4, 687–693.

Kelly, J. A. et al. (1994). The effects of HIV/AIDS intervention groups for high-risk women in urban clinics. *American Journal of Public Health, 84*, 12, 1918–1922.

Khabbaz, R. F. et al. (1990). Seroprevalence and risk factors for HTLV-I/II infection among female prostitutes in the United States. *Journal of the American Medical Association, 263*, 60–64.

Kilpatrick, D. G., Resnick, H. S., Saunders, B. E., & Best, C. L. (1998). Victimization, posttraumatic stress disorder, and substance use and abuse among women. In C. L. Wetherington & A. B. Roman (Eds.), *Drug addiction research and health of women* (NIH Publication No. 98-4290, pp. 285–307). Rockville, MD: U.S. Department of Health and Human Services, National Institute on Drug Abuse.

Leslie, L. A., & Leitch, M. L. (1989). A demographic profile of recent Central American immigrants: Clinical and service implications. *Hispanic Journal of Behavioral Sciences, 11*, 315–329.

Mann, J. (1991). AIDS: Challenges to epidemiology in the 1990s. In L. C. Chen, J. Sepulveda Amor, & S. J. Segal (Eds.), *AIDS and women's reproductive health.* New York: Plenum.

Marín, B. V., & Gomez, C. A. (1997). Latino culture and sex: Implications for HIV prevention. In J. G. Garcia & M. C. Zea (Eds.), *Psychological interventions and research with Latino populations.* Des Moines, IA: Allyn & Bacon, pp. 73–93.

Marín, B. V., Gómez, C. A., Tschann, J., & Gregorich, S. E. (1997). Condom use in unmarried Latino men: A test of cultural constructs. *Health Psychology, 16*, 458–467.

Marín, B. V., & Marín, G. (1992). Predictors of condom accessibility among Hispanics in San Francisco. *American Journal of Public Health, 79*, 836–839.

Marín, B. V., Tschann, J. M., Gómez, C. A., & Kegeles, S. M. (1993). Acculturation and gender differences in sexual attitudes and behaviors: Hispanic vs. non-Hispanic white unmarried adults. *American Journal of Public Health, 83*, 1759–1761.

Marín, G. (1989). AIDS prevention among Hispanics: Needs, risk behaviors, and cultural values. *Public Health Reports, 104*, 411–415.

Marks, G., Cantero, P. J., & Simoni, P. J. (1998). Is acculturation associated with sexual risk behavior? An investigation of HIV/AIDS positive Latino men and women. *AIDS Care, 10*, 283–295.

Martin, J. (1997). The meanings of macho: Being a man in Mexico City. *Journal of the Royal Anthropological Institute, 3,* 817–818.

Mikawa, J. K., Morones, P. A., Gómez, A., Olsen, D., & Gonzalez-Huss, M. (1992). Cultural practices of Hispanics: Implications for prevention of AIDS. *Hispanic Journal of Behavioral Sciences, 14,* 421–433.

Miller, J. B. (1986). *Toward a new psychology of women.* Boston: Beacon Press.

Miller, L. C., Bettencourt, B. A., DeBro, S. C., & Hoffman, V. (1993). Negotiating safer sex: Interpersonal dynamics. In J. Pryor & G. D. Reeder (Eds.), *The social psychology of HIV infection.* Hillsdale, NJ: Erlbaum, pp. 85–123.

Misovich, S. J., Fisher, J. D., & Fisher, W. A. (1997). Close relationships and elevated HIV risk behavior: Evidence and possible underlying psychological processes. *Review of General Psychology, 1,* 1, 72–107.

Moore, J., Harrison, J. S., Kay, K. L., Deren, S., & Doll, L. S. (1995). Factors associated with Hispanic women's HIV-related communication and condom use with male partners. *AIDS Care, 7,* 415–427.

Nyamathi, A., Bennett, C., Leake, B., Lewis, C., & Flaskerud, J. (1993). AIDS-related knowledge, perceptions, and behaviors among impoverished minority women. *American Journal of Public Health, 83,* 1, 65–71.

Organista, K. C., Organista, P. B., Garcia de Alba, J. E., Castillo Moran, M. A., & Ureta Carrillo, L. E. (1997). Survey of condom-related beliefs, behaviors, and perceived social norms in Mexican migrant laborers. *Journal of Community Health, 22,* 3, 185–198.

Padilla, A., & Salgado de Snyder, N. (1992). Hispanics: What the culturally informed evaluator needs to know. In M. A. Orlandi (Ed.), *Cultural competence for evaluators. A guide for alcohol and other drug abuse prevention practitioners working with ethnic/racial communities.* Rockville, MD: U.S. Department of Health and Human Services, Office for Substance Abuse Prevention.

Peragallo, N. (1996). Latino women and AIDS risk. *Public Health Nursing, 13,* 217–222.

Pérez, A. M. (1998). *Migration and mental health among Dominican immigrants living in New York City: A comparison of two migration-mental health models.* Unpublished doctoral dissertation, Fordham University, New York.

Pleck, J. H., Sonenstein, F. L., & Ku, L. C. (1993). Masculinity ideology: Its impact on adolescent males' heterosexual relationships. *Journal of Social Issues, 49,* 3, 11–29.

Pleck, J. H. (1995). The gender role strain paradigm: An update. In R. F. Levant & W. S. Pollack (Eds.), *A new psychology of men.* New York: Basic Books.

Pulerwitz, J., Gortmaker, S. L., & De Jong, W. (2000). Measuring relationship power in STD/HIV research. *Sex Roles, 42,* 7–8, 637–660.

Quina, K., Harlow, L. L., Morokoff, P. J., Burkholder, G., & Deiter, P. J. (2000). Sexual communication in relationships: When words speak louder than actions. *Sex Roles, 42,* 7–8, 523–549.

Raj, A., & Pollack, R. H. (1995). Factors predicting high-risk sexual behavior in heterosexual college females. *Journal of Sex and Marital Therapy, 21,* 3, 213–224.

Raj, A., Silverman, J., & Amaro, H. (2000). The relationship between sexual abuse and sexual risk among high school students: Findings from the 1997 Massachusetts Youth Risk Behavior Survey. *Maternal and Child Health Journal, 4,* 2, 125–134.

Riehman, K. S., Sly, D. F., Soler, H., Eberstein, I. W., Quadagno, D., & Harrison. (1998). Dual-method use among an ethnically diverse group of women at risk for infection. *Family Planning Perspectives, 30,* 5 , 212–217.

Rogler, L. H. (1994). International migrations: A framework for directing research. *American Psychologist, 49,* 701–708.

Rogler, L. H., Cortés, D. E., & Malgady, R. (1991). Acculturation and mental health status among Hispanics. *American Psychologist, 46,* 585–597.

Romero, G. J., & Arguelles, L. (1993). AIDS knowledge and beliefs of citizen and noncitizen Chicanas/Mexicanas. *Latino Studies Journal, 4,* 79–94.

Romero, G. J., Wyatt, G. E., Chin, D., & Rodriguez, C. (1998). HIV-related behaviors among recently immigrated and undocumented Latinas. *International Quarterly of Community Health Education, 18,* 89–105.

Romero-Daza, N., Weeks, M., & Singer, M. (1998). Much more than HIV!: The reality of life on the streets for drug-using sex workers in inner city Hartford. *International Quarterly of Community Health Education, 18,* 107–119.

Sabogal, F., & Catania, J. A. (1996). HIV risk factors, condom use, and HIV antibody testing among heterosexual Hispanics: The National AIDS Behavioral Surveys (NABS). *Hispanic Journal of Behavioral Sciences, 18,* 367–391.

Sabogal, F., Faigeles, B., & Catania, J. A. (1993). Data from the AIDS Behavioral Surveys: II. Multiple sexual partners among Hispanics in high-risk cities. *Family Planning Perspectives, 6,* 257–262.

Sabogal, F., Pérez-Stable, Otero-Sabogal, R., & Hiatt, R. A. (1995). Gender, ethnic, and acculturation differences in sexual behaviors among Hispanic and non-Hispanic white adults. *Hispanic Journal of Behavioral Sciences, 17,* 139–159.

Salazar, J. G. (2000, March 21). (Manager, National Minority AIDS Coalition.) *Testimony on [Fiscal Year 2000] . . . before the House Appropriations [Subcommittees on] Labor, Health and Human Services, and Education . . . .* Text from Federal Document Clearinghouse Congressional Testimony. Available from Congressional Universe (Online Service). Bethesda, MD: Congressional Information Service.

Sikkema, K. J. et al. (1995). Levels and predictors of HIV risk behavior among women in low-income public housing developments. *Public Health Reports, 101,* 707–713.

Singer, M. (1999). Why do Puerto Rican injection drug users inject so often? *Journal of Anthropology and Medicine, 6,* 1, 31–58.

Stevens, S. J., Estrada, A. L., & Estrada, B. D. (1998). HIV sex and drug risk behavior and behavior change in a national sample of injection drug and crack cocaine using women. *Women's Health, 27,* 1–2, 25–48.

Stevens, S. J., Ruiz, D., Romero, O., & Gama, D. (1995, February). *HIV prevention and education: Street outreach for special populations: The crack addicted and intravenous drug users.* Paper presented at the National Update on AIDS, San Francisco, CA.

Sufian, M., Friedman, S. R., Neaigus, A., Stepherson, B., Rivers-Beckman, J., & Des Jarlais, D. (1990). Impact of AIDS on Puerto Rican intravenous drug users. *Hispanic Journal of Behavioral Sciences, 12,* 122–134.

Sweat, M., & Denison, J. (1995). Reducing HIV incidence in developing countries with structural and environmental interventions. *AIDS, 9,* Suppl. A, S251–S257.

Tawil, O., Verster, A., & O'Reilly, K. (1995). Enabling approaches for HIV/AIDS prevention: Can we modify the environment and modify risk? *AIDS, 9,* 1299–1306.

Wagstaff, D. A. et al. (1995). Multiple partners, risky partners and HIV risk among low-income urban women. *Family Planning Perspectives, 27,* 6, 241–244.

Weeks, M. R., Grier, M., Romero-Daza, N, Puglisi-Vasquez, M. J., & Singer, M. (1998). Street, drugs, and the economy of sex in the age of AIDS. *Women's Health, 27,* 205–229.

Wingood, G. M., & DiClemente, R. J. (1997). The effects of an abusive primary partner on the condom use and sexual negotiation practices of African-American women. *American Journal of Public Health, 87,* 6, 1016–1018.

Worth, D. (1989). Sexual decision-making and AIDS: Why condom promotion among vulnerable women is likely to fail. *Studies in Family Planning, 20,* 297–307.

Wyatt, G. E., Vargas Carmona, J., Burns Loeb, T., Guthrie, D., & Gordon, G. (2000). Factors affecting HIV contraceptive decision making among women. *Sex Roles, 42,* 7–8, 495–521.

Zierler, S., Feingold, L., Laufer, D., Velentgas, P., Kantrowitz-Gordon, I., & Mayer, K. (1991). Adult survivors of childhood sexual abuse and subsequent risk of HIV infection. *American Journal of Public Health, 81,* 5, 572–575.

Zierler, S., & Krieger, N. (1997). Reframing women's risk: Social inequalities and HIV infection. *Annual Review of Public Health, 18,* 401–436.

PART FOUR

# OCCUPATIONAL HEALTH AND THE LATINO WORKFORCE

CHAPTER TWELVE

# OCCUPATIONAL HEALTH AMONG LATINO WORKERS IN THE URBAN SETTING

Rafael Moure-Eraso, George Friedman-Jiménez

This chapter focuses on Latino workers in urban areas, where approximately 88 percent of U.S. Latinos live (1994 data) (Environmental Protection Agency, 1999). Occupational health can be defined as the recognition, diagnosis, treatment, and prevention of work-related injury and illness. Achieving these objectives requires medical surveillance to identify trends and high-risk groups, screening and medical diagnosis and treatment of disease, as well as workplace hazard evaluation, education, and interventions to reduce exposures. A work-related disease is one that is caused or exacerbated by chemical substances, physical conditions, or other hazardous exposures on the job.

The occupational health of Latino workers in the United States is increasingly being recognized as an important area for study as well as for public health and clinical intervention (see the following example for additional information). From a public health perspective, this is an important issue to address for several reasons. The U.S. Latino population is sizeable (see Table 12.1) and growing rapidly, especially in urban areas. Work-related diseases cause substantial morbidity and mortality and are amenable to public health primary prevention interventions, such as the elimination or reduction of the exposures that cause them. Secondary prevention interventions, in the form of surveillance and clinical services, are also an essential part of the public health approach to occupational health. Although occupational diseases can affect members of all racial or ethnic groups and socioeconomic classes, available evidence suggests that Latino workers, along with other minority workers as well as low-income workers, are at higher risk for occupational disease than other workers in the general population. This excess risk is probably due to overrepresentation of Latino workers in the more hazardous occupations and industries.

*Federal Agencies and Occupational Health*

The United States lacks a national system to provide services in occupational health for all workers; even the limited occupational health services that presently exist have not been accessible to large segments of the Latino population, which remain virtually unserved. Three federal agencies lead the U.S. effort to prevent and control occupationally induced morbidity and mortality: the National Institute for Occupational Safety and Health (NIOSH), in the U.S. Department of Health and Human Services, for surveillance, research, and education; the Occupational Safety and Health Administration (OSHA), in the U.S. Department of Labor, for regulation and enforcement; and the Bureau of Labor Statistics (BLS), in the U.S. Department of Labor, for morbidity and mortality data. These federal agencies are also complemented by autonomous state agencies that perform similar functions at the state level.

The resources allocated by the federal government for workers' health are modest: NIOSH, OSHA, and BLS have budgets that are smaller by one order of magnitude than the budgets allocated to other federal agencies with comparable missions, such as the Environmental Protection Agency (EPA) and the Food and Drug Administration (FDA). These allocations have consistently proved inadequate to serve the needs of the U.S. workforce in general. Consequently, the occupational health needs of minority workers, for example, African Americans and Latinos, have been largely unmet with regard to targeted surveillance or primary prevention interventions.

## TABLE 12.1.   1998/99 RACIAL/ETHNICITY DISTRIBUTION OF THE U.S. POPULATION AND CIVILIAN WORKFORCE: ESTIMATED BY THE U.S. CENSUS[a] AND U.S. DEPARTMENT OF LABOR.[b]

| Racial or Ethnic Group | U.S. Civilian Workforce Greater Than 16y (in Thousands)[b] | Percentage[c] | Total U.S. Population (in Thousands)[a] | Percentage[c] |
|---|---|---|---|---|
| Latino | 13,381 | 10 | 34,864 | 12.8 |
| African American | 14,795 | 11 | 31,355 | 11.5 |
| White | 111,863 | 84 | 224,650 | 84.0 |
| Total | 132,684 | 100 | 272,820 | 100.0 |

[a]United States Bureau of the Census (2000). *Projections of the resident population by race.* Washington, D.C.

[b]United States Department of Labor, Bureau of Labor Statistics (1998). *National census of fatal occupational injuries.* Washington, D.C.

[c]Percentages are greater than 100 because Latinos can be classified as Black or White, causing an undetermined overlap.

# Primary and Secondary Prevention

Primary prevention is achieved by the elimination or substantial reduction of risk factors that are known to cause workplace death and disease. These interventions can only be successful with the full participation and cooperation of the groups affected by the hazards—the workers and the companies. A first step is to quantify the dimensions of the problem through hazard surveillance, or collection of systematic data on the prevalence of workplace hazards and populations at risk, followed by specific recommendations for engineering interventions at the point of production to control risk factors. Hazard surveillance should precede disease surveillance for the purposes of primary prevention. (See definitions in the following example.)

*Definitions of Primary and Secondary Prevention*

From an epidemiological point of view, *primary prevention* is defined as prevention of new cases of disease, that is, activities that decrease incidence (new cases) of disease; *secondary prevention* is defined as early detection of disease and effective treatment to decrease morbidity and mortality, that is, decrease prevalence (Last, 1988).

From an engineering point of view, primary prevention encompasses activities aimed at preventing the *possibility* of disease; it is also referred to as "inherent safety." Secondary prevention encompasses activities that reduce the *probability* of disease; it is also referred to as "mitigation" (Ashford, 1997). Ashford notes that some might argue that primary prevention—defined as preventing the *possibility* of disease—can never be achieved. Since 100 percent safety is impossible, we can only make processes "safer." However, articulating the ideal makes an important point: dramatic, not marginal, changes are required to achieve prevention. Primary prevention defined as above focuses attention on the proper target—the sources of exposure (Ashford, 1997).

Secondary prevention involves the early medical diagnosis and treatment of injury or illness that is successful in achieving recovery and return to work. The data on specific types of morbidity caused by the work environment in the Latino population are very limited, and many Latino workers lack access to available clinical occupational health services. As a result of this lack of epidemiological and surveillance data, programs providing clinical occupational health services to Latino working populations have not been developed adequately. This vicious cycle of "no services therefore no data therefore no services" can be broken by simultaneously developing epidemiological research and surveillance methods that will effectively include Latino workers, and by providing clinical occupational health services accessible and targeted to Latino working populations.

## Environmental Justice

A related topic of growing interest in public health for the Latino population is environmental justice (sometimes considered from the perspective of "environmental injustice"). Environmental justice has focused on the observation that air pollution, hazardous worksites, hazardous waste dumps, and other sources of environmental pollution are likely to be sited in proximity to communities of color (Frumkin, Walker, & Friedman-Jiménez, 1999).

## Minorities as a Percentage of the U.S. Working Population

There are no systematic and reliable sources of data on occupational diseases in the U.S. working population (Herbert & Landrigan, 2000). Recent peer-reviewed estimates of occupational morbidity and mortality experience for the general U.S. population (from 1992), not differentiated by race, are substantial (Leigh, Markowitz, Fahs, Shin, & Landrigan, 1997). Based on the best available denominator data for the U.S. working population, in this chapter we develop an estimate of the numbers of occupational disease deaths and new cases among Latino workers in the United States. Next, using U.S. and New York City aggregate data, we show that Latino workers are disproportionately employed in the more hazardous occupational categories and underrepresented in the less hazardous categories. A description of the "sweatshops" that exist in many urban areas provides an example of workplaces that employ large numbers of Latino workers in hazardous conditions (Moure-Eraso, 1999). Rates of occupational disease are available for selected *industrial categories,* defined as sectors of productive industrial activity, as well as *occupational categories,* which describe specific jobs described by a numerical code (see United States Department of Labor, 1987). However, only the rates by job category are reported by workers' race or ethnic background. After reviewing the evidence that Latino workers are overrepresented in the more hazardous jobs and are at higher risk for occupational diseases, we discuss some of the social, economic, and political factors responsible for this inequitable situation.

The U.S. Bureau of the Census and the Bureau of Labor Statistics (BLS) of the U.S. Department of Labor publish population statistics for each year, based on population projections from the 1990 Census (United States Bureau of the Census, 2000). U.S. Census data for 1998 and current statistics (1998) from the U.S. Department of Labor on U.S. occupational injury and illness experience and characteristics provided the basis for Tables 12.1 to 12.9 (United States Department of Labor, Bureau of Labor Statistics, 1999). The demographic estimates of the U.S. working population by race and ethnicity appear in Table 12.1.

Note in Table 12.1 that Latinos are 10 percent of the civilian workforce (older than sixteen years old) but 12.8 percent of the total population. In contrast, the African American civilian workforce is 11 percent while their proportion in the total population is 11.5 percent. The proportions of Latinos in both columns appear to show a substantial number of young Latinos (less than sixteen years) not yet included in the civilian workforce.

Only 12 percent of the Latino population works in agriculture (data on the employed U.S. civilian population older than sixteen years) (Environmental Protection Agency, 1999). A distribution of the 88 percent Latinos employed in occupations not in the agricultural sector shows that more than 67 percent are in blue collar, low-paying jobs (service, labor, and support and sales), while Whites hold 56 percent of the same jobs (Table 12.2).

The most dramatic difference between the two groups is the proportion of Latinos in professional and managerial occupations (white collar jobs) that is half of the proportion of Whites in the same category (14 percent Latino versus 28 percent White). African Americans follow a similar pattern except that their proportion in the professional and managerial classes is higher (20.2 percent) than that of Latinos. Still the proportion of blue collar workers among African Americans is the highest at 75 percent.

## TABLE 12.2. DISTRIBUTION OF OCCUPATIONS OF EMPLOYED U.S. CIVILIAN WORKERS CLASSIFIED AS LATINOS, AFRICAN AMERICANS, AND WHITES OLDER THAN SIXTEEN YEARS IN 1994 (IN THOUSANDS).

| Occupation | Latinos Number | Latinos Percent | African Americans Number | African Americans Percent | Whites Number | Whites Percent |
|---|---|---|---|---|---|---|
| Professional and managerial | 1,517 | 14.0 | 2,405 | 20.2 | 30,045 | 28.6 |
| Service (household, protective, other) | 2,131 | 19.8 | 2,890 | 23.8 | 13,207 | 12.6 |
| Operators, fabricators, and laborers | 2,474 | 22.9 | 2,677 | 22.0 | 14,416 | 13.7 |
| Sales, administrative, and technical support | 2,639 | 24.0 | 3,637 | 29.9 | 32,232 | 30.7 |
| Other | 2,082 | 19.7 | 537 | 4.4 | 15,253 | 14.5 |
| Total | 10,788 | | 12,146 | | 105,190 | |

*Source:* Modified from Environmental Protection Agency (1999). Table 7.3: *Sociodemographic data used for identifying potentially highly exposed populations.* Washington, D.C.

## Occupational Disease Morbidity Estimate

Early estimation of the magnitude of occupational diseases in the United States showed that numbers of new cases could reach more than 390,000 per year (Ashford, 1976). More recent estimates show a range of 817,015 to 907,385 new cases of occupational disease annually. The newer estimate counted first the occupational deaths distributed among four major disease categories: cancer, coronary heart disease, cerebrovascular disease, and pulmonary disease (Leigh, Markowitz, Fahs, Shin, & Landrigan, 1997) (Table 12.3).

To this number Leigh and colleagues (1997) added cases of nonfatal occupational disease reported by the U.S. Department of Labor Annual Survey of Occupational Illness in 1992, as well as the number of cases reported in the same year by public employees (identified as nonclassified occupational disease in Table 12.3). Because the great majority of cases of occupational disease are not diagnosed as occupational and never become known to the surveillance mechanisms that currently exist, Leigh and colleagues used several indirect approaches to judge the magnitude and severity of the problem. However, the estimate of work-related musculoskeletal disorders, in particular, was likely not corrected sufficiently for known underreporting in administrative record-keeping systems

### TABLE 12.3.  ESTIMATED OCCUPATIONAL DISEASE MORBIDITY IN THE UNITED STATES IN 1992 FOR AFRICAN AMERICAN AND LATINO WORKING POPULATIONS.

| Disease Categories | Estimated Number of Occupational Illnesses Attributed to Occupation[a] (Includes All Races/ Ethnicities) | Estimated Number of New Cases of Occupational Illnesses Attributed to Occupation for African Americans[b] (11 Percent) | Estimated Number of New Cases of Occupational Illnesses Attributed to Occupation for Latinos[b] (10 Percent) |
|---|---|---|---|
| Cancer | 66,790–111,130 | 7,347–12,244 | 6,679–11,113 |
| Coronary heart disease | 36,500–73,000 | 4,015–8,030 | 3,650–7,300 |
| Cerebrovascular disease | 5,050–14,400 | 556–1,584 | 505–1,440 |
| Chronic obstructive pulmonary disease | 150,000 | 16,500 | 15,000 |
| Subtotal | 258,340–348,710 | 28,418–38,358 | 25,834–34,853 |
| Nonclassified occupational illness[c] | 538,675 | 61,454 | 55,867 |
| Total | 817,015–907,385 | 89,872–99,812 | 81,701–90,720 |

[a]Data from Leigh, Markowitz, Fahs, Shin, & Landrigan (1997).

[b]Percentages from United States Department of Labor, Bureau of Labor Statistics (1998). *National census of fatal occupational injuries.* Washington, D.C.

[c]This total includes United States Department of Labor, Bureau of Labor Statistics numbers for *occupational illness for 1992* and *occupational illness reported in 1992* by *U.S. government employees* (see Leigh, Markowitz, Fahs, Shin, & Landrigan, 1997).

(Silverstein, Stetson, Keyserling, & Fine, 1997; Punnett, 1999). Thus, the totals more likely underestimate the true values.

For the purposes of estimating Latino work-related morbidity, we assume that the percentage of disease in Latinos and African Americans corresponds to their percentage in the civilian labor force (10 percent and 11 percent, respectively) (United States Department of Labor, Bureau of Labor Statistics, 1999). Applying the 10 percent estimate, the range of new cases for Latinos would be between 81,701 and 90,720 for the year 1992 (Table 12.3). There is no reason to believe that this yearly estimate has changed since the reported numbers for 1992.

In addition, when other occupational diseases such as occupational asthma (included under chronic obstructive pulmonary disease in Table 12.3) are considered, the morbidity total grows substantially (Milton, Solomon, Rosiello, & Herrick, 1998; Wagner & Wegman, 1999).

A more focused look at the occupations with the greatest number of injuries illustrates the proportion of Latinos in those categories (Table 12.4). The BLS identified the ten job categories with the highest numbers of injuries and illnesses among 1,883,380 cases analyzed in 1997 (United States Department of Labor, Bureau of Labor Statistics, 1999). Latino workers were overrepresented in at least three of the most hazardous job categories: janitors, laborers, and cooks.

## Occupational Mortality Estimations

Work-related fatalities are classified as caused by acute traumatic injury (fatal occupational injury) or fatal occupational disease. The later is generally considered a long-term chronic condition.

**TABLE 12.4.  PERCENTAGE OF LATINOS IN TEN OCCUPATIONS  WITH THE LARGEST NUMBER OF OCCUPATIONAL INJURIES/ILLNESSES: 1997.**

| Occupation | Number of Cases | Latinos (Percent) |
|---|---|---|
| All occupations | 1,833,400 | 10.2 |
| Truck drivers | 145,500 | 6.3 |
| Laborers (nonconstruction) | 106,900 | 11.5 |
| Nurses' aides | 91,300 | 7.6 |
| Janitors and cleaners | 45,800 | 20.0 |
| Laborers (construction) | 45,800 | 17.9 |
| Assemblers | 44,300 | 9.7 |
| Carpenters | 37,100 | 8.2 |
| Cooks | 31,500 | 12.8 |
| Stock handlers | 29,200 | 7.7 |
| Welders and cutters | 28,400 | 8.4 |

*Source:* Data from United States Department of Labor, Bureau of Labor Statistics (1999) *Occupational injuries and illness: 1997.* Washington, D.C.

## Fatal Occupational Injuries

The BLS compiles every year the number of traumatic fatalities by race within the U.S. civilian workforce older than sixteen years of age (United States Department of Labor, Bureau of Labor Statistics, 1998). Traumatic occupational fatalities are deaths that occur during employment or in the course of employment and that are caused by acute incidents related to the victim's occupation. The first three columns of Table 12.5 present these data for 1998. The proportion of fatalities occurring to Latinos (12 percent of 6,026) is greater than the expected proportion corresponding to the percentage of Latino workers in the working civilian population (10 percent of 132,684,000). If the fatality rate were proportionate to the number of Latinos in the workforce, 10 percent or 603 fatalities would be expected, whereas 700 were observed. The ninety-seven deaths in excess over the expected number, or a relative risk (Gardner & Altman, 1989) of 1.18, indicate that Latinos are 18 percent more likely to die a traumatic death from injury on the job than Whites and African Americans combined.

However, since the Latino classification in the BLS includes members of every race (and thus the percentages sum to more than 100 percent), no valid statistical test could be applied to measure differences in fatal occupational injury rates by race or ethnicity. To bring some context to these traumatic fatalities, the BLS reports the event or exposure to which each death is directly attributed, that is, the underlying cause (Table 12.6).

Transportation incidents are by far the principal cause of traumatic occupational fatalities (44 percent), followed by homicide (16 percent) and being struck by objects and equipment in work settings (15 percent) (United States Department of Labor, Bureau of Labor Statistics, 1998). Unfortunately, the BLS statistics only provide the distribution of all deaths by race and ethnicity, without stratification by event or exposure. In order to have a benchmark, the number of traumatic deaths were estimated within each race and ethnicity by event or exposure, assuming the same percentages as the total number of deaths. These numbers are

### TABLE 12.5. OCCUPATIONAL TRAUMATIC FATALITIES FOR THE WHITE, AFRICAN AMERICAN, AND LATINO WORKING POPULATIONS.[a]

| Race/ Ethnicity | Fatal Injuries | Percentage | U.S. Civilian Workers | Percentage | Rate/100,000 |
|---|---|---|---|---|---|
| White | 5,016 | 83 | 111,863,000 | 84 | 4.484 |
| African American | 591 | 10 | 14,795,000 | 11 | 3.995 |
| Latino[b] | 700 | 12 | 13,381,000 | 10 | 5.231 |
| Total | 6,026 | 100 | 132,684,000 | 100 | 4.541 |

[a]United States Department of Labor, Bureau of Labor Statistics (1998). *National census of fatal occupational injuries.* Washington, D.C.

[b]Percentages are greater than 100 because Latino workers may also be categorized as Black or White, causing an undeterminated overlap.

## TABLE 12.6.   OCCUPATIONAL TRAUMATIC FATALITIES BY EVENT OR EXPOSURE,[a] 1998: LATINO, AFRICAN AMERICAN, AND WHITE POPULATIONS.

| Event or Exposure | BLS 1998 | Percentage of Events | Estimation of Fatalities by Race/Ethnicity[c] Latinos | African Americans | Whites |
|---|---|---|---|---|---|
| Transportation incidents | 2,630 | 44 | 308 | 260 | 2,207 |
| Assault or violence | 960 | 16 | 112 | 94 | 803 |
| Contact with objects or equipment | 949 | 15 | 105 | 89 | 754 |
| Falls | 702 | 12 | 84 | 70 | 603 |
| Exposure to electricity or toxins | 572 | 9 | 63 | 53 | 456 |
| Other | 213 | 3 | 28 | 25 | 193 |
| Totals (from Table 12.5)[b] | 6,026 | | 700 | 591 | 5,016 |

[a]United States Department of Labor, Bureau of Labor Statistics (1998). *National census of fatal occupational injuries.* Washington, D.C. The distribution of *Percentage of Events* was obtained by BLS over all races and ethnicities. BLS reported the distribution race and ethnicity of all the 6,026 fatalities as *Percentage of Events* (see third column) with no breakdown by race or ethnicity.

[b]Sum totals (last row) are greater than 6,026 because Latino workers may also be identified as Black or White, causing an undetermined overlap.

[c]The estimation of numbers of deaths by event and by race or ethnicity was done based on the *Percentage of Events* of all fatalities; that is, calculation of estimate of transportation fatalities of Latinos: $700 \times 0.44 = 308$.

thus only an approximation, because the distribution of occupational titles differs between African Americans, Whites, and Latinos.

Recent studies have calculated estimates of fatal injury lifetime risk accumulated over the life of the worker (Myers, Kisner, & Fosbroke, 1998). The National Institute for Occupational Safety and Health (NIOSH) published recently (1998) a study comparing experiences of the highest working lifetime risks by race and ethnicity that permits a direct comparison between Latinos, African Americans, and Whites (Table 12.7).

All comparisons were made between lifetime risks of African Americans and Whites in the same occupation and industry categories. In Table 12.7 the descending list of the highest fatal working lifetime risk for Latinos, in five occupations within five industries, is compared with the same occupation or industry lifetime risk experiences of African Americans and Whites. Latinos had the highest lifetime risk of fatalities by homicide among cashiers in gas stations and guards in security services, and also the highest lifetime risk of fatality by collision as truck drivers. Latinos also had the second-highest lifetime risk of homicide as cab drivers and employees of grocery stores (Myers, Kisner, & Fosbroke, 1998).

## Fatal Occupational Diseases

Fatal occupational disease is defined as death due to a disease that is either caused or exacerbated by substances, physical conditions, or other hazardous exposures on the job. The best available estimates of fatal occupational disease in the

**TABLE 12.7. HIGHEST WORKING LIFETIME FATALITY RISK FOR HOMICIDES AND TRANSPORTATION INCIDENTS FOR LATINO, AFRICAN AMERICAN, AND WHITE WORKERS: ACCUMULATED DATA FROM 1992 TO 1996 FOR DEATHS GREATER THAN FIVE.[a]**

| Industry | Occupation | Event | *Latinos* | | *African Americans* | | *Whites* | |
|---|---|---|---|---|---|---|---|---|
| | | | Number of Deaths | Lifetime Risk[b] | Number of Deaths | Lifetime Risk[b] | Number of Deaths | Lifetime Risk[b] |
| Cab or transportation | Driver | Homicide/shooting | 46 | 49.5 | 137 | 66.7 | 120 | 40.7 |
| Gas station | Cashier | Homicide/shooting | 12 | 13.1 | 6 | 4.5 | <5 | NA |
| Grocery store | Employee | Homicide/shooting | 52 | 12.2 | 30 | 7.2 | 13 | 33.5 |
| Security service | Guard | Homicide/shooting | 31 | 9.5 | 41 | 4.5 | <5 | NA |
| Truck or transportation | Driver | Collision | 28 | 4.9 | 42 | 4.2 | <5 | NA |

[a]Modified from Myers, Kisner, & Fosbroke (1998).

[b]Working lifetime risk (WLTR) in units of death per 1,000 (forty-five-year working lifetimes):

$$WLTR = [1 - (1 - R)^y] \times 1000$$

where $R$ = ratio of the average annual number of work-related fatal injuries among workers in a given group to average annual employment in that group; $y$ = years of exposure to work-related fatal injury risk. Working lifetime is assumed to start at age twenty and end at age sixty-five.

U.S. general population were published recently by Leigh and colleagues (1997). Their estimates considered six groups of occupational diseases—cancers, cardiovascular, renal, chronic respiratory diseases, and pneumoconioses, in all of which occupational exposures were the prime contributor to death—and they exclude occupational injuries (Table 12.8). They estimated that 46,800 to 73,600 deaths occur annually in the United States due to occupational diseases (Table 12.9).

These estimates are similar to and more conservative than the previously published estimates of 100,000 deaths annually (Ashford, 1976). Using the BLS estimate for 1999 (United States Department of Labor, Bureau of Labor Statistics, 2000) that 12 percent of the traumatic fatalities in the U.S. civilian workforce were of Latino workers (Table 12.5), we can estimate that some 5,000–9,000 Latinos die from occupational diseases annually. The same 1997 estimates by Leigh and colleagues of deaths by occupational disease are distributed by cause of death using the percentages of death for traumatic fatalities (12 percent for Latinos; 10 percent for African Americans). The results appear in Table 12.8.

# Quality of Data on Latino Workers

All the data generated by federal agencies on morbidity and mortality are based on reported counts for a limited number of workers in the private sector only (excluding self-employed workers). For any overall estimation, adjustments (that is,

## TABLE 12.8. ESTIMATED FATAL WORK-RELATED ILLNESS DISTRIBUTED BY DISEASE.[a]

| Causes of Death | Estimation of Number of Deaths Attributed to Occupation[a] (all Races and Ethnicities) | Number of Deaths of Latinos Attributed to Occupation (12 Percent)[b] | Number of Deaths of African Americans Attributed to Occupation (10 Percent)[b] |
|---|---|---|---|
| Cancer | 31,025–51,706 | 3,723–6,204 | 3,103–5,171 |
| Cardiovascular and cerebrovascular disease | 5,092–10,185 | 611–1,222 | 509–1,019 |
| Chronic respiratory diseases | 9,154 | 1,099 | 915 |
| Pneumoconioses | 1,136 | 136 | 114 |
| Nervous system disorders | 269–806 | 32–96 | 27–89 |
| Renal disorders | 223–689 | 27–83 | 22–76 |
| Total | 46,800–73,600 | 5,520–8,832 | 4,680–7,360 |

[a]Data from Leigh, Markowitz, Fahs, Shin, & Landrigan (1997).

[b]Percentages of working population in 1998 from United States Department of Labor, Bureau of Labor Statistics (1998). *National census of fatal occupational injuries.* Washington, D.C.

## TABLE 12.9. ESTIMATED FATAL WORK-RELATED DISEASE FOR THE WHITE, AFRICAN AMERICAN, AND LATINO WORKING POPULATIONS.

| Race or Ethnicity | Fatal Work-Related Disease Range[b] | Percentage[a,c] |
|---|---|---|
| Whites | 38,844–73,600 | 83 |
| African Americans | 4,680–7,360 | 10 |
| Latinos | 5,148–8,096 | 12 |
| Total | 46,800–73,600 | 100 |

[a]United States Department of Labor, Bureau of Labor Statistics (1998). *National census of fatal occupational injuries.* Washington, D.C. Percentages of traumatic fatalities as reported by Bureau of Labor Statistics for 1998.

[b]Modified from Leigh, Markowitz, Fahs, Shin, & Landrigan (1997).

[c]Percentages are greater than 100 because of an undetermined overlap of racial classifications (Latinos can be double-counted as Whites or Blacks).

using additional data sources) need to be made to arrive at total counts for the entire workforce. Unreported and uncounted cases generally lead to underestimation of occupational morbidity and mortality. A second estimation is required because of the inadequate recording of race and ethnicity, necessitating the assumption that the risk of occupational disease and injury is the same in the U.S. Latino workforce as in the general U.S. workforce. Because evidence strongly suggests that Latinos are overrepresented in the more hazardous jobs and are at higher risk, the true numbers are likely to be even higher.

Landrigan and Markowitz (1989) estimated the degree of underreporting by comparing independently generated estimates of occupational disease mortality and incidence with the actual numbers of cases reported by the Workers' Compensation Board. In New York State, only 3 to 5 percent of the estimated number of deaths due to occupational diseases was reported by the Workers' Compensation Board as being of occupational etiology. Similarly, 11 to 38 percent of the estimated number of incident cases of occupational disease were reported by the Workers' Compensation Board as occupational.

Many of the estimated 95 to 97 percent of occupational disease deaths and 62 to 89 percent of incident cases of occupational disease that were not reported as occupational probably represent unrecognized epidemics. Certainly they represent many lost opportunities to properly treat and prevent occupational disease. In many of these cases the correct diagnosis is missed entirely, and in other cases, it is made too late in the disease process for primary or secondary prevention to be possible.

A survey of unionized garment workers in New York City demonstrated the magnitude of underreporting to Workers' Compensation of both occupational diseases and occupational injuries (Herbert, Luo, Marcus, Landrigan, Plattus, & O'Brien, 1989). Only four of forty-two workers (10 percent) told by an occupational physician that their illness was work-related had filed for Workers' Compensation. In the same survey, only nineteen of sixty-two workers (31 percent) injured on the job filed for Workers' Compensation. Of these sixty-two injured workers, six of the thirteen White workers (46 percent), three of the eight African American workers (37 percent), ten of the thirty-nine Latino workers (26 percent), and neither of the two Asian workers (0 percent) filed for Workers' Compensation. This study was done using highly trained occupational physicians in a union occupational health clinic with the active cooperation of the union, and reported rates are probably much better than usual. In spite of the limitations of this survey, it suggests that reported rates of occupational injury and disease are likely to underestimate population prevalence or incidence of occupational health problems. In addition, the study suggests that the sensitivity of surveillance mechanisms based on Workers' Compensation case reports may be lower for occupational diseases than for occupational injuries and even lower for Latino workers than for White workers.

## Costs of Occupational Morbidity and Mortality

Missed and delayed diagnosis of occupational disease produce substantial and avoidable costs (see summary following). These costs and social burdens contribute to the rising costs of medical insurance. The missed diagnoses are not reported as occupational diseases and are thus invisible to the occupational health surveillance system that might be in place, delaying recognition and resolution of the problem of work-related disease.

*Summary of Hidden Costs and Burdens of Unrecognized Occupational Disease.*

Costs

- Suffering, disability, and death.
- Economic hardship, job loss, continued unemployment.
- Prolonged duration of disease.
- Profession of acute reversible disease to chronic irreversible disease that persists even after exposure ends.
- Time lost from work, decreased productivity, and low morale of workers.
- Inappropriate diagnostic testing and medical or surgical treatment.
- Increased burden on an already overloaded health care system.

Economic Social Burden

- Families of workers.
- Employers (who pass costs onto consumers).
- City, state, and federal governments (who pass costs onto taxpayers, for example, of Welfare or Medicaid).
- Union benefit funds.
- Medical insurance companies (who pass costs onto their other clients).
- Medical care organizations and providers.

Leigh and colleagues (1997) estimated that the total cost of occupational morbidity and mortality in the United States reaches $171 billion per year: $65 billion in direct costs plus $106 billion in indirect costs. The grim share of this cost from the Latino working population is approximately 12 percent of $171 billion, or $21 billion dollars each year.

# Work-Related Diseases in Latino Workers

Which work-related diseases occur in Latino workers in urban areas of the United States? Incidence, prevalence, and mortality data for specific work-related diseases have not been compiled. However, some examples of work-related diseases, which occur in industries and occupations that employ many Latino workers, are listed in the following summary. Most of these are drawn from the list of *occupational sentinel health events* (Rutstein et al., 1983; Mullan & Murthy, 1991). Occupational sentinel health events are diseases or other causes of disability or death (with ICD-9 [*International Classification of Diseases, 9th Revision*] codes) that satisfy defined criteria for literature-supported associations with specific toxic substances, industries, or occupations. The importance of an occupational sentinel health event is that it serves as a warning signal that a preventable injury or illness has occurred, meaning that industrial hygiene or ergonomic evaluation and modification of the workplace is needed. Preventive interventions in the workplace include substitution of toxic materials with nontoxic or less toxic materials, low-ering of exposures with engineering controls such as ventilation, or brief reduc-tion of exposures using personal protective equipment such as respirators. The examples following are presented in order to facilitate creation of surveillance programs by identifying the industrial sector, the hazardous exposure, and the as-sociated occupational disease. They may also facilitate planning appropriate oc-cupational health measures such as clinical evaluations, preventive interventions, and educational services. Most of the occupational disease–exposure associations have been listed by NIOSH (Mullan & Murthy, 1991) as occupational sentinel health events; the remainder have been reported in the occupational medicine literature and are marked with an asterisk (*). Because our knowledge of occupational diseases is constantly growing, the list is most likely incomplete. Due to the multicausal nature of many of the diagnoses, this list can only be a general guide. In individual cases, a detailed occupational health clinical evaluation (as discussed in several occupational medicine textbooks, such as LaDou, 1990; Rosenstock & Cullen, 1996; Levy & Wegman, 1999; Rom, 1998) is obtained once a work-related disease is suspected, in order to clinically confirm or rule out work-relatedness. In addition, sixteen reviews of clinical evaluation for specific occu-pational diseases have recently been published in the *American Journal of Industrial Medicine* (vol. 37, pp. 1–142, January 2000).

*Some Examples of Work-Related Diseases.*

*Note:* This list is meant to assist in recognition of occupational diseases and is neither exhaustive nor definitively diagnostic. Actual diagnosis of occupational disease should be done in consultation with an occupational physician. Most of these conditions and exposures have been designated as *occupational sentinel health events* (Mullan & Murthy, 1991). Those which have not are well documented in the clinical literature and are preceded by an asterisk.

*Work-related asthma.* Workers exposed to a variety of airborne dusts or chemi-cal fumes and vapors (Rom, 1998)

*Pulmonary tuberculosis (TB).* Health care workers; *shelter workers; *prison workers; *other workers exposed on the job to persons with active TB; workers with silicosis

*Pulmonary asbestosis (parenchymal pulmonary fibrosis with or without pleural scarring).* Asbestos workers with substantial asbestos exposure more than fifteen years ago

*Acute bronchitis, pneumonitis, and pulmonary edema.* Manufacturing workers exposed to airborne irritants including ammonia, chlorine, nitrogen oxides, sulfur dioxide, cadmium, and trimellitic anhydride

*Hypersensitivity pneumonitis.* Workers (such as agricultural workers or *office workers) exposed to organic dusts from molds, fungi, bacteria, and other sources

*Silicosis.* Sandblasters and other workers exposed to silica dust

*Carpal tunnel syndrome.* Meat packers and processors, *typists, *garment workers, *supermarket checkers, and *factory workers

*Raynaud's phenomenon.* Workers exposed to vibrations or vinyl chloride

*Occupational cancers.* Lung cancer in workers exposed to asbestos, polycyclic aromatic hydrocarbons, arsenic, chromate, or nickel dust, ionizing radiation and radon, Bis(chloromethyl)ether, as well as welders and smelter, foundry, rubber reclamation, and steel workers

> Malignant mesothelioma in persons with asbestos exposure (even low doses, especially more than thirty years ago)
>
> Leukemia or aplastic anemia in workers exposed to benzene or ionizing radiation
>
> Bladder cancer in workers exposed to aromatic amine dyes
>
> Laryngeal cancer in asbestos-exposed workers
>
> *Nasopharyngeal, *oropharyngeal, and *brain cancer in *formaldehyde-exposed workersp
>
> Nasal cancer in furniture makers and woodworkers
>
> *Angina and *myocardial infarction
>
> Workers exposed to *carbon disulfide, *carbon monoxide, or *methylene chloride
>
> *Cardiac arrhythmias
>
> Workers exposed to *halogenated hydrocarbon solvents or *anticholinesterase insecticides

*Toxic neuropathy.* Workers exposed to lead, *n*-hexane, methyl-*n*-butyl ketone, carbon disulfide, acrylamide, ethylene oxide, or arsenic

*Toxic encephalitis.* Workers exposed to lead or mercury

*Parkinson's disease.* Workers exposed to manganese, carbon monoxide, or *carbon disulfide

*Noise-induced hearing loss.* Air hammer operators, musicians, factory workers, and others exposed to loud sounds

*Contact dermatitis.* Workers who have skin contact with irritant or allergenic liquids or dusts

*"Sick building syndrome"*. Fatigue, headache, mucous membrane irritation, chest tightness, irritability, and other nonspecific symptoms in workers in centrally ventilated buildings with sealed windows and inadequate ventilation

*Cataracts*. Workers exposed to infrared light, microwaves, ionizing radiation, trinitrotoluene, naphthalene, or ethylene oxide

*Hepatitis B, non-A, non-B hepatitis (NANB), and—rarely—HIV infection.* Health care workers' injuries from contaminated sharp instruments

## Latino Workers' Risk of Occupational Disease and Injury

Table 12.4 shows the blue-collar occupations with the highest number of occupational illness and injury nationwide. These recent data (1997) show how the percentage of injuries and illness exceeded the representation of Latino workers in three categories (janitors, laborers, and cooks) (United States Department of Labor, Bureau of Labor Statistics, 1999). Another approach to judging the magnitude of the problem of occupational disease in Latino workers is to examine data on the rates of occupational disease in various industries and the presence of Latinos in these.

Analysis of an independent data set using the 1980 Census data (United States Bureau of the Census, 1980) reveals a similar pattern (Table 12.10). It is difficult to rank the occupational categories more quantitatively than "higher risk" and "lower risk." The two white-collar industries have the lowest rates of occupational diseases, and the blue-collar industries have the higher rates of occupational diseases, in terms of incident cases as well as lost workdays (Table 12.10). Compared to White workers, Latino (then called "Spanish origin") workers are greatly overrepresented in the two most numerous high-risk occupational categories: operators, factory workers, and laborers (30.4 percent of Latino workers versus 11.4 percent of White workers were in this category) and service occupations (19.6 percent of Latino workers versus 10.4 percent of White workers were in this category). Following the national pattern again, Latinos are underrepresented in both of the lower-risk occupational categories: managerial and professional people (10.8 percent of Latino workers in this category versus 30.2 percent of White workers) and technical, sales, and clerical employees (29 percent of Latino workers in this category versus 39 percent of White workers). The patterns of employment at both the national and New York City levels support the hypothesis that Latino workers tend to work in jobs with higher-than-average risk for occupational disease.

Several bodies of evidence independent of the job distribution data discussed previously suggest that disproportionate employment in high-risk jobs concretely translates into increased risk of occupational diseases and injuries.

A study based on data from the state of California concluded that African American and Latino workers are at greater risk of occupational illnesses and

**TABLE 12.10. DISTRIBUTION OF OCCUPATIONS FOR WHITE, AFRICAN AMERICAN, AND LATINO ("SPANISH ORIGIN") POPULATIONS OF NEW YORK CITY: 1980 U.S. CENSUS.**

| | Whites | African Americans | Latinos |
|---|---|---|---|
| **Higher-risk occupations** | | | |
| Operators, fabricators, and laborers | 11.40 percent | 17.80 percent | 30.40 percent |
| Service occupations | 10.40 percent | 24.40 percent | 19.60 percent |
| Crafts and foremen | 8.50 percent | 6.70 percent | 9.70 percent |
| Farming | 0.40 percent | 0.50 percent | 0.50 percent |
| **Lower-risk occupations** | | | |
| Technical, sales, and clerical | 39.00 percent | 36.10 percent | 29.00 percent |
| Managerial and professional | 30.20 percent | 14.50 percent | 10.80 percent |
| Total (in thousands) | 2,160 | 826 | 616 |

*Source:* United States Bureau of the Census (1980). *Public use microdata, 5 percent sample.* Prepared for the Center for Puerto Rican Studies, Hunter College, City University of New York.

*Note:* Percentages are *column* percentages and represent distributions of jobs within racial or ethnic groups.

injuries than are White workers (Robinson, 1989). Latino men had more than a 100 percent increase in the risk of work-related acute illness or injury compared with White men, while African American men had a 41 percent increase compared with White men. Latino women had a 49 percent increase over the risk of White women, and African American women had a 31 percent increase over the risk of White women. All 95 percent lower confidence limits of the study's calculated odds ratio were less than 1. Statistical adjustment for educational level and potential years of work experience reduced the excess risks but did not eliminate them, suggesting that part of the excess risk can be explained by differences in these factors and the rest cannot. However, the unadjusted excess risks represent actual elevations in risk from all contributing factors, including educational factors and potential years of work experience, and are more useful for public health inference and action than the adjusted excess risks.

Two studies of occupational injuries from the New Jersey Department of Health show patterns consistent with and more extreme than the California studies. In the first, 200 fatal occupational injuries in construction workers were reported to the New Jersey Fatal Occupational Injury Surveillance registry from 1983 to 1989 (Sorock, O'Hagan Smith, & Goldoft, 1993). Fatality rates were three times higher for construction workers than for all workers combined. Fatality rates for Latino workers (in this case defined as born in a Spanish-speaking country) and African American workers were 34.8 per 100,000 employees per year and twenty-four per 100,000 employees per year, respectively. In contrast, the fatality rate for American-born White construction workers was 10.6 per 100,000 employees per year. Thus, rates for Latino and African American construction workers were 3.3 and 2.3 times higher than the rate for American-born White construction workers. Interestingly, only 6 percent of all the deaths had been reported to Workers' Compensation. Fatality rates for U.S.-born Latinos were not reported, and it is not stated explicitly whether they were included in or excluded from the U.S. White and U.S. African American categories.

The second study (Sorock, Smith, & Hall, 1993) was a telephone survey of individuals who had been hospitalized previously for finger amputations. Of 637 persons invited to participate, 355 were contacted and 228 were interviewed. Of those interviewed, 134 (59 percent) said their injury occurred at work. Age-adjusted rates of hospitalized occupational finger amputations were 52.8 for Latino men, 28.9 for African American men, and 9.5 for White men, per 100,000 employees per year. The relative risks were 5.6 and 3.0 for Latino and African American men, respectively, compared to White men. Ethnic classification was by self-report for both numerators and denominators. Although the absolute rates for women were lower, a similar pattern was found. Age-adjusted rates for women were 7.4 for Latino women, 3.5 for African American women, and 1.2 for White women, yielding relative risks of 6.2 and 2.9 for Latino women and African American women, respectively, compared to White women. Two weaknesses of this study were the low response rate (36 percent) and the use of 1980 Census data to generate denominators for the rates. The 1980 Census data clearly undercounted the Latino population, which had grown substantially during the 1980s. This would produce a spuriously elevated rate when this undercount was used as a denominator. However, it is extremely unlikely that this alone could account for a sixfold elevation in rates of hospitalized occupational finger amputations. In spite of its weaknesses, this study is consistent with the pattern of higher risks of occupational diseases among Latino workers seen in the other bodies of evidence.

A study of California adults with elevated blood lead levels provides additional insights (Maizlish & Rudolph, 1993). Of 149 adults reported directly by laboratories to the California Adult Blood Lead Registry with lead levels above sixty micrograms per deciliter ($\mu$g/dl), 46 percent were classified as Latino. This is the level at which OSHA legally mandates removal of a worker from the job, although toxic effects in adults have been documented at levels of twenty-five $\mu$g/dl and probably occur at even lower levels. The industries accounting for the largest numbers of reported cases were automobile radiator repair, lead battery manufacturing, brass and copper foundries, and gun firing ranges. Household contamination with lead was documented for at least one participant, an automobile radiator repair worker.

In a companion study (Bellows & Rudolph, 1993), 275 radiator service companies were enrolled in a lead-poisoning prevention project conducted by the California Department of Health. The percentage of companies that voluntarily performed blood lead screening on their employees was increased from 9 percent to 95 percent by this project. Of the individuals participating in the screening program, 60 percent had Latino surnames; 22 percent of the study participants had blood lead levels above forty $\mu$g/dl and 6 percent had levels above sixty $\mu$g/dl.

This study demonstrates the potential for successful recruitment of employers in an occupational health screening program, and it also suggests that Latino workers are overrepresented in this high-risk industry.

Some parental occupations and toxic exposures have been associated with cancer in the children of exposed individuals (Savitz & Chen, 1990). Associations that have been reported with consistency include childhood brain cancer with paternal exposure to hydrocarbons, paints, and the chemical and petroleum industries, and childhood leukemias with paternal paint exposures. Maternal occupational exposures have been less well studied, but consistent associations between leukemia and a variety of chemicals have been reported.

The asbestos abatement industry is potentially a safe, low-risk industry, provided proper preventive methods and personal protective equipment are used. Published data on this industry and ethnicity of workers has not been found in a search of the literature. However, in New Jersey, about one-third of asbestos abatement workers take their certification exam in Spanish and many more are Latino. One of this chapter's authors has lectured to more than 2,000 Latino workers in a training program for certification and recertification as asbestos handlers. In informal classroom discussions, many Latino students already working as asbestos abatement workers reported flagrant noncompliance with protective regulations by their employers. The violations included being forced to reuse the same disposable clothing for three or more days, refusal by the employer to supply fresh filter cartridges for respirators, and lack of showers on the job. These practices, clear violations of the OSHA asbestos standard, undoubtedly lead to significant asbestos exposure and convert a potentially safe industry into a hazardous one.

## Sweatshops in the Garment Industry

"Sweatshops" have been discussed in two documents published recently by the U.S. General Accounting Office (GAO) (1988), where they are formally defined as "businesses that regularly violate *both* safety or health *and* wage or child labor laws" and are also defined more loosely as "chronic labor law violators." Construction firms, farms, and homework (such as piecework apparel or electronics manufacturing in the home) are included in this definition.

Sweatshops are hazardous workplaces by definition. The occupational hazards encountered in sweatshop work in the garment industry include ergonomic hazards (for instance, repetitive motions, awkward working postures, vibrating tools such as fabric cutters, or falls from ladders), airborne hazards (for instance, high concentrations of dust, poorly ventilated dry-cleaning solvents, or fumes from glues and fabric treatments like formaldehyde), temperature extremes, and skin contact with irritant and allergenic substances. Occupational diseases and injuries prevalent among apparel sweatshop workers include musculoskeletal or cumulative trauma disorders like back, neck, and shoulder pain and carpal tunnel syndrome (Punnett, Robins, Wegman, & Keyserling, 1985; Sokas, Spiegelman, & Wegman, 1989), contact dermatitis, occupational asthma and bronchitis, vibration-induced Raynaud's phenomenon, and acute and chronic toxicity from solvents and other toxic chemicals.

A poll of fifty-three federal enforcement officials, published by the U.S. GAO (1988), showed that sweatshops were reported in significant numbers in forty-seven of the fifty-states, most commonly in the apparel, restaurant, and meat processing industries. Major concentrations were found in large cities, with New York having been the most intensively studied. At the national level, Latinos were thought to make up the majority of sweatshop workers in both restaurant and apparel industries, followed by Asian and African Americans.

No national estimates of numbers of sweatshop workers have been published, but local estimates from several sources have been reported. In New York, the director of the Apparel Industry Task Force of the New York State Department of Labor estimated that 4,500 of the 7,000 apparel factories and shops in New York City were sweatshops and that more than 50,000 workers were employed in this sector. Other sources estimated the number of apparel sweatshops at 3,000, also with more than 50,000 workers (United States General Accounting Office, 1988). In New Orleans, an estimated 25 percent of the 100 apparel firms (employing 5,000 workers) were multiple labor law violators. The only available estimate for restaurant workers comes from an official in Chicago, who estimated that half of the 5,000 restaurants there (employing 25,000 workers) were chronic labor law violators (United States General Accounting Office, 1988).

Sweatshops have proliferated because of social and economic factors that continue to be prevalent. The reasons for the existence of sweatshops cited by more than 50 percent of the federal officials (United States General Accounting Office, 1988) were as follows (in decreasing order of response):

1. Available supply of an immigrant workforce.
2. The labor-intensive nature of the industries.
3. The low profit margin in these industries.
4. Too few inspectors.
5. Weak or non-existent unions.
6. Inadequate penalties for infractions.

Not mentioned but probably important is the fact that these industries require skills that are either already possessed by a large proportion of the immigrant workforce or can be learned on the job with little formal training. This does not imply that these are low-skilled jobs; Fernández-Kelly (1983) gave a graphic description of the high level of skill and productivity needed even to approach earning the minimum wage in a piecework payment system. Sweatshops have also been identified as a system of production that invariably inflicts violence on minorities, either traumatic, violent deaths and injuries (from fires, explosions, accidents, and other causes), or chronic, occupational diseases that although extended in time are not less severe (Moure-Eraso, 1999).

### *Maquiladora* Industry as Modern Sweatshops

Closely related to sweatshops are *maquiladoras,* manufacturing and assembly factories along the Mexican side of the United States–Mexico border. The *maquiladora* produces a variety of goods (from television sets to computer boards and wire harnesses) exclusively earmarked for export to the United States. More than one million workers are employed in this industry (Cedillo, 1999). These workers are exclusively Mexican citizens working in the Mexican side of the frontier. The community and occupational health impacts have been studied only in the 1990s following the explosive growth of *maquiladoras.* A community-based study of 267 *maquiladora* workers, mostly female, in the cities of Matamoros and Reynosa found evidence of musculoskeletal disorders related to working conditions (pace of work, poor workplace design, and ergonomic hazards). Acute health effects were also identified compatible with chemical exposures. Although other chronic diseases were not apparent, the high presence of musculoskeletal disorders was a striking result for a very young workforce (average age, twenty-five years) (Moure-Eraso, Wilcox, Punnet, MacDonald, & Levenstein, 1994; Moure-Eraso, Wilcox, Punnet, MacDonald, & Levenstein, 1997).

# Barriers to Prevention of Occupational Diseases

The evidence presented strongly suggests that occupational disease in the Latino workforce is a common, severe, and preventable problem. In order to suggest rational solutions to the problem, it is helpful to explore critically some of the barriers to prevention of occupational diseases as well as some of the reasons that Latino workers tend to be overrepresented in hazardous jobs.

In principle, all occupational diseases are preventable. Prevention depends upon identifying the causal exposure(s), and eliminating or reducing these exposures until no more workers get sick. Effective prevention requires timely identification and elimination or control of the causative exposures. It is clearly preferable to try to prevent the disease from occurring at all, rather than allowing it to occur and then trying to rehabilitate the person and provide monetary compensation for damage already done.

Several types of barriers currently exist to prevent implementation of effective prevention strategies. A lack of scientific understanding of the causal agents and their mechanisms is one important barrier, and research must be ongoing to identify hazardous agents and work situations. For example, only about 10,000 of the 60,000 commercially used chemicals have been tested for toxicity in animals (LaDou, 1990), and very few of these have been studied epidemiologically in humans. Understanding of the cellular and molecular mechanisms of toxicity is clearly an important component in developing new approaches to treatment and prevention of occupational disease. Even so, results of epidemiological studies can often be used to effectively prevent occupational disease even without detailed knowledge of the mechanisms involved. An example is the identification of asbestos-related diseases using epidemiological methods. This knowledge led to the reduction in asbestos-related disease through regulation and decreased use of asbestos in the United States. Other situations may not be so clear-cut and may require more sophisticated epidemiological techniques (such as preventive intervention trials) or basic understanding of the toxicology to definitively identify the causative agent.

Although an incomplete understanding of the biomedical and epidemiological etiological agents causing specific occupational diseases are important factors, the main barriers to prevention have been economic, political, legislative, and social in nature. Frequently, workers cannot afford to turn down a job simply because it is hazardous. Similarly, they often are unable to leave a job they know is hazardous, because they do not have the financial resources to stop working for the time required to find another job, to retrain for another job, or to apply for and receive Workers' Compensation payments. It is an unfortunate fact that Workers' Compensation payments for occupational diseases generally take more than six months and often more than a year to begin, even in the most clearly documented cases. Although this barrier affects relatively affluent workers as well, it affects workers with less financial resources more severely. In addition, the threat of prolonged unemployment weighs heavily on members of communities where jobs are scarce. The need to continue supporting a family frequently serves as an irresistible pressure on workers to endure concrete physical discomforts or more abstract elevated risks of occupational diseases. As a result, workers in these circumstances may present with advanced- or late-stage occupational diseases and may be resistant to quitting their jobs even when strongly counseled to do so by a physician. This economic and bureaucratic trap is a major barrier to successfully preventing occupational illness in Latino workers.

Employers who are ethical, well informed about occupational health, and sensitive to the particular needs of their workforces can play a key role in providing safe and healthy workplaces. Labor and management health and safety committees can be helpful in raising issues and resolving them before serious health effects occur. Employers sometimes believe that improvement of working conditions will be prohibitively expensive and will not make the investment, even if their workers are getting sick from exposures on the job. In spite of this common perception that safe and healthy working conditions cost too much, sometimes the cost of directly eliminating the hazard is less than the combined long-term costs of decreased productivity due to time lost from work and low morale, increased Workers' Compensation premiums, and fines from enforcing agencies like OSHA or the EPA. Sometimes a "win–win" solution can be found that improves the working conditions without incurring unmanageable costs and which may even increase productivity (Friedman-Jiménez & Claudio,1998).

Lack of access to comprehensive clinical occupational health services is another barrier to effective recognition and prevention of occupational diseases. Access is difficult for most workers, but particularly so for Latino workers. Evidence for this is indirect, as direct measures of access to these services have not been published. The increased risk of occupational disease combined with poor access to clinical, preventive, and educational occupational health services suggests that the public health impact of interventions to correct this situation would be particularly great.

Overcoming the socioeconomic and political barriers to prevention may prove to be an even greater challenge for Latino workers than for White workers. It will not occur until the problem is recognized and adequate additional resources are committed to a rational solution.

## A Comprehensive Approach to Addressing Occupational Disease in Latino Workers

The evidence strongly suggests that preventable occupational diseases cause substantial mortality and morbidity in the U.S. Latino population and that this problem is not being recognized or addressed adequately. Admittedly, the evidence is fragmented and of variable quality, but it is more than sufficient to drive us to begin addressing this problem now. The economic and noneconomic costs of not addressing the problem are great. OSHA has not been effective in reliably identifying hazardous exposure situations or epidemics of occupational disease, as we have seen previously in the section on sweatshop inspections. We need to address the problem directly and break the cycle of "no services equals no data equals no services" by making comprehensive occupational health services more accessible to Latino workers and simultaneously documenting the epidemics with careful clinical, epidemiological, and surveillance studies of working populations that include significant numbers of Latino workers. In order to facilitate this process, recommendations are offered in the following sections for a comprehensive approach to addressing this problem. These recommendations fall into five categories: primary prevention intervention approaches; clinical occupational health services; educational approaches; research and surveillance; unionization and organization of workers; and legislation and regulation of hazardous workplace exposures. In order to have a significant impact on the occupational health of Latino workers, efforts must be made in all five areas. Although occupational diseases may disproportionately affect Latino workers, the aim of preventive programs should be to reduce hazards for *all* workers, not simply redistribute the hazards more "equitably." These recommendations are intended to supplement broader ongoing efforts to improve health and safety conditions in the workplace.

## Primary Prevention and Intervention Approaches

Occupational health professionals are looking more and more to primary prevention interventions as the way to evolve from a paradigm of *control* of occupational exposures to a new one of *prevention* (Moure-Eraso, 1999; Quinn, Kriebel, Geiser, & Moure-Eraso, 1998). For example, traditional industrial hygiene has at the top of the hierarchy of engineering interventions the fabrication of local exhaust ventilation systems to "control" chemical exposures in work environments. Such strategies are proving to be very problematic in the long run. The "ventilated" (exhausted) toxic substance extracted from the worksite becomes an environmental contaminant in the community. This method of control generates toxic pollutants (gases or tiny particles) that need to be treated as either a hazardous waste or an air pollutant. In environmental science, that approach is defined as an "end of pipe" solution equivalent to waste disposal. New strategies of engineering interventions are being developed that avoid this type of risk transfer. The most obvious one for primary prevention purposes is raw material substitution. If this is not a viable option, toxics use reduction or source reduction by process changes is the strategy of choice (Moure-Eraso, 1999; Ellenbecker, 1996). Housing in minority communities is often clustered around factories and emitters of pollutants. Risk shifting from the point of production can be avoided or at least mitigated by primary prevention strategies such as substitution, source reduction, closed-loop recycling, improvement of maintenance, process modernization, reformulation of products, and improvements of housekeeping and training changes (Moure-Eraso, 1999; Ellenbecker, 1996). All these interventions need to occur at the point of production and with full participation of the parties involved, namely, workers and companies in conjunction with occupational health professionals.

## Clinical Occupational Health Services

Access to comprehensive clinical occupational health services is probably the major determinant of the success of medical treatment for occupational diseases, as well as of surveillance and secondary prevention programs. In New York City and other urban areas in the United States, working Latinos have even less access to these services than does the general working population. Access is determined mainly by the existence of local occupational health clinics and primary care providers knowledgeable in occupational medicine, as well as existence of other referral sources such as concerned unions, and workers and businesses aware of occupational health. Occupational diseases are usually only recognized when the diagnoses are specifically considered by clinicians with some training in occupational medicine or when suggested by an educated worker or patient.

Comprehensive occupational health services should include the following:

1. Diagnosis and symptomatic treatment of the medical condition.

2. Judging whether the medical condition is work related and identifying the causative exposure(s) as specifically as possible.

3. Evaluation of workplace conditions, including inspection of the workplace if necessary and feasible.

4. The capability to mount a group medical screening of coworkers from the same workplace with similar exposures, if indicated.

5. Education of the worker or patient as well as the employer and union regarding occupational hazards.

6. Recruitment of the cooperation of the employer and, if the workforce is organized, the union in addressing health and safety issues on the job.

7. Removal or control of the hazardous exposure by materials substitution, engineering controls, personal protective equipment, or (if this proves impossible) removal of the worker from the workplace.

8. Filing Workers' Compensation applications when appropriate.

9. If necessary, *and with the workers' informed consent,* reporting hazardous workplaces to OSHA, NIOSH, EPA, the state Department of Environmental Protection (DEP), or the appropriate regulatory or research agency.

10. Reporting all cases to the appropriate surveillance program, if one exists (for example, the Occupational Disease Registry of the New York State Department of Health, or the NIOSH Sentinel Event Notification System for Occupational Risks (SENSOR) program (Baker, et al., 1977).

11. Facilitating vocational rehabilitation and job retraining for workers disabled by occupational diseases (for instance, workers with allergic sensitizations to substances present at the worksite).

12. Educating primary care providers about recognition, basic management, and referral of their patients with likely occupational diseases.

Clinical services for most Latinos begin with primary care providers in the Latino communities, including community-based practitioners and community health centers as well as staff of hospital outpatient departments and emergency rooms. The majority of primary care providers have never been trained to recognize occupational diseases and do not know how to or where to refer a patient they think may have an occupational disease. Education of hospital-based providers is important, but education of the community-based providers is crucial, because they are often the first or only accessible source of health care and advice. If the first-contact providers do not recognize the occupational etiology of the illness, it is unlikely that the correct diagnosis will be made at all. They should have a basic knowledge of those diagnoses they might encounter that are likely to be work related, the *occupational sentinel health events* discussed earlier. Appropriate referral channels must be made accessible to them to follow up on possible work-related diagnoses. The Association of Occupational and Environmental Clinics (AOEC), based in Washington, D.C., is a network of occupational and environmental health clinics across the United States and currently has more than sixty clinics available for referrals from primary care providers.

## Educational Approaches

Much is already known about workplace hazards and prevention (see Rom, 1998; Rosenstock & Cullen, 1996; LaDou, 1990; Levy & Wegman, 1999; DiNardi, 1998). Application of this knowledge to improve public health requires effective education of professionals, workers, and employees.

Comprehensive, widespread culturally and linguistically appropriate occupational health education programs should be targeted at and accessible to workers in specific industries and occupations. To be accessible to Latino workers, these programs need to be in Spanish and English and should include "right to know" education, other health and safety training, and Spanish translations of relevant material safety data sheets (MSDSs). An excellent book by Kimball (1990) that lists and reviews 289 Spanish-language occupational health and safety materials for workers is a useful aid in planning and conducting worker education programs for Spanish-speaking Latino workers. Literature on empowerment approaches to worker health and safety education (Wallerstein & Weinger, 1992; Wallerstein & Rubinstein, 1993) emphasizes active involvement of workers in creating solutions to health problems in their own workplaces.

Employers are often not well versed in health and safety issues, even those related to hazardous substances or conditions in their own facilities. Educational programs to make them aware of appropriate health and safety practices and to sensitize them to workers' concerns and perspectives will facilitate improvements in health and safety conditions. However, many corporate and union health and safety departments have been downsized or eliminated in recent years. Occupational health programs in academic centers or in the community (for example, committees for occupational safety and health [COSH]) could play increasingly important roles in meeting occupational health training needs.

Limitation of job opportunities due to lack of education is important as an independent factor and, in combination with other factors, in increasing risk of occupational disease in Latino workers. Improvement of both the quality of education and the numbers of high school and college graduates in Latino communities would help lower the risk of occupational disease in Latino workers by opening up opportunities for less hazardous jobs as well as by empowering workers to improve their working conditions.

## Research and Surveillance

Sufficient evidence exists already to justify beginning to address the problem of occupational disease in Latino workers immediately. Nevertheless, in order to allow this issue to compete successfully with other high-priority issues for funding as well as research and clinical talent, objectives of this research would be (1) to determine which occupational health issues are most pressing, (2) to document the extent and severity of the problem, and (3) to develop effective and practical solutions.

NIOSH has called on the occupational health community to develop a National Occupational Research Agenda (NORA) to address the financial and human challenges brought about by the large burden of work-related disease injury and death. This agenda has developed twenty-one research priorities that include categories of special importance to the Latino community. Of these, special populations at risk, occupational health services, social and economic consequences of workplace illness and injuries, and innovative methods of hazards and health surveillance are four of the research topics particularly relevant to the needs of the Latino working community (National Occupational Research Agenda, 1998). NIOSH has organized periodic meetings with more than 500 organizations and individuals to provide it with input into development and guidance of research programs under NORA.

Improving access of Latino workers to clinical occupational health services would help greatly in documenting the prevalences and incidences of currently undiagnosed occupational diseases in Latinos. For example, a successful statewide network of occupational health clinics coordinated by and reporting to the New York State Department of Health and supported by funds from Workers' Compensation was started in 1989. State and federal occupational disease surveillance programs should include standardized ethnic classifications and should provide data on Latino workers.

In 1984, the collection of data on occupational disease in the United States was described as "fragmented, unreliable and seventy years behind communicable disease surveillance" (Sixtieth Report by the Committee on Government Operations, 1984). Both occupational disease surveillance and communicable disease surveillance have advanced since 1984, but a large gap remains.

Principles of effective occupational health surveillance have been well summarized by Markowitz (see Rom, 1998) who wrote that "[o]ccupational health surveillance entails systematic monitoring of health events and exposures in working populations in order to prevent and control occupational hazards and associated diseases and injuries." He went on to list four essential components of occupational health surveillance:

1. To gather information on cases of occupational diseases and injuries and on workplace exposure.
2. To distill and analyze the data.
3. To disseminate organized data to necessary parties, including workers, unions, employers, government agencies, and the public.
4. To intervene on the basis of data to alter the factors that produced these health events and hazards (see the previous section on primary prevention interventions).

Consensus among authorities on occupational health surveillance is that *intervention* must be an integral part of any surveillance program, in addition to the first three components listed. It is clear from these principles that accessible occupational health clinical and educational services are necessary and prerequisite to the establishment of an effective program of occupational health surveillance.

## Unionization and Organization of Workers, Legislation, and Regulation of Hazardous Workplace Exposures

Ideally, employers provide healthy and safe working conditions without intervention from the outside. Some companies have identified worker health and safety as a priority and have inhouse occupational medicine departments or have hired consultants to provide occupational health services. However, it is fairly common that the employer does not voluntarily provide healthy and safe working conditions. In these situations, a union can facilitate the process of improving the health and safety conditions in the workplace.

Organized workers are better able to avoid or reduce toxic and dangerous exposures in the workplace, with less vulnerability to being fired by an unscrupulous employer. Health and safety regulatory laws do not effectively prevent an employer from firing an individual worker for becoming sick from his or her job, filing for Workers' Compensation, requesting appropriate protective equipment, or simply complaining about dangerous working conditions. The protections under the law that do exist are frequently circumvented when the employer asserts that the worker was terminated for economic or other non-health-related reasons; the burden of proof rests on the worker to demonstrate otherwise.

Like other workers in the United States, currently only about one in six Latino workers is a member of a union. Organizing Latino workers can be a crucial step in improving compliance with OSHA guidelines and bringing about safe and healthy working conditions, as we saw in the garment industry example. A strong union health and safety committee can often be especially effective in facilitating this process, especially when management cooperates and forms a labor–management health and safety committee.

## Conclusions

The available evidence is inadequate to enable us to quantify the prevalence and incidence of occupational diseases and injuries in Latino working populations (although more and more sound estimates are becoming available) (see Leigh, Markowitz, Fahs, Shin, & Landrigan, 1997) at national or state levels. However the current estimates suggest that the overall risk of occupational diseases and injuries among Latino workers is beyond that which should be expected. In spite of obvious inadequacies, the currently available evidence is certainly sufficient to justify primary prevention interventions in the occupations for which we have identified morbidity and mortality excesses. It also warrants a greatly accelerated continuation of the investigation of the problem, specifically including Latino workers and high-risk industries that employ Latino workers.

Local epidemics of specific occupational diseases among Latino workers in particular industries have occurred and undoubtedly continue to occur. These epidemics are sometimes severe and would be readily observed if we looked for them.

It is clear that primary prevention interventions are needed in the workplace, such as substitution of problem chemicals, process changes to address the sources of chemical and physical hazards, and other engineering interventions. In addition, secondary prevention interventions must be conducted, including a rapid and substantial increase in clinical, preventive, and educational occupational health services accessible to Latino workers. Because most occupational diseases remain undiagnosed and unreported by the current medical care system, improving the recognition, diagnosis, and reporting of occupational diseases by primary care, subspecialist, and occupational medicine providers is critical. Recognition and clinical diagnosis of occupational diseases are prerequisite to adequate reporting, so improving access to clinical occupational health services is a necessary step in this process.

Although the focus of this chapter has been Latino workers, it is clear that in order to adequately address the problems of occupational disease and injury among Latino workers, any solution must address these problems among high-risk workers of all races and ethnicities, while ensuring that Latino workers are meaningfully included in the process. Addressing local epidemics haphazardly, when and if they happen to be discovered, will never be an adequate solution to this problem. A more humane, scientifically valid, and ultimately cost-effective strategy for addressing this problem is an integrated program of occupational health surveillance, accessible clinical occupational health services, careful epidemiological research, worker and health care provider education, collaboration with cooperative employers, unionization of Latino workers, legislative reform, and improved enforcement of regulatory standards.

# References

Ashford, N. (1976). *Crisis in the workplace: Occupational disease and injury.* Cambridge MA: MIT Press.

Ashford, N. (1997). Industrial safety: The neglected issue in industrial ecology. *Journal of Cleaner Production, 5,* 1, 115–121.

Baker, E. L. et al. (1977). Lead poisoning in children of lead workers: Home contamination with industrial dust. *New England Journal of Medicine, 296,* 5, 260–261.

Bellows, J., & Rudolph, L. (1993). The initial impact of a workplace lead-poisoning prevention program. *American Journal of Public Health, 83,* 3, 406–410.

Cedillo, L. (1999). *Psychosocial risk factors among women workers in the Maquiladora industry in Mexico.* Unpublished dissertation, University of Massachusetts, Lowell.

DiNardi, S. R. (1998). The occupational environment: Its evaluation and control. Fairfax, VA: American International Health Alliance.

Ellenbecker, M. J. (1996). Engineering controls as an intervention to reduce workers exposure. *American Journal of Industrial Medicine, 29,* 303–307.

Environmental Protection Agency. (1999, July). *Sociodemographic data used for identifying potentially highly exposed populations* (EPA/600/R-99/060). Washington, D.C.: Author.

Fernández-Kelly, M. P. (1983). *Maquiladoras:* The view from the inside. In Fernández-Kelly, M. P., *For we are sold, I and my people: Women and industry in Mexico's frontier.* Albany: State University of New York Press.

Friedman-Jiménez, G., & Claudio, L. (1998). Environmental justice. In W. N. Rom (Ed.), *Environmental and occupational medicine* (3rd ed.). Philadelphia: Little, Brown & Company.

Frumkin, H., Walker, E. D., & Friedman-Jiménez, G. (1999). Minority workers and communities. *Occupational Medicine, 14,* 3, 495–519.

Gardner, M. J., & Altman, D. G. (Eds.). (1989). *Statistics with confidence.* London: British Medical Journal Publishers.

Herbert, R., & Landrigan, P. J. (2000). Work related death: A continuing epidemic. *American Journal of Public Health, 90,* 541–545.

Herbert, R., Luo, J., Marcus, M., Landrigan, P. J., Plattus, B., & O'Brien, S. (1989). *The failure of workers' compensation statistics to monitor work-related illness in garment workers.* Abstract of paper presented at the American Public Health Association annual meeting.

Kimball, A. (1990). *A workers' sourcebook: Spanish language health and safety materials for workers [La Fuente Obrera: Materiales de salud y seguridad en español para trabajadores].* Labor Occupational Safety and Health Program, Center for Labor Research and Education, Institute of Industrial Relations, University of California, Los Angeles.

LaDou, J. (1990). *Occupational medicine.* Norwalk, CT: Appleton & Lange.

Landrigan, P. J., & Markowitz, S. (1989). Current magnitude of occupational disease in the United States: Estimates from New York State. *Annals of the New York Academy of Science, 572,* 27–45.

Last, J. M. (1988). *A Dictionary of Epidemiology* (2nd ed.). New York: Oxford University Press, 103–105.

Leigh, J. P., Markowitz, S. B., Fahs, M., Shin, C., & Landrigan, P. J. (1997). Occupational injury and illness in the United States: Estimates of costs, morbidity and mortality. *Archives of Internal Medicine, 157,* 1557–1568.

Levy, B. S., & Wegman, D. H. (Eds.). (1999). *Occupational health: Recognizing and preventing work-related disease* (3rd ed.). Philadelphia: Lippincott Williams & Wilkins.

Maizlish, N., & Rudolph, L. (1993). California adults with elevated blood lead levels, 1987 through 1990. *American Journal of Public Health, 83,* 3, 402–405.

Milton, D. K., Solomon, G. M., Rosiello, R. A., & Herrick, R. F. (1998). Risk and incidence of asthma attributable to occupational exposure among HMO members. *American Journal of Industrial Medicine, 33,* 1, 1–10.

Moure-Eraso, R. (1999). Sweatshops. In R. Gottesman (Ed.), *Violence in America: An encyclopedia* (Vol. 2). New York: Scribner, pp. 243–244.

Moure-Eraso, R., Wilcox, M., Punnet, L., MacDonald, C., & Levenstein, C. (1994). Back to the future: Sweatshop conditions on the Mexico–U.S. border: I. Community health impact of *maquiladora* industrial activity. *American Journal of Industrial Medicine, 25,* 311–320.

Moure-Eraso, R., Wilcox, M., Punnet, L., MacDonald, C., & Levenstein, C. (1997). Back to the future: Sweatshop conditions on the Mexico-U.S. border: II. Occupational health impact of *maquiladora* industrial activity. *American Journal of Industrial Medicine, 31,* 587–599.

Mullan, R. J., & Murthy, L. I. (1991). Occupational sentinel health events: An updated list for physician recognition and public health surveillance. *American Journal of Industrial Medicine, 19,* 775–799.

Myers, J. R., Kisner, S. M., & Fosbroke, D. E. (1998). Lifetime risk of fatal occupational injuries within industries, by occupation, gender, and race. *Human and Ecological Risk Assessment, 4,* 6, 1291–1307.

National Occupational Research Agenda. (1998). Center for Disease Control and Prevention (CDC) NIOSH. DHHS (NIOSH). Publication No. 98–141. Cincinnati.

Punnett, L. (1999). The costs of work-related musculoskeletal disorders in automotive manufacturing. *New Solutions: A Journal of Environmental and Occupational Health Policy, 9,* 4, 403–406.

Punnett, L., Robins, J. M., Wegman, D. H., & Keyserling, W. M. (1985). Soft tissue disorders in the upper limbs of female garment workers. *Scandinavian Journal of Work Environment and Health, 11,* 417.

Quinn, M. M., Kriebel, D., Geiser, K., & Moure-Eraso, R. (1998). Sustainable production: A proposed strategy for the work environment. *American Journal of Industrial Medicine, 34,* 297–304.

Robinson, J. C. (1989). Exposure to occupational hazards among Hispanics, African-Americans and non-Hispanic Whites in California. *American Journal of Public Health, 79,* 5, 629–630.

Rom, W. N. (1998). *Environmental and occupational medicine* (2nd ed.). Boston: Little, Brown.

Rosenstock, L., & Cullen, M. (1996). *Clinical occupational medicine.* (Saunders Blue Book Series). Philadelphia: Saunders.

Rutstein, D. D. et al. (1983). Sentinel health events (occupational): A basis for physician recognition and public health surveillance. *American Journal of Public Health, 9,* 198–221.

Savitz, D., & Chen, J. (1990). Parental occupation and childhood cancer: Review of epidemiologic studies. *Environmental Health Perspectives, 88,* 325–337.

Silverstein, B. A., Stetson, D. S., Keyserling, W. M., & Fine, L. J. (1997). Work-related musculoskeletal disorders: Comparison of data sources for surveillance. *American Journal of Industrial Medicine, 31,* 600–608.

Sixtieth Report by the Committee on Government Operations, U.S. House of Representatives. (1984, October 5). *Occupational illness data collection: Fragmented, unreliable and seventy years behind communicable disease surveillance.* H.R. 98–1144.

Sokas, R. K., Spiegelman, D., & Wegman, D. H. (1989). Self-reported musculoskeletal complaints among garment workers. *American Journal of Industrial Medicine, 15,* 197–206.

Sorock, G. S., O'Hagan Smith, E., & Goldoft, M. (1993). Fatal occupational injuries in the construction industry, New Jersey, 1983–1989. *Journal of Occupational Medicine, 35,* 9, 916–921.

Sorock, G. S., Smith, E., & Hall, N. (1993). An evaluation of hospital discharges data for surveillance of nonfatal occupational injuries. *American Journal of Industrial Medicine, 3/23,* 3, 427–437.

United States Bureau of the Census. (2000). *Projections of the resident population by race.* Washington, D.C.: U.S. Department of Commerce.

United States Bureau of the Census. (1980). *Public use microdata, 5 percent sample.* Prepared for the Center for Puerto Rican Studies, Hunter College, University of New York.

United States Department of Labor. (1987). *Standard Industrial Classification Manual* (1987 ed.). Washington, D.C.: Author. (Paperback version issued by the Office of the President, Bureau of Management and Budget.)

United States Department of Labor, Bureau of Labor Statistics. (1999). *Occupational injuries and illness, 1997.* Washington, D.C.: Author.

United States Department of Labor, Bureau of Labor Statistics. (1998). *National census of fatal occupational injuries.* Washington, D.C.: Author.

United States Department of Labor, Bureau of Labor Statistics. (1992). *Annual Bulletins* (1980–1990). Data compiled by D. Kotelchuck & R. Phillips, Environmental and Occupational Health Sciences Program, Hunter College, City University of New York.

United States General Accounting Office. (1988). *"Sweatshops" in the U.S.: Opinions on their extent and possible enforcement options.* Briefing report to the Honorable Charles E. Schumer, House of Representatives (GAO/HRD-88–130BR).

Wagner, G., & Wegman, D. H. (1999). Comments on: Risk and incidence of asthma attributable to occupational exposure among HMO members. *American Journal of Industrial Medicine, 35,* 2, 206.

Wallerstein, N., & Rubinstein, H. L. (1993). *Teaching about job hazards: A guide for workers and their health providers.* Washington, D.C.: American Public Health Association.

Wallerstein, N. B., & Weinger, M. (Eds.). (1992). Special issue on empowerment approaches to worker health and safety education. *American Journal of Industrial Medicine, 22,* 5, 619–783.

CHAPTER THIRTEEN

# HEALTH AND OCCUPATIONAL RISKS OF LATINOS LIVING IN RURAL AMERICA

Kathryn Azevedo, Hilda Ochoa Bogue

Nationwide, Latinos living in rural areas are an important component of the rural economy in the United States. Rural Latinos play a prominent role in the agricultural, meat, poultry, fishery, and mining industries, as well as in other occupations (United States Department of Agriculture, 1995; Rochín & Marroquin, 1997). Yet, like other working poor people in the United States, they struggle to meet the basic needs of their families, doing work that remains arduous and low paying and that entails substantial occupational health risks. In the United States, research studies continue to document the hardships experienced by this hardworking group (Azevedo, 2000; Bade, 1993, 1999; Barger & Reza, 1987, 1994; Commission on Security and Cooperation in Europe, 1993; Griffith & Kissam, 1995; Johnston, 1985; Palerm, 1992, 1994, & 1995; Rosenberg, Stierman, Gabbard, & Mines, 1998; Taylor, Martin, & Fix, 1997; Wells, 1996).

"Rural Latinos" in this chapter refers to those persons self-identified as Latinos—with roots from any Latin American nation or the Commonwealth of Puerto Rico—living and/or working in a rural area within the United States. Although no one knows with certainty how many Latinos are living in rural America, it is estimated that the figure ranges from one million to five million. One commonly cited approximation of the total number is some 4.2 million Latino agricultural workers and their dependents (Quandt, Arcury, Austin, & Saavedra, 1998; Dever, 1993). Latinos residing in rural America are not a homogeneous group; on the contrary, they comprise a mosaic of subgroups with different characteristics shaped, for example, by their ethnic background, language, place of origin, cultural beliefs, nationality, and level of acculturation (Rochín & Marroquin, 1997). Moreover, some of these residents speak languages other than Spanish, such as Mixteco, Zapoteco, Trique, Quiché, Kanjobal, and Tarascan. These rural residents are concentrated in the states of California, Florida, Colorado, and Texas (Bade, 1999; Taylor, Martin, & Fix, 1997; Villarejo, 1999). Each Latino subgroup has specific assets, needs, and characteristics that need to be considered.

This chapter examines key characteristics and health barriers experienced by Latino rural residents. More specifically, the chapter provides a brief overview of the industries that employ Latinos, examines rural Latino housing concerns, and discusses health and medical conditions. In addition, the last section presents approaches to addressing the many challenges to providing medical services to Latinos living and working in rural America.

## Profile of Latinos in Rural America

Gaining an understanding of the dynamics of rural America provides an important context for evaluating the conditions of Latinos living and working in these regions. Rural America accounts for 83 percent of the nation's land and more than sixty million people. Rural America is composed of 2,288 nonmetropolitan counties (see the next subsection), has 21 percent of the population, and generates 14 percent of the nation's earnings (United States Department of Agriculture, 1995). More than 800 rural counties have high poverty rates. The elderly are more concentrated in rural than in urban regions of the country. Over the last four decades of the twentieth century, rural employment saw a shift from farming to services and manufacturing jobs. More specifically, the largest share of rural employment originates from the services sector, which employs 50.6 percent of all rural workers. These jobs include employment related to recreation, retirement, financial services, insurance, real estate, retail stores, dry cleaners, restaurants, and telecommunications (United States Department of Agriculture, 1995). Other employment sectors are identified in Table 13.1.

Even though agriculture operations and related businesses are the largest single user of land in many areas, data from both farm operator and farmworker households reveal that both groups also rely heavily on nonfarm rural employment (United States Department of Agriculture, 1995; United States Department of Labor, 2000).

### TABLE 13.1.   SOURCES OF RURAL EMPLOYMENT.

| Service Sector | Government | Manufacturing | Farming | Construction | Mining | Agriculture, Forestry, and Fisheries |
|---|---|---|---|---|---|---|
| 50.60 percent | 17.20 percent | 16.90 percent | 7.60 percent | 4.90 percent | 1.90 percent | 0.90 percent |

*Source:* United States Department of Agriculture (1995); United States Department of Labor (2000).

## The Rural Latino Population

Rural Latinos represent the fastest-growing segment of the rural population in most nonmetropolitan areas in the United States (Rochín & Marroquin, 1997). There continues to be debate, however, on the definition of rural. According to the U.S. Bureau of the Census, rural residents are defined as those who live in counties outside metropolitan areas. Rural counties include small cities with less than 50,000 residents. These areas are designated as "nonmetro." However, if a county includes a city within its geographic boundary that has more than 50,000 persons, the entire county will be designated as urban. This definition of rural is problematic in states like California, where county geographic boundaries cover vast areas of land. As a consequence, large agricultural areas are often designated as urban rather than rural nonmetro counties (Villarejo, 1999; Rochín & Marroquin, 1997; Taylor, Martin, & Fix, 1997). More specifically, according to Villarejo (of the California Institute for Rural Studies in Davis), "1.6 million rural Californians, out of a total of 2.2 million, have been reclassified as metro county residents, and are no longer counted as rural for many Federal policy purposes" (1999, p. 10). Therefore, the actual numbers of rural Latino residents are subject to debate because of a systematic undercount of rural Latino residents working in agriculture in so-called urban counties due to inconsistencies in geographic boundaries and unique population concentration patterns.

Researchers from the Julian Samora Research Institute in East Lansing, Michigan, and the California Institute for Rural Studies report that socioeconomic as well as demographic characteristics link rural Latinos together when they are compared to non-Latinos and urban Latinos. Census data, for example, indicates that by 1990 Latinos grew by more than 30 percent from 1.8 million to 2.4 million. Furthermore, 76.9 percent of rural Latino residents residing in the United States are of Mexican origin and account for the majority of those employed in agriculture and related industries (Garcia & Gonzalez Martinez, 1999; Rochín & Marroquin, 1997). Rural Latino residents not only include agricultural workers but self-employed persons who own small businesses in these areas. Rural Latinos are also making inroads into the farm entrepreneurial population, where they may be self-employed as independent contractors in agriculture or owners of small stores, restaurants, beauty salons, and the like (Rochín & Marroquin, 1997). Moreover, in 1992 Latinos owned and operated more than 20,000 farms covering twelve million acres, with a total of some $2.4 billion in market value of agricultural products sold (United States Census of Agriculture, 1992; Rochín & Marroquin, 1997).

## Employment Sector Patterns Among Latinos in Rural America

Many rural Latino residents are employed as hired workers in agriculture and are concentrated in the states of California, Florida, and Texas where they account for 38 percent of farm labor expenditures (Rochín & Marroquin, 1997). However, rural Latinos also have sizable populations in Michigan, Minnesota, Iowa,

Pennsylvania, Nebraska, and Kansas. According to government statistics, in 1994 the hired farm labor force was 51 percent White, 42 percent Latino, and 8 percent African American and other ethnic and racial groups (Rochín & Marroquin, 1997).

One unique aspect of hired farm labor is the need to migrate from one job to another as the crop seasons change throughout the year. According to the 1997–1998 National Agricultural Workers Survey (NAWS) of the U.S. Department of Labor (2000), 56 percent of Latino agricultural workers migrated for employment. The migratory patterns of agricultural workers are referred to in the literature as "streams." Three major streams are described as the East Coast, the Midwest, and the West Coast streams. Characteristic of each stream is a "homebase" downstream, where these laborers reside and work when they are not traveling (Dever, 1993; Benavides-Vaello & Setzler, 1994) (see Figure 13.1).

The formal educational level of Latino agricultural workers averages six years; the average yearly income for individual Latino agricultural workers is reportedly $7,500 representing an average of twenty-four weeks in farm labor a year. Among hired Latino agricultural workers, 52 percent are not authorized to work legally in the United States (United States Department of Labor, 2000). These data are revealing in that Latino agricultural workers interviewed reported that they are employed for half of the year in agriculture and the other half of the year in other types of employment. Other research reports that 8 percent of Mexican

## FIGURE 13.1.   THE MAJOR MIGRANT STREAMS.

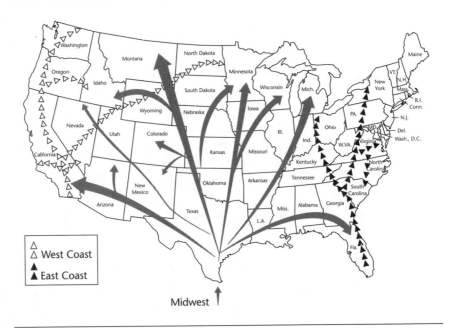

*Source:* National Migrant Resource Project (1992). NMRP is now renamed the National Center for Farmworker Health Inc.

Americans that work in farming, forestry, or fishing jobs, whereas 2 percent of Puerto Ricans and 1 percent of Cubans on the U.S. mainland (Sanchez-Bane, 1994) work in these industries.

Latinos have resided in most regions of the Southwest for hundreds of years. However, more recently, Latinos, mainly from Mexico, have moved into Midwestern states as more stable jobs in produce, poultry, and meatpacking houses have become available in these rural areas of the country. Large-scale meat industrial processing plants such as those of Manford, Swift Armour, and IBP (Iowa Beef Packers) offer year-round employment at the minimum salary of $6 per hour (Rochín & Marroquin, 1997). These plants, which employ large numbers of Latinos from Mexico, operate assembly-line production processes that have given rise to numerous health concerns.

As Latinos have become concentrated in rural areas, researchers are reporting greater poverty, lower salaries, and lower educational attainment of rural Latinos when compared to Latinos employed in urban areas (Rochín & Marroquin, 1997; Taylor, Martin, & Fix, 1997). California has experienced the fastest increase in the concentration of rural Latinos workers, most notably in the Central Valley and Southeastern desert regions of the state (Rochín & Marroquin, 1997; Palerm, 1995; Taylor, Martin & Fix, 1997; Villarejo, 1999; Azevedo, 2000).

# Housing Conditions Among Rural Latinos

The housing and living conditions experienced by Latinos vary and influence the medical conditions reported among these rural residents. In California, for example, there is some subsidized housing with running water, electricity, and other modern commodities (State of California, Employment Development Department, 1994). Nevertheless, there are also some rural Californians who live in less desirable mobile home units on and around Native American lands in isolated areas near the Salton Sea (Azevedo, 2000). Similarly, in Colorado there are "migrant camps" owned by private employers that can be better described as large dormitory rooms that accommodate some fifty to hundred agricultural workers each. The unit may have bunk beds, one shower and restroom, and a small kitchen with a cook who prepares the food for the workers. Other "migrant camps" have family units, with one or two rooms where farmworker families can be accommodated; those units may have a small kitchen and a restroom and shower. Yet there are some rural Latino residents living in their cars or under bridges (National Advisory Council of Migrant Health, 1995; Slesinger & Ofstead, 1993). In Texas, along the Rio Grande Valley, there is also a mix of living arrangements from home ownership to very modest mobile units, to "las Colonias"—squatter settlements—communities that lack running water, sewage systems, or electricity. In Florida, rural Latino residents also experience great variation in the available housing, from very modest mobile units, to crowded "migrant camps," to the modern, well-planned facilities of the Everglades Community Association in south Dade County, where hundreds live in comfortable, well-built, single-family houses near a community health clinic (Housing Assistance Council, 1994; Rural Community Assistance Program, 1992; National Advisory Council on Migrant Health, 1995; Margolis, 1981).

Unfortunately, in rural areas throughout the United States, poor sewage, contaminated water, no drainage infrastructure for water runoff, open pools of water in which insects breed in large numbers, improper garbage and sewage disposal, wild dogs, burning trash, incorrect electrical connections, and improperly installed propane tanks can be observed. These conditions have implications that seriously compromise the health and safety of rural Latino residents and their children (Azevedo, 2000; National Advisory Council on Migrant Health, 1995; Mobed, Goid, & Schenker, 1992; Rural Community Assistance Program, 1992; Ciesielski & Seed, 1990; Wilt, 1986, 1996).

# Health and Medical Conditions Among Rural Latinos

Information available on the health conditions and health status of rural Latino residents is limited. The systematic collection of comprehensive data on morbidity patterns of Latino agricultural workers, who represent a demographically younger patient population than the general U.S. population, was recently conducted (Dever, 1993). To date, there has not been a systematic, epidemiological, nationwide profile of the health status of rural Latinos in the United States. Rather, there have been several smaller-scale community and regional studies that document the medical conditions reported by agricultural laborers.

Latino agricultural workers suffer from a multitude of health problems that are related to the consequences of primary and secondary occupational hazards. Primary occupational hazards include pesticide exposure, sun exposure, injuries, and poor field sanitation. Secondary occupational hazards result from structural and institutional barriers such as difficulties in obtaining health care services, exclusion from traditional workers' benefits, lack of enforcement of health and safety standards, lack of adequate housing, and the lack of access to clean water (Sakala, 1987).

Pesticide exposure is a major health problem because both pesticide applicators and other field workers receive significant doses without adequate protection, despite a multitude of laws regulating their use nationwide. Acute clinical conditions that have been documented to be associated with pesticide exposure include systemic toxicity, dizziness, nausea, headache, and death. Long-term consequences include Bell's palsy, Guillain–Barré syndrome, Parkinson's disease, aplastic anemia, hemolytic anemia, pseudotumor cerebri, asthma, chloracne, toxic epidermal necrolysis, deafness, azoospermia, stillbirth, premature birth, hemorrhagic cystitis, pancreatisis, diabetes, and porphyria (Quant, Arcury, Austin, & Saavedra, 1998; Ciesielski, Loomis, Dana, Mims, & Aver, 1994; Gamsky, McCurdy, Wiggins,

Samuels, Berman, & Shenker, 1992; Krieger et al., 1990; Mehler, O'Malley, & Krieger, 1992; Osorio, Ames, Rosenberg, & Mengle, 1991, Sakala, 1987).

The children of farmworkers are also at risk since they can receive secondary exposure from residue on clothes or windblown pesticide drift. The U.S. Environmental Protection Agency (EPA) has estimated that at least 300,000 Latino agricultural workers each year experience acute injuries as a result of pesticide exposure (University of California Institute for Mexico and the United States, 1995).

Moreover, exposure to heat and sun causes acute heat exhaustion, heat stroke, skin cancers, and eye cataracts in the long term. Many injuries to rural Latino residents can also be attributed to unsafe transportation, which is a serious problem. In addition, poor field sanitation results in prolonged urine retention and consequently, urinary tract infections are twenty times the national average (Sakala, 1987; National Advisory Council on Migrant Health, 1987).

Dever (1993) tested the hypothesis that Latino migrant and seasonal agricultural workers differ in health problems from the rest of the Latino population and the general population. The data confirm that Latino agricultural workers have more clinic visits for diabetes, medical supervision of children, ear infections, pregnancy, hypertension, contact dermatitis, and eczema than both the general population and the Latino population in urban areas (Dever, 1993). Dever's assertion that Latino agricultural workers display an infectious disease cycle is supported by earlier research.

Multiple surveys indicate that Latino agricultural workers experience greater levels of parasitic diseases, chronic diarrhea, heart disease, gross gum disease, diabetes, kidney injuries, muscular skeletal injuries (especially the back), tooth decay, hearing loss, hunger, uncorrected vision defects, nutritional deficits, anemia, and lower rates of childhood immunization (Bade, 1999; Thu, 1998; Griffith & Kissam, 1995; Achata, 1993; Dever, 1993; Atkin, 1993; Rust, 1990; Scheder, 1988; Littlefield & Stout, 1987; Sakala, 1987; Wilt, 1986; Alvarez, 1985; Ashabranner, 1985; Daniel, 1982; Mines & Kearney, 1982; Bissell, 1976; Galarza, 1964). Moreover, HIV infection and tuberculosis are significant for certain segments of this mobile population (National Advisory Council on Migrant Health, 1995; Jones, Rion, Hollis, Longshore, Leverette, & Ziff, 1991).

Research on maternal child health issues for rural Latino residents are difficult to generalize, because there are no national epidemiological studies that provide baseline data. Case studies indicate that children of Latino agricultural workers suffer disproportionately higher rates of infant mortality and morbidity (Ruducha, 1989; Slesinger, Christensen, & Cautley, 1989; Rodriguez, 1993). Slesinger and colleagues (1989) reported that infant mortality among migrant farmworker women in California was thirty per 1,000, as opposed to fourteen per 1,000 births characteristic in the general U.S. population. Other studies that did not factor in migration report different findings. In one study, 1,040 pregnant women in California were followed throughout pregnancy and the sample was divided into three groups—women in agriculture, women working outside agriculture, and women not working at all. The incidence of low birth weight and mean birth weight did not vary significantly by work status (Coye, 1990). Another study indirectly supports these findings. Hayes-Bautista, Baezconde-Garbanati, Schink, and Hayes-Bautista (1994) report that analysis of Health Data from the Statistic Branch of California shows that California's 7.7 million Latinos demonstrate "a strong health profile" that has been deemed the "epidemiological paradox." According to this statewide statistical data set, in 1989 the infant mortality rate for Latinos was 7.9 per 1,000 births. By comparison, the rate was 7.8 for Whites and substantially lower than that of 18.2 infant deaths per 1,000 births for African Americans (Hayes-Bautista, Baezconde-Garbanati, Schink, & Hayes-Bautista, 1994). Moreover, Villarejo (1999), in summarizing these studies states, "[D. E.] Hayes-Bautista and [S.] Guendelman and [J. V.] Palerm have studied birth outcomes among successive generations of Mexican immigrant women. Both groups find that unhealthful birth outcomes and low birth weight babies are less prevalent among recent immigrant women than among non-Latino U.S.-born California residents, more prevalent among their U.S.- born daughters, and even more prevalent among their second-generation granddaughters (p. 10)." Given these findings, some researchers are beginning to question the utility of using aggregate Latino birth outcomes to gauge future Latino health priorities—especially because rural Latino children are burdened with infections and poor dental health, Latino adolescents with early pregnancy, and adults are increasingly vulnerable to a vast array of occupational illness syndromes (Balcazar, 2000).

The presence of domestic violence in the lives of rural Latina residents is an issue that cannot be ignored. The Migrant Clinicians Network (1996) published the results of one of the first nationwide research projects on domestic violence rates among 524 adult migrant women. Some 19.8 percent of the respondents reported physical abuse within the previous year. This rate is consistent with figures nationwide. Overall, the health, illness, and disease profile of rural Latino residents is complicated because many medical conditions are compounded by the effects of occupational and environmental conditions.

Research highlighting the occupational and environmental hazards associated with rural Latinos engaging in other nonagricultural employment sectors reveals that overall Latinos are overrepresented in the more hazardous occupations and industries in the United States (Friedman-Jiménez & Ortiz, 1994; see also Chapter Twelve). More specifically, Latinos in rural areas also work in the labor-intensive meat, poultry, and fruit packing industries that have high turnover due to hand, eye, and other repetitive motion injuries (Rochín & Marroquin, 1997).

While it is important to acknowledge that there have been some improvements in the working conditions of farmworkers with respect to portable bathrooms in the fields, the use of umbrellas as protection from the sun, and better access to drinking water, pesticide-related illness continues to plague rural Latino residents nationwide (Villarejo, 1999; Quandt, Arcury, Austin, & Saavedra, 1998; Ciesielski, Loomis, Mims, & Auer, 1994; Dever, 1993; Mehler, O'Malley, & Krieger, 1992; Krieger et al., 1990). Moreover, new occupational syndromes are beginning to emerge as food processors strive to achieve assembly-line efficiency. Because many rural workers engage in more than one type of rural employment, the risk for injuries increases. Multiple chemical exposures and repetitive motions aggravate occupational risks, and their effects over time may be cumulative. In addition to these risks, rural Latinos face confusing public and private medical insurance provisions, restrictive immigrant legislation, and linguistic and cultural barriers that affect access and use of medical services.

# Accessing Medical Services for Rural Latinos

Rural Latinos face significance barriers to accessing medical services, despite the presence of the Community and Migrant Health Program.

## Community and Migrant Health Program

Rural Latino residents, including farmworkers, can receive primary health care services though the Community and Migrant Health Program (CMHP) authorized by the Public Health Service Act, §§329, 330, and 329 (United States Congress, 1982). Under the CMHP, rural residents receive primary care services on a sliding fee scale based on the Federal Poverty Family Income Guidelines (Johnston, 1985; Martin & Martin, 1994). The CMHP has two components: health-center-based programs and voucher programs. The former are located at community and migrant health centers. The latter provide health services to Latino agricultural workers where there are no health centers available. In such cases, the voucher program contracts with private providers to provide health services to those Latino agricultural workers who are eligible for the program.

Today there are approximately 144 community and migrant health centers across the country, supported by numerous satellite clinics, which provide the following: prenatal, primary prevention, dental, nutrition, family planning, and emergency on after-hours care; health education; HIV care; pharmacy services; and other clinical services (Rural Community Assistance Program, 1992). For fiscal year 2000, the appropriation for these consolidated health center programs was $91.5 million dollars (Mata, 2000). Although federal funding is granted to more than 400 clinic sites nationwide, where there are approximately 500,000 clinic visits per year, it is estimated that only some 13 to 20 percent of the farmworkers utilize these health care services (Benavides-Vaello & Setler, 1994; National Migrant Resource Program, Inc., 1990; Stilp, 1994; Wilt, 1993; Rust, 1990). Therefore, despite the introduction of the CMHP and the political commitments to providing health care to Latino agricultural workers as well as other low-income rural residents, this population continues to be one of the most underserved groups in the United States due to inadequate levels of funding. Based on analyses made by Stilp (1994), the average dollar amount available in 1993 to provide services for each agricultural worker was $12.87 per year. This restricted amount of spending results in limited resources for transportation, outreach, and staffing.

Many levels of federal and state health care policy decisions determine how community and migrant health centers operate throughout the United States. Bilingual and bicultural medical practitioners remain a critical need in rural communities throughout the country. Inadequate management of medical record data also burdens community and migrant health centers in rural areas. Data are regularly entered but are not easily extracted for meaningful analysis. This is an increasingly salient issue, as many of the clinics are becoming affiliated with managed care providers that require detailed productivity reports (Azevedo, 2000).

Another challenge facing community and migrant health centers is the recent loss of the Federally Qualified Health Center (FQHC) reimbursement rate and the lack of increase in federal appropriations, while there continues to be an increase in numbers of rural Latino residents with no health insurance. For example, in 1980 the FQHC rate served five million people with an appropriation rate of $360 million. In contrast, however, by 1995 the number of people served increased to 9.3 million while the budget remained at only $247 million (National Association of Community Health Centers, 1997). Unless the capacity of community and migrant health centers can be maintained at a secure level, rural Latinos will face increasing challenges to meeting their health care needs. This potentially could increase the use of emergency rooms in the few remaining rural hospitals for both urgent and nonemergency conditions. The continued provision of uncompensated care at these emergency rooms will undoubtedly aggravate the plight of already vulnerable rural hospitals throughout the United States. Legislative and regulatory interventions are needed in order to ensure and retain a health care delivery system that delivers responsive and quality care to Latinos and other rural residents who lack health insurance (National Rural Health Association, 2000).

## Federal and State Legislation Impacting Rural Latino Immigrants

Since the welfare-reform legislation of 1996 (the Illegal Immigration Reform and Immigration Responsibility Act of 1996, passed by Congress at the end of July and signed by President Clinton on August 22) gave states the option to restrict Medicaid for documented immigrants, rural Latino residents who are legal residents (but not citizens) have faced restrictions (Medicare and Medicaid, 1996b; Rosenbaum & Darnell, 1996; Super, Parrott, Steinmetz, & Mann, 1996). The legislation states that federally allocated Medicaid dollars cannot be spent on immigrants who have come to the United States after August 22, 1996. This results in an additional loss of income for many community and migrant health centers. In California, recent legislation is responding to these federal policies by infusing state-only funding into publicly subsidized programs for recent and undocumented immigrants. Nevertheless, at the local level, advocates are concerned about the sustainability of this new allocation of resources by the state.

However, recent legislative changes throughout the nation reflect an anti-immigrant stance. For example, in California, the passing of Proposition 187 by voters on November 4, 1994, which made undocumented persons ineligible for public social services, public health care, and public school education, created a great deal of confusion among Spanish-speaking residents about who qualified for what services. Other state laws that have repealed affirmative action laws and restructured bilingual education significantly impact rural Latino children living in isolated rural areas. This type of legislative action creates a perception that it is risky to use public services, especially since some of the laws cited have consequences that affect the immigration application processes.

The cumulative effects of these different types of legislative actions discourage some rural Latino residents from applying for subsidized health insurance programs. New concerns emerge regarding Medicaid programs because "public charge" and "sponsor liability" provisions complicate immigration applications. More specifically, if a sponsored immigrant uses federal Medicaid or state Child Health Insurance Programs (CHIPs) and the immigrant's sponsor (usually a family member) signed the I-864 affidavit of support on or after December 19, 1997, their sponsor may be responsible for paying these costs to the U.S. government. This is what is meant by the term "sponsor liability": the person who sponsored the immigrant will be liable for these expenses, which are known as the "public charge." Because these new immigrants are barred from using these federally sponsored public health insurance programs for five years, the sponsor would not have to worry about this liability for these five years (California Primary Care Association, 2000). However, the sponsor liability clause is not well understood by most Latinos, rural or nonrural. Consequently, this has served as a powerful deterrent to their applying for government-subsidized programs in general. Thus, what will happen to these families if they are low income and in need of continuous subsidized primary health care remains a critical concern. Although there have been recent attempts to clarify public charge legislation, the guidelines are still not clear. Confusion about these laws leads rural Latino residents to seek medical services in Mexico, to delay treatment for non-life-threatening conditions, or both.

## Cultural Considerations

In addition to the above political and socioeconomic barriers, there are cultural considerations that must be taken into account when we are examining medical care use among rural Latino residents. A broad range of sociocultural processes involved in access to medical services for rural Latinos has been discussed in various forms elsewhere throughout this book. Some Latinos use traditional remedies such as massage, creams, or herbs. Others use herbal preparations in combination with over-the-counter remedies and prescription medications (Bogue-Ochoa, McCormack, Parson, & Fisher, 1993; McVea, 1995; Licona, 1994; Nall, 1967).

Despite the use of traditional medicine, studies consistently show that "the mechanisms which limit access to health care focus primarily on an individual's

ability to pay for services" (Chavez, 1986, see also Palerm, 1992). As Chavez point-
edly states, "access to health care services is dependent upon factors which are
economically and politically determined; . . . cultural factors may add to the problem of access to health services for a given subgroup in a community, but cultural
beliefs are not a major *cause* of limited access" (1986, p. 345). Moreover, Slesinger
(1992) posits that the use of traditional versus biomedical health services among
farmworkers "depended more on structural conditions such as geographic location and availability of folk or clinical medical services and on the nature of the
illness to be cured than any specific characteristics of individuals" (p. 233).
Theoretical orientations that explain the minimal levels of health care access
among poor populations as a function of individual cultural attributes tend to
blame the poor when factors limiting access are more largely determined by factors
beyond a person's control.

This is not to say, however, that cultural barriers are not important. For example, cultural perceptions of illness, sickness, and disease influence when a
person decides to seek care. More specifically, cultural beliefs and structural barriers may work in a synergistic fashion to limit access to rural medical services. For
example, some rural Latino residents will seek medical services only if they visi-
bly exude blood or experience pain that interferes with their ability to work. These
beliefs, along with the strong work ethic among Latinos, operate in conjunction
with structural constraints such as the lack of sick time and limited health insurance to further restrict preventive health-seeking behaviors. Therefore, the interventions designed to tackle these problems need to address structural barriers in
a culturally competent manner. On the individual level, rural Latino residents still
face significant barriers because provisions in public and private medical insurance programs are difficult to understand. The following subsection examines
medical insurance issues that confront many rural Latino residents.

## Medical Insurance Concerns for Latinos Living in Rural America

Structural access variables inherent in public and private health insurance
programs for rural Latino residents restrict use of medical services. These forces,
which are embedded in sociocultural processes, explain who seeks medical services, why they do so, what type of care they receive, how they access it, and where
they go for these services.

The percentage of rural Latino households nationwide covered by public or
private comprehensive medical and dental insurance is unknown. Case studies
show that only a small percentage of rural Latino families have medical insurance
for the entire family. For rural Latino residents with private insurance, dependent
coverage may be limited. For those covered by public programs, family members who are undocumented are eligible only for restrictive Medicaid benefits (Azevedo, 2000; Villarejo, 1999; California Primary Care Association, 2000;
Medi-Cal Policy Institute, 1999a). Although regardless of coverage rural Latinos
do usually seek treatment when they are very sick, they may have to delay seeking

such treatment because of inability to pay if they have no insurance or have not met their deductible (Chavez, 1986).

Among rural Latino residents who are eligible for public health insurance (Medicaid), actual use is restricted by lack of awareness of how these programs work and by the difficult and confusing application process and eligibility procedures (Azevedo, 2000; Villarejo, 1999; California Primary Care Association, 2000; Medi-Cal Policy Institute, 1999b). For a person to become eligible for Medicaid, he or she must complete a very detailed application process and meet property, income, institutional, residence, and citizenship requirements (Medi-Cal Policy Institute, 1999b). Use of public coverage is also restricted by difficulties in transferring caseloads and eligibility information when households migrate between counties for employment. Moreover, travel between states presents challenges to those, especially migrating Latino agricultural workers, who have county-specific Medicaid coverage or geographically limiting, employee-based medical insurance. Quarterly recertification under the Medicaid programs remains a major obstacle to actual use of these programs by eligible rural Latinos and their dependents. Of serious concern is eligibility for "presumptive Medicaid" (a new state option). It permits state Medicaid eligibility employees to enroll applicants temporarily, relying on the applicant's declaration that his or her income is below the Medicaid income eligibility limits, and also to enroll children in state CHIPs. However, eligibility provisions are different in each state and there is no reciprocity between states (Mizeur, 2000). Thus, potential and realized access to care for non-life-threatening emergencies and for specialized care can be restricted by each state's interpretation of its legal responsibilities to persons covered by various forms of Medicaid.

Private U.S.-based medical insurance companies, such as Transwestern and Western Growers, which cover agricultural firms, pay 100 percent of medical costs if their employees go to Mexico for medical care (Azevedo, 2000). Those who live close to the Mexican border appreciate this binational health coverage. Nevertheless, many private insurance programs available to family members of those working in rural areas face barriers that include high deductibles, caps on coverage, limitations on dependent coverage, and fear of retribution from their employer, which restrict the use of these programs. Also, the time needed to travel in order to obtain care from approved medical providers restricts rural residents' use of private insurance (Azevedo, 2000; Villarejo, 1999; California Primary Care Association, 2000; Medi-Cal Policy Institute, 1999a). Latinos often find the use of private insurance problematic when they are migrating, because of the confusion over qualified providers. The requirement to meet a medical insurance deductible is difficult not only because of cost but also because it is difficult to ascertain what portion of the deductible has been paid when visiting a clinic away from home. For example, if a member of a rural Latino resident family seeks care in a clinic while migrating and the medical insurance company office is closed, he or she may be asked to pay the deductible again (Azevedo, 2000). For those private insurance programs that offer coverage for care and treatment in Mexico, distance to the border may become an access issue during migration. Moreover, in some states, having private insurance coverage may disqualify some low-income rural Latinos from the more comprehensive coverage that public Medicaid insurance programs offer.

## Lessons Learned from Effective Programs

The use of community health workers has become an important part of community-oriented primary health care outreach to the rural poor. These programs have received much attention and have been funded by a variety of international health and development agencies as one way to address the inequitable health care in rural areas. The utility and sustainability of these programs have been debated. Nevertheless, lay health worker programs have become essential components of rural health care delivery systems worldwide (Warrick, Wood, Meiester, & De Zapien, 1992; Werner, 1977; New & New, 1975; Thomason & Kolehmainen-Aiken, 1991; Bastien, 1990; Kuhn et al., 1990; Vaughan, 1980; Gagnon, 1991). In the United States, however, the use of lay health workers has been less extensive. Community health workers have been used as a part of outreach efforts for patients in tuberculosis treatment programs, AIDS education, needle exchange programs, and the like, but primarily in major urban areas (Azevedo, 1997; Warrick, Wood, Meiester, & De Zapien, 1992). More recently, however, community health workers in rural areas throughout the United States have been trained in small grassroots programs to conduct outreach among Spanish-speaking rural residents, especially farmworkers.

One such program is known as the East Coast Program, which hires and trains health care professionals to outreach to migrant Latino agricultural workers and travel with them throughout the Eastern stream. This program facilitates continuity of care, especially among those migrant Latino agricultural workers with chronic conditions such as high blood pressure and diabetes. AmeriCorps, another new outreach strategy for rural Latino residents, focuses its attention on teaching rural Latino residents about pesticide safety. The Camp Aide program, based in Monroe, Michigan, is a lay community health education program targeted toward farmworkers in Texas, Michigan, and Florida. This program strives to increase access to health care, while promoting leadership development among farmworkers trained as lay health promoters. These community workers are trained to provide community outreach, first aid, language translation, culturally competent health education, and referrals to health and human service organizations, as well as to facilitate the scheduling of clinic appointments and to advocate for improving health conditions in the community (United States Department of Health and Human Services, 1997; Murphy, 1995; Murillo, 1995). On the West Coast, *Lideres Campesinas* and the Coachella Valley Health Care Connection have pioneered programs that reach rural Latino residents in isolated rural areas of Southeastern California. *Lideres Campesinas* focuses its outreach efforts on farmworker women subjected to domestic violence, as well as AIDS and other health issues (Street & Orozco, 1992). The Coachella Valley Health Care Connection focuses its efforts on educating women on the importance of prenatal care and immunization programs for rural residents living in the poorest sections of Riverside County, California.

Although there has not been a systematic evaluation of those programs, they are viewed as effective. For example, the Camp Aide Program and the *Lideres Campesinas* (Street, 1992) were assessed by the USDHHS Bureau of Primary Health Care as *models that work*. A recent evaluation of the latter program concluded that varying degrees of personal empowerment were exhibited by the *"promotores"* participating in the program (Booker, Robinson, Kay, Najera, & Stewart, 1997). The program has been profiled in a number of publications. When well managed, these programs bring information and resources into the homes of Latino rural residents in a culturally appropriate manner. Lay community health workers are often able to address a problem before it reaches crisis proportions. Furthermore, these lay community health workers are able to teach concepts of preventative public health and increase effective utilization of maternal and child health services (United States Department of Health and Human Services, 1997; Warrick, Wood, Meiester, & De Zapien, 1992). In summary, effective outreach programs targeting rural Latinos are those that:

- Utilize people from the community to be served.
- Provide training and appropriate salaries.
- Offer flexible work schedules.
- Achieve financial program stability.
- Promote networking and foster self-advancement.
- Encourage healthy traditions and enhance cultural pride.

Utilizing people from the community opens doors because lay health workers frequently know key informants or community gatekeepers. Community health workers speak the language of the target group. They are familiar with the cultural expectations, health practices, and health-seeking behaviors or the target community. Because they know their community, they can determine the best time and most accepted methods of information dissemination to conduct successful outreach activities. When properly trained and with clear expectations of their performance and accountability, lay workers can be very effective peer educators. Although these workers should not substitute for trained professionals who are lacking in underserved areas, they can promote use of health care services and serve as a cost-effective bridge between rural Latino residents and medical providers.

# Recommendations for Future Research, Policies, Education, and Training

Based on existing evidence, the following eight measures are recommended in order to diminish the structural constraints that rural Latinos experience when they try to use health care services.

1. *Improve the Medicaid application and eligibility process.* Medicaid eligibility processes are cumbersome in many rural regions throughout the United States. Applications are long, and translations in Spanish need improvement. Files are purged, thrown away, and clients have to fill out the same forms repeatedly. Therefore, we strongly recommend that state agencies simplify the process by shortening the application and developing a uniform eligibility application that can be used nationwide. Therefore these recommendations are suggested to facilitate continuous eligibility for rural workers:

- Determine eligibility based on a household's annual income, and eliminate the assets tests. Because Medicaid benefits are tied to income, rural families usually lose Medicaid benefits during peak season.
- Allow for continuity of care by offering clients the option to pay monthly premiums if a family's income rises by increasing the share of costs instead of removing them from Medicaid.
- Medicaid clients in many states must reapply every forty-five days. This represents an undue burden. Determine eligibility for Medicaid by encouraging states to exercise the twelve-month continuous eligibility option.
- Make Medicaid programs portable by developing interstate and intercounty reciprocity agreements. As a result, when a migrant moves to another county or state, the case can be transferred along with his or her eligibility.
- Enforce Medicaid's outstationing requirements so that rural residents have the opportunity to apply for these programs in more convenient locations closer to home.
- Expand Medicaid funding for dental clinics in rural areas serving large concentrations of rural residents. Allocate additional funding for mental health services, especially culturally appropriate substance abuse treatment programs and family violence intervention programs in the rural areas where people live.

2. *Fund and train community health workers about medical insurance.* Rural Spanish-speaking residents need a direct liaison between themselves, clinic providers, and other advocacy groups. In addition to this health education, train and adequately fund community health workers to understand both private and public medical insurance programs in the states in which they work. These workers, in turn, can inform rural residents and their family members about their options and how to select the most appropriate insurance program for their family's needs.

3. *Establish a committee to examine binational medical insurance practices.* Binational efforts between Mexico and the United States need to be strengthened. A binational commission should be established to examine the potential consequences when private U.S. medical insurance plans operate in Mexico. More specifically, issues of true portability, medical quality, and medical liability need to be examined in order to ensure that rural Latino residents who are U.S. citizens or permanent residents understand their rights and obligations when they seek medical care service outside the United States.

4. *Direct adequate resources to improve rural medical education.* Develop a nationwide *comprehensive* medical school curriculum, similar to the Rural Medical Education Program developed by the Illinois College of Medicine at Rockford, as well as national rural residency standards. Currently, pre- and postdoctoral training opportunities are limited for those interested in rural medicine (Stearns, Stearns, Glasser, & Londo, 2000). Augment the support for the National Health Training Corps.

5. *Encourage rural clinic data management research.* Medical schools, public health schools, schools of social science, and schools of computer science need to collaborate to effectively automate medical data for community and migrant health centers so that such data can be extracted for meaningful analysis. These data should also include documentation of the actual number and type of health care providers that do and do not accept Medicaid clients in rural areas with severe medical service personnel shortages.

6. *Consider ambulatory and urgent care clinics in isolated rural areas.* Rural Latino residents utilize services primarily when they are very sick. Perhaps the concept of a primary health care clinic should be modified. Rural Latino residents need urgent care or ambulatory medical clinics in addition to preventative primary health care clinics. Indeed, the very design of community clinics in isolated rural areas may well need to be reexamined, given the reality that rural hospitals are closing nationwide. In many geographic areas of rural America, facilities that can handle emergency, trauma, and urgent medical problems, such as childbirth, are several hours away from rural population concentrations.

7. *Encourage the development of more ergonomic rural work environments.* Many rural work environments mass produce and package food in assembly-line fashion. The ergonomic design of this type of work environment—whether in the fields or in a packinghouse—needs improvement in order to enhance worker safety. Moreover, occupation and health and safety regulations in place need to be effectively enforced.

8. *Make more accurate the definition of "rural."* Because federal health policy provides supplementary resources to designated rural areas (Villarejo, 1999), more accurate ways of determining just what a *rural area* is must be devised in order to prevent more agricultural areas from being classified as urban metropolitan areas despite the fact that they actually remain rural in character.

# Conclusions

The *Healthy People 2010* campaign strives to achieve broad access to quality health services, eliminate racial and ethnic disparities in health status, and improve the availability and distribution of health-related information. Ultimately we need to increase our efforts to develop the infrastructure for rural health delivery, especially because rural hospitals are closing and access to all types of medical services is becoming more and more limited. Steps that can help achieve this goal include improving the Medicaid application and eligibility process, encouraging the development of outreach programs, examining binational medical insurance strategies, strengthening efforts to improve rural medical education nationwide, supporting clinical data management research efforts, improving the design of the rural health care delivery system, improving the ergonomics of the rural work environment, and defining more accurately the definition of modern rural America.

In summary, significant barriers limit access and use of health services among rural Latinos nationwide. First, the CMHC system is still underfunded, relative to the increased need for these services. Second, federal and state legislation restricts the use of public health insurance programs for certain categories of Latino immigrants. Third, private medical insurance regulations can be confusing and may actually cover less than Medicaid programs. Finally, cultural considerations, including language limitations, decrease access and use of appropriate health care services (Bade, 1999; Ochoa-Bogue, McCormack, Parson, & Fisher, 1993; National Advisory Council on Migrant Health, 1993, 1995; National Migrant Resource Program, Inc., 1990; Slesinger, 1992; Slesinger & Ofstead, 1993; Wilt, 1986). Ultimately, rural Latino residents face these significant barriers—often in the absence of reliable information. Community outreach is an important way to bridge the gap between rural Latino residents and those committed to providing health services to this population.

# References

Achata, C. (1993). Immunization of Mexican migrant farm workers' children on site at a day care center in a rural Tennessee county: Three successful summers. *Journal of Health and Social Policy, 4,* 4, 89–101.

Alvarez, M. (1985). Health conditions of Mexican women immigrants: A review of the literature on border health. *Salud Fronteriza, 1,* 3, 48–52.

Ashabranner, B. (1985). *Dark harvest migrant Latino agricultural workers in America.* New York: Dodd, Mead.

Atkin, S. B. (1993). *Voices from the fields.* Boston: Little, Brown.

Azevedo, K. (1997). *TB outreach activities in Los Angeles County* (TB Notes, No. 2). Atlanta, GA: Centers for Disease Control and Prevention, pp. 13–15.

Azevedo, K. (2000). *Health care access among California farmworker households in the desert Southwest.* Doctoral dissertation. University of California, Irvine.

Bade, B. (1993). *Problems surrounding health care service utilization for Mixtec migrant Latino agricultural workers families in Madera, California.* Davis: California Institute for Rural Studies.

Bade, B. (1999, September 16 & 17). *Is there a doctor in the field?: Underlying conditions affecting access to health care for California Latino agricultural workers and their families.* Paper presented at the Conference on Expanding Health Care Access for California's Latino Agricultural Workers, Sacramento. California Policy Research Center, California Program on Access to Care (CPAC).

Balcazar, H. (2000, July 5). *Latino health: Families, women, and children.* Paper presented at a session of the National Council of La Raza 2000 Annual Conference, San Diego, CA.

Barger, W. K., & Reza, E. (1987). Community action and social adaptation: The farmworker movement in the Midwest. In *Collaborative research and social change*. Boulder, CO: Westview Press, pp. 55–75.

Barger, W. K., & Reza, E. M. (1994). *The farm labor movement in the Midwest: Social change and adaptation among migrant Latino agricultural workers*. Austin: University of Texas Press.

Bastien, J. (1990). Community health workers in Bolivia: Adapting to traditional roles in the Andean community. *Social Science and Medicine, 30*, 3, 281–287.

Benavides-Vaello, S., & Setzler, H. (1994). *Migrant and seasonal Latino agricultural workers: Health care accessibility*. (Working Paper No. 76). University of Texas at Austin, Lyndon B. Johnson School of Public Affairs.

Bissell, K. A. (1976). *The migrant farmworker: A multi-disciplinary discussion module.* Washington, D.C.: Catholic University of America, Institute for Multidisciplinary Graduate Research.

Booker, V. K., Robinson, J. G., Kay, B. J., Najera, L. G., & Stewart, G. (1997). Changes in empowerment: The effects of participation in lay health promotion program. *Health Education and Behavior, 24*, 4, 452–464.

California Primary Care Association. (2000). *Questions and answers about sponsor liability.* Sacramento, CA: Author. Available from: http://www.cpca.org

Chavez, L. R. (1986). Mexican immigration and health care: A political economy perspective. *Human Organization, 45*, 4, 344–352.

Ciesielski, S., Loomis, D. P., Mims, S. R., & Auer, A. (1994). Pesticide exposures, cholinesterase depression and symptoms among North Carolina migrant Latino agricultural workers. *American Journal of Public Health, 84*, 3, 446–451.

Ciesielski, S., Seed, J. R., & Ortiz, J.C. (1992). Intestinal parasites among North Carolina migrant farmworkers. *American Public Health Association, 82*, 1258–1262.

Ciesielski, S., Loomis, D. P., Dana, P., Mims, S. R., & Auer, A. (1994). Pesticide exposures, cholinesterase depression and symptoms among North Carolina migrant Latino agricultural workers. *American Journal of Public Health, 84*, 3, 446–451.

Commission on Security and Cooperation in Europe. (1993, May). *Implementation of the Helsinki Accords: Migrant Latino agricultural workers in the United States*. Washington, D.C.: U.S. Government Printing Office.

Coye, F. L. (1990). Birthweight of infants born to Hispanic women employed in agriculture. *Archives of Environmental Health, 45*, 1, 46–52.

Daniel, C. E. (1982). *Bitter harvest: A history of California Latino agricultural workers, 1870–1941.* Berkeley: University of California Press.

Dever, A. (1993). *Migrant health status: Profile of a population with complex health problems* [Monograph Series]. Austin, TX: Migrant Clinicians Network.

Friedman-Jiménez, G., & Ortiz, J. S. (1994). Occupational health. In M. Aguirre-Molina & C. Molina (Eds.), *Latino health in the U.S.: A growing challenge*. Washington, D.C.: American Public Health Association.

Gagnon, A. (1991). The training and integration of village health workers. *Bulletin of the Pan American Health Organization, 25*, 2, 127–138.

Galarza, E. (1964). *Merchants of labor: The Mexican bracero story*. Charlotte, NC and Santa Barbara, CA: McNally & Loftin.

Gamsky, T., McCurdy, S., Wiggins, P., Samuels, S., Berman, B., & Shenker, M. (1992). Epidemiology of dermatitis among California farm workers. *Journal of Occupational Medicine, 34*, 3, 304–310.

Garcia, V., & Gonzalez Martinez, L. (1999). *Guanajuatense and other Mexican immigrants in the United States: New communities in non-metropolitan and agricultural regions*. (JSRI Research Report No. 47). East Lansing: Michigan State University, Julian Samora Research Institute.

Griffith, D., & Kissam, E. (1995). *Working poor Latino agricultural workers in the United States.* Philadelphia: Temple University Press.

Hayes-Bautista, D. E., Baezconde-Garbanati, L., Schink, W. O., & Hayes-Bautista, M. (1994, October). Latino health in California 1985–1990: Implications for family practice. *Family Medicine, 26,* 556–562.

Housing Assistance Council. (1994). *Taking stock of rural poverty and housing for the 1990s.* Available from: http://www.ruralhome.org

Johnston, H. E. (1985). *Health for the nation's harvesters.* Farmington Hills, MI: National Migrant Worker Council.

Jones, J. L., Rion, P., Hollis, S., Longshore, S., Leverette, W. B., & Ziff, L. (1991). HIV-related characteristics of migrant workers in rural South Carolina. *Southern Medical Journal, 84,* 9, 1088–1090.

Krieger, R. et. al. (1990). Gauging pesticide exposure of handlers (mixers/loaders/applicators) and harvesters in California agriculture. *La Medicina del Lavaro, 81,* 6, 474–479.

Kuhn, L. et al. (1990). Village health-workers and GOBI-FFF: An evaluation of a rural programme. *South African Medical Journal, 77,* 471–475.

Licona, V. (1994). Panel IV: Ethic-related issues blending traditional and modern. In conference, *A Shared Vision: Building Bridges for Rural Health Access, National Rural Health Association,* pp. 121–123.

Littlefield, C., & Stout, C. L. (1987). A survey of Colorado's migrant Latino agricultural workers: Access to health care. *International Migration Review, 21,* 3, 688–708.

Margolis, R. J. (1981). *Homes of the brave: A report on migrant farmworker housing.* Washington, D.C.: Rural America.

Martin, M., & Martin, A. (1994). The endless quest helping America's farm workers. Boulder, CO: Westview Press.

Mata, A. (2000, May 4–7). *Directors update.* Paper presented at the 2000 National Farmworker Health Conference, Portland, OR.

McVea, K. L. (1995, March/April). *Self-injection among North Carolina migrant farmworkers.* Austin, TX: Migrant Clinicians Network.

Medi-Cal Policy Institute. (1999a, July). *Medi-Cal County data book.* Oakland, CA: Author.

Medi-Cal Policy Institute. (1999b, July). *Understanding Medi-Cal: The basics.* Oakland, CA: Author.

Medicare and Medicaid. (1996b). Welfare reform bill restricts Medicaid coverage for immigrants. *Medicare and Medicaid Guide, 918,* Pt. 1, 1–11.

Mehler, L. N., O'Malley, M. A., & Krieger, R. L. (1992). Acute pesticide morbidity and mortality: California. In *Reviews of Environmental Contamination and Toxicology.* New York: Springer-Verlag, pp. 51–66.

Migrant Clinicians Network. (1996, April). *Domestic violence and migrant farmworker women: 1996 Final Report.* Austin, TX: Author.

Mines, R., & Kearney, M. (1982). *The health of Tulane County Latino agricultural workers.* Sacramento, CA: State of California, Department of Health Services.

Mizeur, H. R. (2000, May 4–7). *Making Medicaid and CHIP work for migrant and seasonal farmworkers and their families.* Paper presented at the 2000 National Farmworker Health Conference, Portland, OR.

Mobed, K., Goid, E., & Schenker, M. (1992, September). Cross-cultural medicine a decade later occupational health problems among migrant and seasonal farm workers. *Western Journal of Medicine, 157,* 367–372.

Murillo, R. (1995). *Consejeras de salud y acción.* (National Migrant Resource Program.) *Migrant Health Newsline, 2,* 5.

Murphy, M. (1995). Lay health programs: Public health service that works. (National Migrant Resource Program). *Migrant Health Newsline, 2,* 5.

Nall, F. C. (1967). Social and cultural factors in the responses of Mexican-Americans to medical treatment. *Journal of Health and Social Behavior, 4,* 299–308.

National Advisory Council on Migrant Health. (1993) (1995). *Losing ground: The condition of farmworkers in America: Recommendations of the National Advisory Council on Migrant Health.* Bethesda, MA: Health Resources and Services Administration.

National Association of Community Health Centers. (1997). *Access to community health care: A national and state data book.* Washington, D.C.: Author.

National Migrant Resource Program, Inc. (1990). *Migrant and seasonal farmworker health objectives for the Year 2000.* Austin, TX: Author.

National Migrant Resource Program, Inc. (1992). Proceedings of the 1992 Migrant Stream Forums. Portland, Oregon; South Padre Island, Texas, and Philadelphia, Pennsylvania. Comprehensive program to improve the supply of rural family physicians. *Family Medicine, 32,* 1, 17–21.

National Rural Health Association. (2000). *Legislative and regulatory agenda.* Kansas City, MO: Author.

New, P.K.-M., & New, M. L. (1975). The links between health and political structure in new China. *Human Organization, 34,* 237–251.

Ochoa-Bogue, H., McCormack, K., Parson, P. N., & Fisher, K. (1993). Health care needs of Mexican migrant farmworkers in rural Illinois: An exploratory study. The Health Educator. *Journal of Eta Sigma Gamma, 25,* 1.

Osorio, A. M., Ames, R. G., Rosenberg, J., & Mengle, D. C. (1991). Investigations of a fatality among parathion applicators in California. *American Journal of Industrial Medicine, 20,* 533–546.

Palerm, J. V. (1992). Cross-cultural medicine a decade later: A season in the life of a migrant farm worker in California. *Western Journal of Medicine, 157,* 3, 362–366.

Palerm, J. V. (1994). *Immigrant and migrant farm workers in the Santa Maria Valley, California.* Berkeley: University of California, Survey Research Center.

Palerm, J. V. (1995). *Policy implications of community studies. Changing face of rural California.* Pacific Grove: University of California, Riverside.

Quandt, S., Arcury, T., Austin, C., & Saavedra, R. (1998). Latino agricultural workers and farmer perceptions of farmworker agricultural chemical exposure in North Carolina. *Human Organization, 57,* 3, 359–368.

Rochín, R. I., & Marroquin, E. (1997, June). *Rural Latino resources.* East Lansing: Michigan State University, Julian Samora Research Institute.

Rodriguez, R. (1993). Violence in transience: Nursing care of battered migrant women. *AWHONN's Clinical Issues, 4,* 3, 437–441.

Rosenbaum, S., & Darnell, J. (1996). *Preliminary report: An analysis of the Medicaid and health related provisions of the Personal Responsibility and Work Opportunity Reconciliation Act of 1996.* Berkeley: University of California, Center for Health Policy Research.

Rosenberg, H., Stierman, A., Gabbard, S., & Mines, R. (1998). *Who works on California farms: Demographic and employment findings from the National Agricultural Workers Survey.* (Agricultural and Natural Resources Publication 21583). Berkeley: University of California, Agricultural Personnel Management Program.

Ruducha, J. (1989). *Determinants of health status and use of health services by migrant children.* Baltimore, MD: Johns Hopkins University.

Rural Community Assistance Program. (1992). *The MESA environmental health resource manual.* Available from: http://www.rcap.org

Rust, G. (1990). Health status of migrant Latino agricultural workers: A literature review and commentary. *American Journal of Public Health, 80,* 10, 1213–1217.

Sakala, C. (1987). Migrant and seasonal Latino agricultural workers in the United States: A review of health hazards, status, and policy. *International Migration Review, 21,* 3, 659–687.

Sanchez-Bane, M. (1994). *Economic health of the Hispanic community.* Conference Proceedings: A Shared Vision—Building Bridges for Rural Health Access. Kansas City, MO: National Rural Health Association.

Scheder, J. C. (1988). A sickly-sweet harvest: Farmworker diabetes and social equality. *Medical Anthropology Quarterly, 2,* 3, 251–277.

Slesinger, D. P. (1992). Health status and needs of migrant farm workers in the United States: A literature review. *Journal of Rural Health, 8,* 3, 227–234.

Slesinger, D., Christensen, B., & Cautley, E. (1989). Health and mortality of migrant farm children. *Social Science and Medicine, 23,* 65–74.

Slesinger, D. P., & Ofstead, C. (1993). Economic and health needs of Wisconsin migrant farm workers. *Journal of Rural Health, 9,* 2, 138–147.

State of California, Health and Welfare Agency. (1994). *Farm Worker Services Coordinating Council: A status report—Improving services for California's farm worker community.* Sacramento, CA: Author.

Stearns, J. A., Stearns, M. A., Glasser, M., Londo, R. A. (2000). Illinois RMED: A comprehensive program to improve the supply of rural family physicians. *Family Medicine, 32,* 1, 17–21.

Stilp, F. J. (1994). The migrant health program in the United States: A personal view from the front line. *Migration World Magazine, 22,* 4, 13–21.

Street, R. S. (1992). Organizing for our lives: New voices from rural communities. Troutdale, OR: New Sage Press; Sacramento: California Rural Legal Assistance.

Super, D. A., Parrott, S., Steinmetz, S., & Mann, C. (1996). *The new welfare law.* Washington, D.C.: Center of Budget and Policy Priorities.

Taylor, J. E., Martin, P. I., & Fix, M. (1997). *Poverty amid prosperity: Immigration and the changing face of rural California.* Washington, D.C.: Urban Institute Press.

Thomason, J. A., & Kolehmainen-Aiken, R.-L. (1991). Distribution and performance of rural health workers in Papua New Guinea. *Social Science and Medicine, 32,* 2, 159–165.

Thu, K. M. (1998). The health consequences of industrialized agriculture for farmers in the United States. *Human Organization, 57,* 3, 335–341.

United States Census of Agriculture. (1992). *Summary data.* Table 17, p. 23. Washington, D.C.: U.S. Bureau of the Census.

United States Congress. (1982). Public Health Service Act, §§329, 320, 000.

United States Department of Agriculture. (1995, February). *Understanding rural America.* (Agricultural Information Bulletin No. 170). Economic Research Service. Washington, D.C.: U.S. Government Printing Office.

United States Department of Health and Human Services. (1997, October). *Camp Health Aid Program (CHAP). Strategy transfer guide—Models that work.* Washington, D.C.: Author.

United States Department of Labor. (2000, March). *Findings from the National Agricultural Workers Survey (NAWS), 1997–1998: A demographic and employment profile of United States Latino agricultural workers.* Washington, D.C.: Author.

University of California Institute for Mexico and the United States. (1997). Latinos in California. Report of Activities Funded by the University of California Committee on Latino Research 1990–1995.

Vaughan, J. P. (1980). Barefoot or professional? Community health workers in the third world: Some important questions concerning their function, utilization, selection, training and evaluation. *Journal of Tropical Medicine and Hygiene, 83,* 3–10.

Villarejo, D., (1999). *Health care status to health care among California's hired farm workers.* Davis: California Institute for Rural Studies.

Warrick, L. H., Wood, A., Meiester, J., & De Zapien, J. G. (1992). Evaluation of a peer health worker prenatal outreach and education program for Hispanic farmworker families. *Journal of Community Health, 17,* 1, 13–26.

Wells, M. J. (1996). *Strawberry fields: Politics, class, and work in California agriculture.* Ithaca, NY: Cornell University Press.

Werner, D. (1977). *The village health worker: Lackey or liberator?* Palo Alto, CA: Hesperian Foundation.

Wilt, V. A. (1986). *The occupational health of migrant and seasonal Latino agricultural workers in the United States.* Washington, D.C.: Farmworker Justice Fund.

Wilt, V. A. (1996). *Farmworker health and safety: An annotated bibliography.* Washington, D.C.: Rural Community Assistance Program & the Farmworker Justice Fund.

PART FIVE

# ALCOHOL, TOBACCO, AND OTHER DRUG USE AMONG LATINOS

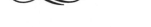

# CHAPTER FOURTEEN

# ALCOHOL USE AND ALCOHOL-RELATED PROBLEMS AMONG LATINOS IN THE UNITED STATES

Raul Caetano, Frank Hector Galvan

A major problem for Latinos in the United States is the high level of alcohol consumption per capita among both adolescents and adults. Death rates linked to such alcohol-related conditions as cirrhosis and other chronic liver diseases are unacceptably high among Latinos. Moreover, high-risk behaviors such as alcohol-impaired driving and its consequences are matters of great concern to Latino communities and to society at large. Although the incidence of intimate partner violence (IPV) is also high among Latinos, the relationship between such violence and excessive drinking is complex and requires careful analysis. Generally, problems stemming from high-risk drinking and chronic alcohol consumption beset Latino communities across the nation.

This chapter describes the effects of such drinking by Latino adolescents and adults (defined as those eighteen years of age or older), the problems associated with excessive alcohol consumption, and the prevention efforts that have been developed to minimize alcohol problems among individuals in this ethnic group in the United States. Most of the research to be reviewed has been conducted since publication of the review of alcohol-related issues among Latinos by Aguirre-Molina and Caetano (1994). The present review is also focused on epidemiological data collected from household samples in the U.S. population. These data are collected with random sample methodology and thus are representative of drinking that happens in the United States generally. There has been important research on clinical samples of Latinos (for example, Arciniega, Arroyo, Miller, & Tonigan, 1996; Arroyo, Westerberg, & Tonigan, 1996), but this and ethnographic research is not reviewed here. The data to be analyzed in this chapter come from a variety of sources. Adolescent data come from the Youth Risk Behavior Survey (YRBS) (United States Department of Health and Human Services, 1998), the National Alternative High School Youth Risk Behavior Survey (Alternative YRBS) (United States Department of Health and Human Services, 1999), and the National Health Interview Survey—Youth Risk Behavior Survey (NHIS–YRBS) (Adams, Schoenborn, Moss, Warren, & Kahn, 1992). Adult data come from the 1995 National Alcohol Survey conducted by the Alcohol Research Group and from the 1995 National Couples Study of Intimate Partner Violence. These two studies oversampled Latinos in the U.S. household population, thus providing important data that enable us to analyze drinking patterns and problems in this ethnic group. Most of the trends analyses focusing on adults described here have been discussed in a number of published papers reporting trends in alcohol consumption and problems among U.S. Latinos between 1984 and 1995 (Caetano & Clark, 1998a, 1998b, 1999). Results reporting on alcohol-related IPV have been reported in another series of papers based on the 1995 National Couples Study (Caetano, Cunradi, Schafer, & Clark, in press-a; Caetano, Schafer, & Cunradi, in press-b; Caetano, Schafer, Clark, Cunradi, & Raspberry, 2000; Cunradi, Caetano, Clark, & Schafer, 1998, 1999).

Most of the results are presented for all Latinos as a group, that is, without distinction of national origins. This should not be seen as implying that there is no national diversity among Latinos. The grouping of Latinos without recognition of national origin is a limitation that arises from most of the alcohol research conducted with this ethnic group in the United States. Even when Latinos have been oversampled in surveys of the U.S. general population, the relatively small number of Cubans, Puerto Ricans, and other Latinos in these samples makes it very difficult to conduct analyses that are specific to these national groups. Mexican Americans are the exception just because they are the largest Latino national group in the United States; general population samples therefore do not have to be very large to yield a group of Mexican Americans that is large enough to generate accurate results. Thus, more alcohol research has been conducted among Mexican Americans than among any other Latino group. A few federal surveys such as the National Household Survey on Drug Abuse, conducted by the Office of Applied Studies of the Substance Abuse and Mental Health Services Administration (SAMHSA) (1999), and the National Longitudinal Epidemiological Survey, conducted by the National Institute on Alcohol Abuse and Alcoholism (Stinson, Yi, Grant, Chou, Dawson, & Pickering, 1998) have samples that are large enough to yield a considerable number of Latinos in many national groups. Some analyses focusing on Latinos have been done using data from these surveys (for example, Dawson, 1998). Unfortunately, however, these analyses are not consistent enough and detailed enough to create a body of literature providing information of public health importance about alcohol use among Latino national groups with relative small proportional representation in the U.S. general population.

# Alcohol Use Among Latino Adolescents

Until the 1990s, population-based estimates of the prevalence of alcohol consumption and related problems among Latino youth were not available. Beginning in 1991, the Centers for Disease Control and Prevention (CDC) started national surveys to monitor various adolescent health behaviors in the U.S. population (Adams, Schoenborn, Moss, Warren, & Kann, 1992). These include the YRBS (United States Department of Health and Human Services, 1998), a national probability sample of high school students in grades nine through twelve conducted every other year; the National Alternative High School Youth Risk Behavior Survey (Alternative YRBS) (United States Department of Health and Human Services, 1999), conducted among students in grades nine through twelve who attend alternative high schools because they were expelled from regular high school due to behavioral problems or are at high risk for failing or dropping out of regular high school; and the NHIS–YRBS (Adams, Schoenborn, Moss, Warren, & Kann, 1992), a national household-based interview of youth twelve to twenty-one years of age. Unlike the YRBS and the Alternative YRBS, the NHIS–YRBS includes out-of-school youth (9 percent among school-age youth ages twelve to nineteen for the survey conducted in 1992) and separates data collected for Latinos into three categories: All Latinos, Mexican Americans, and Other Latinos.

Tables 14.1 and 14.2 present data from the 1997 YRBS (United States Department of Health and Human Services, 1998), the 1998 Alternative YRBS, and the 1992 NHIS–YRBS (United States Department of Health and Human Services, 1999) on the percentage of youth who report drinking alcohol. Overall, Latino students in the 1997 YRBS were significantly more likely than African American students to have consumed alcohol in their lifetime, to report current alcohol use, and to report episodic heavy drinking, but did not differ significantly from White students in any of these categories (see part (a) of Table 14.1). When the 1998 Alternative YRBS data were used, overall the Latino students were significantly more likely than African American students to have consumed alcohol in their lifetime, to report current alcohol use, and to report episodic heavy drinking (see part (b) of Table 14.1). The Latino students were significantly less likely than White students to report lifetime alcohol use but did not differ significantly from them on current alcohol use and episodic heavy drinking. Additionally, in all three categories of alcohol consumption for each ethnic group, the students attending alternative high schools reported higher levels of alcohol use than the students attending regular high schools. The data from the 1992 NHIS–YRBS reveal that, overall, Latino youth are intermediate between White and African American youth in rates of lifetime alcohol use, current alcohol use, and episodic heavy drinking (Table 14.2).

## TABLE 14.1. PERCENTAGE OF HIGH SCHOOL STUDENTS WHO DRANK ALCOHOL.

### (a) Youth Risk Behavior Survey, 1997.

| | Lifetime Alcohol Use[a] | | | Current Alcohol Use[b] | | | Episodic Heavy Drinking[c] | | |
|---|---|---|---|---|---|---|---|---|---|
| | Female | Male | Total | Female | Male | Total | Female | Male | Total |
| White | 79.9 (±2.9) | 82.4 (±2.0) | 81.3 (±2.1) | 51.6 (±4.8) | 56.0 (±2.8) | 54.0 (±3.0) | 32.9 (±3.2) | 41.6 (±3.1) | 37.7 (±2.3) |
| African American | 73.8 (±3.4) | 72.2 (±2.8) | 73.0 (±2.4) | 34.9 (±3.5) | 39.2 (±4.5) | 36.9 (±2.9) | 11.5 (±2.8) | 21.0 (±3.0) | 16.1 (±2.0) |
| Latino | 82.1 (±3.8) | 83.9 (±3.6) | 83.1 (±2.3) | 50.7 (±3.9) | 56.7 (±6.5) | 53.9 (±3.8) | 28.8 (±4.2) | 40.0 (±6.1) | 34.9 (±3.4) |

### (b) National Alternative High School Youth Risk Behavior Survey, 1998.

| | Female | Male | Total | Female | Male | Total | Female | Male | Total |
|---|---|---|---|---|---|---|---|---|---|
| White | 96.7 (±1.6) | 96.0 (±1.5) | 96.3 (±1.2) | 66.8 (±7.5) | 74.2 (±7.0) | 71.1 (±6.2) | 52.2 (±6.8) | 63.3 (±6.2) | 58.7 (±5.7) |
| African American | 80.7 (±5.0) | 83.6 (±3.9) | 82.1 (±3.2) | 46.9 (±7.9) | 57.0 (±5.8) | 51.8 (±5.1) | 22.2 (±4.9) | 34.7 (±3.8) | 28.4 (±3.3) |
| Latino | 92.9 (±2.1) | 93.3 (±2.5) | 93.1 (±1.9) | 60.1 (±4.3) | 67.2 (±8.1) | 63.9 (±5.3) | 46.2 (±4.7) | 57.5 (±7.5) | 52.4 (±5.2) |

[a]Ever had at least one drink of alcohol.

[b]Drank alcohol on greater than or equal to one of the thirty days preceding the survey.

[c]Drank five or more drinks of alcohol in a row on at least one occasion on greater than or equal to one of the thirty days preceding the survey.

*Note:* 95 percent confidence intervals are given in parentheses.

*Sources:* (a) United States Department of Health and Human Services (1998); (b) United States Department of Health and Human Services (1999).

**TABLE 14.2. PERCENTAGE DISTRIBUTION OF YOUTH 12–21 YEARS OF AGE WHO DRANK ALCOHOL, NATIONAL HEALTH INTERVIEW SURVEY—YOUTH RISK BEHAVIOR SURVEY, 1992.**

| | Lifetime Alcohol Use[a] | | | Current Alcohol Use[b] | | | Episodic Heavy Drinking[c] | | |
|---|---|---|---|---|---|---|---|---|---|
| | Female | Male | Total | Female | Male | Total | Female | Male | Total |
| White | 71.0 | 69.3 | 70.1 | 47.8 | 47.9 | 47.8 | 26.2 | 32.7 | 29.5 |
| African American | 61.7 | 62.6 | 62.2 | 35.7 | 40.2 | 38.1 | 10.1 | 18.9 | 14.5 |
| Latino | | | | | | | | | |
| Total | 61.7 | 66.9 | 64.4 | 36.8 | 46.4 | 41.6 | 15.4 | 28.4 | 22.1 |
| MA[d] | 59.1 | 68.4 | 64.0 | 35.2 | 48.9 | 42.4 | 15.8 | 30.0 | 23.4 |
| Other[e] | 65.7 | 64.3 | 65.0 | 39.0 | 42.2 | 40.5 | 15.0 | 25.5 | 20.1 |

[a]Ever had at least one drink of alcohol.

[b]Drank alcohol on greater than or equal to one of the thirty days preceding the survey.

[c]Drank five or more drinks of alcohol within a couple of hours greater than or equal to one of the thirty days preceding the survey.

[d]MA includes youth reported as Mexican/Mexicano, Mexican American.

[e]Other Latino includes youth reported as Puerto Rican, Cuban, other Latin American, other Spanish, or multiple Latino origin.

*Note:* Gender categories include non-Latino racial groups not shown separately and unknown if of Latino origin.

*Source:* Adapted from Adams, Schoenborn, Moss, Warren, & Kann (1992).

## Alcohol-Related Problems

As noted earlier, alcohol consumption among adolescents can be associated with a number of related problems. The 1997 YRBS, the 1998 Alternative YRBS, and the 1992 NHIS–YRBS all provide data on the prevalence of specific alcohol-related problems experienced by Latino adolescents, such as riding with a driver who had been drinking alcohol, driving after drinking alcohol, and using alcohol or drugs at the time of sexual intercourse. Data from the 1997 YRBS reveal that, overall, Latino students (42.8 percent) were significantly more likely than African American students (33.5 percent) to have ridden with a driver who had been drinking alcohol and to have driven after drinking alcohol (18.1 percent versus 9.4 percent). Among currently sexually active students, the Latino students (25.3 percent) are intermediate between the White students (26 percent) and African American students (18.1 percent) in the rates of reported alcohol or drug use at their last sexual intercourse and did not differ significantly from either of them.

Overall, Latino students (53.5 percent) in the 1998 Alternative YRBS did not differ significantly from the African American students (45.2 percent) or White students (53.6 percent) in their rates of having ridden with a driver who had been drinking alcohol, nor in the rates of driving after drinking alcohol (23.4 percent, 19.1 percent, and 28.3 percent, respectively). Among currently sexually active students, the Latino students (38.5 percent) are intermediate between the White students (43.1 percent) and African American students (35.3 percent) in the rates of reported alcohol or drug use at their last sexual intercourse and did not differ significantly from either of them. Youth in the 1992 NHIS–YRBS reported approximately similar rates of riding with a driver who had been drinking alcohol (25.2 percent, Whites; 26.1 percent, African Americans; 24.6 percent, Latinos), and driving after drinking alcohol (31.2 percent, Whites; 26.1 percent, African Americans; 26.8 percent, Latinos). Among those eighteen to twenty-one years of age who have ever had sexual intercourse, the Latino youth (16.4 percent) are intermediate between the White youth (18.8 percent) and African American youth (12.7 percent) in reported rates of having used alcohol or drugs before their last sexual intercourse.

## Predictors of Alcohol Use

Several studies have identified predictors of drinking among young Latinos by utilizing a multivariate framework. Sokol-Katz and Ulbrich (1992) reported that males and older adolescents had significantly more alcohol consumption than females and younger adolescents. More alcohol consumption was reported by Mexican adolescents living in single-parent homes than those in two-parent homes, Cuban adolescents who took the interview in English than those who took it in Spanish, Puerto Rican adolescents living in a city than those living in suburbs, and Mexican adolescents living in higher-income households than those living in lower-income ones.

Dusenbury, Epstein, Botvin, and Diaz (1994) found significant predictors of current alcohol use to include several demographic and social influence variables. Gender was a significant predictor, with males being 2.54 times more likely to drink currently than females. Dominican (1.98 odds) and Colombian (1.92 odds) students were more likely to drink than were Puerto Rican students. Students who reported that some or all of their friends drank were 23.3 times more likely to drink than those who reported that none of their friends drank. Even those who reported that only a few of their friends drank were still 8.44 times more likely to drink than those who reported that none of their friends drank. Both parents' and friends' attitudes emerged as significant predictors. The odds of drinking were 2.21 times higher for students whose parents had neutral or favorable as opposed to negative attitudes toward the adolescent's drinking, and two times higher for those whose friends had neutral or favorable attitudes toward the adolescent's drinking.

Based on a sample of 207 Los Angeles public junior high school Latino students (85 percent born in the United States), Alva and Jones (1994) found alcohol users to be more likely to be in a higher grade and to have a lower self-concept than nonusers. Alcohol users also were more likely to ascribe greater benefits to the consumption of alcohol, such as believing that alcohol helps a person to feel like an adult and also to get over feelings of sadness. Additionally, those students whose friends did not use alcohol were more likely to be in a lower grade, have a higher self-concept, and ascribe fewer benefits to alcohol consumption.

Vega, Zimmerman, Warheit, Apospori, and Gil (1993) studied predictors of lifetime alcohol use in a Miami sample of 6,760 sixth- and seventh-grade boys of which 45 percent were Latinos. The Latinos were divided into those of Cuban and "other Latino" (Nicaraguan, Salvadoran, Colombian, Puerto Rican, Dominican, and Venezuelan) descent. For both the Cubans and the "other Latino" group, significant predictors of lifetime alcohol use included perceived peer substance use, peer approval for substance use, low family pride, a willingness to engage in nonnormative behavior, family substance use problems, and parents' smoking. Additionally, for the "other Latino" group, other predictors were the presence of delinquent behavior, low self-esteem, and a previous suicide attempt.

# Trends in Drinking Patterns Among Latino Adults: 1984–1995

The data for the analysis of trends in drinking patterns come from two national surveys of U.S. Latinos conducted by the first author at the Alcohol Research Group, Berkeley, California. Latinos who participated in these surveys were selected through a multistage area probability[1] procedure from among individuals eighteen years of age or older living in households in the forty-eight contiguous United States both in 1984 and in 1995. A total of 1,453 Latinos were interviewed in 1984, for a 72 percent response rate. The sample interviewed in 1995 comprised 1,585 Latinos, and the response rate was 77 percent. Both in 1984 and in 1995 data were collected by trained interviewers in face-to-face interviews that averaged one hour. Interviews were conducted using standardized questionnaires in respondents' homes.

Latino respondents were so identified by self-identification. In both surveys, respondents who selected "Black of Hispanic origin (Latino, Mexican, Central or South American, or any other Hispanic origin)" and "White of Hispanic origin (Latino, Mexican, Central or South American, or any other Hispanic origin)" were classified as Latinos. Respondents who selected the category "Black, not of Hispanic origin" were identified as African Americans. Finally, subjects who selected "White, not of Hispanic origin" were identified as Whites.

---

[1]The quantity–frequency index used to classify subjects' drinking in Table 14.3 was based on questions assessing drinking in the twelve months previous to the survey interview. The categories in the index are defined as follows: *frequent heavy drinker*, drinks once a week or more often and has five or more drinks at a sitting at least once a week or more often (a drink is a one ounce of spirits, a four-ounce glass of wine, or a twelve-ounce can of beer); *frequent drinker*, drinks once a week or more often and may or may not drink five or more drinks at a sitting less than once a week but at least once a year; *less frequent drinker*, drinks one to three times a month and may or may not drink five or more drinks at least once a year; *infrequent drinker*, drinks less than once a month but at least once a year, and does not drink five or more drinks at a sitting; *abstainer*, drinks less than once a year or has never drunk.

# TABLE 14.3. DRINKING PATTERNS BY AGE: 1984–1995 (PERCENTAGES).

| | Men[a] (Age, Years) | | | | | | | | | | | |
|---|---|---|---|---|---|---|---|---|---|---|---|---|
| | 18–29 | | 30–39 | | 40–49 | | 50–59 | | 60+ | | All | |
| | 1984 | 1995 | 1984 | 1995 | 1984 | 1995 | 1984 | 1995 | 1984 | 1995 | 1984 | 1995 |
| | (n = 202) | (n = 267) | (n = 169) | (n = 215) | (n = 90) | (n = 123) | (n = 60) | (n = 83) | (n = 77) | (n = 76) | (n = 599) | (n = 764) |
| Abstain | 22 | 32 | 17 | 26 | 24 | 38 | 22 | 44 | 30 | 60 | 22 | 35 |
| Infrequent drinking | 9 | 13 | 5 | 9 | 12 | 11 | 8 | 13 | 21 | 13 | 10 | 12 |
| Less frequent drinking | 14 | 27 | 18 | 24 | 38 | 15 | 44 | 9 | 24 | 12 | 22 | 21 |
| Frequent drinking | 37 | 11 | 33 | 20 | 15 | 13 | 11 | 19 | 21 | 12 | 30 | 15 |
| Frequent heavy drinking | 17 | 17 | 26 | 21 | 10 | 23 | 16 | 16 | 3 | 3 | 17 | 18 |

| | Women[b] | | | | | | | | | | | |
|---|---|---|---|---|---|---|---|---|---|---|---|---|
| | 18–29 | | 30–39 | | 40–49 | | 50–59 | | 60+ | | All | |
| | 1984 | 1995 | 1984 | 1995 | 1984 | 1995 | 1984 | 1995 | 1984 | 1995 | 1984 | 1995 |
| | (n = 276) | (n = 255) | (n = 229) | (n = 231) | (n = 126) | (n = 147) | (n = 85) | (n = 79) | (n = 113) | (n = 105) | (n = 831) | (n = 817) |
| Abstain | 41 | 54 | 46 | 48 | 40 | 57 | 48 | 65 | 79 | 73 | 47 | 57 |
| Infrequent drinking | 35 | 16 | 22 | 14 | 19 | 23 | 7 | 14 | 11 | 2 | 24 | 14 |
| Less frequent drinking | 12 | 18 | 48 | 25 | 22 | 13 | 15 | 16 | 5 | 8 | 16 | 17 |
| Frequent drinking | 10 | 7 | 8 | 12 | 16 | 7 | 24 | 4 | 6 | 17 | 11 | 9 |
| Frequent heavy drinking | 2 | 6 | 2 | 2 | 2 | 1 | 6 | 1 | 0 | 0 | 2 | 3 |

[a]Differences across age groups in 1984 and 1995 are statistically significant, chi square $p < .05$.
[b]Differences across age groups in 1984 and 1995 are statistically significant, chi square $p < .01$.

Note: Numbers of the samples (n) are shown in parentheses.

Results from this trends analysis for Latino men showed an increase in abstention, a decrease in rates of frequent drinking, but stability in frequent heavy drinking (Table 14.3). As a result of these trends, in 1995 Latino men had rates of abstention that were 1.5 times higher than those for White men, and Latino men had rates of frequent heavy drinking that were similar to those of White men (Caetano & Clark, 1998a). The increase in abstention rates in 1995 from 1984 and the stability of frequent drinking between these two data points was confirmed in a multivariate analysis controlling for sociodemographic factors. Data by age showed an increase in abstention in all age groups, but particularly for men fifty years of age and more, for whom rates doubled. Less frequent drinking increased among younger men but decreased among men fifty years of age and older. Frequent drinking decreased in all groups with the exception of men fifty to fifty-nine years of age. There is a decrease in the rate of frequent heavy drinking among men thirty to thirty-nine years of age and an increase among those forty to forty-nine years of age.

Among Latino women, trends in drinking patterns between 1984 and 1995 show less variation than trends among men. The largest variation in rates is associated with the trend for increased abstention, which is seen together with a decrease in the rate of infrequent drinking. Finally, the rate for frequent heavy drinking among women was also stable between 1984 and 1995. The age-specific trends among Latino women showed that all drinking patterns tended to be mixed (see Table 14.3), with rates being stable, increasing, or decreasing depending on the age group. For instance, abstention increases in the youngest age group and among women forty to forty-nine and fifty to fifty-nine years of age, but it is stable among women thirty to thirty-nine and those sixty years of age and older. Frequent heavy drinking increases slightly among the youngest group, decreases among women fifty to fifty-nine years of age, and is stable in all other age groups.

Among Latino men in the United States, data by national group showed a considerable increase in abstention among Puerto Ricans, Cubans, and "other Latinos" (Table 14.4). The increase in abstention rates for Mexican American men is smaller in magnitude. There was also a considerable decrease in less frequent drinking for Puerto Rican and Cuban men and a decrease in frequent drinking for Mexican Americans and men of "other Latino" nationality. Frequent heavy drinking remained stable among Mexican American men and Cuban men but decreased among Puerto Ricans. Among women, there was an increase in abstention for Mexican Americans and Puerto Ricans, but stability for Cubans and a decrease for women of "other Latino" nationality. Trends for infrequent, less frequent, and frequent drinking were group specific. For instance, infrequent drinking decreased among Mexican Americans, Puerto Ricans, and Cubans but remained stable among women of "other Latino" nationality. In general, rates for frequent heavy drinking were stable in all groups. These results must be interpreted very cautiously, given the relatively small number of Latinos of Puerto Rican, Cuban, and "other" nationalities interviewed in the sample.

# TABLE 14.4. DRINKING PATTERNS BY NATIONAL GROUP AND GENDER: 1984–1995 (PERCENTAGES).

## Men

| | Mexican Americans | | Puerto Ricans | | Cubans | | Other Latinos | |
|---|---|---|---|---|---|---|---|---|
| | 1984 | 1995 | 1984 | 1995 | 1984 | 1995 | 1984 | 1995 |
| | (n = 410) | (n = 503) | (n = 78) | (n = 75) | (n = 45) | (n = 43) | (n = 66) | (n = 129) |
| Abstain | 27 | 31 | 19 | 58 | 12 | 39 | 9 | 38 |
| Infrequent drinking | 8 | 10 | 4 | 10 | 31 | 10 | 12 | 14 |
| Less frequent drinking | 14 | 23 | 41 | 10 | 40 | 17 | 23 | 23 |
| Frequent drinking | 32 | 13 | 15 | 15 | 11 | 28 | 41 | 16 |
| Frequent heavy drinking | 18 | 23 | 16 | 7 | 5 | 6 | 15 | 10 |

## Women

| | Mexican Americans | | Puerto Ricans | | Cubans | | Other Latinos | |
|---|---|---|---|---|---|---|---|---|
| | 1984 | 1995 | 1984 | 1995 | 1984 | 1995 | 1984 | 1995 |
| | (n = 539) | (n = 477) | (n = 141) | (n = 116) | (n = 50) | (n = 52) | (n = 104) | (n = 141) |
| Abstain | 46 | 57 | 35 | 66 | 42 | 46 | 69 | 55 |
| Infrequent drinking | 23 | 16 | 29 | 11 | 31 | 16 | 14 | 13 |
| Less frequent drinking | 14 | 17 | 24 | 14 | 15 | 31 | 10 | 18 |
| Frequent drinking | 14 | 7 | 9 | 5 | 11 | 7 | 3 | 13 |
| Frequent heavy drinking | 2 | 3 | 2 | 4 | 0 | 0 | 4 | —* |

*0.5 percent or less.

Note: Numbers of the samples (n) are shown in parentheses.

# Trends in Norms and Attitudes Toward Drinking: 1984–1995

The general trend for less drinking in the United States should be associated with an increased conservatism in norms and attitudes toward drinking. Evidence in support of this hypothesis comes from trend analyses of survey data by Hilton (1991) and Greenfield and Room (1997). The former reported on U.S. drinking data for the period 1979 to 1984, whereas the latter reported a trend for more restrictive situational norms between 1979 and 1990. However, the data for drinking among Latinos is not uniformly indicative of less drinking, as seen in Tables 14.3 and 14.4. An increase in the rate of abstention exists side by side with stability in frequent heavy drinking. This mixed trend is reflected in the trends for norms supporting "any drinking" in 1984 and 1995. These trends were first reported by Caetano and Clark (1999).

For this analysis, Latino respondents were presented with the nine drinking situations and asked to indicate "how much drinking is all right" by selecting one of the four response categories: (1) no drinking; (2) one or two drinks; (3) enough to feel the effects but not drunk; and (4) getting drunk is sometimes all right. Respondents' answers to the three latter categories were combined so as to represent the proportion allowing any drinking in each situation. Among men, three items out of the nine showed more support for drinking in 1995 than in 1984 (drinking by a man at a bar, drinking by a woman at a bar, and drinking with a couple of coworkers out to lunch), and two items showed less support for any drinking in 1995 than in 1984 (drinking when at a friend's home, drinking when with friends after work). Among Latino women, norms became more liberal when applied to coworkers drinking at lunch. Norms became more conservative in three situations: drinking at a party at someone else's home, drinking when at a friend's home, and drinking when with friends after work.

Variation in attitudes among Latino men and women between 1984 and 1995 also showed a mixture of increased liberalism and conservatism. There was an increase in the proportion of Latino men who agreed that "getting drunk is an innocent way of having fun" and that "it is good to get drunk once in a while." On the other hand, Latino men became more conservative in their attitudes toward drinking by a woman at a bar and toward seeing drinking as a way of being friendly. Latino women showed more liberal attitudes with regards to items such as "getting drunk is an innocent way to have fun," "drinking is one of the pleasures of life," "drinking brings out the worst in people," and "it is good to get drunk once a while." They showed more conservative attitudes in the items "there is nothing good to be said about drinking" and "drinking is a way of being friendly."

# Alcohol-Related Mortality and Morbidity

Alcohol consumption is related to a number of medical conditions, both directly and indirectly. Of all alcohol-related deaths reported in the United States in 1988, 17 percent were directly attributed to alcohol, 38 percent were from medical conditions indirectly attributed to alcohol, and 45 percent were from injuries indirectly attributed to alcohol (Miller, 1999). Alcohol consumption is said to be a major contributor in 41 percent to 95 percent of deaths from liver cirrhosis and alcohol hepatitis (National Institute on Alcohol Abuse and Alcoholism, 1999). Cirrhosis is also reported to account for 75 percent of all deaths due to medical causes among alcoholics (Miller, 1999). Medical conditions that are sometimes indirectly related to alcohol consumption include heart disease and cancer (National Institute on Alcohol Abuse and Alcoholism, 1999).

Data on the leading causes of death in the United States in 1997 for Latinos as well as for Whites and African Americans, using Latinos as the reference group, show that diseases of the heart and malignant neoplasm are the two highest leading causes of death for all three groups. Deaths from chronic liver diseases including cirrhosis constitute the eighth-leading cause of death for Latinos, whereas they do not appear among the ten leading causes of death for either Whites or African Americans. In 1996, the death rate for alcohol-related liver cirrhosis was 13.3 deaths per 100,000 for Latino males, 8.3 for African American males, 5.2 for White males, and 3.1 for African American females (National Institute on Alcohol Abuse and Alcoholism, 1999). Between 1991 and 1996, a decrease in the death rate for alcohol-related liver cirrhosis of 29.5 percent was seen for African American females, 21.7 percent for African American males, 7.6 percent for Latino males, and no change for White males (National Institute on Alcohol Abuse and Alcoholism, 1999).

## Alcohol-Related Intimate Partner Violence

The results described in the paragraphs below have been reported by Caetano and colleagues (in press-a, in press-b, 2000) and Cunradi and colleagues (1998; also Cunradi, Caetano, Clark, & Schafer, 1999), and are based on the analysis of the National Couples Study of 1995. This sample was a representative group of White, African American, and Latino couples (married and cohabiting) - living in the continental United States. A total of 1,925 eligible couples eighteen years of age and older were identified in the survey, and 1,635 couples participated, for a response rate of 85 percent. Among these couples who were interviewed there were 555 who were White, 358 who were African American, and 527 who were of Latino origin. The analyses here are restricted to the 555 White couples whose both members self-identified as White, and the 527 couples whose both members self-identified as Latino. This sample is somewhat unusual in that reports were obtained from both partners, this project therefore providing a methodological advancement over previous studies that relied on one person's report to serve as a proxy for the other partner's report.

The individuals selected to participate in the study were asked about the occurrence during the past year of eleven violent behaviors that they may have perpetrated against their partners or that their partners may have perpetrated against them. The violence items were adapted from the Conflict Tactics Scale, Form R (Straus, 1990) and included the following: threw something; pushed, grabbed, or shoved; slapped; kicked, bit, or hit; hit or tried to hit with something; beat up; choked, burned, or scalded; forced sex; threatened with a knife or gun; and used a knife or gun. Separate analyses were conducted for male-perpetrated violence (male-to-female partner violence, MFPV) and female-perpetrated violence (female-to-male partner violence, FMPV). For both of these variables, violence was considered as present when at least one of the partners reported a violent incident. Following an affirmative response, the respondent was then asked if he or she or his or her spouse was drinking during the incident. In addition, questions were asked about exposure to violence in childhood and adolescence. Participants reported whether any of the following acts had been perpetrated against them during childhood or adolescence by a parent or other caregiver: hit with something; beaten up; choked, burned, or scalded; threatened with a knife or gun; and had a knife or gun used against them.

Overall rates of MFPV (Table 14.5) were higher among Latinos than among Whites. Likewise, rates of specific MFPV events were generally higher for Latinos than for Whites. Overall rates of FMPV were higher among Latinos than among Whites. Rates of specific types of FMPV events were higher than comparable MFPV events, independent of ethnicity. Rates for most of these events were higher among Latinos than among Whites.

Drinking during the event was more common among men than among women, independent of which gender perpetrated the violence (Table 14.6). Drinking during the event was equally common among Whites and Latinos. More than one-quarter each of the White and Latino men reported drinking during MFPV incidents. Between one-quarter and one-third of all men were drinking during incidents of FMPV. There were significant differences in the proportion of White and Latino women who reported drinking during FMPV. The rate among White women was about four times higher than the rate among Latino women. When the effect of sociodemographic variables, personality factors (impulsivity), attitudes toward IPV, experience of victimization by violence during childhood, experience of violence among parents or guardians during childhood, and alcohol problems was controlled for in multivariate analysis, the difference between Whites and Latinos in rates of violence disappeared. Further, the effect of alcohol consumption on partner violence also disappeared. Alcohol problems, however, remained predictive of IPV, but in specific ways: female alcohol-related problems (but not male alcohol-related problems) were associated with IPV among White couples; among Latino couples, there was no longer a strong relationship between alcohol problems and IPV.

Finally, a separate analysis focused on acculturation and its relationship with IPV. Acculturation was assessed with a scale composed of twelve items covering the following areas: ability to speak English; use of English with family, neighbors, and at work; easiness of relationships with Whites and Latinos; opinions

# TABLE 14.5. PREVALENCE OF INTIMATE PARTNER VIOLENCE BY RACE OR ETHNICITY.

(a) Percentage Reporting Any Intimate Partner Violence in Previous Twelve Months.

| Male-to-Female Partner Violence (MFPV) | | | Female-to-Male Partner Violence (FMPV) | | |
|---|---|---|---|---|---|
| Whites | African Americans | Latinos | Whites | African Americans | Latinos |
| (n = 555) | (n = 358) | (n = 527) | (n = 555) | (n = 358) | (n = 527) |
| 11 | 23 | 17** | 15 | 30 | 21** |

(b) Percentage Reporting Each Type of Event.

| | Male-to-Female Partner Violence (MFPV) | | | Female-to-Male Partner Violence (FMPV) | | |
|---|---|---|---|---|---|---|
| Event | Whites | African Americans | Latinos | Whites | African Americans | Latinos |
| 1. Throw something | 4.1 | 5.4 | 5.8 | 9.5 | 22.1 | 13.0** |
| 2. Push, shove, grab | 9.4 | 19.7 | 13.0* | 10.5 | 21.3 | 13.0* |
| 3. Slap | 1.5 | 7.8 | 5.5* | 0.3 | 9.7 | 6.4 |
| 4. Kick, bite, hit | 0.7 | 4.1 | 2.6** | 2.7 | 9.9 | 5.0* |
| 5. Hit with something | 0.9 | 5.1 | 4.2** | 3.8 | 15.8 | 7.5** |
| 6. Beat up | 0.3 | 1.4 | 2.2 | 0.0 | 2.1 | 1.3** |
| 7. Choke | 0.4 | 2.7 | 1.9 | 0.1 | 1.4 | 0.7 |
| 8. Burn | 0.4 | 0.2 | 0.0 | 0.0 | 1.2 | 0.2 |
| 9. Force sex | 0.5 | 1.7 | 1.9 | 0.4 | 2.9 | 1.0* |
| 10. Threaten with knife/gun | 0.4 | 0.6 | 0.7 | 0.1 | 3.1 | 0.9* |
| 11. Use knife/gun | 0.3 | 0.2 | 0.4 | 0.3 | 0.09 | 0.5 |

*$p < .05$, **$p < .01$.

# TABLE 14.6. CORRESPONDENCE BETWEEN INTIMATE PARTNER VIOLENCE AND ALCOHOL CONSUMPTION.

(a) *Percentage of Individuals Drinking During Intimate Partner Violence.*

| | Male-to-Female Partner Violence (MFPV) | | | Female-to-Male Partner Violence (FMPV) | | |
|---|---|---|---|---|---|---|
| | Whites | African Americans | Latinos | Whites | African Americans | Latinos |
| Men | 29.4 | 41.4 | 29.1 | 27.1 | 33.7 | 28.4 |
| Women | 11.4 | 23.6 | 5.4* | 14.7 | 22.4 | 3.8** |

(b) *Percentage of Intimate Partner Violence Perpetrators among Abstainers and Selected Drinkers.*

| | Whites | African Americans | Latinos |
|---|---|---|---|
| | (n = 527) | (n = 358) | (n = 527) |
| Male-to-female partner violence (MFPV) | | | |
| Male quantity/frequency abstainer | 6 | 18 | 17 |
| Drinks 5 or more drinks on occasion at least once a week | 19 | 40 | 24 |
| Female-to-male partner violence (FMPV) | | | |
| Female quantity/frequency abstainer | 12 | 25 | 17 |
| Drinks at least once a week | 19 | 57 | 21 |

*Chi-square. Whites × African Americans × Latinos, $p < .05$.

**Chi-square. Whites × African Americans × Latinos, $p < .001$.

Note: Chi-square analysis was conducted among ethnic groups.

Source: Adapted from Caetano et al. (in press-b).

about interethnic marriage; preference for Latino media (books, TV, and radio); preference for Latino music; proportions of friends who are Latinos; proportion of current church congregation who are Latinos; proportion of people in the neighborhood who are Latinos; proportion of people in the neighborhood "where you grew up" who were Latinos; and proportion of people in the parties "you usually go to" who are Latinos. Scores on the scale were divided into three groups representing low, medium, and high levels of acculturation. The cutoff points for these groupings were based on data collected in a 1984 national survey of Latinos, and they forced roughly 33 percent of the respondents to fall into each group.

Latino couples with at least one medium-acculturated couple member were three times more likely to experience MFPV than couples with two low-acculturated partners (Caetano, Schafer, Clark, Cunradi, & Raspberry, 2000). Acculturation status was not associated with FMPV. This result, indicating that medium-acculturation couples are more at risk to be involved in violent relationship than couples at other levels of acculturation, is in disagreement with the results of Kantor, Jasinski, and Aldarondo (1993). These authors suggest that IPV is more frequent among those individuals highly acculturated to U.S. society. According to Kantor and colleagues (1993), Latinos high in acculturation may experience stressful life conditions in which their experience of poverty runs counter to economic aspirations for betterment, resulting in frustration and ultimately provoking incidents of IPV.

# Trends in Alcohol-Related Problems: 1984–1995

Chronic excessive drinking as well as acute alcohol intoxication may lead to a number of problems that range from severe chronic illnesses such as liver cirrhosis and alcohol dependence to alcohol-impaired driving, job-related problems, and family-related problems. Alcohol surveys have assessed rates of many types of alcohol-related problems among Latinos. Both in 1984 and 1995, Latino respondents were presented with a comprehensive list of twenty-nine social and dependence alcohol-related problems and asked to report whether or not they had experienced each of these problems in the twelve months prior to the interview. The items included in the surveys reflect twenty years of cumulative experience in the measurement of alcohol-related problems and address fourteen specific problem areas: salience of drinking, impaired control, withdrawal, relief drinking, tolerance, binge drinking, belligerence, accidents, health-related problems, work-related problems, financial problems, problems with the police, problems with the spouse, and problems with persons other than the spouse.

Results from analyses of the data showed that prevalence of most problems increased among Latino men, while among Latino women problem such prevalence was stable. Table 14.7 shows these data for the five most frequent

# TABLE 14.7. ALCOHOL PROBLEMS AMONG LATINOS BY NATIONAL GROUP: 1984–1995 (PERCENTAGES).

| | Mexican Americans | | Puerto Ricans | | Cubans | | Other Latinos | | All | |
|---|---|---|---|---|---|---|---|---|---|---|
| **Men** | 1984 | 1995 | 1984 | 1995 | 1984 | 1995 | 1984 | 1995 | 1984 | 1995 |
| | (n = 407) | (n = 494) | (n = 77) | (n = 74) | (n = 45) | (n = 42) | (n = 65) | (n = 142) | (n = 599) | (n = 767) |
| Salience | 11 | 12 | 6 | 9 | 3 | 2 | 6 | 7 | 7 | 10 |
| Impairment of control | 11 | 16 | 6 | 3 | 1 | 7 | 4 | 12 | 6 | 13 |
| Belligerence | 7 | 13 | 1 | 5 | 3 | 3 | 2 | 5 | 5 | 11 |
| Family | 9 | 17 | 6 | 2 | 2 | 4 | 1 | 10 | 7 | 14 |
| People | 7 | 11 | 5* | 2 | 3 | 2 | 4 | 4 | 6 | 8 |
| **Women** | | | | | | | | | | |
| | (n = 534) | (n = 477) | (n = 140) | (n = 116) | (n = 50) | (n = 52) | (n = 104) | (n = 141) | (n = 833) | (n = 706) |
| Salience | 4 | 5 | 1 | 4 | 2 | 0 | 2 | 4 | 3 | 4 |
| Impairment of control | 4 | 5 | 1 | 5* | 0 | 0 | 1 | 2 | 0 | 4 |
| Belligerence | 4 | 3* | 1 | 4 | 2 | 0 | 3 | 2 | 3 | 3 |
| Family | 1 | 5 | 1 | 5 | 2 | 0 | 1 | 2 | 1 | 4 |
| People | 4 | 4 | 2 | 3* | 0 | 0 | 6 | 4 | 3 | 3 |

*(0.5 percent or less.)

Note: Numbers of the samples (n) are shown in parentheses.

alcohol-related problems for men in 1984 and 1995 by Latino national group and for all national groups together. Data for 1984 differ somewhat from previous reports using the same data because of recent reanalysis using different statistical software and different weighting methods. Data for all Latino men together show an increase in most problem types between 1984 and 1995, as reported by Caetano and Clark (1998b). When data are divided into Latino national groups, it can be seen that most of the increase in problem rates among men has occurred among Mexican Americans. Among women, problem rates are low and for the most part stable, as predicted.

## Alcohol Prevention Interventions

Alcohol prevention interventions have common characteristics, independent of the ethnicity of target populations. In general, prevention interventions in the alcohol field are based on two theoretical approaches: the environmental model (Holder, 1998) and the risk-factor model (Hawkins, Catalano, & Miller, 1992), which also may include attention to resilience factors. For the most part, environmental approaches are not directed to a specific population group but aim at reducing the amount of alcohol available for consumption in the community. Examples of environmental interventions targeting particular groups are those aimed at raising the legal drinking age from eighteen to twenty-one as well as those seeking to discourage the sales of alcoholic beverages to minors. Examples of environmental approaches applied to prevention that are not directed to specific population groups are taxation, lowering blood alcohol concentration (BAC) levels under which it is legal to drive (Hingson, 1993; Hingson, Howland, & Levinson, 1988), and implementing community intervention to reduce alcohol-related trauma (Holder, Saltz, Grube, Voas, Gruenewald, & Treno, 1997). Environmental approaches can also target a particular community or geographic area. An example is the attempt by community groups to control the number of liquor stores in their neighborhoods.

Environmental interventions have become an important approach to the prevention of alcohol problems, given the considerable research evidence that now exists indicating that environmental factors that increase alcohol availability contribute to an increase in the prevalence of alcohol-related problems. For instance, alcohol outlet density (the number of locations selling alcohol in a particular community) in Latino neighborhoods has received some attention in the literature. Alaniz, Cartmill, and Parker (1998) found that in San Jose, California, Latino neighborhoods had 4.56 alcohol outlets per 1,000 people in comparison to the predominantly White neighborhoods with 0.94 outlets per 1,000 people. Alcohol outlet density is of particular importance because it has been associated with alcohol consumption (Scribner, Cohen, & Fisher, 2000), violence (Alaniz, Cartmill, & Parker, 1998; Alaniz, 1998; Cohen,

Scribner, & Farley, 2000; Scribner MacKinnon, & Dwyer, 1995), arrests for alcohol-impaired driving (Scribner, MacKinnon, & Dwyer, 1994), alcohol-related motor vehicle crashes (Scribner, MacKinnon, & Dwyer, 1994), traffic fatalities (Cohen, Scribner, & Farley, 2000), and cirrhosis deaths (Scribner, MacKinnon, & Dwyer, 1994).

Another environmental factor is the advertising of alcohol to Latino populations. Spanish-language advertising by the nation's top three domestic brewers increased from $26.3 million in 1996 to $31 million in 1997 ("Sobering Facts," 1999). Additionally, Latino and African American neighborhoods have been found to have proportionately more billboards promoting alcoholic beverages than do White and Asian American neighborhoods (Altman, Schooler, & Basil, 1991). Advertising to Latinos often incorporates images drawing from Latino mythology, history, tradition, culture, language, and nationalism (Alaniz & Wilkes, 1995). Such blending of alcohol with Latino cultural symbols attempts to normalize alcohol consumption for this population.

Some Latino organizations have attempted to curtail the presence of both alcohol outlets and alcohol advertisements in their communities (Alaniz, 1998) as well as the sponsorship of community events by the alcohol industry ("Sobering Facts," 1999). Such attempts to curtail alcohol advertisements directed to Latinos have been described as elitist and condescending ("Sobering Facts," 1999), and an infringement of the advertisers' constitutional rights (Ringold, 1995). However, environmental factors do have a role in shaping both community norms and individual behavior (Alaniz, Cartmill, & Parker, 1998; Cohen, Scribner, & Farley, 2000). Efforts by Latino community members to alter individual behavior and its negative consequences through interventions on the environmental level should be seen as being as valid as campaigns led by the U.S. Surgeon General to alter smoking and sexual practices deemed to have negative consequences for both an individual and the community at large.

Alcohol prevention interventions based on the risk-factor model have been more directed at adolescents than adults. Based on the fact that drinking by those under twenty-one is illegal, these programs try to prevent any use of alcohol, independent of its frequency or of the amount drunk per occasion. Interventions targeting youth are for the most part school-based. This literature on school-based prevention intervention has been reviewed by Moskowitz (1989), who concluded that approaches that rely solely on educational interventions are not effective strategies for inducing long-lasting changes in alcohol-related behavior.

Interventions targeting adults do not try to prevent any use of alcohol, but rather are usually focused on specific problem behaviors. In the recent past, many of these interventions have targeted drinking and driving (Hingson, Howland, & Levinson, 1988) and drinking during pregnancy (Casiro, Stanwick, Pelech, Taylor, & Manitoba Medical Association, 1994; Dufour, Williams, Campbell, & Aitken, 1994; Hankin, 1994; Kaskutas & Graves, 1994). Warning labels drawing the public's attention to the dangers of drinking are directed at the population at large. Evaluations of the effect of these warning labels indicate that they are supported by the public (Hilton & Kaskutas, 1991) and that they reach a target population of young heavy drinkers. Such warning labels may have a limited effect on knowledge and specific alcohol-related behaviors (Greenfield, Graves, & Kaskutas, 1993). However, because these labels are in English and not in Spanish, their impact on many U.S. Latinos is minimized because a large proportion of them have little or no ability to understand English.

A recent search of the literature beginning in 1992 did not unveil any published outcome-based comprehensive evaluation of either environmental or "risk factor-based" interventions with a special focus on Latinos (Caetano, Clark, & Raspberry, 1998). Thus, the previously identified (Ames & Mora, 1988; Caetano, 1992; Singer, Davison, & Yalin, 1987) lack of prevention research focused on this ethnic group continues to date. However, the literature search showed that a number of programs are being implemented across the country, many of which reach Latinos in the school-based population and in the community. For instance, Cervantes and Peña (1998) identified twenty-three Latino high-risk youth programs funded by the Center for Substance Abuse Prevention (CSAP). The search of the literature also revealed the existence of two groups of papers of importance for alcohol prevention with Latinos. The first group comprises conceptual papers focusing on topics relevant to the development of evaluation of prevention interventions with minority groups (Casas, 1992; Cervantes & Peña, 1998; Colon, 1998; Delgado, 1996; Padilla & Snyder, 1992; Schinke, Moncher, Palleja, Zayas, & Schilling, 1988). The second group reports results from the evaluation of program effectiveness (for example, Forgey, Schinke, & Cole, 1997; Tobler & Stratton, 1997). These papers either report on a particular program or provide results from meta-analyses of series of school-based interventions.

## Conceptual and Methodological Literature

This literature suggests that specific knowledge about the culture and the predictors of alcohol problems among Latinos is needed to develop interventions in this minority group. The cultural identity and distinctiveness of Latinos must be recognized and understood so that both prevention strategies are culturally appropriate and thus effective. Some of these papers discuss issues such as cultural competence or sensitivity (Casas, 1992; Cervantes & Peña, 1998; Colon, 1998; Padilla & Snyder, 1992). Cultural competence has been defined as the ability to include cultural factors of importance to a certain ethnic group (language, acculturation, family values, and community attitudes) into evaluation designs (Cervantes & Peña, 1998; Orlandi, Weston, & Epstein, 1992). Attention has also focused on the cultural characteristics of ethnic minority groups judged of importance to prevention. These include gender roles, stress due to racism or poverty, stress due to immigration and acculturation, family involvement, and birthplace.

Authors discussing prevention among Latinos identify concepts such as *familialism, simpatia, respeto,* and *machismo* (Marin, 1990) as important to consider when developing prevention interventions with this ethnic group. *Familialism* is described as a strong orientation to close emotional bonds within the family as well as a strong sense of obligation to provide economic as well as emotional support to family members. This circle is frequently increased by others (such as *compadres* and *comadres*) linked to the family though baptism and other religious rituals. Thus, appeals to Latinos' strong family orientation and family involvement in prevention efforts would, ideally, increase the effectiveness of prevention efforts. *Simpatia* and *respeto* are identified as concepts emphasizing the establishment of smooth and pleasant social relations (*simpatia*) characterized by deference and respect (*respeto*) for the individual. The use of data collection instruments that are culturally appropriate and have been validated among Latinos is another important methodological consideration (Cervantes & Peña, 1998).

## The Literature on Program Effectiveness

A number of meta-analyses of prevention research have been published (Tobler, 1986, 1994; Tobler & Stratton, 1997). Some of these analyses show that only a small number of programs are offered to ethnic minority populations. Tobler (1986) reported that only nineteen school-based programs out of a total of 415 had a focus on minorities. In other analyses, the effect on ethnic minorities has been assessed by grouping programs offered to "special populations" (for example, see Tobler, 1994), that is, programs that were implemented in schools with more than 50 percent minority or problem students. Thus, even when a significant effect for such programs is reported, as did Tobler (1986, 1994), it is impossible to know which "special" group is the focus of the programs that showed effectiveness. More recently, Tobler (1998) expanded previous meta-analyses of prevention interventions with school-based populations. Results of these meta-analyses showed that programs delivered to predominantly minority populations were about one and a half times more effective than programs delivered to predominantly White populations. Interactive programs were more effective in minority populations than in nonminority populations. Unfortunately, the most effective programs—those that were interactive—had a success rate of only 7 percent.

One of the few attempts to compare the effectiveness of a general school-based prevention intervention and an ethnic-specific approach was reported by Botvin, Schinke, Epstein, and Diaz (1994) and Forgey, Schinke, and Cole (1997). The study was conducted in six public junior high schools in New York City with predominantly minority populations (88 to 100 percent). A life skills training approach was compared to a culturally focused approach and to an information-only control group. While the content of the two experimental programs was the same, the cultural approach used "mythic and contemporary" story contexts to impart information. The first follow-up results were at four months after the intervention (Botvin, Schinke, Epstein, & Diaz, 1994); other follow up results were obtained at two years after intervention (Forgey, Schinke, & Cole, 1997). Based on two-year follow-up data, Forgey and colleagues (1997) reported that students in both interventions drank alcohol less often, were drunk less often, and had lower intentions to drink than students in the control group. Students who had been given the culturally focused intervention drank less and intended to drink less than students in the life skills intervention group and in the control group. A problem in interpreting these results arises from the selection of students in the general life skills intervention and culturally focused intervention groups. According to Botvin and colleagues (1994) the general life skills approach was implemented with all students in a classroom while the culturally focused intervention was given to "targeted high-risk students" and also involved group counseling with professionally trained individuals and peers. The use of different selection criteria for assembling these two groups plus the use of group counseling with one group and not the other probably rendered the comparisons invalid.

Finally, Dent, Sussman, Ellickson, Brown, and Richardson (1996) examined arguments against and for the generalizability of current prevention programs across ethnic groups. Arguments in support of generalizability included those based on the following: strong evidence that current programs work versus little evidence that they do not work, thus making it premature to switch entirely to new programs; evidence that "social influences" prevention programs may be effective across ethnic groups; current programs are interactive, thus taking into account participants' experiences and backgrounds; evidence that the substance use initiation is similar across ethnic groups; costs associated with the implementation of ethnic-specific programs; and the difficulty of implementing several different programs in schools where the student body is ethnically diverse. Arguments in support of program specificity were based on the following: an intuitive sense that differences in culture and history across ethnic groups are important influences in substance use and must be taken into account; evidence that interventions directed at the majority population may be less effective with minorities and may not reach ethnic groups; information that schools in minority areas may lack funds to support programs and other public institutions may give priority to health care delivery rather than prevention; evidence that media usage may vary across ethnic groups and may not be the same as that which is effective in the general population; information that ethnic communities may be more willing to pay attention to and use prevention messages and materials that are ethnic specific; and information that generic programs may fail to address important ethnic-specific risk factors for substance use. After weighing the evidence, Dent and colleagues (1996) conclude that the need for ethnic-specific programs is debatable.

## Summary and Conclusions

Research continues to indicate that levels of alcohol consumption and associated problems are unacceptably high among U.S. Latinos. Data on Latino adolescents indicates that about 80 percent have already used alcohol before the age of eighteen and that about one-third have engaged in episodic heavy drinking. Rates for high-risk behaviors such as drinking and driving or riding with a driver who has had too much to drink are also unacceptably high among Latino youth. The evidence of alcohol consumption and alcohol-related problems among Latino youth reinforces the need for effective intervention programs with this population. The findings from the 1997 YRBS (United States Department of Health and Human Services, 1998), the 1998 Alternative YRBS (United States Department of Health and Human Services, 1999), and the 1992 NHIS–YRBS (Adams, Schoenborn, Moss, Warren, & Kann, 1992) on the percentage of youth who report drinking alcohol before age thirteen point to the need to implement prevention programs at an early age. This is consistent with the findings of other studies that argue for the need to implement prevention interventions early in life (Flannery, Vazsonyi, Torquati, & Fridrich, 1994; Grunbaum, Basen-Engquist, & ElSouki, 1996; Vega, Zimmerman, Warheit, Apospori, & Gil, 1993; Warheit, Vega, Khoury, Gill, & Elfenbein, 1996). Given the strong role of friends and peers in influencing alcohol consumption noted above, prevention programs should include interventions that address these social influences to drink through the teaching of personal and social skills to effectively address peer pressure, such as assertiveness, decision making, problem solving, making responsible choices, and reducing stress (Alva & Jones, 1994; Dusenbury, Epstein, Botvin, & Diaz, 1994; Epstein, Botvin, Diaz, & Schinke, 1995; Flannery, Vazsonyi, Torquati, & Fridrich, 1994). Prevention programs should also teach adolescents about the health and other related consequences of drinking. Developing prevention programs that address all forms of substance abuse may be more efficient than interventions addressing only alcohol use, because alcohol consumption has been found to correlate with other drug use and problem behaviors among adolescents (Dusenbury, Epstein, Botvin, & Diaz, 1994).

Not surprisingly, the picture among Latino adults is not very different. As discussed by Caetano and Clark (1998a), the reduction in per capita consumption in the United States may be occurring among Latinos through a switch from lighter drinking patterns to abstention, with stability in the rate of frequent heavy drinking. Stability of such a drinking pattern puts Latinos at a high risk for problem development, which should be a concern to public health professionals and to all those interested in the prevention of alcohol-related problems among this ethnic group in the United States.

The occurrence of intimate partner violence (IPV) is also too high among Latinos. However, the relationship between drinking, alcohol problems, and IPV must be interpreted with caution. The presence of alcohol during a partner violence event does not necessarily mean that alcohol is the cause of the violence. The violence could have occurred, and many times it does, without alcohol in the picture. All together, the research evidence suggests that the occurrence of IPV is the result of a constellation of factors that can be summarized as characteristics of the individual (say, drinking or alcohol problems), of their relationship with their partner (say, how long they have been together), and the social environment (say, poverty level). Individuals who are heavy drinkers are certainly at an increased risk for perpetration of or victimization by IPV. Individuals with alcohol problems also seem to be at an increased risk for IPV. However, the occurrence of IPV in couples where both members are heavy drinkers or where one member has an alcohol problem may not necessarily be caused by the drinking or the problem. In some cases (for instance, in Whites and Latinos), after researchers control for the effect of differences in socioeconomic background, personality variables and other factors eliminate the association between problems and IPV. In this case, alcohol problems are not the cause of IPV but just a marker, useful in identifying a population that for other reasons has an increased risk of developing violent relationships.

Regarding prevention efforts, it is fair to say that there continues to be a dearth of such interventions with Latinos. The lack of prevention efforts directed at the adult population of Latinos is puzzling if one considers the results of the trend analysis presented here. The evidence is clear: The trends analyses indicate that patterns of high-risk drinking such as frequent heavy drinking (drinking five or more drinks at a sitting once a week or more often) are more frequent and more stable among Latinos than, for example, Whites. This is a strong indication that Latinos, especially men, should be targets for prevention interventions designed to minimize such risky drinking patterns. Further, there has been a considerable increase in alcohol problem prevalence among Latino men.

Most of the prevention interventions reviewed in the literature are directed at the adolescent population and are school-based and universal; that is, they offer interventions to all those who are eligible in the target population independent of ethnic identification. This emphasis on school-based populations may be misguided. The effectiveness of this approach in promoting prolonged change in cognitions or behavior is still controversial. School-based interventions do not reach the dropout population, which is rather high among Latinos. Still, in spite of the obvious limitations of the existing universal, school-based approaches, there also are reasons why these programs are defensible when integrated with other preventive interventions directed at other systems in the environment. Offering the same intervention to students of all ethnic groups is an integrational approach in an environment that strives to be integrative. If programs are interactive—as they should be because of evidence suggesting that such programs are more effective than noninteractive ones—prevention activities may provide opportunity for students of different ethnic groups to interact and learn from one another.

The prevention research literature also lacks clarity regarding whether interventions need to be culturally specific or culturally sensitive. Interventions that are culturally specific, that is, are developed and implemented with a particular ethnic group in mind, should also perforce be culturally sensitive in regard to that particular ethnic group. Interventions that are culturally sensitive need not be specific; that is, they may be based on the same theoretical model or they may address the same factors of risk addressed by interventions directed to the majority population. The difference is that they may incorporate elements of ethnic culture (language, media preference, cultural icons, and the like) that would make them more acceptable, increase their penetration, and thus also increase their effectiveness when applied to majority populations.

Prevention interventions based on the environmental model, including alcohol policies aimed at reducing consumption, are still underutilized, although they are effective and perhaps more so than traditional educational approaches. These interventions are also cost effective and can be effective not only with majority groups but also with ethnic minority populations such as Latinos. There is a need to further develop these interventions both nationally and locally, but especially at the local level. It is at the local community level that issues related to billboard advertisement of alcohol, number of alcohol outlets, hours of sale, and sale of alcoholic beverages to minors can be addressed most effectively.

Finally, we enter the year 2001 with estimates of tremendous growth in the U.S. Latino population. Relatively soon, by the year 2050, about one in four Americans will be of Latino origin. At the same time problems arising from excessive alcohol consumption continue to be highly prevalent in Latino communities across the nation. It is therefore urgent for health care and public health professionals in general to focus their attention on issues related to alcohol and to increase efforts to minimize this problem among Latinos. By effectively addressing the problems associated with alcohol consumption in Latino communities, we can help ensure the well-being of Latinos in the United States.

# Acknowledgments

Work on this chapter was supported by Grant R37-AA10908 from the National Institute on Alcohol Abuse and Alcoholism to the Houston School of Public Health, University of Texas. Data collection was also supported by Grants RO1-AA10013 and AA-05595 (National Alcohol Research Center Grant) from the National Institute on Alcohol Abuse and Alcoholism to the Alcohol Research Group, Public Health Institute, Berkeley, California.

# References

Adams, P. F., Schoenborn, C. A., Moss, A. J., Warren, C. W., & Kann, L. (1992). *Health risk behaviors among our nation's youth: United States, 1992.* [Vital Health Statistics, No. 10, 1992]. Hyattsville, MD: National Center for Health Statistics.

Aguirre-Molina, M., & Caetano, R. (1994). Alcohol use and alcohol-related issues. In C. W. Molina & M. Aguirre-Molina (Eds.), *Latino health in the U.S.: A growing challenge.* Washington, D.C.: American Public Health Association, pp. 393–424.

Alaniz, M. L. (1998). Alcohol availability and targeted advertising in racial/ethnic minority communities. *Alcohol Health and Research World, 22,* 286–289.

Alaniz, M. L., Cartmill, R. S., & Parker, R. N. (1998). Immigrants and violence: The importance of neighborhood context. *Hispanic Journal of Behavioral Sciences, 20,* 155–174.

Alaniz, M. L., & Wilkes, C. (1995). Reinterpreting Latino culture in the commodity form: The cases of alcohol advertising in the Mexican American community. *Hispanic Journal of Behavioral Sciences, 17,* 430–451.

Altman, D. G., Schooler, C., & Basil, J. D. (1991). Alcohol and cigarette advertising on billboards. *Health education research: Theory and practice, 6,* 487–490.

Alva, S. A., & Jones, M. (1994). Psychosocial adjustment and self-reported patterns of alcohol use among Hispanic adolescents. *Journal of Early Adolescence, 14,* 432–448.

Ames, G., & Mora, J. (1988). Alcohol problem prevention in Mexican American populations. In M. J. Gilbert (Ed.), *Alcohol consumption among Mexicans and Mexican Americans: A binational perspective.* University of California, Los Angeles: Spanish Speaking Mental Health Research Center, pp. 253–280.

Arciniega, L. T., Arroyo, J. A., Miller, W. R., & Tonigan, J. S. (1996, November). Alcohol, drug use and consequences among Hispanics seeking treatment for alcohol-related problems. *Journal of Studies on Alcohol, 6,* 613–618.

Arroyo, J. A., Westerberg, V. S., & Tonigan, J. S. (1996). *Comparison of treatment utilization and outcome for Hispanics and non-Hispanic Whites.* Albuquerque: University of New Mexico.

Botvin, G. J., Schinke, S. P., Epstein, J. A., & Diaz, T. (1994). Effectiveness of culturally focused and generic skills training approaches to alcohol and drug abuse prevention among minority youths. *Psychology of Addictive Behaviors, 8,* 2, 116–127.

Caetano, R. (1992). *The prevention of alcohol-related problems among U.S. Hispanics: A review.* (DHHS Publication No. [SMA]95-3042). Bethesda, MD: National Institute on Alcohol Abuse and Alcoholism, Center for Substance Abuse Prevention.

Caetano, R., & Clark, C. (1998a). Trends in alcohol consumption patterns among Whites, Blacks and Hispanics: 1984–1995. *Journal of Studies on Alcohol, 59,* 659–668.

Caetano, R., & Clark, C. (1998b). Trends in alcohol-related problems among Whites, Blacks, and Hispanics: 1984–1995. *Alcoholism: Clinical and Experimental Research, 22,* 2, 534–538.

Caetano, R., & Clark, C. (1999). Trends in situational norms and attitudes toward drinking among Whites, Blacks, and Hispanics: 1984–1995. *Drug and Alcohol Dependence, 54,* 45–56.

Caetano, R., Clark, C. L., & Raspberry, K. (1998, October 21 & 22). *Preventing alcohol-related problems among U.S. Hispanics and Blacks: An update.* Paper presented at the National Institute on Alcohol Abuse and Alcoholism Extramural Scientific Advisory Board Meeting on Prevention, Washington, D.C.

Caetano, R., Cunradi, C. B., Schafer, J., & Clark, C. L. (in press-a). Intimate partner violence and drinking patterns among White, Black and Hispanic couples in the U.S. *Journal of Substance Abuse, 16.*

Caetano, R., Schafer, J., Clark, C. L., Cunradi, C. B., & Raspberry, K. (2000). Intimate partner violence, acculturation, and alcohol consumption among Hispanic couples in the United States. *Journal of Interpersonal Violence, 15,* 1, 3–45.

Caetano, R., Schafer, J., & Cunradi, C. (in press-b). Alcohol-related intimate partner violence among Whites, Blacks and Hispanics. *Alcohol Research and Health.*

Casas, J. M. (1992). A culturally sensitive model for evaluating alcohol and other drug abuse prevention programs: A Hispanic perspective. In M. A. Orlandi, R. Weston, & L. G. Epstein (Eds.). *Cultural competence for evaluators: A guide for alcohol and other drug abuse prevention practitioners working with ethnic/racial communities* (OSAP Cultural Competence Series I). Rockville, MD: U.S. Department of Health and Human Services, pp. 75–116.

Casiro, O. G., Stanwick, R. S., Pelech, A., Taylor, V., & Manitoba Medical Association, C.H.C. (1994). Public awareness of the risks of drinking alcohol during pregnancy: The effects of a television campaign. *Canadian Journal of Public Health, 85,* 1, 23–27.

Cervantes, R. C., & Peña, C. (1998). Evaluating Hispanic/Latino programs: Ensuring cultural competence. *Alcoholism Treatment Quarterly, 16,* 1/2, 109–131.

Cohen, D. A., Scribner, R. A., & Farley, T. A. (2000). A structural model of health behavior: A pragmatic approach to explain and influence health behaviors at the population level. *Preventive Medicine, 30,* 146–154.

Colon, E. (1998). Alcohol use among Latino males: Implications for the development of culturally competent prevention and treatment services. *Alcoholism Treatment Quarterly, 16,* 1/2, 147–161.

Cunradi, C., Caetano, R., Clark, C., Schafer, J. (1998, September 27). *Neighborhood poverty as a predictor of intimate partner violence.* Paper presented at American College of Epidemiology, San Francisco, CA.

Cunradi, C. B., Caetano, R., Clark, C. L., & Schafer, J. (1999). Alcohol-related problems and intimate partner violence among White, Black and Hispanic couples in the U.S. *Alcoholism: Clinical and Experimental Research, 23,* 9, 1492–1501.

Dawson, D. A. (1998). Beyond Black, White, and Hispanic: Race, ethnic origin and drinking patterns in the United States. *Journal of Substance Abuse, 10,* 4, 321–339.

Delgado, M. (1996). Implementing a natural support system AOD project: Administrative considerations and recommendations. *Alcoholism Treatment Quarterly, 14,* 2, 1–14.

Dent, C. W., Sussman, S., Ellickson, P., Brown, P., & Richardson, J. (1996). Is current drug abuse prevention programming generalizable across ethnic groups? *American Behavioral Scientist, 39,* 7, 911–918.

Dufour, M. C., Williams, G. D., Campbell, K. E., & Aitken, S. S. (1994). Knowledge of FAS and the risks of heavy drinking during pregnancy, 1985 and 1990 [NIAAA Epidemiologic Bull. No. 33]. *Alcohol Health and Research World, 18,* 1, 86–92.

Dusenbury, L., Epstein, J. A., Botvin, G. J., & Diaz, T. (1994). Social influence predictors of alcohol use among New York Latino youth. *Addictive Behaviors, 19,* 4, 363–372.

Epstein, J. A., Botvin, G. J., Diaz, T., & Schinke, S. P. (1995). The role of social factors and individual characteristics in promoting alcohol use among inner-city minority youths. *Journal of Studies on Alcohol, 56,* 39–46.

Flannery, D. J., Vazsonyi, A. T., Torquati, J., & Fridrich, A. (1994). Ethnic and gender differences in risk of early adolescent substance use. *Journal of Youth and Adolescence, 23,* 195–213.

Forgey, M. A., Schinke, S., & Cole, K. (1997). School-based interventions to prevent substance use among inner-city minority adolescents. In D. K. Wilson, J. R. Rodriguez, & W. C. Taylor (Eds.), *Health-promoting and health compromising behaviors among minority adolescents.* Washington, D.C.: American Psychological Association, pp. 251–267.

Greenfield, T. K., Graves, K. L., & Kaskutas, L. A. (1993). Alcohol warning labels for prevention: National survey findings. *Alcohol, Health and Research World, 17,* 1, 67–75.

Greenfield, T. K., & Room, R. (1997). Situational norms for drinking and drunkenness: Trends in the U.S. adult population, 1979–1990. *Addiction, 92,* 1, 33–47.

Grunbaum, J. A., Basen-Enquist, K., & ElSouki, R. (1996). Tobacco, alcohol, and illicit drug use among Mexican-American and non-Hispanic White high school students. *Substance Use and Misuse, 31,* 10, 1279–1310.

Hankin, J. R. (1994). FAS prevention strategies: Passive and active measures. *Alcohol Health and Research World, 18,* 1, 62–66.

Hawkins, J. D., Catalano, R. F., & Miller, J. Y. (1992). Risk and protective factors for alcohol and other drug problems in adolescence and early adulthood: Implications for substance abuse prevention. *Psychological Bulletin, 112,* 1, 64–105.

Hilton, M. E. (1991). Trends in U.S. drinking patterns: Further evidence from the past twenty years. In W. B. Clark & M. Hilton (Eds.). *Alcohol in America: Drinking practices and problems.* Albany: State University of New York Press, pp. 121–148.

Hilton, M. E., & Kaskutas, L. A. (1991). Public support for warning labels on alcoholic beverage containers. *British Journal of Addiction, 86,* 1323–1333.

Hingson, R. (1993). Prevention of alcohol-impaired driving. *Alcohol Health and Research World, 17,* 1, 28–34.

Hingson, R. W., Howland, J., & Levinson, S. (1988). Effects of legislative reform to reduce drunken driving and alcohol-related traffic fatalities. *Public Health Reports, 103,* 659–667.

Holder, H. D. (1998). *Alcohol and the community: A systems approach to prevention.* Cambridge, MA: Cambridge University Press.

Holder, H. D., Saltz, R. G., Grube, J. W., Voas, R. B., Gruenewald, P. J., & Treno, A. J. (1997). A community prevention trial to reduce alcohol-involved accidental injury and death: Overview. *Addiction, 92,* Suppl. 2, S155–S172.

Kantor, G. K., Jasinski, J., & Aldarondo, E. (1993). *Incidence of Hispanic drinking and intra-family violence.* San Antonio, TX: Research Society on Alcoholism.

Kaskutas, L. A., & Graves, K. (1994). Relationship between cumulative exposure to health messages and awareness and behavior-related drinking during pregnancy. *American Journal of Health Promotion, 9,* 2, 115–124.

Marín, B. V. (1990). Hispanic drug abuse: Culturally appropriate prevention and treatment. In R. R. Watson (Ed.), *Drug and alcohol abuse prevention.* Clifton, NJ: Humana Press, pp. 151–165.

Miller, N. S. (1999). Mortality risks in alcoholism and effects of abstinence and addiction treatment. *Addictive Disorders, 22,* 371–383.

Moskowitz, J. M. (1989). The primary prevention of alcohol problems: A critical review of the research literature. *Journal of Studies on Alcohol, 50,* 1, 54–88.

National Institute on Alcohol Abuse and Alcoholism. (1999). *Liver cirrhosis mortality in the United States, 1970–96* (Surveillance Rep. No. 52). Bethesda, MD: Author.

Orlandi, M. A., Weston, R., & Epstein, L. G. (Eds.). (1992). *Cultural competence for evaluators: A guide for alcohol and other drug abuse prevention practitioners working with ethnic/racial communities.* (OSAP Cultural Competence Series I). Rockville, MD: U.S. Department of Health and Human Services, Office of Safety and Asepsis Procedures.

Padilla, A. M., & Snyder, N.S.D. (1992). Hispanics: What the culturally informed evaluator needs to know. In M. A. Orlandi, R. Weston, & L. G. Epstein (Eds.), *Cultural competence for evaluators: A guide for alcohol and other drug abuse prevention practitioners working with ethnic/racial communities.* (OSAP Cultural Competence Series I). Rockville, MD: U.S. Department of Health and Human Services, Office of Safety and Asepsis Procedures, pp. 117–146.

Ringold, D. J. (1995). Social criticisms of target marketing. *American Behavioral Scientist, 38,* 578–592.

Schinke, S. P., Moncher, M. S., Palleja, J., Zayas, L. H., & Schilling, R. F. (1988). Hispanic youth, substance abuse, and stress: Implications for prevention research. *International Journal of the Addictions, 23,* 8, 809–826.

Scribner, R. A., Cohen, D. A., & Fisher, W. (2000). Evidence of a structural effect for alcohol outlet density: A multilevel analysis. *Alcoholism: Clinical and Experimental Research, 24,* 188–195.

Scribner, R. A., MacKinnon, D. P., & Dwyer, J. H. (1994). Alcohol outlet density and motor vehicle crashes in Los Angeles County cities. *Journal of Studies on Alcohol, 55,* 447–453.

Scribner, R. A., MacKinnon, D. P., & Dwyer, J. H. (1995). The risk of assaultive violence and alcohol availability in Los Angeles County. *American Journal of Public Health, 85,* 335–340.

Singer, M., Davison, L., & Yalin, F. (1987). *Alcohol use and abuse among Hispanic adolescents: State of knowledge, state of need–Conference proceedings.* Hartford, CT: Hispanic Health Council.

Sobering facts: Heavy drinking by some Mexican American men is taking a severe toll on families—Cultural sensitivity has held back discussion in the community. (1999, March 21). *Los Angeles Times.*

Sokol-Katz, J. S., & Ulbrich, P. M. (1992). Family structure and adolescent risk-taking behavior: A comparison of Mexican, Cuban, and Puerto Rican Americans. *International Journal of the Addictions, 27,* 1197–1209.

Stinson, F. S., Yi, H., Grant, B. F., Chou, P., Dawson, D. A., & Pickering, R. (1998). Drinking in the United States: Main findings from the 1992 National Longitudinal Alcohol Epidemiologic Survey (NLAES). *U.S. alcohol epidemiological data reference manual.* (NIH Publication 99-3519). Bethesda, MD: National Institute on Alcohol Abuse and Alcoholism.

Straus, M. A. (1990). The conflict tactics scales and its critics: An evaluation and new data on validity and reliability. In M. A. Straus & R. J. Gelles (Eds.), *Physical violence in American families: Risk factors and adaptations to violence in 8,145 families.* (Chap. 4). New Brunswick, NJ: Transaction Books.

Substance Abuse and Mental Health Services Administration. (1999). *Summary of findings from the 1998 National Household Survey on Drug Abuse.* (Series H-10). Rockville, MD: Author.

Tobler, N. S. (1986). Meta-analysis of 143 adolescent drug prevention programs: Quantitative outcome results of program participants compared to a control or comparison group. *Journal of Drug Issues, 16,* 4, 537–567.

Tobler, N. S. (1994). Meta-analytical issues for prevention intervention research. In W. Bukowski (Ed.), *Advances in data analysis for prevention intervention research* (NIDA Research Monograph 142). Rockville, MD: U.S. Department of Health and Human Services, National Institute on Drug Abuse, pp. 5–68.

Tobler, N. S. (1998). *A meta-analysis of school-based prevention programs.* Rockville, MD: Substance Abuse and Mental Health Services Administration, Center for Substance Abuse Prevention.

Tobler, N. S., & Stratton, H. H. (1997). Effectiveness of school-based drug prevention programs: A meta-analysis of the research. *Journal of Primary Prevention, 18,* 1, 71–128.

United States Department of Health and Human Services. (1998). *Youth Risk Behavior Surveillance: United States, 1997* [47 (SS-3)]. Rockville, MD: Centers for Disease Control and Prevention.

United States Department of Health and Human Services. (1999). *Youth Risk Behavior Surveillance: National Alternative High School Youth Risk Behavior Survey, United States, 1998* [48(SS07)]. Rockville, MD: Centers for Disease Control and Prevention.

Vega, W. A., Zimmerman, R. S., Warheit, G. J., Apospori, E., & Gil, A. G. (1993). Risk factor for early adolescent drug use in four ethnic and racial groups. *American Journal of Public Health, 83,* 2, 185–189.

Warheit, G. J., Vega, W. A., Khoury, E. L., Gill, A. A., & Elfenbein, P. H. (1996). A comparative analysis of cigarette, alcohol, and illicit drug use among an ethnically diverse sample of Hispanic, African American, and non-Hispanic White adolescents. *Journal of Drug Issues, 26,* 901–922.

CHAPTER FIFTEEN

# TOBACCO USE AMONG LATINOS

Gerardo Marín

As early as 1964, the U.S. Surgeon General's Report stated that tobacco use was an important source of illness (for example, cancer, chronic pulmonary obstructive disease, coronary heart disease, and stroke). Subsequent reports by the Surgeon General have further emphasized that the effects of tobacco use can be easily prevented by quitting smoking. This warning was also mentioned in the 1998 Surgeon General's Report (United States Department of Health and Human Services, 1998) where evidence was presented for the relationship between cigarette smoking and impaired health status among Latinos[1] and other ethnic groups. Nevertheless, the addictive nature of tobacco and a large number of social, economic, and psychosocial factors have contributed to worrisome patterns of tobacco consumption among Latinos and the consequent threats to their health.

This chapter briefly summarizes various aspects of tobacco use among Latinos including predictors of consumption, epidemiological information, and efforts at developing culturally appropriate preventive approaches. The 1998 Report of the Surgeon General (United States Department of Health and Human Services, 1998) provides a more detailed analysis of tobacco use among Latinos and the other major ethnic minority groups (African Americans, American Indians [lately also called Native Americans], Native Alaskans [the Inuit and other

---

[1]The term "Latino" is used in this chapter instead of "Hispanic" in order to maintain editorial consistency with the rest of the book. Nevertheless, the reader should be aware of the fact that much epidemiological data have been collected using "Hispanic" as the operational label. For a discussion of these issues, see Hayes-Bautista and Chapa (1987), Marín and Marín (1991), and Trevino (1987).

groups], Asian Americans, and Native Hawaiians and other Pacific Islanders). That report constitutes the most comprehensive analysis to date of tobacco use among Latinos and should be consulted by those wishing to gain a comprehensive understanding of the issues involved. This chapter attempts to highlight issues of concern to students, researchers, policymakers, and practitioners alike. The chapter first analyzes possible predictors and correlates of tobacco use, followed by a brief discussion of the epidemiological information currently available on tobacco use by Latinos. The chapter concludes with a review of prevention efforts among Latino populations and a brief analysis of policy implications.

## Predictors of Initiation and Continued Use

As might be expected for a complex behavior such as tobacco use, there are a number of variables that affect initiation as well as continuation of use. In the case of tobacco smoking, the social environment including some macrosocial variables (such as targeted advertising and low amounts of sales taxes) can be expected to support or even reinforce tobacco use as well as certain variables more closely related to the individual (such as personality and psychosocial variables, normative expectancies, and addiction). Unfortunately, most research in the field tends to concentrate on one set or subset of variables ignoring the role of other types of predictors or their interaction. The literature for Latinos is equally flawed. For example, some authors emphasize the role of macrosocial variables such as the historical significance of tobacco smoking, the economic role of the tobacco industry in supporting Latino communities and their activities, and the role of advertising and product promotion in initiating and maintaining the behavior of cigarette smoking among Latinos. Others suggest that certain psychosocial and personality variables act as predictors or determinants of cigarette smoking such as the need for thrill seeking, negative self-esteem, and risk taking. A third set of variables are related to an individual's social context and includes the presence of role models who smoke, supportive norms for cigarette smoking, and low religiosity. One further set of possible predictors is the presence of risk behaviors such as drug use, sexual promiscuity, alcoholic beverage use, and truancy that often may go together with cigarette smoking (particularly among the youth) and that may provide social and psychological support for cigarette smoking. Also relevant to continued use of cigarettes is the fact that tobacco is an addictive substance that may have differential effects among certain individuals; this differential rate of absorption, distribution, and elimination may make it even more difficult for those individuals to quit. The rest of this section reviews briefly the evidence for these assumptions.

An initial concern of studies in the area of predictors of initiation is the age when youth start using cigarettes or other tobacco products. Data from various surveys tend to show that Latino youth start smoking cigarettes during their late teen years. For example, the Hispanic Health and Nutrition Examination

Survey (HHANES) showed that cigarette smoking initiation rates were highest for Mexican American, Cuban, and Puerto Rican youths between the ages of fifteen and nineteen (Escobedo, Anda, Smith, Remington, & Mast, 1990). This implies that prevention interventions must occur during the early teen years (probably before the age of fourteen) and that significant work in "inoculating" Latino youth against tobacco use must occur early in their lives. Further research (for example, by Anderson & Burns, 2000) shows that initiation patterns vary not just by gender but also by ethnicity, requiring gender- and ethnicity-targeted research in order to understand epidemiological patterns as well as for developing preventive strategies.

## Macrosocial Variables

There are a number of societal circumstances that can have an effect in the initiation or continuation of tobacco use. The growing of tobacco has played an important role in the economies of many Latin American countries, and it is possible that these economic realities may have produced attitudes and norms that are supportive of tobacco use (United States Department of Health and Human Services, 1998). As a matter of fact, the 1992 Surgeon General's Report (United States Department of Health and Human Services, 1992) includes a detailed account of the role of tobacco in Latin American economies. In the United States, the tobacco industry has played an important role in supporting the economic advancement of ethnic groups (United States Department of Health and Human Services, 1998)—whether by providing employment, placing advertising in ethnic media, funding community agencies and organizations, or supporting civic and cultural events. Latinos have indeed benefited from these resources in activities as varied as tobacco advertising in Latino media (when legal), funding provided to organizations (such as the Congressional Latino Caucus), supporting community events such as *Cinco de Mayo* festivals, and promoting cultural events such as Miami's Calle Ocho festival or the *Copa Nacional* (a soccer championship). These investments and endorsements can be expected to produce positive reactions toward tobacco, and—in a manner similar to advertising—they help create and support a norm of acceptability for tobacco products that goes beyond mere brand recognition.

The 1994 Surgeon General's Report (United States Department of Health and Human Services, 1994) considered cigarette advertising as an important promoter of cigarette smoking, given that it can encourage experimentation, prevent quitting, and support increased consumption (Centers for Disease Control, 1990) and there are data to confirm this concern (for example, see Evans, Farkas, Gilpin, Berry, & Pierce, 1995). Latinos have indeed been exposed to targeted tobacco advertising not only in newspapers and magazines but also in outdoor media (United States Department of Health and Human Services, 1998). For example, a study of San Diego outdoor advertising found high proportions of billboard advertising tobacco in ethnic neighborhoods (Elder, Edwards, & Conway, 1993). Overall, 4.7 percent of billboards in Latino neighborhoods advertised tobacco products, as compared with 1.1 percent in White areas. These factors are important because there is evidence that supports the notion that less acculturated Latinos tend to be influenced by radio and billboard advertisements whereas more acculturated Latinos report being influenced by magazine advertisements, brochures, and product labels in making purchasing and behavioral decisions (Webster, 1992). Promotional items (clothing or hard goods with tobacco brand names or logos), which are another type of advertising, also have been shown to have an effect in triggering initiation of tobacco use (Biener & Siegel, 2000).

## Psychosocial and Personality Variables

Among the relevant variables here are attitudes and expectancies that are shared by Latinos and that may influence the initiation and continued use of tobacco. There is a body of research that shows that cigarette smoking among Latinos is a social event supported by important cultural norms such as *simpatia* (concern for smooth interpersonal relations), *personalismo* (value placed on personal relationships), and *familialism* (influence of relatives on a person's behavior and values) (Felix-Ortiz & Newcomb, 1996; Marín, Marín, Pérez-Stable, Sabogal, & Otero-Sabogal, 1990; Marín, Marín, Pérez-Stable, Otero-Sabogal, & Sabogal, 1990). These cultural norms support the influence of cigarette-smoking role models and enhance the social power of relatives and friends who use tobacco products by promoting behavioral imitation and acquiescence to suggestions of engaging in smoking. In addition, these attitudes and expectancies are influenced by the culture in which the individual resides so that acculturation produces modifications in expectancies held by individuals undergoing the process of culture learning implicit in acculturation (Marín, Marín, Otero-Sabogal, Sabogal, & Pérez-Stable, 1989). There is also evidence to show that certain cultural values (such as *respeto*, or respect for others) play a role in preventing cigarette smoking, particularly among Latino girls (Mermelstein & Tobacco Control Network Writing Group, 1999). There is still a need to analyze how these cultural values and social scripts interact by supporting or preventing cigarette smoking among Latinos. Unfortunately, little attention has been paid to these issues in the extant tobacco control literature.

The role of psychosocial expectancies in cigarette smoking has been analyzed in a series of studies conducted with adult Latinos (for example, Marín, Marín, Otero-Sabogal, Sabogal, & Pévez-Stable, 1989; Marín, Marín, Pérez-Stable, Sabogal, & Otero-Sabogal, 1990). In general, those studies showed that adult Latino smokers worried about the bad example they were providing their children by smoking and that this and the concern for damaging their health were important predictors of quitting smoking. Indeed, Latino smokers felt that by quitting smoking they would improve family relations, feel better, and taste food better. Data from San Francisco Latinos also showed that those smokers who thought they were highly addicted tended to report lower levels of self-efficacy in quitting and heavy smokers tended to exhibit lower self-efficacy (Sabogal, Otero-Sabogal, Pérez-Stable, Marín, & Marín, 1989).

Studies among Latino adolescents have shown a variety of psychosocial and personality variables that tend to be related to cigarette smoking experimentation and initiation. For example, Felix-Ortiz and Newcomb (1992) found that low academic achievement, poor law abidance, limited religiosity, and depression were associated with cigarette-smoking frequency among Latino boys. Studies carried out in the New York City area have shown that tobacco use is related to poor self-esteem and risk taking and other psychosocial difficulties among Latino adolescents (Bettes, Dusenbury, Kerner, James-Ortiz, & Botvin, 1990).

Research with Latino adults show that cigarette smoking tends to be related to depression (Escobedo, Kirch, & Anda, 1996; Lee & Markides, 1991; Pérez-Stable, Marín, Marín, & Katz, 1990). For example, the study by Pérez-Stable and colleagues among Mexican Americans in San Francisco showed that smokers had a 70 percent greater risk for showing depressive symptoms (measured by the Center for Epidemiologic Studies—Depression Scale [CES-D]) than nonsmokers. This finding is of particular significance because it supports the notion that prevention efforts need to address approaches to moderating or controlling depression as part of an integrated smoking prevention and cessation campaign.

## Social Context

The presence of parents, siblings, or peers who smoke has been proposed as an important variable in determining cigarette-smoking initiation and maintenance among adolescents. Studies among Latinos have shown that the perceived normative support provided by siblings, parents, or peers who smoke is an important predictor of tobacco use initiation and continued use (for example, Cowdery, Fitzhugh, & Wang, 1997; Dusenbury, Kerner, Baker, Botvin, James-Ortiz, & Zauber, 1992; Dusenbury, Epstein, Botvin, & Diaz, 1994; Mermelstein & Tobacco Control Network Writing Group, 1999). The supporting role of other smokers in an individual's social environment has also been shown to be relevant among Latino adults with data from the HHANES (Coreil, Ray, & Markides, 1991). There is also some evidence regarding adults (particularly members of extended families) serving not just as a role model but also as an initiator of cigarette smoking among Latino adolescents (Mermelstein & Tobacco Control Network Writing Group, 1999). Preventive approaches directed at minimizing the role of the social context (or inoculating against its effect) are of particular relevance among Latino adolescents because they have been found to be at high risk (higher than most other ethnic groups) for cigarette smoking initiation (Unger, Palmer, Dent, Rohrbach, & Johnson, 2000).

## Acculturation

Also of relevance is the possible role that the level of acculturation may have in supporting the initiation of tobacco use. The argument suggests that acculturation (the culture learning process that individuals living in multicultural societies undergo) produces psychological stresses that in turn support tobacco use as a coping mechanism. These psychological reactions are often called *acculturative stress*. Unfortunately, the data are not that clear, but some evidence exists showing that Latino youth who may be facing more acculturative stress (manifested, for example, by low English-language ability) indeed tend to be more likely to smoke cigarettes (see, for instance, Felix-Ortiz & Newcomb, 1996). Other researchers have found that more acculturated Latino youth tend to be more likely to smoke (Smith, McGraw, & Carrillo, 1991), whereas other studies have found no relationship between acculturation and tobacco use among Latino youth (for example, Bettes, Dusenbury, Kerner, James-Ortiz, & Botvin, 1990). The difficulties in predicting the role of acculturation on youth tobacco use probably derive from methodological limitations of the studies such as the way in which acculturation was measured (using unidimensional scales or instruments of poor psychometric properties), the use of proxy variables to measure acculturation (say, language of survey, linguistic proficiency), and the presence of confounding variables (for example, length of residence) and poor methodologies (improper measures of tobacco use as compared to experimentation, irregular use, and so on). Nevertheless, the evidence seems to point to the presence of a relationship that needs to be better understood.

## Risk Behaviors

The literature on tobacco use among Latino youth tends to support a constellation effect of risk behaviors being associated with cigarette smoking (Newcomb, Maddahian, Skager, & Bentler, 1987; Felix-Ortiz & Newcomb, 1992; An, O'Malley, Schulenberg, Bachman, & Johnston, 1999; Vega, Zimmerman, Warheit, Apospori, & Gil, 1993). Behaviors such as drug use, alcoholic beverage use, poor school performance or dropping out of school, gang membership or criminal behavior, truancy, sexual activity, and cigarette smoking have often been proposed as being closely related and often found in the same individuals. Various studies (including Escobedo, Reddy, & DuRant, 1997; Felix-Ortiz & Newcomb, 1992; Vega, Zimmerman, Warheit, Apospori, & Gil, 1993) have found that these problem behaviors are associated with cigarette smoking among Latino youth, although at times the type of behaviors changes according to the individual's gender. Indeed, the assumption in some studies is that what is important is the actual number of risk factors rather than the specific behaviors. A problem with this assumption, of course, is that it makes it difficult to design preventive strategies, as it is seldom possible to address so many risk behaviors in one intervention and they may not all be of equal significance. Nevertheless, this approach is important in that it provides fairly objective indicators to help determine individuals at risk not just for cigarette smoking but also for other deviant behaviors. An additional problem with this approach is the lack of consistency in findings. For example, while the literature seems to support the notion that poor school performance or dropping out of school tends to be associated with cigarette or tobacco use (Felix-Ortiz & Newcomb, 1992, among others), there is also evidence that the relationship may not be as clear (Chavez, Edwards, & Oetting, 1989). The need for better data on the role of risk factors is of significance because some Latino adolescents seem to experience some risks at a higher rate than other adolescents. For example, Latinos show a high rate of school dropout and an important proportion (14 percent) leave school by Grade four, well before the grades (sixth to eighth) when tobacco use initiation is most frequent (United States General Accounting Office, 1994).

## Differences in Addictive Nature of Tobacco

The fact that many smokers find it difficult to quit because of an addiction to nicotine has been established for a number of years (United States Department of Health and Human Services, 1988). Researchers have proposed that there may be genetically-determined differences in the way nicotine affects an individual (Benowitz, Pérez-Stable, Herrera, & Jacob, 1995; Hughes, 1986) and that behavioral patterns (for example, how deep a cigarette is inhaled) may also affect the level of nicotine present in the body of a smoker (Benowitz, Pérez-Stable, Herrera, & Jacob, 1995). Data from the Hispanic Health and Nutrition Examination Survey (HHANES) showed that nicotine levels were unusually high among Latinos who had reported smoking a low number of cigarettes (Pérez-Stable, Marín, Marín, Brody, & Benowitz, 1990). While these differences could be due to underreporting of cigarette smoking, they could also be showing differential absorption of nicotine by Latinos (Henningfield, Cohen, & Giovino, 1990).

Another indicator of tobacco addiction often used in the literature is the amount of time an individual waits in the morning before lighting the first cigarette. A study of San Francisco Bay Area patients (Vander Martin, Cummings, & Coates, 1990) showed that Latinos were the least likely to need a cigarette within fifteen minutes of waking up compared to other ethnic groups. Data from the 1987 National Health Interview Survey (NHIS) analyzed for the Surgeon General's Report showed that the number of cigarettes smoked in a day was related to how long an individual could wait before smoking the first cigarette in the day and that, in general, Latinos did not differ from Whites in the proportion of smokers who smoked their first cigarette ten or thirty minutes after waking up (United States Department of Health and Human Services, 1998). For example, among individuals smoking one to fourteen cigarettes per day, 11.3 percent of Latinos and 11.1 percent of Whites reported smoking their first cigarette within ten minutes of awakening. The corresponding figures for smoking within thirty minutes of awakening were 26.2 percent for Latinos and 27.1 percent for Whites.

# Patterns of Tobacco Use

In general, the prevalence of cigarette smoking among adult Latinos has decreased over the last ten to fifteen years of the twentieth century (United States Department of Health and Human Services, 1998). Nevertheless, there are indications that certain Latino subgroups have not decreased their prevalence of cigarette smoking or that, indeed, an increase in prevalence may be occurring. A difficulty with establishing solid parameters on cigarette smoking prevalence among Latinos is the somewhat incomplete sources of information available as well as the poor quality of some data, particularly when investigators are trying to analyze the role of such important variables as acculturation in prevalence rates. The data from the HHANES are now quite old (collected between 1982 and 1984) and national surveys (for example, NHIS, Monitoring the Future [MTF] Survey, and Teenage Attitudes and Practices Survey [TAPS]) usually do not include enough Latinos to provide strong estimates of the prevalence of tobacco use among Latinos. Nevertheless, until better data are collected, researchers and policymakers must rely on what is available, being cognizant of the limitations inherent in the data because of methodological concerns (limited samples, unreliable data, poor sampling) as well as conceptual issues (such as inadequate operationalization of ethnicity and acculturation).

An analysis of the NHIS from 1978 through 1995 (United States Department of Health and Human Services, 1998) showed a decrease in general prevalence from 30.1 percent (for data from 1978 through 1980) to 18.9 percent (for data for 1994 and 1995). These results resemble other analyses that have looked at birth cohorts among Cuban in the United States, Mexican Americans, and Puerto Ricans (Escobedo & Remington, 1989). Nevertheless, the decline is less steep in the first five years of the decade of the 1990s: 21.5 percent for 1990 and 1991 surveys, 20.5 percent for 1992–1993; and 18.9 percent for 1994–1995.

There are some intriguing differences in prevalence rates when data from various surveys are compared. The HHANES showed that cigarette smoking prevalence for Latino men ranged from 41.3 percent for Puerto Ricans to 43.6 percent for Mexican Americans (Escobedo & Remington, 1989), whereas the combined data for the NHIS from 1983 through 1985 showed a prevalence of 31.6 percent for Latino men (United States Department of Health and Human Services, 1998). The same was true for Latino women, for whom the NHIS estimate was lower. Obviously, the comparison of results across surveys with different sampling techniques, different methodologies, and somewhat different time frames is not totally appropriate, but the difference in estimates is nevertheless worrisome and indicative of the need for better data about the health status of Latinos.

Despite the aforementioned limitations in the data, Latinos seem to have one of the lowest overall rates of cigarette smoking prevalence among various ethnic groups (United States Department of Health and Human Services, 1998). Indeed, comparisons with the 1994 and 1995 NHIS data carried out for the 1998 Surgeon General's Report showed that the prevalence of cigarette smoking was highest among Native Americans (American Indians, 36 percent), with Latinos showing one of the lower rates (18 percent) and African Americans (26.5 percent) and Whites (26.4 percent) reporting higher prevalence rates. Only Asian Americans (14.2 percent) showed lower prevalence rates than Latinos.

An important trend in cigarette smoking among adult Latinos in the United States is the fact that they tend to smoke few cigarettes per day, fewer than Whites.

The 1994 and 1995 NHIS data (United States Department of Health and Human Services, 1998), for example, showed that 65 percent of Latino smokers reported smoking less than fifteen cigarettes per day, as compared to 35.3 percent of White smokers. This pattern is similar to that found among the other major ethnic groups in the United States cigarettes (United States Department of Health and Human Services, 1998). The NHIS data also show that Latino women tend to show a somewhat higher proportion of adult smokers smoking less than fifteen cigarettes per day (for example, 68.8 percent in 1994 and 1995) than Latino men (62.4 percent).

The use of pipes and the smoking of cigars seem to be of somewhat lesser significance than cigarette smoking among Latinos. For example, aggregated NHIS data for 1987 and 1991 showed 1.1 percent of all Latinos reporting cigar smoking and 0.5 percent reporting pipe smoking (United States Department of Health and Human Services, 1998). There are some subgroup differences in these NHIS data. For example, Cuban men in the United States reported cigar smoking in higher proportions (2.5 percent) than Mexican Americans (1.5 percent) and Puerto Ricans (1.3 percent). More recent data (1996) included in the 1998 Surgeon General's Report showed that a large proportion (26.2 percent) of Latino adolescents (aged fourteen to nineteen years) reported smoking a cigar during the year previous to the survey, as compared with 28.9 percent of White respondents and 19.3 percent of African American adolescents.

Smokeless tobacco use among Latino high school seniors seems to have increased from 4.4 percent in 1987 to 8.1 percent in 1996, as reported in the 1998 Surgeon General's Report (United States Department of Health and Human Services, 1998), although the Youth Risk Behavior Survey (YRBS) data for 1995 showed 4.4 percent of Latino high school students reporting use of smokeless tobacco in the month previous to the survey. The 1995 YRBS showed that male Latino adolescents used smokeless tobacco in lower proportions (5.8 percent) than Whites (25.1 percent), although among teen females, Latinas (3.1 percent) reported using smokeless tobacco in larger proportions than did White adolescents (2.5 percent).

The analysis of NHIS data on cigarettes conducted for the 1998 Surgeon General's Report (United States Department of Health and Human Services, 1998) showed that the proportion of Latino adult "ever smokers" (that is, those who had smoked) who reported having quit has increased in recent years. Data for the 1978 through 1980 NHIS showed that 35 percent of adult Latino ever smokers had quit (35.5 percent for men and 34.2 percent for women) compared with 46.2 percent for the 1994 and 1995 NHIS (48.2 percent for men and 43.1 percent for women). The highest rates of Latino ever smokers reporting having quit are found among those with a college education (71.1 percent for the 1994 and 1995 NHIS), as compared with those with high school education (44.5 percent), and among those over the age of fifty-five (68.1 percent for the 1994 and 1995 NHIS), as compared with those aged thirty-five to fifty-four (49.6 percent).

Data are presented below in terms of various sociodemographic variables that seem to have an effect on cigarette-smoking prevalence among Latinos. As mentioned earlier, the data are limited because of various methodological problems in the studies, but they serve as indicators of the extent of the problem and of areas that need to be taken into consideration in the development of preventive efforts.

## Gender

In general, Latino men report higher prevalence of cigarette smoking than do Latino women. For example, in the 1994 and 1995 NHIS data, 22.9 percent of men and 15.1 percent of women reported smoking cigarettes (United States Department of Health and Human Services, 1998).

## Age

Latino youth smoke cigarettes in proportions that are of considerable concern to public health officials. Data from the Monitoring the Future (MTF) survey of high school seniors show that Latino youth report daily cigarette smoking at a rate lower than Whites but higher than African Americans and this pattern has remained fairly stable since around 1982 (Giovino, 1999). Data from 1985 to 1989 for the MTF (Bachman, Wallace, O'Malley, Johnston, Kurth, & Neighbors, 1991) among high school seniors showed fairly high proportions of individuals reporting smoking cigarettes during the previous month among Mexican American males (23.8 percent) and Mexican American females (18.7 percent). In addition, the 1995 Youth Risk Behavior Survey-YRBS (Centers for Disease Control and Prevention, 1996) showed that 34 percent of Latino high school students reported smoking cigarettes during at least one day in the previous month compared to 38.3 percent of Whites. Of particular concern is the statement made by the 1998 Surgeon General's Report asserting that rates of cigarette smoking among Latino youth have increased in the last decade of the twentieth century (United States Department of Health and Human Services, 1998). The report bases its conclusion on data from various surveys including the MTF and the YRBS. For example, results from the YRBS show 34 percent of Latino high school students reporting smoking cigarettes in 1995 compared to 25.3 percent in 1991.

Interestingly, little difference in prevalence is usually found between younger adults (eighteen to thirty-four years) and older adults (thirty-five to fifty-four years) among Latinos. In the 1994 and 1995 NHIS data (United States Department of Health and Human Services, 1998), 19.8 percent of both age groups reported smoking cigarettes. In previous surveys, the older adults had reported a somewhat higher prevalence than the younger adults, usually between two and four percentage points. Nevertheless, the NHIS data and the HHANES results (Haynes, Harvey, Montes, Nickens, & Cohen, 1990) show that Latinos aged fifty-five or more tend to report cigarette smoking at much lower proportions (for example, 14.3 percent in the 1994 and 1995 NHIS). Latino women of reproductive age seem to be reporting cigarette smoking in lower proportions than their predecessors. For example, aggregated NHIS data (United States Department of Health and Human Services, 1998) showed that 16.4 percent of Latino women of reproductive age reported current cigarette smoking in the 1994–1995 data compared with 25.5 percent for the 1978–1980 data.

## Level of Education

Level of education seems to have little relationship to cigarette-smoking prevalence among Latinos with the exception of those with a college education, who report smoking at a much lower rate than the rest of the population. For example, in the 1994 and 1995 NHIS data (United States Department of Health and Human Services, 1998), Latinos with a college education reported a cigarette-smoking prevalence of 8.7 percent whereas those respondents with high school education (21.6 percent) and those with less than high school education (20.2 percent) reported much higher prevalence. These differences by level of education resemble those found in the HHANES data, where Latinos with higher levels of education reported lower levels of cigarette smoking (Haynes, Harvey, Montes, Nickens, & Cohen, 1990).

## Acculturation

As noted earlier, the process of culture learning as a function of exposure to a multicultural society is often labeled *acculturation*. Current ideas regarding acculturation define the concept as a multidimensional phenomenon whereby individuals learn aspects (such as values, norms, behaviors, expectancies, and attitudes) of the new culture(s) while retaining some parts or all of the culture of origin. Generally, acculturation is related to length of residence in the new culture, so that newcomers or recently immigrated individuals can be expected to be low in acculturation (actually in "biculturalism"), although this relationship is not always an exact linear function.

The relationship between acculturation and prevalence of cigarette smoking is less clear than what has been reported above for other sociodemographic variables. The HHANES data (Haynes, Harvey, Montes, Nickens, & Cohen, 1990) showed that acculturation was related differentially across genders. Among Mexican American women, the less acculturated reported a lower prevalence of cigarette smoking (19 percent) than the more acculturated (28 percent). Among Mexican American men, the HHANES data showed that there were no differences in prevalence due to acculturation. Community-wide surveys in San Francisco (Marín, Marín, Pérez-Stable, & Hauck, 1994) showed that the less acculturated Latino men reported cigarette smoking at a higher proportion (38.7 percent) in 1986 than the more acculturated (28.7 percent), with the pattern being reversed among Latinas (13.9 percent of the less acculturated and 23.1 percent of the more acculturated reporting cigarette smoking). A subsequent community-wide smoking cessation program (*Programa Latino Para Dejar de Fumar*—Hispanic Smoking Cessation Program) conducted by the same authors in San Francisco had an effect of lowering total prevalence within three years of the program, so that in 1989 some 24.2 percent of the less acculturated Latinos and 24.4 percent of the more acculturated Latino men reported cigarette smoking. Among Latino women, the more acculturated (19.5 percent) continued reporting greater prevalence rates than the less acculturated Latino women (9.9 percent). Data from the 1990 California Tobacco Survey (Navarro, 1996) showed that the less acculturated Latinos also showed the lowest rates of cigarette-smoking prevalence. Acculturation may also be related to patterns of cigarette smoking. Navarro (1996) found that the less acculturated Latinos in the 1990 California Tobacco Survey reported smoking cigarettes on a daily basis less often that the more acculturated respondents and were also less likely to smoke fifteen or more cigarettes per day.

There are different suggestions as to the relationship between acculturation and cigarette smoking. Navarro (1996) has suggested that the level of urban experiences of the respondents may influence cigarette smoking so that those immigrants coming from rural Latin American countries would be less likely to smoke cigarettes than those immigrating from urban centers.

## Preventive Approaches to Tobacco Use

A number of preventive interventions and strategies have been designed to control tobacco use among Latinos. These include primary prevention approaches to curtail initiation or experimentation, smoking cessation programs, as well as community-wide or government-imposed macrosocial approaches such as advertising controls, increases in taxes, and limitations on access to tobacco products. Some of these interventions have been designed for the community at large, such as the increases in tobacco-related taxes imposed by various states or the limitations imposed on the type of tobacco product advertising. Others, usually primary and tertiary interventions, have been designed for Latinos or have been adapted from strategies originally designed for non-Latinos. This section first describes some macrosocial approaches and the possible or documented effects on Latinos, and attention is later given to preventive interventions directed at individuals.

The last few years have seen an increase in the design of preventive strategies that are directed at changing the social climate or normative circumstances of cigarette smoking. Concerns for environmental tobacco smoke and its effects (see Hovell, Zakarian, Wahlgren, & Matt, 2000, for example) have produced limitations in the number and types of places where smokers can use cigarettes or other tobacco products. Other macrosocial interventions have included new taxes, limits in advertising, controls on sales to minors, and limitations in access to cigarette vending machines. While these actions should have similar effects among Latinos and non-Latinos, the level of implementation seems to differ. For example, Latino adolescents report that they are asked less frequently to show proof of age for purchasing tobacco products than non-Latinos (Centers for Disease Control and Prevention, 1996), and Latino adolescents as well as other ethnic minority adolescents seem to have no difficulty in purchasing (illegally) single cigarettes from neighborhood shopkeepers (Klonoff, Fritz, Landrine, Riddle, & Tully-Payne, 1994). While there is strong support for macrosocial controls on tobacco use (such as limiting places where cigarette smoking can take place) among Latinos (United States Department of Health and Human Services, 1998) there is little evidence as to how these regulations are being enforced in Latino neighborhoods. Nevertheless, Latinos are aware of societal influences to control tobacco use, as in the case of awareness of warning labels on cigarette packages and advertising (Marín, 1994), where awareness is higher among acculturated Latinos.

A large number of school-based primary prevention programs have been designed to prevent the use of tobacco products and in some cases of other substances. In general, these programs have been "ethnicity blind," targeting all adolescents without paying attention to cultural differences. This approach runs counter to the principles of cultural appropriateness of interventions (as described later) and can be expected to be of limited effectiveness. Indeed, a review of school-based interventions (Glynn, 1989) concluded that ethnic minority children could be expected to benefit the least from these types of approaches. Evaluations of some of these programs have shown differential results based on ethnicity, with Latino youth showing limited effects (for example, Elder et al., 1993; Granham, Johnson, Hansen, Flay, & Gee, 1990), although some programs such as the modified Life Skills Training have shown positive results (Botvin, Dusenbury, Baker, James-Ortiz, Botvin, & Kerner, 1992).

An important consideration in designing preventive approaches to cigarette smoking is the need to convince prospective smokers or quitters that tobacco is an addictive substance. This may not be a problem among Latinos, as data from a national sample reported in the 1998 Surgeon General's Report (United States Department of Health and Human Services, 1998) showed that large proportions of Latinos consider cigarette smoking as a habit (25.1 percent), an addiction (26.3 percent), or both (38.4 percent).

Latino-specific cessation programs have been designed for individual use as well as for groups. Self-help approaches have relied heavily on the production of materials to inform and motivate smokers to quit. An important example is the manual *Rompa con el Vicio* ("Break the Habit") produced in San Francisco and based on large numbers of studies that identified culture-specific attitudes, norms, values, and expectancies of Latino smokers (Marín, Marín, Otero-Sabogal, Sabogal, & Pérez-Stable, 1989; Marín, Pérez-Stable, Otero-Sabogal, Sabogal, & Marín, 1989; Marín, Marín, Pérez-Stable, Otero-Sabogal, & Sabogal, 1990). The manual is a twenty-four-page, four-color brochure that describes the health effects of cigarette smoking as well as the unpleasant social consequences associated with tobacco use (such as bad breath), possible methods for quitting, approaches to deal with depression and social pressures to smoke, and relapse prevention. Previous version of this manual showed that 21 percent of smokers reading the manual quit smoking within two and a half months, although the proportion of nonrelapsers declined to 18.6 percent after eight months (Pérez-Stable, Sabogal, Marín, Marín, & Otero-Sabogal, 1991).

Experiences in California (Pierce et al., 1994) show that Latinos use cessation hotlines at a fairly high rate (approximately 20 percent) when they are advertised in Spanish and services are provided both in English and in Spanish. Nevertheless, a more recent study (Zhu, Anderson, Johnson, Tedeschi, & Roeseler, 2000) found that Latinos are underrepresented in the proportion of smokers who call a hotline (14.9 percent), in comparison to the proportion of Latinos who are smokers when Spanish-language promotion is not appropriate. Group approaches to smoking cessation have not been shown to be effective (for example, Pérez-Stable, Marín, & Marín, 1993), probably because of logistic difficulties (such as accessing facilities, special child care needs, transportation costs, or availability), affordability, embarrassment (talking to other members of the community about a problem), and lack of Spanish-language services (Glynn, 1989; Lichtenstein & Glasgow, 1992).

Another approach to tobacco use prevention has been the design of community-wide interventions that include a variety of approaches and strategies. One of the initial efforts was carried out by Stanford University and targeted Latino communities in Northern California. The project used electronic and print mass media, direct mailings, contests, physician-directed activities, and school-based interventions trying to decrease the presence of risk factors for cardiovascular disease. Spanish-language radio and newspaper articles were used in communities with large Latino populations. In general, a large number of Latinos reported being asked by a physician to quit smoking (approximately 33 percent), although this proportion was higher among Whites (approximately 51 percent) but there were no overall differences in the experimental and control communities (Frank, Winkleby, Altman, Rockhill, & Fortmann, 1991). The use of self-help materials for smoking cessation differed significantly among Latinos, with a substantial proportion of the women (approximately 31 percent) reporting using the materials in contrast to no men reporting the same behavior. Another Northern California program targeting Latino smokers but this time using culturally appropriate materials reported more encouraging results (Marín, Marín, Pérez-Stable, & Hauck, 1994; Pérez-Stable, Marín, & Marín, 1993; Marín & Pérez-Stable, 1995). The *Programa Latino Para Dejar de Fumar* ("Hispanic Smoking Cessation Program") utilized multimedia approaches to motivate and support smokers as they quit, including the use of the manual *Rompa con el Vicio* ("Break the Habit"), radio and television programming, personal consultation, and other outreach efforts. The program showed a number of significant results. There was an increase in the level of information held by members of the community, a decrease in prevalence, and important increases in program awareness and participation in the program's activities (Marín, Marín, Pérez-Stable, & Hauck, 1994; Marín & Pérez-Stable, 1995).

Other community-wide projects have shows results of importance such as *A Su Salud* ("To Your Health") in Texas (Amezcua, McAlister, Ramirez, & Espinoza,

1990; Ramirez & McAlister, 1988), "For You and Your Family," a California program targeting pregnant women (Otero-Sabogal & Sabogal, 1991), and the Great American Smokeout, annually sponsored by the American Cancer Society. What these and other smaller programs seem to demonstrate is that multifaceted approaches that are sensitive to cultural norms and values and that integrate culturally appropriate strategies tend to produce notable results.

## Implications for Research, Policy, and Practice

There is ample evidence that tobacco use is a problem of significance among Latinos in the United States. Of particular concern is the large proportion of Latino youth who are smoking tobacco products and the salient presence of risk factors that have been identified in the literature as supporters of this addiction. The data summarized above support the need for not only better information about tobacco use among Latinos but also for targeted culturally appropriate preventive interventions directed at Latino youth. These are areas of concern that must become a priority not only for practitioners and researchers but also for policymakers and funding sources. The overall youth of the Latino population makes it essential for large-scale preventive efforts to be designed and implemented before we face a more serious health crisis as our population ages and we start seeing the deleterious health effects of tobacco use.

While data on Latinos and tobacco use are available and some excellent studies can be found in the literature, overall the findings are of limited significance due to a number of methodological limitations of the research projects that produced them. These limitations have been identified by the 1998 Surgeon General's Report on tobacco and they deserve to be summarized here. First is the problem that most of the data have limited generalizability because many of the studies have been conducted in a select number of metropolitan areas (New York, Miami, Los Angeles, San Francisco), ignoring Latinos who live in smaller towns or in other parts of the country. Second, studies conducted with Latino youth have tended to rely on captive populations of children attending schools (primarily public schools), ignoring those in parochial or rural schools as well as school dropouts. A third serious methodological limitation of most studies with Latinos is the noncomparability of constructs and instruments. Although the argument is frequently made that appropriate crosscultural research requires culturally appropriate instruments and the use of relevant constructs (see Marín & Marín, 1991; Triandis & Marín, 1983), few studies have actually tried to use comparable instruments or constructs. For example, attitudinal instruments are developed for one ethnic group and used with members of a different ethnic group without ascertaining whether the attitudinal object has the same meaning and significance in the latter group. This process produces the methodological problem of differential instrumentation, an outcome similar to the proverbial comparison of apples with oranges.

One other methodological problem of importance among studies investigating the use of tobacco among Latinos is the aggregation of data across subgroups, genders, acculturation groups, and other variables of relevance. This approach, which is becoming somewhat less common, makes it difficult to identify the differences that may exist within specific Latino subgroups (such as differences between those of Mexican and of Cuban heritage in the United States) or across genders or acculturation levels. Finally, mention must be made of the lack of longitudinal data regarding tobacco use among Latinos. Despite their usefulness in explaining causal links between variables (Conrad, Flay, & Hill, 1992), very few studies have followed Latino respondents for more than a year.

Policymakers and government agencies must realize that a phenomenon as complex as tobacco use, which is produced and supported by multiple causes, requires multipronged approaches to properly modify its prevalence among a community. These approaches should try to modify the social environment or climate and be properly evaluated (Flay, Petraitis, & Hu, 1999). Indeed, evidence from California (for example, Siegel et al., 2000) shows that an aggressive and comprehensive tobacco control campaign can have an effect in lowering tobacco use prevalence across all populations in the state. Unfortunately, most approaches to curtail tobacco use among Latinos have been either short-lived or not properly developed. For examples, despite evidence that the media is an important resource in tobacco control (Worden, 1999; Siegel & Biener, 2000), few programs have used print and electronic media extensively and seldom have they used culturally appropriate interventions.

An important consideration in the development of prevention strategies is the cultural relevance of the constructs utilized, the methodologies included, and the strategies chosen to be part of the study or the intervention. This concern is of particular significance in the area of tobacco use, where culture-specific attitudes, norms, and values have indeed been identified for Latinos (see Marín, Marín, Pérez-Stable, Otero-Sabogal, & Sabogal, 1990). As argued elsewhere (Marín, 1993), a culturally appropriate intervention must of necessity meet three criteria: (1) it must reflect the ethnic group's attitudes, values, and norms that are of relevance to the behavior; (2) it must consider the group's basic values or cultural characteristics that differentiate the group from other ethnic groups in terms of what is valued and considered of value such as the social script of *simpatia* among Latinos (Triandis, Marin, Lisansky, & Betancourt, 1984) or the cultural value of *familialism* (Sabogal, Marin, Otero-Sabogal, Marín, & Pérez-Stable, 1987), as defined earlier; and (3) a culturally appropriate intervention must consider those strategies that are acceptable and credible to members of the community (for example, Marín, 1996). Taking these principles into consideration in the development of an intervention will of necessity increase its acceptability and the likelihood of being effective.

In summary, two general findings can be presented here as a result of the extant literature on tobacco use among Latinos. First, there is a dire need for better-designed studies that can analyze the predictors of tobacco use initiation and continued use among Latinos. These studies should probably be longitudinal in nature, have a sound theoretical basis, and be designed in a culturally appropriate fashion by following the suggestions made by crosscultural methodologists (for example, Brislin, Lonner, & Thorndike, 1973; Marín & Marín, 1991; Stanfield & Rutledge, 1993). Second, the outcomes of previous studies point toward the importance of certain variables in explaining the initiation and maintenance of tobacco use among Latinos. In particular, the literature seems to support the notion that attention should be given to the design of targeted ethnic-specific interventions to ameliorate the stressful experiences of migration, support the improvement of school performance as well as the prevention of school dropouts, change the normative perceptions regarding the use of tobacco among Latinos, and endorse the process of biculturalism as a way to diminish acculturate conflicts. These concerns must also inform all public health policies designed to prevent the use of tobacco among Latinos.

More and better-designed studies should provide a clearer indication of group-specific correlates of tobacco use as well as of the "universality" of other correlates. The outcome of an increased pool of good-quality studies will help program designers and public health policymakers in the development of large-scale prevention campaigns as well as of culturally appropriate targeted interventions. The end result will be the lowering of tobacco use prevalence among Latinos and so will contribute to their improved health. Indeed, the scale of the problem requires the active participation of researchers, policymakers, and community health activists and providers who, working within the framework of cultural sensitivity and appropriateness, can move Latinos toward improved health and longer life expectancy.

## Acknowledgments

This chapter benefited significantly from the author's role as Senior Scientific Editor of the 1998 Surgeon General's Report on tobacco use. The author wishes to thank once more the contributions made to that publication by a large number of researchers and by the staff of the Centers for Disease Control and Prevention (CDC). The results analyzed as part of that process as well as the comments and discussions during the preparation of that report shaped the author's thinking about tobacco use among Latinos and are frequently reflected in this chapter. Preparation of this chapter was partially funded by Grants 6PT-6001 and 6RT-0407 from the Tobacco-Related Disease Research Program in California.

## References

Amezcua, C., McAlister, A., Ramirez, A., & Espinoza, R. (1990). *A Su Salud:* Health promotion in a Mexican-American border community. In N. Bracht (Ed.), *Health promotion at the community level.* Newbury Park, CA: Sage, pp. 257–277.

An, L. C., O'Malley, P. M., Schulenberg, J. E., Bachman, J. G., & Johnston, L. D. (1999). Changes at the high end of risk in cigarette smoking among U.S. high school seniors, 1976–1995. *American Journal of Public Health, 89,* 699–705.

Anderson, C., & Burns, D. M. (2000). Patterns of adolescent smoking initiation rates by ethnicity and sex. *Tobacco Control, 9,* Suppl. II, ii4–ii8.

Bachman, J. G., Wallace, J. M., Jr., O'Malley, P. M., Johnston, L. D., Kurth, C. L., & Neighbors, H. W. (1991). Racial/ethnic differences in smoking, drinking, and illicit drug use among American high school seniors, 1976–89. *American Journal of Public Health, 81,* 372–377.

Benowitz, N. L., Pérez-Stable, E., Herrera, B., & Jacob, P. (1995). African American–Caucasian differences in nicotine and cotinine metabolism [abstract]. *Clinical Pharmacology and Therapeutics, 57,* 2, 159.

Bettes, B. A., Dusenbury, L., Kerner, J., James-Ortiz, S., & Botvin, G. J. (1990). Ethnicity and psychosocial factors in alcohol and tobacco use in adolescence. *Child Development, 61,* 557–565.

Biener, L., & Siegel, M. (2000). Tobacco marketing and adolescent smoking: More support for a causal inference. *American Journal of Public Health, 90,* 407–411.

Botvin, G. J., Dusenbury, L., Baker, E., James-Ortiz, S., Botvin, E. M., & Kerner, J. (1992). Smoking prevention among urban minority youth: Assessing effects on outcome and mediating variables. *Health Psychology, 11,* 290–299.

Brislin, R., Lonner, W., & Thorndike, R. (1973). *Cross-cultural research methods.* New York: Wiley.

Centers for Disease Control and Prevention. (1990). Cigarette advertising—United States, 1988. *MMWR [Morbidity and Mortality Weekly Report], 39,* 16, 261–265.

Centers for Disease Control and Prevention. (1996). Accessibility of tobacco products to youths aged 12–17 years—United States, 1989 and 1993. *MMWR [Morbidity and Mortality Weekly Report], 45,* 6, 125–130.

Centers for Disease Control and Prevention. (1997). Cigar smoking among teenagers—United States, Massachusetts, and New York, 1996. *MMWR [Morbidity and Mortality Weekly Report], 46,* 20, 433–440.

Chavez, E. L., Edwards, R., & Oetting, E. R. (1989). Mexican American and White American school dropouts' drug use, health status, and involvement in violence. *Public Health Reports, 104,* 594–604.

Conrad, K., Flay, B., & Hill, D. (1992). Why children start smoking cigarettes: Predictors of onset. *British Journal of Addiction, 87,* 1711–1724.

Coreil, J., Ray, L. A., & Markides, K. S. (1991). Predictors of smoking among Mexican-Americans: Findings from the Hispanic HANES. *Preventive Medicine, 20,* 508–517.

Cowdery, J. E., Fitzhugh, E. C., & Wang, M. Q. (1997). Sociobehavioral influences on smoking initiation of Hispanic adolescents. *Journal of Adolescent Health, 20,* 46–50.

Dusenbury, L., Epstein, J. A., Botvin, G. J., & Diaz, T. (1994). The relationship between language spoken and smoking among Hispanic–Latino youth in New York City. *Public Health Reports, 109,* 421–427.

Dusenbury, L., Kerner, J. F., Baker, E., Botvin, G., James-Ortiz, S., & Zauber, A. (1992). Predictors of smoking prevalence among New York Latino youth. *American Journal of Public Health, 82,* 55–58.

Elder, J. P., Edwards, C., & Conway, T. L. (1993). *Independent evaluation of Proposition 99–funded efforts to prevent and control tobacco use in California.* [Annual Report]. Submitted to the California Department of Health Services, Tobacco Control Section. San Diego, CA: San Diego State University, Graduate School of Public Health.

Elder, J. P. et al. (1993). The long-term prevention of tobacco use among junior high school students: Classroom and telephone interventions. *American Journal of Public Health, 83,* 1239–1244.

Escobedo, L. G., Anda, R. F., Smith, P. F., Remington, P. L., & Mast, E. E. (1990). Sociodemographic characteristics of cigarette smoking initiation in the United States: Implications for smoking prevention policy. *Journal of the American Medical Association, 264,* 1550–1555.

Escobedo, L. G., Kirch, D. G., & Anda, R. F. (1996). Depression and smoking initiation among U.S. Latinos. *Addiction, 91,* 113–119.

Escobedo, L. G., Reddy, M., & DuRant, R. H. (1997). Relationship between cigarette smoking and health risk and problem behaviors among U.S. adolescents. *Archives of Pediatrics and Adolescent Medicine, 151,* 66–71.

Escobedo, L. G., & Remington, P. L. (1989). Birth cohort analysis of prevalence of cigarette smoking among Hispanics in the United States. *Journal of the American Medical Association, 261,* 66–69.

Evans, N., Farkas, A., Gilpin, E., Berry, C., & Pierce, J. P. (1995). Influence of tobacco marketing and exposure to smokers on adolescent susceptibility to smoking. *Journal of the National Cancer Institute, 87,* 1538–1545.

Felix-Ortiz, M., & Newcomb, M. D. (1992). Risk and protective factors for drug use among Latino and white adolescents. *Hispanic Journal of Behavioral Sciences, 14,* 291–309.

Felix-Ortiz, M., & Newcomb, M. D. (1996). Cultural identity and drug use among Latino and Latina adolescents. In G. J. Botvin, S. P. Schinke, & M. A. Orlandi (Eds.), *Drug abuse prevention with multiethnic youth.* Thousand Oaks, CA: Sage, pp. 147–165.

Flay, B. R., Petraitis, J., & Hu, F. B. (1999). Psychosocial risk and protective factors for adolescent tobacco use. *Nicotine and Tobacco Research, 1,* S59–S65.

Frank, E., Winkleby, M. A., Altman, D. G., Rockhill, B., & Fortmann, S. P. (1991). Predictors of physicians' smoking cessation advice. *Journal of the American Medical Association, 266,* 3139–3144.

Giovino, G. A. (1999). Epidemiology of tobacco use among U.S. adolescents. *Nicotine and Tobacco Control, 1,* S31–S40.

Glynn, T. J. (1989). Essential elements of school-based smoking prevention programs. *Journal of School Health, 59,* 181–188.

Graham, J. W., Johnson, C. A., Hansen, W. B., Flay, B. R., & Gee, M. (1990). Drug use prevention programs, gender, and ethnicity: Evaluation of three seventh-grade Project SMART cohorts. *Preventive Medicine, 19,* 305–313.

Hayes-Bautista, D. E., & Chapa, J. (1987). Latino terminology: Conceptual bases for standardized terminology. *American Journal of Public Health, 77,* 61–68.

Haynes, S. G., Harvey, C., Montes, H., Nickens, H., & Cohen, B. H. (1990). Patterns of cigarette smoking among Hispanics in the United States: Results from HHANES 1982–84. *American Journal of Public Health 1990, 80,* Suppl., 47–54.

Henningfield, J. E., Cohen, C., & Giovino, G. A. (1990). Can genetic constitution affect the "objective" diagnosis of nicotine dependence? [editorial] *American Journal of Public Health, 80,* 1040–1041.

Hovell, M. F., Zakarian, J. M., Wahlgren, D. R., & Matt, G. E. (2000). Reducing children's exposure to environmental tobacco smoke: The empirical evidence and directions for future research. *Tobacco Control, 9,* Suppl. II, ii40–ii47.

Hughes, J. R. (1986). Genetics of smoking: A brief review. *Behavior Therapy, 17,* 335–345.

Klonoff, E. A., Fritz, J. M., Landrine, H., Riddle, R. W., & Tully-Payne, L. (1994). The problem and sociocultural context of single-cigarette sales. *Journal of the American Medical Association, 271,* 618–620.

Lafromboise, T., Coleman, H.L.K., & Gerton, J. (1993). Psychological impact of biculturalism: Evidence and theory. *Psychological Bulletin, 114,* 395–412.

Lee, D. J., & Markides, K. S. (1991). Health behaviors, risk factors, and health indicators associated with cigarette use in Mexican Americans: Results from the Hispanic HANES. *American Journal of Public Health, 81,* 859–864.

Lichtenstein, E., & Glasgow, R. E. (1992). Smoking cessation: What have we learned over the past decade? *Journal of Consulting and Clinical Psychology, 60,* 518–527.

Marín, B. V., Marín, G., Pérez-Stable, E. J., & Hauck, W. W. (1994). Effects of a community intervention to change smoking behavior among Hispanics. *American Journal of Preventive Medicine, 10,* 340–347.

Marín, B. V., Marín, G., Pérez-Stable, E. J., Otero-Sabogal, R., & Sabogal, F. (1990). Cultural differences in attitudes toward smoking: Developing messages using the theory of reasoned action. *Journal of Applied Social Psychology, 20,* 478–493.

Marín, G. (1993). Defining culturally appropriate community interventions: Hispanics as a case study. *Journal of Community Psychology, 21,* 149–161.

Marín, G. (1994). Self-reported awareness of the presence of product warning messages and signs by Hispanics in San Francisco. *Public Health Reports, 109,* 275–283.

Marín, G. (1996). Perceptions by Hispanics of channels and sources of health messages regarding cigarette smoking. *Tobacco Control, 5,* 30–36.

Marín, G., & Marín, B. V. (1991). *Research with Hispanic populations.* Newbury Park, CA: Sage.

Marín, G., Marín, B. V., Otero-Sabogal, R., Sabogal, F., & Pérez-Stable, E. J. (1989). The role of acculturation in the attitudes, norms, and expectancies of Hispanic smokers. *Journal of Cross-Cultural Psychology, 20,* 399–415.

Marín, G., Marín, B. V., Pérez-Stable, E. J., Sabogal, F., & Otero-Sabogal, R. (1990). Cultural differences in attitudes and expectancies between Hispanic and non-Hispanic white smokers. *Hispanic Journal of Behavioral Sciences, 12,* 422–436.

Marín, G., & Pérez-Stable, E. J. (1995). Effectiveness of disseminating culturally appropriate smoking-cessation information: *Programa Latino Para Dejar de Fumar. Journal of the National Cancer Institute Monographs, 18,* 155–163.

Marín, G., Pérez-Stable, E. J., Otero-Sabogal, R., Sabogal, F., & Marín, B. V. (1989). Stereotypes of smokers held by Hispanic and White non-Hispanic smokers. *International Journal of the Addictions, 24,* 203–213.

Mermelstein, R., & Tobacco Control Network Writing Group. (1999). Explanations of ethnic and gender differences in youth smoking: A multi-site, qualitative investigation. *Nicotine and Tobacco Research, 1,* S91–S98.

Navarro, A. M. (1996). Cigarette smoking among adult Latinos: The California Tobacco Baseline Survey. *Annals of Behavioral Medicine, 18,* 238–245.

Newcomb, M. D., Maddahian, E., Skager, R., & Bentler, P. M. (1987). Substance abuse and psychosocial risk factors among teenagers: Associations with sex, age, ethnicity, and type of school. *American Journal of Drug and Alcohol Abuse, 13,* 413–433.

Otero-Sabogal, R., & Sabogal, F. (1991). *La mujer: La familia y el cigarrillo.* San Francisco: American Lung Association of San Francisco.

Pérez-Stable, E. J., Marín, B. V., & Marín, G. (1993). A comprehensive smoking cessation program for the San Francisco Bay Area Latino Community: *Programa Latino Para Dejar de Fumar. American Journal of Health Promotion, 7,* 430–442, 475.

Pérez-Stable, E. J., Marín, B. V., Marín, G., Brody, D. J., & Benowitz, N. L. (1990). Apparent underreporting of cigarette consumption among Mexican American smokers. *American Journal of Public Health, 80,* 1057–1061.

Pérez-Stable, E. J., Marín, G., Marín, B. V., & Katz, M. H. (1990). Depressive symptoms and cigarette smoking among Latinos in San Francisco. *American Journal of Public Health, 80,* 1500–1502.

Pérez-Stable, E. J., Sabogal, F., Marín, G., Marín, B. V., & Otero-Sabogal, R. (1991). Evaluation of *"Guia Para Dejar de Fumar,"* a self-help guide in Spanish to quit smoking. *Public Health Reports, 106,* 564–570.

Pierce, J. P. et al. (1994). *Tobacco use in California: An evaluation of the Tobacco Control Program, 1989–1993.* La Jolla: University of California, San Diego.

Ramirez, A. G., & McAlister, A. L. (1988). Mass media campaign—*A Su Salud. Preventive Medicine, 17,* 608–621.

Sabogal, F., Marín, G., Otero-Sabogal, R., Marín, B. V., & Pérez-Stable, E. J. (1987). Hispanic familism and acculturation: What changes and what doesn't? *Hispanic Journal of Behavioral Sciences, 9,* 397–412.

Sabogal, F., Otero-Sabogal, R., Pérez-Stable, E. J., Marín, B. V., & Marín, G. (1989). Perceived self-efficacy to avoid cigarette smoking and addiction: Differences between Hispanics and non-Hispanic Whites. *Hispanic Journal of Behavioral Sciences, 11,* 136–147.

Siegel, M., & Biener, L. (2000). The impact of an antismoking media campaign on progression to established smoking: Results of a longitudinal youth study. *American Journal of Public Health, 90,* 380–386.

Siegel, M. et al. (2000). Trends in adult cigarette smoking in California compared with the rest of the United States, 1978–1994. *American Journal of Public Health, 90,* 372–379.

Smith, K. W., McGraw, S. A., & Carrillo, J. E. (1991). Factors affecting cigarette smoking and intention to smoke among Puerto Rican–American high school students. *Hispanic Journal of Behavioral Sciences, 13,* 401–411.

Stanfield, J. H., & Rutledge, M. (1993). *Race and ethnicity in research methods.* Newbury Park, CA: Sage.

Trevino, F. (1987). Standardized terminology for Hispanic populations. *American Journal of Public Health, 77,* 69–72.

Triandis, H. C., & Marín, G. (1983). Etic plus emic versus pseudo-etic: A test of a basic assumption of contemporary cross-cultural psychology. *Journal of Cross-Cultural Psychology, 14,* 489–500.

Triandis, H. C., Marín, G., Lisansky, J., & Betancourt, H. (1984). *Simpatia* as a cultural script of Hispanics. *Journal of Personality and Social Psychology, 47,* 1363–1375.

Unger, J. B., Palmer, P. H., Dent, C. W., Rohrbach, L. A., & Johnson, C. A. (2000). Ethnic differences in adolescent smoking prevalence in California: Are multi-ethnic youth at higher risk? *Tobacco Control, 9,* Suppl. II, ii9–ii14.

United States Department of Health and Human Services. (1988). *The health consequences of smoking: Nicotine addiction. A report of the Surgeon General.* (DHHS Publication No. [CDC] 88-8406). Rockville, MD: DHHS, Public Health Service, Centers for Disease Control, Center for Health Promotion and Education, Office on Smoking and Health.

United States Department of Health and Human Services. (1992). *Smoking and health in the Americas. A 1992 report of the Surgeon General.* (DHHS Publication No. [CDC] 92-8419). Atlanta, GA: DHHS, Centers for Disease Control, National Center for Chronic Disease Prevention and Health Promotion, Office on Smoking and Health.

United States Department of Health and Human Services. (1994). *Preventing tobacco use among young people. A report of the Surgeon General.* (DHHS Publication No. [CDC] 94-0000). Atlanta, GA: DHHS, Public Health Service, Centers for Disease Control and Prevention, National Center for Chronic Disease Prevention and Health Promotion, Office on Smoking and Health.

United States Department of Health and Human Services. (1998). *Tobacco use among U.S. racial/ethnic minority groups—African Americans, American Indians and Alaska Natives, Asian Americans and Pacific Islanders, and Latinos: A report of the Surgeon General.* (DHHS Publication No. [CDC] 98-0000). Atlanta, GA: DHHS, Centers for Disease Control and Prevention, National Center for Chronic Disease Prevention and Health Promotion, Office on Smoking and Health.

United States General Accounting Office. (1994, July). *Latinos' schooling: Risk factors for dropping out and barriers to resuming education.* (GAO/PEMD-94-24). Gaithersburg, MD: GAO, Program Evaluation and Methodology Division.

Vander Martin, R. V., Cummings, S. R., & Coates, T. J. (1990). Ethnicity and smoking: Differences in White, Black, Hispanic, and Asian medical patients who smoke. *American Journal of Preventive Medicine, 6,* 194–199.

Vega, W. A., Zimmerman, R. S., Warheit, G. J., Apospori, E., & Gil, A. G. (1993). Risk factors for early adolescent drug use in four ethnic and racial groups. *American Journal of Public Health, 83,* 185–189.

Webster, C. (1992). The effects of Hispanic subcultural identification on information search behavior. *Journal of Advertising Research, 32,* 5, 54–62.

Worden, J. K. (1999). Research in using mass media to prevent smoking. *Nicotine and Tobacco Research, 1,* S117–S121.

Zhu, S.-H., Anderson, C. M., Johnson, C. E., Tedeschi, G., & Roeseler, A. (2000). A centralized telephone service for tobacco cessation: The California experience. *Tobacco Control, 9,* Suppl. II, ii48–ii55.

CHAPTER SIXTEEN

# LATINO DRUG USE

## Scope, Risk Factors, and Reduction Strategies

Andres G. Gil, William A. Vega

The United States has the highest rates of illicit drug use of any nation in the developed world (Alderete, Vega, Kolody, & Aguilar-Gaxiola, 2000). In the calendar year 1998 there were 542,544 emergency room episodes in the United States where the primary reason for medical attention was drug ingestion (Substance Abuse and Mental Health Services Administration, 1998b). Between 1991 and 1998 emergency room admissions for drug use problems among Latinos in the United States increased by 80 percent.

Drug abuse is a major public health problem that reduces the productivity and quality of life of the American population. Drug users have inferior physical and mental health, and they are more likely to have problems with educational attainment and employment, an unstable family life, and heightened probability of criminal justice system involvement (Newcomb & Bentler, 1988). Latinos who live in the United States share this vulnerability. Latinos are particularly at risk for drug dependency and addiction because of poverty, minority status, and residential concentration in areas with wide drug distribution and drug abuse.

Understanding patterns of drug use problems in the U.S. Latino population is complicated by differences among Latino ethnic subgroups across and within regions. Another factor affecting Latino drug use is immigration. Two of every five Latinos are immigrants, and their familiarity with illicit drugs is very different than that of U.S.-born Latinos. Drug use rates in Latin America are very low, and attitudes and beliefs about drug use there are more intolerant than in the United States (Caetano & Medina-Mora, 1988). In this chapter, a model of adolescent drug use vulnerability is employed to evaluate how these factors influence Latinos. Additionally, epidemiological and intervention information is presented, and the implications for prevention and treatment are discussed.

## Risk and Protective Factors

There are specific durable patterns of risk that affect Latino drug use. Sociodemographic, cultural, and environmental factors are implicated in the process. Figure 16.1 presents a model of adolescent drug use vulnerability. This model illustrates the variance in lifestyles among Latinos and the segmentation that takes place in their personal experiences within the United States. The internal composition of the Latino population consists of groups and individuals with distinctive cultural and historical backgrounds. Latinos who immigrated or migrated (in the instance of Puerto Ricans) as children have had quite different formative experiences with regard to drug use than individuals who came to the United States as adults because the younger immigrants matured in an environment where drug use was more acceptable. In turn, U.S.-born Latinos are more likely than immigrants to have peers who have ambiguous or even supportive attitudes concerning drug use. Thus, it can be anticipated that the exposure to risk factors and the effects of risk factors on substance use varies with the personal history of the individual, including immigration history, and his or her personal characteristics. Women generally have lower frequency of drug use than men. Age is important because most people initiate illicit drug use before reaching their middle twenties. Early drug experimentation greatly increases the risk of continuance, progression to other drugs, and addiction (Vega, Alderete, Kolody, & Aguilar-Gaxiola, 2000). Conversely, those who do not use drugs during their youth or early adulthood, such as most adult immigrants, are unlikely ever to do so.

Figure 16.1 illustrates overlapping processes of social adaptation to local environments, social incorporation of Latino youth into local institutions, peer groups, and public life, and the challenges of child rearing for low-income

### FIGURE 16.1.  ACCULTURATIVE MODEL OF LATINO ADOLESCENT SUBSTANCE USE.

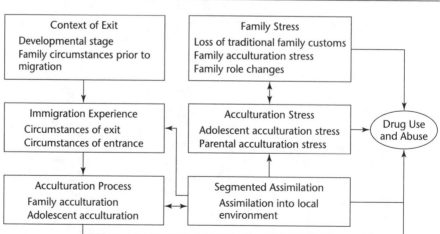

families in different types of social circumstances (Vega & Gil, 1999). A good deal of research in the past decade has focused on disentangling how these factors and experiences are related to drug use for U.S.-born and immigrant Latinos.

## Acculturation and Acculturation Stress

Acculturation and acculturation stress independently influence Latinos, especially adolescents (Lopez & Guarnaccia, 2000). Acculturation is the process of acquiring and selectively adapting new cultural information and behaviors either to supplement or replace one's culture of origin (Vega & Gil, 1998). Many studies have unequivocally shown that social integration into American society (assimilation) and adopting U.S. behaviors and customs (acculturation) increases drug use (Amaro, Whitaker, Coffman, & Heeren, 1990; Burnam, Hough, Karno, Escobar, & Telles, 1987). Immigrants' risk of drug use is affected by how long they have lived in the United States and their degree of assimilation into American culture (Vega, Gil, & Wagner, 1998). Similarly, Vega, Kolody, Aguilar-Gaxiola, Alderete, and Catalano (1998) have shown that length of residence in the United States correlated with markedly increased substance abuse rates (using DSM-III-R lifetime criteria; American Psychiatric Association, 1987) among Mexican Americans. The rates were 0 percent among immigrants who were in the United States less than thirteen years, 1.8 percent for those living in the United States more than thirteen years, and 3.4 percent among those born in the United States. The above authors found that trends for drug dependence also differed in the three groups, with the rates being 3 percent, 5.3 percent, and 13.8 percent, respectively. The same study reported that the abuse and dependence rates of the Mexican immigrant group with less than thirteen years in the United States were similar to those of a group of residents in Mexico City. The U.S.-born group may be at higher risk of drug abuse due to poverty and minority status than due to acculturation per se. Paradoxically, poverty is not a risk factor for immigrants (Burnam, Hough, Karno, Escobar, & Telles, 1987; Vega & Gil, 1998). This is because immigrants in poverty usually are not highly assimilated into U.S. culture. This protects them against drug use (Vega, Alderete, Kolody, & Aguilar-Gaxiola, 1998).

Acculturation stress derives from negative personal experiences with the dominant culture that threaten a person's positive self-image and cognitive–emotional functioning. Conflicts about behavioral expectations with authority figures or peers, problems with language competency and literacy, and exposure to racism and pejorative remarks about one's ethnic identity in the United States are all causes of acculturation stress (Vega & Gil, 1998). They are especially consequential for adolescents because they influence identity development, acquisition of social skills, and personal efficacy. Latino youth who are turned off to school due to such negative experiences and so drop out, often feeling that their ethnic culture and personal identity are marginal in American society, are much more vulnerable to becoming illicit drug users (Chavez & Swaim, 1992). Use of drugs under these circumstances might be seen as both a product of risk factors and a coping response.

Risk factors occur in unique combinations and are additive in their effects on drug use: more risk factors produce a higher prevalence of drug use (Vega, Zimmerman, Warheit, Apospori, & Gil, 1993; Newcomb, Maddahian, & Bentler, 1986). For example, Latino youth whose parents are immigrants are less likely to have witnessed illegal drug use in the home. However, if they do experience substance abuse problems in the home, it is a risk factor for their own drug use (Vega & Gil, 1998). There are also specific risk factors that are particularly problematic for Latino adolescents, such as low family cohesiveness, changes in family structure, and high levels of family acculturation stress (Gil & Vega, 1996; Gil, Vega, & Biafora, 1998). The environment and its demographic composition are also contributory factors. For both immigrant and U.S.-born Latinos, the risk of drug dependency increases in deteriorating inner-city neighborhoods where young people routinely experience multiple risk factors such as violence, gangs, and drug distribution networks. One recent study demonstrated that highly acculturated (English-speaking U.S.-born) Latinas were less likely to use alcohol during pregnancy if they lived in low-acculturation (linguistically isolated and predominantly immigrant) residential areas rather than high-acculturation areas (Finch, Boardman, Kolody, & Vega, 2000). Another study showed that living in rural rather than small town or urban areas of California uniquely decreased the odds of illicit drug use among immigrants and native-born adults of Mexican origin, after the investigators controlled for other risk factors (Vega, Alderete, Kolody, & Aguilar-Gaxiola, 1998).

Greater and more intense involvement with alcohol and illicit drug use is reported for U.S.-born than for immigrant Latinos, and regular and problem use increases with the amount of time immigrants have lived in the United States (Vega, Gil, & Wagner, 1998; Gil, Wagner, & Vega, 2000). Research with immigrant Latinos has shown that *any* increase in acculturation in either parents or adolescents will increase the likelihood of illicit drug use in adolescents (Vega & Gil, 1998). These differences emphasize that drug use is learned behavior, and this learning is much more likely to occur in the United States than in Latin American countries. This higher risk of socialization into drug use and erosion of antidrug values and attitudes that accompanies U.S. assimilation operates for both genders. Yet, because immigrant males have much higher rates of illicit drug use than females, the proportionate increase in use attributable to U.S. birth is *greater for females*. Acculturation does not increase drug use rates among U.S.-born Latinos because they are already at higher risk due to nativity, minority status, and lifelong residence in the United States. Therefore, two important mechanisms are mediating risk for Latinos: (1) social networks that control definitions of drug use and (2) environmental factors that provide access to opportunity structures or, in their absence, access to drugs and high-risk lifestyles.

Portes and Zhou (1993) describe these different social experiences and corresponding variance in social outcomes as "segmented assimilation." These researchers emphasize the importance of the community and local neighborhood,

magnitude of ethnic enclave development in the region, and personal characteristics, such as skin color, as all being formidable influences on the adjustment
of immigrants, their employment opportunities, and the success of the second
generation in assimilating. The segmented assimilation experience is also important for understanding onset of drug use, abuse, and dependence. For example, a
study of Mexican immigrants reported that those of Amerindian heritage (indigenous groups from southern Mexico, such as Mixtecos) had similar rates of
drug abuse or dependence as other immigrants residing in the same region, but
the risk of drug use and of suicide attempts after long-term residence in the
United States was much higher for those of Amerindian heritage (Alderete, Vega,
Kolody, & Aguilar-Gaxiola, 2000). Even within the immigrant stream in the
United States, those of Amerindian heritage are marginal to Mexican social
networks and discriminated against, and they are much more likely to acculturate
directly from Indian dialects to English. These and other findings have produced
the *acculturation hypothesis,* which in essence states that exposure to U.S. society combined with higher levels of mastery, acceptance, and attitudes congruent with
American society increases the likelihood of drug use among Latino or any other
immigrant group (Glick & Moore, 1990).

## Protective Factors

While acculturation and acculturation stress are related to increased risk for drug
use among immigrants, there are factors associated with traditional Latino cultures that can serve as protective mechanisms for drug use and a variety of other
negative health consequences. Research has demonstrated that maintaining Latino
traditional values and behaviors of familism and family cohesion can be protective in preventing drug initiation or progression to abuse (Gil & Vega, 1996; Gil,
Vega, & Biafora, 1998; Gil, Wagner, & Vega, 2000).

# Prevalence and Trends

In the sections that follow, information is presented about the prevalence of different classes of drug use among Latinos. This is followed by a discussion of Latino
treatment and prevention issues, and we conclude with a consideration of policy
implications.

## Adult Prevalence (National Household Survey)

Table 16.1 presents lifetime prevalence rates for marijuana, cocaine, and illicit
drugs from the 1996 National Household Survey on Drug Abuse. "Illicit drug use"
is defined as any use of marijuana or hashish, cocaine (including crack), inhalants,
hallucinogens (including PCP), or heroin, or any nonmedicinal use of psy-
chotherapeutic drugs. In this chapter we do not address alcohol and tobacco use

## TABLE 16.1.  LIFETIME PREVALENCE AND FREQUENCY OF DRUG USE.[a]

|  | Marijuana | | Cocaine | | Illicit Drug Use | |
|---|---|---|---|---|---|---|
|  | Lifetime | 51+ Days | Lifetime | Past Year | Lifetime | Past Year |
| Latino |  |  |  |  |  |  |
|   Males | 27.3 | 3.5 | 11.9 | 3.3 | 32.2 | 12.2 |
|   Females | 16.5 | 1.6 | 5.0 | 1.5 | 19.6 | 7.0 |
| Latinos | 22.0 | 2.5 | 8.5 | 2.4 | 26.0 | 9.6 |
| African Americans | 29.6 | 3.9 | 8.3 | 2.4 | 32.9 | 13.4 |
| Whites | 34.4 | 2.7 | 11.0 | 1.7 | 36.9 | 10.8 |

[a]Age distribution for the National Household Survey is from twelve years old through adulthood.

*Source:* Adapted from Substance Abuse and Mental Health Services Administration (1996).

because they are reviewed elsewhere in this volume. However, rates for both alcohol and tobacco use are higher than for marijuana and other illicit drugs. Epidemiological studies have shown that Latino youth and other ethnic groups tend to progress from alcohol and tobacco use to marijuana and other illicit drugs—and drug use problems (Vega & Gil, 1998). Nevertheless, prevalence rates for illicit drug use are much lower than for alcohol or tobacco use (Vega, Alderete, Kolody, & Aguilar-Gaxiola, 2000).

As shown in Table 16.1, Latino males report higher rates of lifetime marijuana, cocaine, and illicit drug use than their female counterparts. In comparison to Whites and African Americans, Latinos report lower rates of marijuana or all illicit drug use. Looking at more intensive use of marijuana (fifty-one or more days in the past year), Latinos also report rates that are lower than that of Whites. Past year use of all illicit drugs is lowest among Latinos, yet past year cocaine use is higher for both Latinos and African Americans than for Whites. As for lifetime cocaine use rates, those of Latinos and African Americans are rather similar, and both are lower than that of Whites.

The most widely used illicit drug among Latinos in the United States is marijuana. This is also true of Whites and African Americans. As for polydrug use, marijuana and alcohol tend to be the most common multiple drugs used (Earleywine & Newcomb, 1997) across all groups, and individuals that move into the use of other illicit drugs, such as cocaine and crack, tend to be polydrug users (Smart, 1991). However, no information is available as to possible ethnic or racial differences in polydrug use because surveys have not addressed ethnic differences in this area.

Figures 16.2 and 16.3 illustrate trends in current (past month) use of marijuana and other illicit drugs among Latinos, Whites, and African Americans during the 1990s. In terms of marijuana use, it appears that there have been minor reductions in the rates for Whites, small increases among Latinos, and large increases among African Americans—especially from 1993 to 1996.

## FIGURE 16.2. PAST MONTH USE OF MARIJUANA THROUGH THE 1990s.

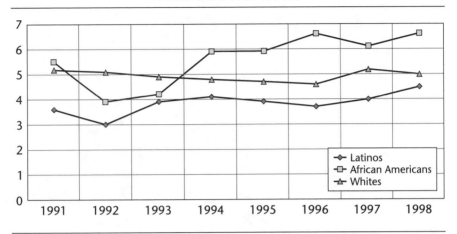

*Source:* Substance Abuse and Mental Health Services Administration (1996).

## FIGURE 16.3. PAST MONTH USE OF ANY ILLICIT DRUG THROUGH THE 1990s.

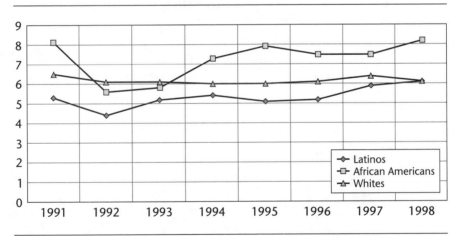

*Source:* Substance Abuse and Mental Health Services Administration (1996).

The trend in current illicit drug use shows that Latinos are catching up with Whites and that there have been more dramatic increases among African Americans since 1993.

## Age Cohort Prevalence

Figures 16.4 and 16.5 illustrate marijuana use of various age cohorts. What is important about these graphs is that the younger age cohorts, between twelve and seventeen years old, report similar rates among Latinos, African Americans,

## FIGURE 16.4.   LIFETIME USE OF MARIJUANA BY AGE AND ETHNICITY.

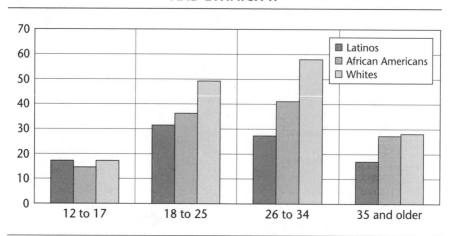

*Source:* Substance Abuse and Mental Health Services Administration (1996).

## FIGURE 16.5.   PAST MONTH USE OF MARIJUANA BY AGE AND ETHNICITY.

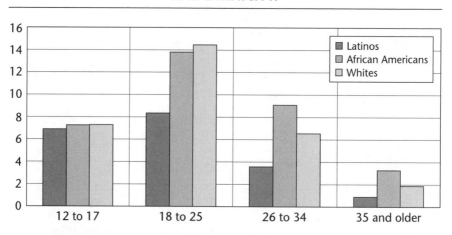

*Source:* Substance Abuse and Mental Health Services Administration (1996).

and Whites. The next age cohorts of eithteen to twenty-five years old show dramatically higher rates of use for African Americans and Whites. However, the rates among Latinos are only slightly higher than those for the younger cohorts. As rates decline for older cohorts, the decreases are sharper for the Latino group. While these graphs pertain only to marijuana use, findings from the National Household Survey on Drug Abuse show similar patterns of results for illicit drug use throughout the 1990s (1991–1998).

Data from the National Co-morbidity Study (Kessler, Nelson, McGonagle, & Liu, 1996), the only national mental health survey ever conducted in the United States, showed higher rates of drug abuse or dependence rates for Latinos in comparison to Whites and African Americans. This result may be explained by excepting Spanish speakers (predominantly immigrants) from the sample. This is indicated by findings of the Mexican American Prevalence and Services Survey (MAPSS), which reported a rate of 3 percent for drug dependence for immigrants who had lived in the United States less than thirteen years, a higher rate of 5.3 percent for those who had lived in the United States for thirteen years or longer, and the highest rate for U.S.-born Mexican Americans (13.8 percent) (Vega, Kolody, Aguilar-Gaxiola, Alderete, Catalano, & Caraveo-Anduaga, 1998).

The findings from these data presented in Table 16.1 and Figures 16.2 through 16.5, as well as the MAPSS study, suggest that drug use among Latinos is equal to or lower than that among Whites. However, the trends shown in Figures 16.2 and 16.3 demonstrate that Latinos have been catching up to the levels of use of Whites during the 1990s. Moreover, the younger cohorts of Latinos (Figures 16.4 and 16.5) are identical in their rates of drug use to those of Whites. This constitutes a serious public health challenge in terms of drug abuse and dependence and negative health consequences, as cohorts of Latinos move through their developmental trajectories into adulthood.

It is important to consider inherent weaknesses of surveys such as the National Household Survey in the examination of Latino drug use patterns in the United States. To reiterate, the U.S. Latino population is diverse in terms of nativity, geographic distribution, and race, and surveys that fail to examine subgroup and regional differences are inherently deficient. The fact is that prevalence rates will vary across Latino groups as a result of geographic and nativity variations. And apparent lower rates of drug use in comparison to other groups in the United States "mask" higher rates among the U.S.-born Latinos. Moreover, given the intensive immigration of Latinos to the United States, prevalence data should be examined in terms of trends and cohorts; regrettably, these types of data are not available from national surveys.

## Youth Prevalence (Monitoring the Future Surveys)

Table 16.2 presents lifetime prevalence rates for adolescent substance use among Latino, White, and African American tenth and twelfth graders. These prevalence data derive from the Monitoring the Future study (Johnston, O'Malley, & Bachman, 1999). In this survey, the term "illicit drug use" is defined as follows: any use of LSD (lysergic acid diethylamide) or other hallucinogens, crack, other cocaine, or heroin, or any use of other narcotics, amphetamines, barbiturates, or tranquilizers not under a doctor's order.

Reflecting the higher rates of drug use among younger cohorts in the National Household Survey (Figures 16.4 and 16.5), drug use among young Latinos appears to be as high or higher than that of Whites. Latinos report the highest

**TABLE 16.2.   ANNUAL PREVALENCE OF DRUG USE AMONG TENTH AND TWELFTH GRADERS IN 1998.**

| | Marijuana | | Cocaine | | Use of Any Illicit Drug Other than Marijuana | |
|---|---|---|---|---|---|---|
| | Tenth Grade | Twelfth Grade | Tenth Grade | Twelfth Grade | Tenth Grade | Twelfth Grade |
| Latinos | 34.4 | 37.2 | 8.3 | 6.7 | 17.5 | 17.5 |
| African Americans | 26.9 | 30.0 | 1.0 | 0.9 | 4.7 | 7.1 |
| Whites | 34.2 | 39.9 | 4.7 | 6.3 | 19.7 | 23.1 |

*Source:* The Monitoring the Future Study, 1975–1998, University of Michigan, Ann Arbor; table adapted from Johnston, O'Malley, & Bachman (1999).

rates of marijuana and cocaine use in tenth grade, while African Americans report the lowest. Cocaine use is also highest among twelfth-grade Latino youth. However, even in cases where Latinos' rates were the highest, they were very close to those reported by Whites. As was the case with adults, these prevalence rates fail to capture regional and acculturation-influenced differences. And, because it is a school-based survey, dropouts and institutionalized youth are excluded, and these are groups that are at highest risk of illicit drug use. The younger age cohorts (twelve to seventeen years old) in the National Household Survey reported earlier can include these groups because it studied a population sample.

Figures 16.6 and 16.7 illustrate the complexity of interpreting drug use prevalence data among Latinos based on national surveys. The data for each of the states in these graphs derive from state public school surveys. Although it is difficult to compare these data across states because of sampling and measurement inconsistencies, it is apparent that while the trends are similar across states and the national data (of Monitoring the Future), there appear to be regional differences. For example, note the much higher rates of cocaine use in New Jersey for the combined Grades 7–12 in comparison to those of California (Figure 16.7). These differences can be a result of urban and rural differences, but just as likely there may be differences in proportions of immigrants, as well as acculturation differences among students attending schools in each of the states in a given year.

## Stages of Youth Drug Use

The examination of drug use prevalence rates fails to illustrate the additional dimension that there are various stages of drug use. Among younger age groups, prevalence of lifetime drug use at a given time can reflect the different stages of use. For example, lifetime use at age fourteen can represent initial

### FIGURE 16.6.    MARIJUANA USE AMONG LATINO YOUTH
### (NATIONAL AND STATE DATA).

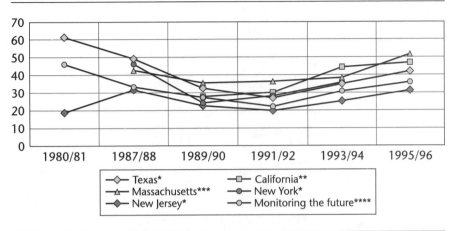

*Grades 7–12;  **Grade 11;  ***Grades 9–12;  ****Annual prevalence for twelfth graders.

experimental use of drugs, as well as occasional or even frequent use related to substance abuse and/or dependence. Most adolescents in the United States experiment with drug use, and the majority do not progress to stages of abuse and dependence. However, given economic and criminal justice inequalities and lack of treatment services, Latino youth that use alcohol heavily are at high risk for drug abuse or dependence as adults (Vega, Alderete, Kolody, & Aguilar-Gaxiola, 2000). In turn, they are also at risk for long mandatory prison sentences for drug-related offenses. Additionally, the age of initiation of drug use is critical in terms of associated negative sequelae of drug dependence, mental health disorders, and other social problems. The younger the individual is when drug use begins, the higher the probability that he or she will develop substance abuse and dependence later in life.

This overview of prevalence rates of drug use points to the conclusion that overall rates of drug use among Latinos appear to be lower or similar to those of Whites. As already noted, important factors are hidden or masked in these general population surveys. These studies were not designed to address issues associated with acculturation levels, specific geographic regions, various Latino ethnic and racial subgroups, or age cohorts. For example, current age-specific data point to future problems in terms of treatment needs and health consequences of drug use, as it appears that younger cohorts of Latinos in the United States have a higher prevalence and frequency of drug use. Since the proportion of Latino immigrants now approximates that of U.S.-born Latinos, the lower use rates of new immigrants tends to offset the higher rates of U.S.-born Latinos. This offset is more likely for adults than for adolescents, because only 15 percent of Latino adolescents are immigrants but 45 percent of all Latino adults in the United States are immigrants.

FIGURE 16.7.   COCAINE USE AMONG LATINO YOUTH (STATE
AND NATIONAL DATA).

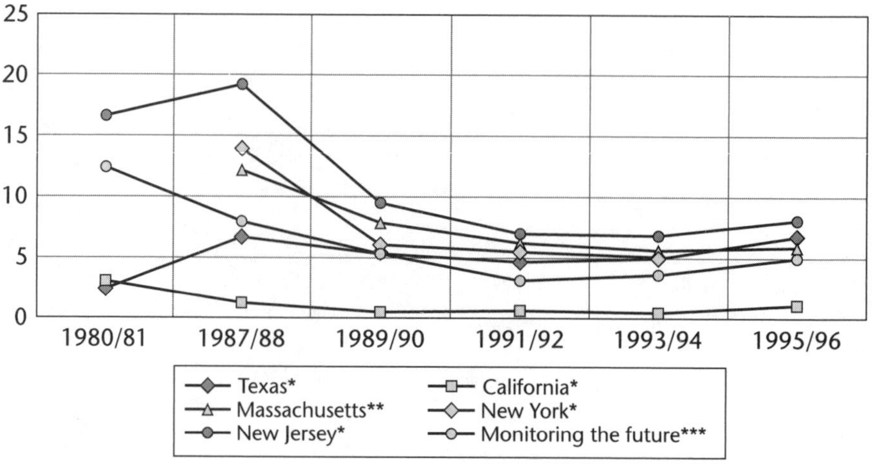

*Grades 7–12; **Grades 9–12; ***Annual prevalence for twelfth graders.

One of the major difficulties in examining Latino youth drug use is the fact that national surveys such as Monitoring the Future fail to distinguish national origin, nativity, and acculturation differences. This factor may be involved in the disparity between the findings of Monitoring the Future and the state surveys. This creates a situation in which there are no national data that allow for comparisons among the various Latino subgroups (such as Mexican, Puerto Rican, Cuban, or Dominican). Few specific studies have compared Latino subgroups (Vega & Gil, 1998), and these have found more profound differences based on nativity (U.S.-born versus immigrant Latinos) than among subgroups. These omissions reduce the value of these surveys, limiting their ability to inform policy, treatment programs, and services.

## Consequences of Drug Use

Latinos are residentially concentrated in large states that share some of the highest drug use levels in the nation, such as California, New York, Florida, Illinois, and Texas. Higher proportions of Latinos than African Americans or Whites who have used an illicit drug in the past year have also reported health, emotional, or psychological problems (Substance Abuse and Mental Health Services Administration, 1998b). Additionally, African Americans and Latinos using drugs in the previous year report the highest rates of drug dependence (Substance Abuse and Mental Health Services Administration, 1998a). These factors co-occur with lower levels of treatment in any given year for Latinos (Substance Abuse and Mental Health Services Administration, 1998a, 1998b).

The Treatment Episode Data Set (TEDS) (Substance Abuse and Mental Health Services Administration, 1998b) indicates that in 1996 and 1997 Latinos represented 10.6 percent and 10.7 percent of all substance abuse admissions, respectively. Note that while Latinos represented the lowest proportion of admissions for most other drugs, heroin appears to be a serious problem. In 1996, 24.3 percent of heroin-related admissions were attributed to Latinos, with proportions for African Americans (24.5 percent) also being disproportionate. In 1997, Latinos were the group with the highest proportion of heroin-related admissions (32 percent). Moreover, the U.S. Medical Examiners' report (Substance Abuse and Mental Health Services Administration, 1998c) indicates that 52 percent of all deaths attributed to drug abuse among Latinos resulted from heroin use.

The epidemiological data presented here show that younger age cohorts tend to use more drugs. However, drug use in the younger cohort is more like that of African Americans and Whites than was the case for older Latinos. These epidemiological trends may be reflected in data from the Drug Abuse Warning Network (Substance Abuse and Mental Health Services Administration, 1998c) showing that the majority of drug-related deaths occur in the thirty-five to forty-four age cohorts for all ethnic groups but that in the younger cohorts the proportions of drug-related deaths are higher for Latinos. For example, more than one-quarter of all drug-related deaths occur in the twenty-six to thirty-four age group for Latinos (27.2 percent) compared with 22.4 percent for Whites and 18.8 percent for African Americans of that age group. The differences become more dramatic with the younger age cohorts. Those aged eighteen to twenty-five years represent 13.1 percent of all deaths for Latinos, 6.5 percent for African Americans, and 1.3 percent for Whites. Among the forty-five to fifty-four age group the proportions are reversed, with Latinos having the lowest percentage of drug-related deaths and African Americans the highest.

Drug abuse is a drain on the health, social stability, and economic vitality of the Latino population. The impact of this drain is magnified by poverty and the marginality of two-fifths of Latino children. Low-income Latino parents are not well prepared to address the problem of drug abuse; they often lack the time, information, and resources. Low-income Latino neighborhoods are targets for drug traffickers, and there is widespread support in American youth culture for experimentation with drugs. Fortunately, most people who experiment with drugs in adolescence and early adulthood do not become addicted and largely stop using illicit drugs in their mid-twenties as transitions into marriage, family life, and work occur. However, those who do become drug dependent create hardships for themselves, their families, and their communities.

The intimate connection of drug abuse problems with the criminal justice system poses a particularly acute issue for Latinos. One impact of tougher mandatory minimum sentencing nationally has been that two-thirds of adult prisoners are directly or indirectly linked to drug use. No ethnic or racial population in the United States has a larger proportion of people in the age group at highest risk for drug use and incarceration than Latinos. Although males are much more likely than females to be arrested and imprisoned, Latinas who are imprisoned (primarily U.S. born) are more likely than men to be sentenced for drug-related behavior (Vega, in press). Because a high percentage of these women are likely to have children and to be in their childbearing years, their endangerment or absence has ramifications for the well-being of entire families. This underscores the importance of expanding treatment options, such as drug courts, which have been shown to reduce subsequent drug use and rearrest rates (Belenko, 1999). However, the use of youth drug courts is endangered by evidence of differential sentencing based on race or ethnicity. In essence, the juvenile system can currently be viewed as in flux. Forces from both the political left and right feel that the system is too harsh or too soft on perpetrators, respectively (Ratner, 1999). The evidence is that minority youth charged with drug offenses are more likely to receive greater restrictions than similarly situated Whites (Lieber & Stairs, 1999) and that, overall, youth residing in urban areas and in single-mother households are more likely to be referred to court and to receive secure placement (DeJong & Jackson, 1998).

Prison surveys have demonstrated that 49 percent of state prisoners are under the influence of alcohol or other drugs at the time they commit their offense and that 80 percent of federal prisoners and 81 percent of state prisoners possess all or some of the following characteristics: regular use of illegal drugs (at least weekly for one month); being under the influence of alcohol or other drugs at the time of the offense; incarcerated for alcohol abuse violations; commitment of the crime to obtain money for drugs; and a history of alcohol abuse (Wald, Flaherty, & Pringle, 1999). Importantly, inroads have been made to demonstrate the effectiveness of treatment in reducing (1) further use of alcohol and other drugs, (2) commitment of additional criminal acts, and (3) the subsequent costs to society (Wald, Flaherty, & Pringle, 1999). Moreover, in-prison therapeutic community treatment (ITC), especially when followed by residential aftercare, has been found to be effective in reducing postrelease recidivism rates (Hartman, Wolk, Johnston, & Colver, 1997; Hiller, Knight, & Simpson, 1999). The critical issue is that although surveys such as the National Institute of Justice's 1992 Drug Use Forecasting (DUF) program showed that 50–80 percent of arrestees in the twenty-four DUF cities tested positive for one or more drugs after arrest and that the rates of drug use were especially high for minorities and women, the evidence is that this high need for treatment is not being met (Falkin, Prendergast, & Anglin, 1994).

We should be encouraged that the overall rates of drug abuse or dependence among Latino adults are lower than for the general U.S. population. However, the restructuring of federal and state laws has resulted in a situation where most prisoners serving time today were arrested for drug-related offenses. Those who use drugs are likely to also distribute them so they are vulnerable to long prison terms for sales. Due to the obvious bias of the criminal justice system toward disproportionate incarceration of low-income people, Latinos who use illicit drugs are much more likely to face incarceration in their lifetime. With few drug treatment options available in the community, prison replaces treatment for many Latinos, and treatment is rarely available in prison. It is Latino immigrants who continue to afford the cultural vitality and anti-drug-conduct expectations that currently offer the best hope of insulating Latinos from the river of drugs flowing through every American city.

## Intervention Strategies

The challenge in developing substance abuse interventions for Latinos is addressing similarities and differences among the various Latino groups in the United States. There are two possible strategies to pursue in the development of interventions that are ethnic or group specific. One is to develop interventions that apply equally to all populations, regardless of ethnic or racial background. The other strategy is to develop interventions that are tailored to specific ethnic or racial groups. While there are similarities in the etiology of drug use across ethnic or racial groups, there are factors specific to Latino youth simply based on their migration, settlement, and assimilation experiences that are not widely shared with other American youth. Moreover, despite similarities in the etiology of drug use, ethnic or racial groups present cultural characteristics and values that may require attention to unique factors in the "process" of intervention.

There is a serious shortfall of information about the treatment of drug use and abuse among ethnic or racial minorities. Among Latinos, we know very little about the effects of factors such as nativity and acculturation on treatment effectiveness. Based on the epidemiological literature, we believe that acculturation, acculturation stress, nativity, immigration history, and family factors are important variables to be considered in the implementation of treatment and assessment of its effectiveness. There is a critical need to empirically evaluate the influence of these variables on treatment effectiveness. A necessary approach is to address these and other ethnic-specific factors in the context of amenability to treatment. That is, these variables should be conceptualized as treatment process factors, which are considered within the context of an intervention strategy that applies to all ethnic or racial groups. Currently a program funded by the National Institute on Alcoholism and Alcohol Abuse (NIAAA) has been implemented in Miami, Florida, by E. F. Wagner, A. G. Gil, and colleagues in which the impact of these factors is being tested in interventions with Latino youth involved in the juvenile justice system. Historically, Jose Szapocznik and colleagues have effectively used family structural systems therapy in programs addressing substance abuse problems in Latino families (see Santisteban, Coatsworth, Perez-Vidal, Mitrani, Jean-Gilles, & Szapocznik, 1997) and at the University of New Mexico's Center for Alcoholism, Substance Abuse, and Addictions (CASAA) intervention efficacy has been demonstrated with programs for highly acculturated Latinos.

## Treatment Delivery

The 1997 National Household Survey (Substance Abuse and Mental Health Services Administration, 1997) reported that drug treatment was received by an average of 3.7 percent of Latino illicit drug users who had health and psychological problems and drug dependence. The rates for marijuana users were also very low at 2.2 percent. Certainly socioeconomic factors, complications around legal-documented residence for immigrants, a shortage of Spanish-language health care providers, and lower health insurance availability influence these low rates of treatment utilization. Additionally, ethnicity and acculturation are likely to impact multiple aspects of the alcohol and other drugs (AOD) treatment process (Collins, 1993). The contrast between endemic drug use in the United States and minimal use in Latin America points to the importance of sociocultural factors in explaining different patterns of drug use in different environments (Vega, Gil, & Wagner, 1998). The acculturation model presented at the outset of this chapter provides a logical, theoretically grounded approach for the development of AOD treatment approaches. It addresses the variance in pathways to drug use and social experiences that either support or sanction drug use, examining these pathways in the context of family, social network, and ecological environments.

Several factors contribute to lower service utilization among Latinos. These include shortages of bilingual and bicultural health care providers, and language and institutional barriers that undermine Latino cultural emphasis on social ties (Giachello, 1994). A broader problem is that most intervention approaches currently available were not developed for Latino groups. The procedures, techniques, and methods of these treatments are based on White-American cultural viewpoints. For example, conventional White-American referral strategies ignore the emphasis on social relations (*personalismo* and *familialism*) of Latino cultures (Smart & Smart, 1995). *Personalismo* refers to the preference in Latino cultures for developing personal relationships as a prelude to personal disclosure; *familialism* refers to the strong influence of relatives on Latinos' behavior and values. This lack of consideration for cultural values, such as avoiding interpersonal conflicts and de-emphasizing negative behaviors in conflictive circumstances (Trandis, Marín, & Betancourt, 1984), has caused Latino families to drop out of programs and interventions that ignore these factors. Latinos tend to need interpersonal connections with therapists, service providers, and institutions in their interactions (Gloria

& Peregoy, 1996). Unresponsiveness to these issues, or lack of cultural competence, have been identified as reasons for underutilization rates and early termination (Sue & Sue, 1990).

## Retention in Treatment Programs

Despite this evidence of low utilization, recent research has shown improved retention in treatment and interventions once Latinos reach service providers (O'Sullivan, Peterson, Cox, & Kirkeby, 1989; Hu, Snowden, Jerrell, & Nguyen, 1991). Furthermore, the matching of Latino clients with therapist and with other Latinos in treatment has resulted in lower dropout rates (O'Sullivan & Lasso, 1992). Perhaps more importantly, knowing where to seek treatment and having more information about programs and services markedly increased the likelihood of utilization (Vega, in press). This new trend of more success in retention may reflect that programs have begun to address the specific needs based on cultural values that have been explored in the literature over the past decade.

## Treatment Components

In community-based approaches, several elements that are unique to Latinos should be addressed as "amenability-to-treatment" factors (in other words, factors that may influence the effectiveness of treatment for Latinos). Acculturation and acculturation stress occurring within Latino families, as well as communication and family cohesiveness, interact with other elements of their social environment such as extended networks and peer groups. Research findings illustrate that U.S.-born and immigrant Latino youth (and their families) present with different needs and strengths, and that treatment programs should be attuned to these differences. For example, family cohesion and *familialism* tend to be lower among U.S.-born than immigrant Latino families (Vega & Gil, 1998).

Brief interventions that address multiple problems and have the goal of early and concrete improvements are more likely to be relevant to the "problem orientation" of Latinos and other similar cultural groups (Santisteban, Coatsworth, Perez-Vidal, Mitrani, Jean-Gilles, & Szapocznik, 1997). This does not mean that Latinos are not interested in long-term future-oriented solutions. It indicates, however, that the views and attitudes of Latinos in relation to psychosocial interventions is that these must address what they perceive as the current problem situation. Often substance abuse problems co-occur with psychiatric disorders and related behavior problems.

The information we have about substance abuse treatment interventions with Latino populations only provides the initial steps in the accumulation of evidence-based treatment knowledge regarding Latinos. We are at a stage in which there is a need to develop and test interventions that are informed by the social, cultural, and environmental circumstances of Latino populations in the United States. While the literature points to the use of brief, community-based, culturally appropriate interventions, there is scant evidence about the types of treatment intervention that are most effective with Latinos or about process elements and variables that need to be manipulated so as to develop effective substance abuse treatments for Latinos. This lack of empirical evidence is not unique to treatment of Latinos. In the area of youth substance abuse, multiple intervention approaches have been developed during the past two decades. Unfortunately, little is yet known about which of these approaches is most effective for which individuals. Clinical demand for adolescent substance abuse prevention and treatment programs has been overwhelming and has far outpaced empirical research to evaluate their effectiveness. The vast majority of currently available substance abuse interventions have not been adequately evaluated as to their effectiveness (Klitzner, Fisher, Stewart, & Gilbert, 1993; Schinke, Botvin, & Orlandi, 1991), and the strongest conclusions that can be drawn about the effectiveness of different interventions is that some intervention is better than none and that no particular intervention is superior to any other (Catalano, Hawkins, Wells, Miller, & Brewer, 1990/91). There are very few controlled studies examining specific treatments most effective for each type of problem (Kendall & Morris, 1991), an empirical gap that is especially pronounced in the areas of AOD problems. Kendall and Morris (1991) suggest the comparison of individual therapy with family-involved therapy as a necessary first step toward understanding what are the most effective interventions for specific problems. This is particularly important with Latinos, for whom the family is preeminent (Vega, 1990).

Well-designed and evaluated interventions are needed. For example, a community-based intervention, mentioned earlier, is being conducted in South Florida (by E. F. Wagner, A. G. Gil, and colleagues) in which individual and family interventions are being examined in terms of their effectiveness with Latino youth. This project, Alcohol Treatment Targeting Adolescents in Need (ATTAIN), will place clinics within Latino communities and will test hypotheses about the effectiveness of the interventions based on acculturation factors and acculturation stress.

## Prevention and Policy Implications

The low median age and projected growth of the Latino population, combined with the consistent high levels of drug use documented in this chapter, accentuate the importance of prevention. Preventive interventions that are effective in reducing rates of first use and persistent use of drugs among Latino populations have an especially high priority. These interventions must be transferable to multiple Latino communities, and implementation must be sufficiently practical that the broad mainstream of communities can support and incorporate them. Because preventive interventions require a significant investment of resources, a key question is whether interventions must be culture specific to be effective. The best information available comes from SAMHSA's recent large-scale community demonstration program that included two dozen communities in which preventive intervention processes were initiated and a similar number of matched controlled communities. Among the intervention communities was El Paso, Texas, a city whose population is nearly 80 percent Latino. The results were mixed: whereas a 3 percent reduction in male substance abuse in intervention communities was reported relative to control communities, adolescent girls did not differ across communities and their substance abuse did not diminish. Another limitation of the study was the short follow-up time, which may not have allowed adequately for the decay of intervention effects. Given the massive expenditure of resources required to produce this ambiguous outcome, it is difficult to be overly enthusiastic in the short term due to an array of organizational and political obstacles. A ray of hope is offered by the finding that results were strongest in communities where a greater total number of intervention activities were initiated and where more people were engaged in the intervention process.

## Policies and Strategies That Make a Difference

Addressing primary determinants of poverty, low educational attainment, and the quality of neighborhoods is fundamental. Latino adolescents who feel good about themselves and are optimistic about their futures in American society are at lower risk for drug addiction. Too often drug and delinquency prevention programs operate in isolated "silos," and they fail to link with (and may even resist cooperation with) other sectors that could extend the power of their interventions. Public and private agencies responsible for developing community assets such as housing, adult literacy, commercial development, job creation, and health care are rarely partners in drug preventive interventions. As a result, these sectors fail to see the relationships of their functions or authority to the general problem of reducing drug use in their community. Federal and state leadership is essential in creating these partnerships, but coalition building requires local community activity.

There are two primary goals of intervention strategies addressing the drug abuse problem. The first is to prevent the initial use of substances or delay their use as long as possible. This includes forestalling initiation of alcohol and cigarette use because these substances usually precede illicit drug use. This minimizes the likelihood of later use or progression to other illicit drugs, and prevents related criminal justice, health, and psychiatric sequelae (Ellickson, Hays, & Bell, 1992). Prevention strategies that involve parents and engage broad sectors of the community in the intervention process are most powerful. Many communities require extensive internal preparation to support interventions of this scale. Too few Latino youth are reached by preventive interventions that go beyond dissemination of information about drug use. Schools are so overwhelmed with instructional obligations that many cannot make a serious time and resource commitment to drug prevention. While drug use is dynamic, with constantly changing popularity cycles of drugs and modes of use, the institutions in charge of preventing drug use are poorly situated to anticipate these changing patterns of drug use behavior and the rapidity of their onset. Drug use prevention is a community responsibility.

The second goal of intervention strategies is early detection of substance use problems and effective referrals. This can occur through schools, the criminal justice system, and primary care doctor's offices. Drug-abusing youth need to be carefully screened for mental health problems, family dysfunction, and parent or sibling drug abuse. Adult drug abusers are often uninsured and have no access to medical treatment for their addiction, other than involuntary treatment through the criminal justice system or self-help groups. Also, there is a high occurrence of psychiatric and substance abuse dual diagnoses. Comorbidity requires specialized treatment protocols that address both problems with a coordinated treatment plan. Due to the fragmentation of services or lack of access to services, this occurs infrequently.

Both goals—constraining first use and detecting, referring, and treating individuals that are drug dependent—require more comprehensive training and availability of culturally and linguistically competent professionals. Many communities have lived with the problem of drug use for so long that they are desensitized. School counselors, teachers, and nurses need continuing education. Primary care physicians and mental health professionals lack training in diagnosing substance abusers. Drug court programs that provide treatment options need rapid deployment, as does drug abuse treatment in correctional facilities. All of these steps, including the key task of increasing the scope of prevention activities in communities, require major resource allocation and careful research or evaluation to identify the level of success or needed changes.

## Conclusion

This chapter has provided an overview of the problem of drug use among Latinos in the United States. Generally, the rate of drug use among U.S. Latinos is lower than that of the White population. However, there is evidence that drug use increases with longer exposure to U.S. society, and that socioeconomic and criminal justice inequalities create vulnerabilities to drug use and its consequences for Latinos in the United States. Moreover, as we look to the future with awareness of the growing numbers of Latinos in this country, we should be concerned that U.S. Latino youth are tending to use more "gateway" drugs, especially marijuana, and that drug use rates for immigrant youth will inevitably increase with acculturation. Therefore, we are presented with the public health challenge of addressing a pattern of drug use among Latino youth that, if unchanged, will produce negative personal and societal consequences in the very near future as the number of Latino youth accelerates dramatically over the next decade.

# References

Alderete, E., Vega, W. A., Kolody, B., & Aguilar-Gaxiola, S. (2000). Effects of time in the United States and Indian ethnicity on DSM-III-R psychiatric disorders among Mexican Americans. *Journal of Nervous & Mental Disease, 188,* 2, 90–100.

Amaro, H., Whitaker, R., Coffman, G., & Heeren, T. (1990). Acculturation and marijuana and cocaine use: Findings from the HHANES 1982–84. *American Journal of Public Health, 80,* 54–60.

American Psychiatric Association. (1987). *Diagnostic and statistical manual of mental disorders* (3rd ed., rev. [DSM-III-R]). Washington, D.C.: Author.

Belenko, S. (1999). Research on drug courts: A critical review 1999 update. *National Drug Court Institute Review, 2,* 1–58.

Burnam, A., Hough, R., Karno, M., Escobar, J., & Telles, C. (1987). Acculturation and lifetime prevalence of psychiatric disorders among Mexican Americans in Los Angeles. *Journal of Health and Social Behavior, 28,* 89–102.

Caetano, R., & Medina-Mora, M. E. (1988). Acculturation and drinking among people of Mexican descent in Mexico and the United States. *Journal of Studies on Alcohol, 49,* 462–471.

Catalano, R. F., Hawkins, J. D., Wells, E. A., Miller, J., & Brewer, D. (1990/91). Evaluation of the effectiveness of adolescent drug abuse treatment, assessment of risks for relapse, and promising approaches for relapse prevention. *International Journal of Addiction, 9A–10A,* 1085–1140.

Center for Substance Abuse Prevention. (1997). *Making prevention work.* Rockville, MD: Author.

Chavez, E. L., & Swaim, R. C. (1992). An epidemiologic comparison of Mexican Americans and White non-Hispanic 8th and 12th grade students' substance abuse. *American Journal of Public Health, 82,* 445–447.

Collins, L. R. (1993). Sociocultural aspects of alcohol use and abuse: Ethnicity and gender. *Drugs and Society, 8,* 89–116.

DeJong, C., & Jackson, K. C. (1998). Putting race into context: Race, juvenile justice processing, and urbanization. *Justice Quarterly, 15,* 487–504.

Earleywine, M., & Newcomb, M. D. (1997). Concurrent versus simultaneous polydrug use: Prevalence, correlates, discriminant validity, and prospective effects on health outcomes. *Experimental and Clinical Psychopharmacology, 5,* 4, 353–364.

Ellickson, P. L., Hays, R. D., & Bell, R. M. (1992). Stepping through the drug use sequence: Longitudinal scalogram analysis of initiation and regular use. *Journal of Abnormal Psychology, 101,* 441–451.

Falkin, G. P., Prendergast, M., & Anglin, M. D. (1994). Drug treatment in the criminal justice system. *Federal Probation, 58,* 3, 31–36.

Finch, B. K., Boardman, J. D., Kolody, B., & Vega, W. A. (2000). Contextual effects of acculturation on perinatal substance exposure among immigrant and native born Latinas. *Social Science Quarterly, 81,* 421–438.

Giachello, A.L.M. (1994). Issues of access and use. In C. W. Molina & M. Aguirre-Molina (Eds.), *Latino health in the U.S.: A growing challenge.* Washington, D.C.: American Public Health Association, pp. 83–111.

Gil, A. G., & Vega, W. A. (1996). Two different worlds: Acculturation stress and adaptation among Cuban and Nicaraguan families. *Journal of Social & Personal Relationships, 13,* 3, 435–456.

Gil, A. G., Vega, W. A., & Biafora, F. (1998). Temporal influences of family structure, and family risk factors on drug use initiation in a multiethnic sample of adolescent boys. *Journal of Youth and Adolescence, 23,* 373–393.

Gil, A. G., Wagner, E. F., & Vega, W. A. (2000). Acculturation, *familialism* and alcohol use among Latino adolescent males: Longitudinal relations. *Journal of Community Psychology, 28,* 4, 443–458.

Glick, R., & Moore, J. (1990). *Drugs in Hispanic communities.* New Brunswick, NJ: Rutgers University Press.

Gloria, A. M., & Peregoy, J. J. (1996). Counseling Latino alcohol and other substance users/abusers. *Journal of Substance Abuse Treatment,* 13, 119–126.

Hartman, D. J., Wolk, J. L., Johnston, J. S., & Colver, C. J. (1997). Recidivism and substance abuse outcomes in a prison-based therapeutic community. *Federal Probation, 61,* 4, 18–25.

Hiller, M. L., Knight, K., & Simpson, D. D. (1999). Prison-based substance abuse treatment, residential aftercare and recidivism. *Addiction, 94,* 6, 833–842.

Hu, T. W., Snowden, L. R., Jerrell, J. M., & Nguyen, T. D. (1991). Ethnic populations in mental health services: Services choice and level of use. *American Journal of Public Health, 81,* 1429–1434.

Johnston, L. D., O'Malley, P. M., & Bachman, J. G. (1999). *National survey results on drug use from the Monitoring the Future Study, 1975–1998* (NIH Publication No. 99-4660). Washington, D.C.: U.S. Department of Health and Human Services, National Institute on Drug Abuse.

Kendall, P. C., & Morris, R. J. (1991). Child therapy: Issues and recommendations. *Journal of Consulting and Clinical Psychology, 59,* 6, 777–784.

Kessler, R. C., Nelson, C. B., McGonagle, K. A., & Liu, J. (1996). Comorbidity of DSM-III—R major depressive disorder in the general population: Results from the U.S. National Comorbidity Survey. *British Journal of Psychiatry, 168,* Suppl 30, 17–30.

Klitzner, M., Fisher, D., Stewart, K., & Gilbert, S. (1993). *Substance abuse: Early intervention for adolescents.* Princeton, NJ: Robert Wood Johnson Foundation.

Lieber, M. J., & Stairs, J. M. (1999). Race, contexts, and the use of intake diversion. *Journal of Research in Crime and Delinquency, 36,* 1, 56–86.

Lopez, S. R., & Guarnaccia, P. J. (2000). Cultural psychopathology: Uncovering the social world of mental illness. *Annual Review of Psychology, 51,* 571–598.

Newcomb, M. D., & Bentler, P. M. (1988). *Consequences of adolescent drug use: Impact on the lives of young adults.* Newbury Park, CA: Sage.

Newcomb, M. D., Maddahian, E., & Bentler, P. M. (1986). Risk factors for drug use among adolescents: Concurrent and longitudinal analyses. *American Journal of Public Health, 76,* 525–531.

O'Sullivan, M. J., & Lasso, B. (1992). Community mental health services for Hispanics: A test of the culture compatibility hypothesis. *Hispanic Journal of Behavioral Sciences, 14,* 4, 455–468.

O'Sullivan, M., Peterson, P. D., Cox, G. B. & Kirkeby, J. (1989). Ethnic populations: Community mental health services ten years later. *American Journal of Community Psychology, 17,* 17–30.

Portes, A., & Zhou, M. (1993). The new second generation: Segmented assimilation and its variants. *Annals of the American Academy of Political and Social Science, 530,* 74–96.

Ratner, R. A. (1999). Juvenile justice: An update. In A. H. Esman et al. (Eds.), *Adolescent psychiatry: Development and clinical studies: Vol. 24. Annals of the American Society for Adolescent Psychiatry.* Hillsdale, NJ: Analytic Press, pp. 143–158.

Santisteban, D. A., Coatsworth, J. D., Perez-Vidal, A., Mitrani, V., Jean-Gilles, M., & Szapocznik, J. (1997). Brief structural/strategic family therapy with African American and Hispanic high-risk youth. *Journal of Community Psychology, 25,* 5, 453–471.

Schinke, S. P., Botvin, G. J., & Orlandi. M. A. (1991). *Substance abuse in children and adolescents: Evaluation and intervention.* Newbury Park, CA: Sage.

Smart, J. F. & Smart, D. W. (1995). Acculturative stress of Hispanics: Loss and challenge. *Journal of Counseling and Development, 73,* 390–396.

Smart, R. G. (1991). Crack cocaine use: A review of prevalence and adverse effects. *American Journal of Drug and Alcohol Abuse, 17,* 1, 13–26.

Substance Abuse and Mental Health Services Administration, Office of Applied Studies. (1996). *1996 National Household Survey on Drug Abuse.* Rockville, MD: Author.

Substance Abuse and Mental Health Services Administration, Office of Applied Studies. (1997). *1997 National Household Survey on Drug Abuse.* Rockville, MD: Author.

Substance Abuse and Mental Health Services Administration, Office of Applied Studies. (1998a). *1998 National Household Survey on Drug Abuse.* Rockville, MA: Author.

Substance Abuse and Mental Health Services Administration Office of Applied Studies. (1998b). *National Admissions to Substance Abuse Treatment Services: The Treatment Episode Data Set (TEDS): 1992–1997* (DHHS Publication No. [SMA] 98-3324). Rockville, MD: Author.

Substance Abuse and Mental Health Services Administration, Office of Applied Studies. (1998c). *Drug Abuse Warning Network: Annual medical examiner's data* (DHHS Publication No. [SMA] 98-3228). Rockville, MD: Author.

Substance Abuse and Mental Health Services Administration, Office of Applied Studies. (1999). *Drug Abuse Warning Network: 07/1999 update.* (DHHS Publication No. [SMA] 98-3244). Rockville, MD: Author.

Sue, D. W., & Sue, D. (1990). *Counseling the culturally different: Theory and practice.* New York: Wiley.

Trandis, H. C., Marín, G., & Betancourt, H. (1984). *Simpatía* as cultural script of Hispanics. *Journal of Personality and Social Psychology, 47,* 1363–1375.

Vega, W. A. (in press). A profile of crime, violence, and drug use among Mexican immigrants. *Perspectives on Crime and Justice: 1999–2000 Lecture Series.*

Vega, W. A. (1990). Hispanic families in the 1980s: A decade of research. *Journal of Marriage and the Family, 52,* 1015–1024.

Vega, W. A., Alderete, E., Kolody, B., & Aguilar-Gaxiola, S. (1998). Illicit drug use among Mexicans and Mexican Americans in California: The effects of gender and acculturation. *Addiction, 93,* 12, 1839–1850.

Vega, W. A., Alderete, E., Kolody, B., & Aguilar-Gaxiola, S. (2000). Adulthood sequelae of adolescent heavy drinking among Mexican Americans. *Hispanic Journal of Behavioral Sciences, 22,* 254–266.

Vega, W. A., & Gil, A. G. (Eds.). (1998). *Drug use and ethnicity in early adolescence.* New York: Plenum.

Vega, W. A., & Gil, A. G. (1999). A model for explaining drug use behavior among Hispanic adolescents. *Drugs and Society, 14,* 57–74.

Vega, W. A., Gil, A. G., & Wagner, E. (1998). Cultural adjustment and Hispanic adolescent drug use. In W. A. Vega & A. G. Gil (Eds.), *Drug use and ethnicity in early adolescence.* New York: Plenum, pp. 125–148.

Vega, W. A., Kolody, B., Aguilar-Gaxiola, S., Alderete, E., Catalano, R., & Caraveo-Anduaga, J. (1998). Lifetime prevalence of DSM-III-R psychiatric disorders in rural and urban Mexican Americans in California. *Archives of General Psychiatry, 55,* 771–778.

Vega, W. A., Zimmerman, R. S., Warheit, G. J., Apospori, E., & Gil, A. G. (1993). Risk factors for adolescent drug use in four racial/ethnic groups. *American Journal of Public Health, 83,* 257–259.

Wald, H. P., Flaherty, M. T., & Pringle, J. L. (1999). Prevention in prisons. In R. T. Ammerman & P. J. Ott (Eds.), *Prevention and societal impact of drug and alcohol abuse.* Mahwah, NJ: Erlbaum, pp. 369–381.

PART SIX

# A NEW HEALTH AGENDA

CHAPTER SEVENTEEN

# LATINO HEALTH POLICY

## A Look to the Future

Marilyn Aguirre-Molina, Angelo Falcón,
and Carlos W. Molina

This book examines Latino health issues from various perspectives and key health issues. Therefore, the purpose of these closing comments is not to cover ground already addressed. To this end, the overarching dilemmas and health issues faced by Latinos in the policy arena are reviewed within an historical context of past attempts to address needs, lessons that can be learned, and new ways of working to address Latinos' needs.

## The Need for Vision and New Strategies for Change

As the Latino population continues to grow dramatically, we find ourselves with more Latino elected and appointed officials, more consumer buying power, more music, more attention to the race and ethnicity of television and film stars . . . and yet the problems persist along with the widespread feeling that nobody's even listening. This need not be the case.

### Efforts to Address Latino Health

If anything distinguishes the health field, it is the abundance of carefully crafted technical reports, studies, and policy recommendations. The last fifteen to twenty years have seen a constant stream of special national initiatives, reports, summits, and task forces to address the health needs of Latinos. Yet the goal of many of these endeavors have yet to be fully actualized.

In the early 1980s, Secretary of Health and Human Services Margaret M. Heckler appointed a Task Force on Black and Minority Health. The result was a series of well-documented, voluminous reports, many of which addressed Latino health concerns (United States Department of Health and Human Services, 1985). They identified needs and developed corresponding recommendations. While the reports were well received because they represented a large-scale effort to produce important documentation on the needs of minority groups, many of the issues and problems identified therein still linger on.

In 1993, then U.S. Surgeon General Dr. Antonia Novello spearheaded a National Hispanic/Latino Health Initiative called Together Organized Diligently Offering Solidarity (TODOS) (United States Office of the Surgeon General, 1993). This initiative convened the leadership in Latino health and health policy for local and regional meetings, advisory groups, and ultimately a national meeting. The initiative, "One Voice, One Vision," resulted in a comprehensive document of clearly defined research, policy, and program recommendations for addressing the needs identified. This occurred at the cusp of changing administrations, thus none of the recommendations were addressed. When President George Bush left office, the Clinton Administration did not pursue the initiative, but choose in the second term of office to address minority issues through the 1998 Department of Health and Human Services' initiative, "Eliminating Ethnic/Racial Disparities in Health" (United States Department of Health and Human Services, 1998). While this effort is more proactive by moving beyond studies, reports, and commissions to actually funding research and programs, it is still not clear what it has or will yield. Moreover, there are no assurances that it will be continued by the George W. Bush Administration.

The United States Department of Health and Human Services initiative, "Healthy People 2000," has now become "Healthy People 2010" (with 467 specific objectives broken into twenty-eight focus areas). After several decades of the "Healthy People" initiative, it is not clear what it has accomplished other than document and track the morbidity and mortality patterns of the American people and minority populations. While this is an important monitoring activity at the national level, corresponding federal program initiatives and funding are not sufficiently linked to achieving the objectives of "Healthy People."

The last year of the twentieth century produced additional studies and recommendations from groups such as the U.S. Commission on Civil Rights (1999). In April 2000, the Congressional Hispanic Caucus released the *Report on Hispanic Health in the United States*. Of the recent efforts to address Latino health priorities, this is one of the more disappointing. The recommendations are void of a strategic implementation plan or mention of a policy agenda that would guide the caucus's work. At the risk of focusing too heavily on the limitations of a report produced by officials who have been elected by Latino communities, the recommendations mirror previous efforts—of limited effect—that have been undertaken over the last twenty years.

If we are to learn from the past, Latinos will need to critically review the history of these ambitious efforts to determine why so little has been accomplished or changed. This process should begin with questioning why progress has not been made. As we progress further into the new century, Latino community advocates, researchers, and health professionals will need to seriously reassess the Latino community's health policy agenda and the strategies pursued. While one can always blame "The System," are we critically examining our own thinking on these issues and the effectiveness of the strategies we endorse within the Latino community?

One of the first things that needs to be reassessed by the Latino community is its vision of society and the corresponding health system. The impact of Reaganism and the New Democrat variation have diminished the expectations of what this society is able to accomplish. This is evident in the health field as report after report and recommendation after recommendation falls victim to an incrementalism and specialization that make their impact on the community increasingly difficult to explain or justify.

While there may be a widespread "silent" consensus among Latino health professionals and advocates on the need for universal health care as a viable course of action, this option does not appear to be in the offing. The existing problems with managed health care that are identified in this book are worthy of serious consideration due to the implications for Latinos. Despite this situation, any consideration of challenging these market approaches to health care are absent from the Latino health agenda. The absence might be explained by the successful influence of the corporate sector to derail the last major health reform effort at the national level in 1993 and its penetration into the culture of many of the major Latino advocacy organizations. (Paprocki, 2000). Regardless of the cause, this absence of discourse is not in the best interest of Latinos.

In the same context of systems reform, Latino advocacy for changes in the health system must look deeper into the state of affairs of this system and its affect on Latinos. For example, in a health system where profits and cost containment are the overriding concern and the prevention of illness is not the priority, what will having Spanish-language interpreters ultimately accomplish? Or will having more Latino doctors, nurses, and administrators in such a system make a difference in the health of Latinos in the long run? In the end, are we promoting illusions of change as opposed to real change? This is not to negate the valid recommendations made by the authors of this book, but to challenge and expand this paradigm of thinking.

## A New Health Agenda

With Latinos becoming one of the largest segments of the population, they will have the opportunity to raise the stakes in setting a new health agenda for this country. A valuable starting point comes from the vision posed by the World Health Organization (2000) that views health systems in the broadest possible way as "all the organizations, institutions and resources that are devoted to producing health actions," (p. xi). The WHO argues that the purpose of the health system is twofold: to improve health *goodness* and *fairness*. They see that health systems must be responsive in the way they "address inequalities, how they respond to people's expectations, and how much or how little they respect people's dignity, rights and freedoms" (p. xi). This is a statement to the effect that health is a basic human right, to be protected by standards set by the international community. This is a perspective that Latino community advocates may need to take more seriously in the health field and other areas. (For its application in terms of the problem of hunger in the United States, see Fox, 2000.)

In addition to a new vision, Latinos will also need to critically reassess the strategies that have been thus far pursued to make the nation's health system more accountable to the needs of the Latino community. This will require that new and difficult questions be asked *within* the Latino community. Are Latinos adequately organized as a community to promote the level of change that is necessary to make the health system responsive? Have Latino national advocacy organizations been working in effective ways? If not, can we, their constituency, enlist them to do so? How are we challenging the corporate sector, especially the insurance companies, private hospitals, pharmaceutical firms, conversion foundations, and others to change their agendas and values without making it easier for them to change ours?

## Conclusion

We have significant resources as a community—that is, a basic infrastructure in the community-based and professional organizations. There is also a growing cadre of committed health professionals who need to be enlisted in more strategic ways to affect the kind of change in the health system that our community requires. Everyday we see courageous Latino community advocates and health professionals working, *contra mar y marea* (against the rough seas and tide), on behalf of their people. The challenge, however, is to more effectively organize *as a community* at the local, statewide, regional, national, and international levels to ensure that Latinos are not only large a segment of the U.S. population but also full participants in the benefits the society has to offer them.

To do so will require asking hard questions of ourselves as well as taking bold risks and actions. Perhaps there is a need to temporarily pause current advocate efforts for redesigns of government policies and programs and to take time to evaluate how well we are working and preparing for the major demographic changes that are emerging (see Chapter One). This would allow for an assessment of the strategies that are being used to hold government accountable, as well as to develop relevant policy approaches. Such a self-assessment could also enable consideration of ways of working with the private sector on the community's own terms. The growing presence and market power of Latinos provide leverage that can be applied for holding this sector accountable for the health of communities, instead of seeing the corporate sector merely as a source of grants. Building on the Latino tradition of self-help, we need to develop strategies based on our strength as a growing and powerful consumer market, as well as as voters and entrepreneurs whose presence is already felt in the labor force and electorate.

To a certain extent, demography is destiny, and being largely poor and working class certainly poses challenges to the Latino community in effecting change. But from the realities of these conditions also flows sources of great although sometimes not so evident strengths—cultural, economic, political, and spiritual—that have resulted in our long-term survival against daunting odds in a largely unwelcoming society. The time seems right to look inward and visualize ourselves as a community that has assets and strengths and that will start to use them in more deliberate and creative ways.

The alternative to this is a very unsatisfying status quo in the health of Latinos. And, as this volume documents so well, this is an unacceptable alternative.

# References

Fox, C. (2000). *Hunger is no accident: New York and federal welfare policies violate the human right to food.* New York: New York City Welfare Reform and Human Rights Documentation Project.

Paprocki, S. L. (2000), *Grants: Corporate grantmaking for racial and ethnic communities.* (A Report from the National Committee for Responsive Philanthropy). Wakefield, RI: Moyer Bell.

United States Commission on Civil Rights. (1999). *The health care challenge: Acknowledging disparity, confronting discrimination, and ensuring equality—Volume I: The Role of Governmental and Private Health Care Programs and Initiatives; and Volume II: The role of federal civil rights enforcement efforts.* Washington, D.C.: United States Commission on Civil Rights.

United States Department of Health and Human Services. (1985, August). *Report of the secretary's task force on black and minority health.* Washington, D.C.

United States Department of Health and Human Services. (1998, October). *Racial and ethnic disparities in health: Response to the President's Initiative on Race.* Washington, D.C.

United States Office of the Surgeon General. (1993, June). *One voice, one vision—Recommendations to the Surgeon General to improve Hispanic/Latino health.* Washington, D.C.: U.S. Office of the Surgeon General.

World Health Organization. (2000). *The world health report 2000—Health systems: Improving performance.* Geneva, Switzerland: World Health Organization.

# NAME INDEX

# SUBJECT INDEX